# Essentials of Anesthesia for Infants and Neonates

# Essentials of Anesthesia for Infants and Neonates

Edited by

**Mary Ellen McCann**
Harvard Medical School, Boston, MA, USA

**Christine Greco**
Harvard Medical School, Boston, MA, USA

**Kai Matthes**
Harvard Medical School, Boston, MA, USA

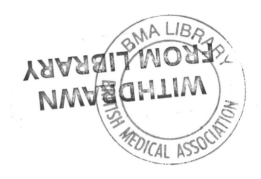

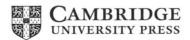
CAMBRIDGE
UNIVERSITY PRESS

# CAMBRIDGE
## UNIVERSITY PRESS

University Printing House, Cambridge CB2 8BS, United Kingdom

One Liberty Plaza, 20th Floor, New York, NY 10006, USA

477 Williamstown Road, Port Melbourne, VIC 3207, Australia

314–321, 3rd Floor, Plot 3, Splendor Forum, Jasola District Centre, New Delhi – 110025, India

79 Anson Road, #06-04/06, Singapore 079906

Cambridge University Press is part of the University of Cambridge.

It furthers the University's mission by disseminating knowledge in the pursuit of education, learning, and research at the highest international levels of excellence.

www.cambridge.org
Information on this title: www.cambridge.org/9781107069770
DOI: 10.1017/9781107707016

First published 2018

Printed in the United Kingdom by Clays, St Ives plc in January 2018.

*A catalogue record for this publication is available from the British Library.*

*Library of Congress Cataloging-in-Publication Data*
Names: McCann, Mary Ellen (Anesthesiologist), editor. | Greco, Christine, editor. | Matthes, Kai, editor.
Title: Essentials of anesthesia for infants and neonates / edited by Mary Ellen McCann, Christine Greco, Kai Matthes.
Description: Cambridge, United Kingdom; New York, NY: Cambridge University Press, 2018. | Includes bibliographical references and index.
Identifiers: LCCN 2017026491 | ISBN 9781107069770 (hardback)
Subjects: | MESH: Anesthesia – methods | Infant | Pain Management – methods
Classification: LCC RD81 | NLM WO 440 | DDC 617.9/6–dc23
LC record available at https://lccn.loc.gov/2017026491

ISBN 978-1-107-06977-0 Hardback

# Contents

v

## Section 4 – Pain Management and Other Newborn and Infant Anesthesia Concerns

# Contributors

Richard Anderson, MD
Massachusetts General Hospital; Harvard Medical School, Boston, MA, USA

T. Anthony Anderson, MD, PhD
Massachusetts General Hospital;
Harvard Medical School, Boston, MA, USA

Philip D. Bailey, DO
The Children's Hospital of Philadelphia, Philadelphia, PA, USA

Dusica Bajic, MD, PhD
Boston Children's Hospital; Harvard Medical School, Boston, MA, USA

Hubert Benzon, MD
Ann & Robert H. Lurie Children's Hospital of Chicago; Northwestern University Feinberg School of Medicine, Chicago, IL, USA

Charles Berde, MD, PhD
Boston Children's Hospital; Harvard Medical School, Boston, MA, USA

Karen Boretsky, MD
Boston Children's Hospital,
Boston, MA, USA

Morgan L. Brown, PhD, MD
Boston Children's Hospital; Harvard Medical School, Boston, MA, USA

Linda A. Bulich, MD
Boston Children's Hospital; Harvard Medical School, Boston, MA, USA

Evan Burke, MD
Hasbro Children's Hospital and Rhode Island Hospital; The Warren Alpert Medical School of Brown University, Providence, RI, USA

Kathleen Chen, MD
Boston Children's Hospital, Boston, MA, USA

Ellen Choi, MD
David Geffen School of Medicine, University of California, Los Angeles, CA, USA

Franklyn Cladis, MD, FAAP
University of Pittsburgh Medical Center, Pittsburgh, PA, USA

Edward Cooper, MD
Boston Children's Hospital, Boston, MA, USA

Joseph P. Cravero, MD
Boston Children's Hospital; Harvard Medical School, Boston, MA, USA

James A. DiNardo, MD
Boston Children's Hospital; Harvard Medical School, Boston, MA, USA

Laura Downey, MD
Boston Children's Hospital, Boston, MA, USA

Elizabeth C. Eastburn, DO
Boston Children's Hospital; Harvard Medical School, Boston, MA, USA

Lynne R. Ferrari, MD
Boston Children's Hospital; Harvard Medical School, Boston, MA, USA

Tiffany Frazee, MD
Children's Hospital Los Angeles; Keck School of Medicine, University of Southern California, Los Angeles, CA, USA

Katherine R. Gentry, MD
Seattle Children's Hospital; University of Washington School of Medicine, Seattle, WA, USA

**Jessica A. George, MD**
Johns Hopkins University, Baltimore, MD, USA

**Christine Greco, MD**
Boston Children's Hospital; Harvard
Medical School, Boston, MA, USA

**Monica Hoagland, MD**
Boston Children's Hospital; Harvard
Medical School, Boston, MA, USA

**Robert S. Holzman, MD, MA (Hon.), FAAP**
Boston Children's Hospital; Harvard
Medical School, Boston, MA, USA

**Vincent Hsieh, MD**
Seattle Children's Hospital; The University of
Washington, Seattle, WA, USA

**Narasimhan Jagannathan, MD**
Ann & Robert H. Lurie Children's Hospital of
Chicago; Northwestern University Feinberg
School of Medicine, Chicago, IL, USA

**Deepa Kattail, MD**
Johns Hopkins University School of Medicine,
Baltimore, MD, USA

**Lauren R. Kelly Ugarte, MA, MD, FAAP**
Boston Children's Hospital; Harvard
Medical School, Boston, MA, USA

**Michael R. King, MD**
Ann & Robert H. Lurie Children's Hospital of
Chicago; Northwestern University Feinberg
School of Medicine, Chicago, IL, USA

**Monica E. Kleinman, MD**
Boston Children's Hospital; Harvard
Medical School, Boston, MA, USA

**Benjamin Kloesel, MD**
University of Minnesota, Minneapolis, MN, USA

**Mary Landrigan-Ossar, MD, PhD**
Boston Children's Hospital; Harvard
Medical School, Boston, MA, USA

**Laura H. Leduc, MD**
The Greenville Health System, Greenville, SC, USA

**Justin Long, MD, FAAP**
Children's Healthcare of Atlanta at Egleston
Children's Hospital; Emory University School of
Medicine, Atlanta, GA, USA

**Anne M. Lynn, MD**
Seattle Children's Hospital; University of Washington
School of Medicine, Seattle, WA, USA

**Thomas J. Mancuso, MD, FAAP**
Boston Children's Hospital; Harvard
Medical School, Boston, MA, USA

**Kai Matthes, MD, PhD**
Boston Children's Hospital; Harvard
Medical School, Boston, MA, USA

**Lynne G. Maxwell, MD**
The Children's Hospital of Philadelphia;
Perelman School of Medicine at the
University of Pennsylvania,
Philadelphia, PA, USA

**Mary Ellen McCann, MD, MPH**
Boston Children's Hospital; Harvard
Medical School, Boston, MA, USA

**Craig D. McClain, MD**
Boston Children's Hospital; Harvard Medical School,
Boston, MA, USA

**Petra M. Meier, MD, DEAA**
Boston Children's Hospital; Harvard Medical School,
Boston, MA, USA

**Arielle Y. Mizrahi-Arnaud, MD**
Boston Children's Hospital; Harvard
Medical School, Boston, MA, USA

**Phil G. Morgan, MD**
Seattle Children's Hospital; The University of
Washington, Seattle, WA, USA

**Bridget L. Muldowney, MD**
University of Wisconsin School of Medicine and
Public Health, Madison, WI, USA

**Charles Nargozian, MD**
Boston Children's Hospital; Harvard
Medical School, Boston, MA, USA

**Viviane G. Nasr, MD**
Boston Children's Hospital; Harvard Medical School, Boston, MA, USA

**Kirsten C. Odegard, MD**
Boston Children's Hospital, Boston, MA, USA

**Raymond Park, MD**
Boston Children's Hospital, Boston, MA, USA

**Shivani S. Patel**
Northwestern University Feinberg School of Medicine, Chicago, IL, USA

**Sharon Redd, MD**
Boston Children's Hospital; Harvard Medical School, Boston, MA, USA

**Lawrence Rhein, MD**
Boston Children's Hospital, Boston, MA, USA

**Samuel Rodriguez, MD**
Boston Children's Hospital, Boston, MA, USA

**Ethan Sanford, MD**
Boston Children's Hospital, Boston, MA, USA

**Puneet Sayal, MD**
Massachusetts General Hospital, Boston, MA, USA

**Annette Y. Schure, MD, DEAA**
Boston Children's Hospital, Boston, MA, USA

**Roby Sebastian**
Nationwide Children's Hospital, Columbus, OH, USA

**Augusto Sola, MD**
New York Medical College, Valhalla, NY, USA; Maimonides University, Buenos Aires, Argentina; Universidad del Norte, Barranquilla, Colombia

**Sulpicio G. Soriano, MD**
Boston Children's Hospital, Boston, MA, USA

**Patcharee Sriswasdi, MD**
Boston Children's Hospital; Harvard Medical School, Boston, MA, USA

**Cornelius A. Sullivan, MD, FACS**
Boston Children's Hospital, Boston, MA, USA

**Kha M. Tran, MD**
The Children's Hospital of Philadelphia, Philadelphia, PA, USA

**Cynthia Tung, MD, MPH**
Boston Children's Hospital; Harvard Medical School, Boston, MA, USA

**Amy Vinson, MD**
Boston Children's Hospital; Harvard Medical School, Boston, MA, USA

**Samuel H. Wald, MD, MBA**
Stanford University, Stanford, CA, USA

**Thomas Weismueller, MD**
Brigham and Women's Hospital, Boston, MA, USA

**Gerhard K. Wolf, MD, PhD**
Ludwig-Maximillians-University, Munich, Germany; Children's Hospital Traunstein, Traunstein, Germany

**Myron Yaster, MD**
University of Colorado Denver; Children's Hospital Colorado, Aurora, CO, USA

# Preface

The mortality of infants in the United States during the last 100 years has decreased from approximately 100 infants for every 1000 births to about 7 infants for every 1000 births. Most of the decline in infant mortality has been due to improvements in medical care, sanitation, improved standards of living, and better nutrition. But relatively speaking, infancy is still the time of highest mortality during childhood. In some studies, almost 10 percent of children will undergo an anesthetic in the first year of life. The leading cause of neonatal death is prematurity, accounting for 30 percent of all deaths in the first month of life. The leading cause of infant death is congenital cardiac disease, with about 25 percent of neonatal deaths attributed to heart defects.

There are great concerns within the pediatric anesthesia community about effects of anesthetic exposure during infancy on long-term neurologic development in humans. Many juvenile animal studies have shown that exposure to a wide variety of general anesthetics and sedatives at a young age lead to widespread neuro-apoptosis and brain cell death. In addition, when these exposed animals are allowed to reach maturity, they demonstrate learning difficulties. Several human studies have shown an association between anesthetic exposure before the age of four years and later neurocognitive deficits. It is not clear that general anesthetic exposure causes learning disabilities or is just a marker for other possible causes, such as the effects of the surgery itself or the underlying reasons that these young children require surgery.

There is ongoing research in humans to try to determine whether general anesthesia is neurotoxic. The epidemiologic studies have been confounded by the effects of surgery and presurgical pathology on the neurodevelopment of babies. Prospective studies examining the effects of general anesthesia on human development have shown that there are great hemodynamic differences between general anesthesia compared with awake regional anesthesia in young infants. Physiologically there are great differences in infants compared to older children and adults, which may not always be intuitive to anesthesiologists who do not routinely care for very young infants. It is very possible that aspects of general anesthesia other than neurotoxicity may predispose young infants to later learning disabilities. Other factors might include overwarming the infants, hypocapnia and hypotension under anesthesia, and hypo- or hyperglycemia. Over the last ten years there has been lots of research that has demonstrated the importance of hemodynamic and other physiologic variables in the care of newborns in critical care nurseries and the operating room.

This textbook focuses on the practical aspects of anesthesia care for our youngest patients. Interwoven through the chapters is information about the development and changing physiology of infants and how this should impact anesthetic practice. The chapters are written by nationally recognized experts in their topics who focus on state-of-the-art, evidence-based practice.

Chapter

1

# The Term Infant

Mary Ellen McCann

## Introduction

The first moment of healthy extrauterine life is usually heralded by a deep breath followed by a cry. Within a few breaths, the color of the infant changes from a mottled dusky blue to a rosy hue and the infant is generally alert, looking around at his new environs. Once he is swaddled and brought to his mother, he may instinctively root and suck even though the mother is not yet able to nourish him. The physiologic changes that occur in the first few minutes of life are astounding. During development, the fetus develops an organ physiology that was adapted to the low-oxygen environment of the maternal circulation and then the first breath of extrauterine life initiates a process of physiologically altering his circulation and respiration. In order to care for neonates during the perioperative period, it is important to understand the physiologic changes that occur during the first few hours, days, and months of life.

## Cardiac

In utero, oxygenated placental blood is divided to pass through either the liver or to the inferior vena cava via the ductus venosus. This oxygenated blood from the inferior vena cave preferentially streams across the right atrium through the foramen ovale into the left atrium. This blood passes through the left ventricle and aorta to supply the myocardium, head, and upper torso. Deoxygenated blood returns to the right atrium via the superior and inferior vena cava and is pumped out into the pulmonary arteries via the right ventricle [1]. About 11 percent of this blood is distributed to the highly resistant pulmonary vascular bed and 89 percent is distributed to the aorta via the ductus arteriosus [2]. Aortic blood then divides to supply the lower extremities and to return to the placenta via the umbilical arteries to be reoxygenated.

Immediately after delivery, with the first breath of life, the expansion of the lungs causes the pulmonary vascular resistance to drop. Concurrently, the umbilical vessels begin to narrow due to traction and the increased oxygen levels in the umbilical artery from the infant breathing the room air. Once these vessels are fully constricted or clamped during delivery, the vascular resistance of the systemic circulation is markedly increased. The result of this is less blood flow through the ductus venosus to the inferior vena cava. The decrease in pulmonary vascular resistance leads to more blood flow to the lungs and higher flows into the left atrium. Thus, the right- and left-sided cardiac pressures begin to reverse, with the left atrium developing higher pressures, which causes the foramen ovale to functionally close. The flow across the ductus arteriosus becomes left-to-right as the pulmonary artery pressure decreases and the system vascular pressure increases. Normally the combination of decreased circulating prostaglandin PGE2 and the increased oxygen levels within the duct lead to functional closure within 2–3 days in greater than 99 percent of term infants [3]. Complete closure does not occur normally until 4–8 weeks, which means that under certain circumstances the ductus arteriosus can reopen. If the vascular resistances of the pulmonary circuit become elevated during this period, it is possible for the foramen ovale to act as a right-to-left shunt, as it did during fetal life. This condition is known as persistent pulmonary hypertension of the newborn and can be exacerbated by hypoxia, acidemia, or primary structural cardiac diseases. Figures 1.1 and 1.2 offer an overview of the circulatory system.

## Neonatal Heart

In a full-term infant, the neonatal cardiac output at 200 ml$^{-1}$ kg$^{-1}$ min$^{-1}$ or greater is roughly double that of adults to meet the metabolic demands of

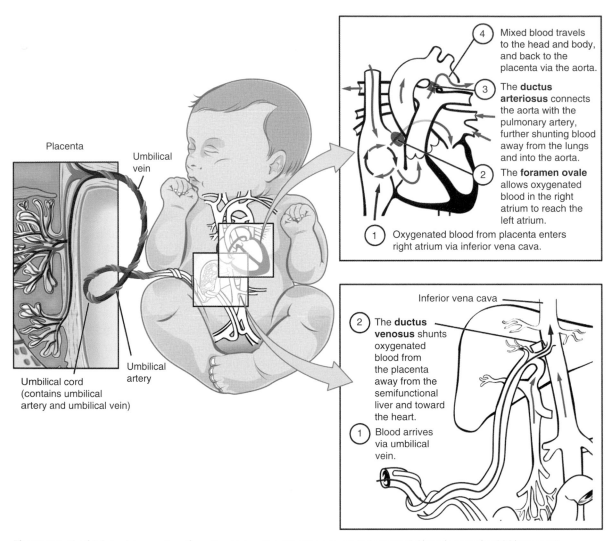

**Figure 1.1** The fetal circulatory system (from Rice University's OpenStax course in Anatomy & Physiology under CCC license 4.0 http://cnx.org/content/col11496/1.6/).

eating, breathing, thermogenesis, and growing [4,5]. Because the myocardium is immature at birth, with a reduced, chaotic arrangement of myofibrils, there is limited compliance at birth [5]. Although filling pressures can increase stroke volume to a small degree, functionally the neonatal heart is primarily dependent on an increase in heart rate to increase cardiac output. At birth the ECG reflects the right-sided dominance of the fetal heart with right axis deviation and R-wave dominance in lead V1 and S-wave dominance in lead V6. After the left ventricle grows and hypertrophies, the ECG assumes the adult configuration of left-sided dominance by about six months of age [5]. Mild congestive heart failure in

young infants is often heralded by sweatiness, tachycardia, tachypnea, difficulties in feeding, and may be missed during a preoperative examination. In cases of moderate to severe congestive failure there will be signs of acidosis, hypothermia, and oliguria. Management consists of diagnosing the underlying physiology, fluid restriction, diuretics, and inotropic agents.

Normal heart rates at birth at rest vary between 104 and 156 (mean $130 \pm 13$ mmHg). The first day of life, the mean systolic blood pressure is 70 mmHg, which rapidly increases over the next three days to 77 mmHg [6]. Mean blood pressure rises by 15 percent over the first month of life [7].

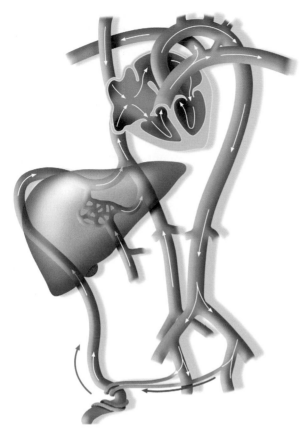

**Figure 1.2** Fetal blood circulation © BSIP/UIG.

## Congenital Cardiac Defects

The most common birth defect in neonates is congenital heart disease (CDH) with a prevalence of between 6 and 13 per 1000 live births [8]. It is 2–3 times more common in premature births compared with full-term births [9]. Critical CDH is defined as lesions requiring surgery or catheterizations within the first year of life, and constitute 15 percent of CDH at birth [10,11]. Approximately 30 percent of critical CDH is diagnosed after initial hospital discharge because the ductus arteriosus is still functioning, masking symptomatology [10,11]. The most common lesions involved include coarctation of the aorta, interrupted aortic arch, aortic stenosis, transposition of the great vessels, and hypoplastic left heart syndrome. Some nondependent duct lesions associated with mild cyanosis such as truncus arteriosus, Tetralogy of Fallot, and total anomalous venous return can be missed during the perinatal period. Missed critical CDH has a high mortality rate, with more than half of patients dying before surgical repair was done [12]. Presentation usually occurs when the ductus arteriosus begins to close and the infants manifest either shock or cyanosis. Careful physical examination of term newborns scheduled for surgery is important, but may not detect all infants with critical CDH. A cardiac murmur is present in many patients with CDH, but in approximately 44 percent of murmur detections in a healthy newborn there is no structural heart disease [13]. A careful physical examination along with a screening pulse oximetry test should be carried out for every preoperative patient. Attention should be paid to abnormal heart rates, precordial activity, S2 splitting, other heart sounds, murmurs, peripheral pulses, and cyanosis. In patients with cyanosis, a hyperoxia test can be done to help discern cardiac from noncardiac causes of decreased oxygen desaturation. In addition to the hyperoxia test, pulse oximeters can be placed both preductally (right hand) and postductally (left limb) to determine whether there is differential saturations. In medical centers with access to echography, a cardiac echo can rapidly determine the structural integrity of the heart.

## Respiratory

The process of extrauterine breathing occurs with fluid being squeezed from the lung during vaginal delivery. The first breath is characterized by high inspiratory negative pressures to overcome the airway resistance of residual fluid in the airways, and pulmonary collapse. With alveolar expansion, the alveolar size increases and the wall tension of the alveolus decreases. Alveolar collapse between breaths is limited by a coating of surfactant that maintains surface tension within the alveolus. Type II pneumocytes are responsible for surfactant production and begin to differentiate at 24 weeks of gestation; however, surfactant synthesis for appropriate pulmonary function is not adequate until 34–36 weeks of gestation [5]. Once oxygenated blood reaches the pulmonary and central circulation, the pulmonary vascular resistance drops and facilitates the transition from fetal to adult circulation.

Neonatal lung mechanics put young infants at a disadvantage compared with older children and adults. The chest wall is exceedingly compliant and the lungs themselves relatively noncompliant; both of which can facilitate lung collapse. In fact, the closing capacity for neonates exceeds functional residual capacity.

Neonates compensate for this by producing auto positive end-expiratory pressure (auto-PEEP) by partial closure of the vocal cords and breathing through the high-resistance nasal passages. The horizontal nature of the ribs and the relatively flat diaphragm make the work of breathing inefficient and increases in minute ventilation are achieved by increasing respiratory rate. Also, infants have a relatively low functional residual capacity compared with adults. Any surgical pathology that decreases the compliance of the abdomen will necessarily affect the ability of the neonate to adequately ventilate. During the first day of life, ventilation flow mismatch accounts for up to 24 percent of cardiac output. This fraction decreases to 10 percent by one week of life [14]. In addition to the disadvantageous lung mechanics, neonates consume twice as much oxygen per kilogram as adults, thus their alveolar ventilation needs to be roughly double that of adults. Because of all these factors, modest decreases in either ventilation or fraction of inspired oxygen ($FiO_2$) will incline neonates to develop hypoxia.

The ventilatory centers of respiration in the brain at birth are not fully developed, and responses to hypoxia are immature in the term neonate. The peripheral chemoreceptors do not respond to hypoxia during the first 48 hours of life because they are effectively suppressed by the rise in $PaO_2$ following delivery and need to be reset [15]. This effect is exacerbated in infants resuscitated with 100 percent $O_2$ in the delivery room [16]. The feedback mechanisms by which the peripheral chemoreceptors send messages to the central centers of ventilation are also not mature, leading to unstable respiratory control mechanisms, especially in sick, unstable neonates.

Apnea and bradycardia is one of the nonspecific signs that a neonate is suffering from stress such as hypoxemia, sepsis, or hypothermia. This apnea can lead to an unstable metabolic state that further increases the risk of apnea and hypoxia. Apnea, which is generally defined as a cessation of breathing for longer than 15 seconds, can also result from airway obstruction, especially in those neonates with congenital abnormalities of the head and neck region or neonates that have been sedated with anesthetic drugs [17]. It is very common for term infants after a general anesthetic to exhibit periodic breathing, which is a breathing pattern in which the tidal volumes become shallower and shallower to the point of brief cessation, and then become deeper again. This pattern is repeated and generally does not lead to oxygen desaturations. Some studies – but not all – have shown an association between anemia and an increased risk of postoperative apnea [18].

# Hematologic

At birth, 50–95 percent of the hemoglobin in an infant is fetal hemoglobin, which has an increased attraction for oxygen compared to adult hemoglobin. Fetal hemoglobin is made up of two alpha chains and two gamma chains, and is gradually replaced by hemoglobin A, which is made up of two alpha chains and two beta chains, by the time the infant is six months old. The fetus lives in a relatively hypoxic zone compared with the maternal environment and compensates for this with a much higher hemoglobin concentration of 19.3 g $dl^{-1}$. Within one week of birth in term infants, hemoglobin levels begin to drop and reach a nadir of about 9–11 g $dl^{-1}$ at about 8–12 weeks of life [19]. Anemia can occur at birth as a result of blood loss before, after, or during delivery. Feto-maternal or twin–twin transfusion, placental abruption, or delayed cord clamping can cause increased blood loss. Decreased erythrocyte production can occur as a result of iron deficiency, or chronic infection. Decreased red blood cell destruction can be caused by Rh and autoimmune hemolytic disease, enzyme abnormalities such as G6 PD, membranopathies such as spherocytosis and elliptocytosis, and hemoglobinopathies such as sickle cell disease, thalassemia, and hemoglobin C disease.

Term infants can also be born with polycythemia, which can lead to a hyperviscous state and complications when the hematocrit is greater than 65 percent [20]. Maternal uterine insufficiency can lead to placental hypoxic state in which the fetus responds with increased red cell production. Postnatally polycythemia can cause decreased blood flow to vital organs including the brain, heart, and lungs, increased bilirubin production, and is associated with hypoglycemia. Treatment is a partial exchange transfusion.

The coagulation profile of neonates also differs from adults. Many of the proteins needed for coagulation are diminished in newborns, including factors II, VII, IX, X, XI, XII; others that promote fibrinolysis are increased, such as thrombomodulin, tPA, and plasminogen activator inhibitor-1 [21,22]. These pro-bleeding tendencies are balanced by an alteration in some procoagulant proteins such as an increase in Von Willibrand factor and a decrease in antithrombin, heparin cofactor II, alpha-2-macroglobulin, protein C, protein S, and plasminogen [22]. The end result is that neonates normally have a prolongation of their prothrombin time (PT), and activated partial thromboplastin time (aPTT), but a shortened bleeding time [21].

Newborns can be adversely affected by low vitamin K levels. Bleeding can occur because of a decrease of the vitamin K-dependent coagulation factors (II, VII, IX, X). Treatment includes prophylactic vitamin K intramuscular injections and fresh frozen plasma transfusions in infants with symptomatic bleeding.

Early thrombocytopenia in the newborn is usually related to maternal–placental factors, and late thrombocytopenia is usually caused by excessive platelet consumption, such as seen in necrotizing enterocolitis and sepsis [23]. Thrombocytopenia is a risk factor for intraventricular hemorrhage even in term infants, so many centers administer platelet transfusions to infants whose levels are below 50 000.

## Thermoregulation

Regulation of body temperature depends on a balance between heat loss and heat generated. Although thermogenesis is suppressed in utero, heat production is actually greater in the fetus than the mother so the heat gradient flows from the fetus to the mother. Humans are a precocial species in regards to thermogenesis, with responses capable of generating heat within minutes of birth. Stimulation of the preoptic chiasma/anterior hypothalamic nuclei from peripheral cutaneous receptors activate non-shivering thermogenesis by sympathetic norepinephrine-secreting nerve fibers that innervate brown adipose tissue and shivering thermogenesis through the posterior hypothalamic nucleus [24].

## Hepatic

During fetal development, the umbilical vein brings blood to the liver. Between 20 to 30 percent of this blood bypasses the liver and is carried directly to the inferior vena cava by way of the ductus venosus [25]. The remaining umbilical vein enters the liver, where some of it joins the portal vein. The ductus venosus typically closes by the first week of life and is then known as the ligamentum venosum.

Liver function is not fully mature until about two years postnatally. Initially, its primary role is to regulate glucose and fatty acid metabolism to maintain a supply of energy for neonates that may not be getting adequate enteral nutrition in the first days of life. It is also responsible for the production of clotting factors and serum proteins, bile synthesis, and the biotransformation of medications and other xenobiotics, as well as the endogenous metabolic byproducts.

Maturation of the many liver functions occurs at differential rates. Albumin synthesis is at adult levels at birth in term infants. The coagulation factors (all are synthesized in the liver except for factor VIII) are initially low at birth but reach adult levels by 2–3 days of life. The expression of the hepatic enzyme uridine diphosphate glucuronyl transferase is poor in the fetus, but by age 2–3 weeks postnatally it reaches adult levels. This enzyme is needed to conjugate bilirubin in order to facilitate biliary excretion into the enteric system. Some of this conjugated bilirubin is then unconjugated by intestinal B glucuronidase and then reabsorbed into the body by way of the enterohepatic circulation. It is very common for term infants to have neonatal jaundice in the first few days to weeks of life because of increased erythrocyte breakdown, deficiencies of their ability to conjugate free bilirubin, and decreased amounts of enteric organisms available to break down unconjugated bilirubin for fecal excretion [26]. Clearance of medications depends on either a drug metabolism pathway or a hepatic transport mechanism. Metabolic pathways are usually divided into phase 1 reactions that involve oxidation, reduction, hydrolysis, cyclization, and decyclization reactions, and phase 2 reactions that involve the addition (conjugation) of polar groups to phase 1 metabolites [25]. Neonates are unable to metabolize medications as rapidly as adults because the cytochrome p450 system (which oxidizes medications) does not reach adult levels until one year of age [27]. For phase 2 metabolism, infants preferentially must use sulfation rather than glucuronidation for conjugation reactions [28]. Table 1.1 summarizes the maturation of liver functions.

## Renal

The kidney matures over the first two years of life. Nephrogenesis is completed by 36 weeks postconception but the nephrons are immature at birth. During fetal development the primary role of the kidney is to maintain amniotic fluid levels and renal blood flow is a very small percentage of the fetal cardiac output. For the first week of life, renal blood flow is only 10 percent

**Table 1.1** Maturation of liver functions

| | Oxidative enzyme activity | Glucuronide conjugation | Sulfate conjugation | Effect on drug metabolism |
|---|---|---|---|---|
| Premature neonates | Decreased oxidative enzyme activity (20–70 percent of adult values for cytochrome p450 activity) | Decreased glucuronide conjugation | Slightly decreased sulfate conjugation | Decreased |
| Neonates | Same as premature infants | Same as premature infants | Slightly decreased from adults | Decreased |
| Infants | Cytochrome p450 reaches adult activity by 6–12 months of age | Reaches adult levels by 24 months of age | Reaches adult levels in early infancy | Decreased |

of cardiac output and does not reach the adult level of 25 percent until 24 months of life [29]. The glomerular filtration rate (GFR) is also diminished for the first two years of life. At birth it is about 40 ml kg$^{-1}$ 1.73 m$^{-2}$ and reaches 66 ml kg$^{-1}$ 1.73 m$^{-2}$ at two weeks of age, which is about one-half of the normal adult GFR [30]. The nephrons for the first few days of life are very immature and allow for some resorption of creatinine, which makes creatinine clearance a poor estimate of GFR during this period. These leaking nephrons rapidly mature and then creatinine levels drop.

One of the main functions of the kidney is to maintain fluid and electrolyte balance. At birth the extracellular volume is approximately 40 percent by body weight; this decreases to about 30 percent at six months of age and 20 percent by one year of age. Term infants generally do not have difficulty maintaining sodium balance, but excessive administration of sodium can overwhelm their kidneys, leading to peripheral edema. Likewise, the term kidney is able to maintain potassium, calcium, and phosphorus balance. Acid–base status is accomplished through ventilation, buffering capacity of serum proteins, bicarbonate-carbonic acids, hemoglobin–oxyhemoglobin and phosphorus, and the renal system. These mechanisms are all mature enough within three days of birth to handle nonrespiratory-induced acid loads.

The kidney also produces renin, which triggers the formation of angiotensin, which is converted to angiotensin II by angiotensin-converting enzyme. This enzyme increases the peripheral vascular resistance and cardiac contractility, leading to an increase in systemic blood pressure. The excretion of renin increases after birth and is higher in infants than older children. The renin angiotensin system, other humoral agents, and an increase in sympathetic activity at birth are responsible for the increase in blood pressure seen over the first weeks of life.

# Neurologic

The neonatal and infancy period represents a time of dramatic brain growth, with the brain size as a neonate being 36 percent of the size of an adult brain and growing to 70 percent of its adult size by one year of age and 80 percent by two years of age [31]. During late gestation, brain development includes gray and white matter myelination, synaptogenesis, pruning, and synaptic modification. These processes continue into early infancy. Although all the cortical layers of cells are present at term and the primary cortical areas such as motor, somatosensory, visual, and auditory cortices are morphologically identifiable, the association cortices are less delineated. There is pronounced gray matter growth in the parietal and occipital areas in the first month of life. The newborn brain still exhibits a small degree of cortical neurogenesis and neuronal migration, but the dramatic brain growth is mainly due to the growth of glia and subsequent myelination during infancy. Abnormal brain growth in infancy is often a harbinger of poor neurocognitive outcomes. Microcephaly can be a result of malnutrition, and macrocephaly has been associated with autism.

MRI and autopsy studies of infants in the first year of life reveal a robust expansion of gray matter by way of elaboration of dendrites, spines, and synapses. Conversely, this is also a time of increased apoptosis or pruning. The pruning process time course begins with the primary cortices followed by the association cortices, and lastly in late childhood by pruning in the frontal lobes.

Along with synaptic pruning, there is remodeling of existing synapses and fine-tuning of neural circuits.

Synaptic remodeling is dependent on the strengthening of certain synaptic pathways and weakening of others. Some of these are time-dependent during infantile maturation, such as the development of binocular vision. Lack of input from an eye with a congenital cataract will lead to potentiation of synapses from the functioning retina and inhibition of synapses from the poorly stimulated retina. This in combination with pruning can lead to permanent visual impairment in infants who get delayed treatment for congenital cataracts.

There is a dramatic increase in the volume of glial cells postnatally, which leads to an increase in myelination during the first year of life. Myelination proceeds in a differential pattern starting with the sensory pathways, then motor and finally association pathways. It also proceeds subcortically before cortically in any given neural pathway. At birth in full-term infants, there are functional networks that include the visual, sensorimotor, and auditory processing networks.

The effects of harmful toxins, illness, and environmental deprivation may be greater in very young infants whose brains are growing rapidly in a time-dependent fashion. The long-term effects of general anesthetics on the neonatal brain have not been adequately characterized yet.

## Dermatologic

The term newborn has a dermis that is 40–60 percent the depth of adult dermis, and a larger surface area to body weight ratio than adults [32]. This means that the infant is more likely to lose heat and body fluids as well as absorb any materials placed on the skin compared to an adult. The pH of adult skin is acidotic at 4.7, which is protective by decreasing the colonization of pathogenic bacteria. At term birth, the pH is 6.0 but decreases to less than 5.0 by four days of age. The skin colonization of neonates resembles adult flora after the first few weeks of life. There are differences between the skin biome of infants delivered vaginally compared with caesarian section, with 60–82 percent of neonatal methicillin-resistant staphylococcus infections occurring in surgically delivered babies [33]. The vernix caseosa is a sebaceous material made from sebum, desquamated skin, water, and lanugo that is present in term infants, which enhances the skin barrier to infection, heat, and fluid loss.

The best type of disinfective skin preparation for surgery has not been determined. Many studies have shown that chlorhexidine in *term* infants can be safely used perioperatively and decreases surgical site infections [34–36]. There is evidence that chlorhexidine absorption does occur and increases after repeated exposures. Povidine iodine is an excellent bacteriocidal agent but causes thyroid suppression secondary to iodine absorption [37]. This effect is greater in premature infants but even in infants less than three months of age, increased levels of serum iodine have been found after skin exposure. Skin rashes and burns have been seen after surgical preparations in term infants exposed to isopropyl alcohol, chlorhexidine, and povidine iodine.

There are several very common rashes seen in term babies. Erythema toxicum neonatorum affects almost 50 percent of term newborns and is heralded by an erythematous macular papular rash with pustules. It usually occurs in the first week of life and lasts a few days. Milia are pinpoint pearly white bumps seen most often on the nose, mouth, or palate which are also seen in 50 percent of neonates and generally resolve by the first month of life. Neonates often get miliaria or heat rash from overbundling. It is caused by occlusion of the sweat ducts and features 1–3 mm vesicles or papules. Treatment is to limit humid or hot environments. Neonates are also susceptible to neonatal acne [38]. This is also self-limited and resolves as circulating maternal hormones diminish.

## Endocrine

There are many endocrine changes that occur perinatally. Normally neonatal blood glucose levels drop in the first few hours of birth, sometimes to levels below 30 mg dl$^{-1}$. A compensatory stress response involving the secretion of epinephrine and cortisol increases the plasma glucose to levels above 40 mg dl$^{-1}$. There are no universally agreed guidelines as to the definition of hypoglycemia in term infants, but many neonatologists consider a plasma glucose of <40 mg dl$^{-1}$ in the first three hours of life, <45 mg dl$^{-1}$ in the first day of life, and <60 mg dl$^{-1}$ after three days of life to be abnormal [39]. Infants who are born of diabetic mothers, large for gestational age, or have suffered severe perinatal stress or asphyxia may have transient hyperinsulinemia. Glucose requirements in excess of 8 mg kg$^{-1}$ min$^{-1}$ in order to maintain normoglycemia suggests a hyperinsulinemic state. Because insulin inhibits ketone body formation, decreases glycogenolysis and gluconeogenesis, and increases peripheral glucose uptake by cells, the brain is very vulnerable to damage such as permanent injury and seizures during hyperinsulinemia.

Thyroid homeostasis is necessary for brain development and growth, cardiac function, and energy balance. Prior to birth, the neonate is primarily dependent on maternal T3 and T4, but postnatally there is a dramatic increase (up to a 50-fold increase) in thyroid stimulating hormone (TSH) over the first 24 hours. It is important to recognize that a TSH in the first day of life in the 60–80 mU/L range is not indicative of thyroid disease [40]. One of the most common causes of abnormally low thyroid hormone levels in term infants is nonthyroidal critical illnesses, but there is no evidence that treating low levels benefits these patients [41,42]. Other causes include excessive iodine intake such as may be seen in iodinated contrast dyes or surgical preparations, and inadequate iodine intake. Congenital hypothyroidism is rare and is usually tested for at birth in the United States. Transient hyperthyroidism occasionally occurs in infants exposed to maternal hyperthyroidism.

At birth the adrenal system is mature, with adrenocorticotropic hormone (ACTH) stimulating the adrenal gland to secrete cortisol. Primary adrenal insufficiency is most often seen in infants that lack the enzyme 21 hydroxylase, which is necessary to synthesize corticosteroids and aldosterone. The symptoms include life-threatening salt wasting, hypotension, and poor growth. Affected infants also have very high levels of 17 hydroxyprogesterone and other adrenal androgens, leading to viralized infants. Female infants will have abnormal external genitalia but male infants may appear normal leading to a delayed diagnosis. Secondary adrenal insufficiency is common in extremely stressed term infants or in infants that have been treated with exogenous steroids. The mortality for infants with known adrenal insufficiency in the setting of sepsis is as high as 86 percent [43]. Treatment with glucocorticoids in infants with known adrenal insufficiency will improve blood pressure. Aldosterone is stimulated by the renin angiotensin system and thus is unaffected by low ACTH levels.

Serum calcium levels are regulated by parathyroid hormone release and special calcium-sensing receptors within the parathyroid glands. Parathyroid hormone (PTH) stimulates bone resorption to mobilize skeletal calcium and conversion of inactive vitamin D to active vitamin D to increase dietary absorption of calcium and phosphate. Transient hypoparathyroidism is seen in infants who are hypomagnesemic and infants born of mothers with diabetes mellitus and hyperparathyroidism [39]. Abnormal thyroid gland development is seen in DiGeorge's syndrome, which can lead to hypocalcemia. Hypercalcemia of the neonate is most commonly iatrogenically caused, but is also seen in patients with Williams syndrome. In this condition, the hypercalcemia usually resolves by one year of age. Infants with Williams syndrome can present with pulmonary artery stenosis and supravalvular stenosis with associated coronary artery abnormalities. Sudden death from this syndrome is rare during infancy but has occurred.

# References

1. Odegard KC, DiNardo JA, Laussen PC. *Anesthesia for Congenital Heart Disease, in Gregory's Pediatric Anesthesia*, 5th edn. Oxford: Wiley-Blackwell; 2012.

2. Mielke G, Benda N. Cardiac output and central distribution of blood flow in the human fetus. *Circulation*. 2001;103:1662–8.

3. Schneider DJ, Moore JW. Patent ductus arteriosus. *Circulation*. 2006;114:1873–82.

4. Walther FJ, Siassi B, Ramadan NA, Ananda AK, Wu PY. Pulsed Doppler determinations of cardiac output in neonates: normal standards for clinical use. *Pediatrics*. 1985;76:829–33.

5. Brusseau R, McCann ME. Anaesthesia for urgent and emergency surgery. *Early Hum Dev*. 2010;86:703–14.

6. Tan KL. Blood pressure in full-term healthy neonates. *Clin Pediatr (Phila)*. 1987;26:21–4.

7. Second Task Force on Blood Pressure Control in Children. Task Force on Blood Pressure Control in Children: National Heart, Lung, and Blood Institute, Bethesda, Maryland. *Pediatrics*. 1987;79:1–25.

8. van der Linde D, Konings EE, Slager MA, et al. Birth prevalence of congenital heart disease worldwide: a systematic review and meta-analysis. *J Am Coll Cardiol*. 2011;58:2241–7.

9. Kenna AP, Smithells RW, Fielding DW. Congenital heart disease in Liverpool: 1960–69. *Q J Med*. 1975;44:17–44.

10. Wren C, Reinhardt Z, Khawaja K. Twenty-year trends in diagnosis of life-threatening neonatal cardiovascular malformations. *Arch Dis Child Fetal Neonatal Ed*. 2008;93:F33–5.

11. Hoffman JI. It is time for routine neonatal screening by pulse oximetry. *Neonatology*. 2011;99:1–9.

12. Chang RK, Gurvitz M, Rodriguez S. Missed diagnosis of critical congenital heart disease. *Arch Pediatr Adolesc Med*. 2008;162:969–74.

13. Ainsworth S, Wyllie JP, Wren C. Prevalence and clinical significance of cardiac murmurs in neonates. *Arch Dis Child Fetal Neonatal Ed.* 1999;80:F43–5.

14. Rennie J, ed. *Robertson's textbook of Neonatology.* 4th ed. Oxford: Elsivier; 2005.

15. Hertzberg T, Lagercrantz H. Postnatal sensitivity of the peripheral chemoreceptors in newborn infants. *Arch Dis Child.* 1987;62:1238–41.

16. Martin RJ, Bookatz GB, Gelfand SL, et al. Consequences of neonatal resuscitation with supplemental oxygen. *Sem Perinatol.* 2008;32:355–66.

17. Craven PD, Badawi N, Henderson-Smart DJ, O'Brien M. Regional (spinal, epidural, caudal) versus general anaesthesia in preterm infants undergoing inguinal herniorrhaphy in early infancy. *Cochrane Database of Syst Rev.* 2003:CD003669.

18. Cote CJ, Zaslavsky A, Downes JJ, et al. Postoperative apnea in former preterm infants after inguinal herniorrhaphy: a combined analysis. *Anesthesiology.* 1995;82:809–22.

19. Kett JC. Anemia in infancy. *Pediatr Rev.* 2012;33:186–7.

20. Rosenkrantz TS. Polycythemia and hyperviscosity in the newborn. *Semin Thromb Hemost.* 2003;29:515–27.

21. Diaz-Miron J, Miller J, Vogel AM. Neonatal hematology. *Semin Pediatr Surg.* 2013;22:199–204.

22. Ignjatovic V, Lai C, Summerhayes R, et al. Age-related differences in plasma proteins: how plasma proteins change from neonates to adults. *PLoS One.* 2011;6:e17213.

23. Kamphuis MM, Paridaans NP, Porcelijn L, Lopriore E, Oepkes D. Incidence and consequences of neonatal alloimmune thrombocytopenia: a systematic review. *Pediatrics.* 2014;133:715–21.

24. Morrison SF, Nakamura K, Madden CJ. Central control of thermogenesis in mammals. *Exp Physiol.* 2008;93:773–97.

25. Grijalva J, Vakili K. Neonatal liver physiology. *Semin Pediatr Surg.* 2013;22:185–9.

26. Dennery PA, Seidman DS, Stevenson DK. Neonatal hyperbilirubinemia. *N Engl J Med.* 2001;344:581–90.

27. Treluyer JM, Cheron G, Sonnier M, Cresteil T. Cytochrome P-450 expression in sudden infant death syndrome. *Biochem Pharmacol.* 1996;52:497–504.

28. Alcorn J, McNamara PJ. Ontogeny of hepatic and renal systemic clearance pathways in infants: part I. *Clin Pharmacokinet.* 2002;41:959–98.

29. Sulemanji M, Vakili K. Neonatal renal physiology. *Semin Pediatr Surg.* 2013;22:195–8.

30. Schwartz GJ, Brion LP, Spitzer A. The use of plasma creatinine concentration for estimating glomerular filtration rate in infants, children, and adolescents. *Pediatr Clin North Am.* 1987;34:571–90.

31. Tau GZ, Peterson BS. Normal development of brain circuits. *Neuropsychopharmacol.* 2010;35:147–68.

32. SYSTOLIC blood pressure determination in the newborn and infant. *Anesthesiol.* 1952;13:648–9.

33. Watson J, Cortes C. Community associated methicillin resistant *Staphylococcus aureus* infection among healthy newborns: Chicago and Los Angeles County, 2004. *JAMA.* 2006;296:36–8.

34. Da Cunha ML, Procianoy RS, Franceschini DT, De Oliveira LL, Cunha ML. Effect of the first bath with chlorhexidine on skin colonization with *Staphylococcus aureus* in normal healthy term newborns. *Scand J Infect Dis.* 2008;40:615–20.

35. Mullany LC, Darmstadt GL, Khatry SK, et al. Topical applications of chlorhexidine to the umbilical cord for prevention of omphalitis and neonatal mortality in southern Nepal: a community-based, cluster-randomised trial. *Lancet.* 2006;367:910–18.

36. Tielsch JM, Darmstadt GL, Mullany LC, et al. Impact of newborn skin-cleansing with chlorhexidine on neonatal mortality in southern Nepal: a community-based, cluster-randomized trial. *Pediatrics.* 2007;119:e330–40.

37. L'Allemand D, Gruters A, Heidemann P, Schurnbrand P. Iodine-induced alterations of thyroid function in newborn infants after prenatal and perinatal exposure to povidone iodine. *J Pediatr.* 1983;102:935–8.

38. Cantatore-Francis JL, Glick SA. Childhood acne: evaluation and management. *Dermatol Ther.* 2006;19:202–9.

39. Wassner AJ, Modi BP. Endocrine physiology in the newborn. *Semin Pediatr Surg.* 2013;22:205–10.

40. Fisher DA, Klein AH. Thyroid development and disorders of thyroid function in the newborn. *N Engl J Med.* 1981;304:702–12.

41. Dimmick S, Badawi N, Randell T. Thyroid hormone supplementation for the prevention of morbidity and mortality in infants undergoing cardiac surgery. *Cochrane Database Syst Rev.* 2004:CD004220.

42. Shih JL, Agus MS. Thyroid function in the critically ill newborn and child. *Curr Opin Pediatr.* 2009;21:536–40.

43. Soliman AT, Taman KH, Rizk MM, et al. Circulating adrenocorticotropic hormone (ACTH) and cortisol concentrations in normal, appropriate-for-gestational-age newborns versus those with sepsis and respiratory distress: cortisol response to low-dose and standard-dose ACTH tests. *Metabolism.* 2004;53:209–14.

# The Preterm Infant

Lauren R. Kelly Ugarte and Thomas J. Mancuso

## Background on the Preterm Newborn

The preterm newborn is defined as a baby born from 22 to 36 weeks postconceptual age (PCA) [1]. More specifically, preterm is defined by the Center for Disease Control as less than 37 completed weeks of gestation, with early preterm being less than 34 weeks of gestation and late preterm being 34–36 weeks [2]. There were 3.95 million live births in the United States in 2011, with the preterm birthrate declining for the fifth year in a row, with a rate of 11.72 percent of all births being younger than 36 weeks, down from 11.99 percent in 2010 [2]. Overall, 0.7 percent of births in 2011 were babies younger than 28 weeks PCA (Figure 2.1) [3].

Categorization of birth age allows for stratification of risk. Data show that survival is least favorable in the smallest and youngest patients. Recently, with greatly improved accuracy in gestational age (GA) measurements, it has become clear that perinatal complications most closely follow GA, not birth weight. In extremely low gestational age newborns (ELGAN) born at 22–28 weeks PCA, there is improved survival with longer gestation as there is about a 6 percent survival to discharge in a 22-week GA newborn and 92 percent for a 28-week GA newborn [1,4]. The survival in very low birth weight patients has increased since the 1980s due to advances in prenatal, obstetric, and neonatal care, and we now see a majority of infants born at 24 weeks GA survive to leave the hospital (Figure 2.2) [4].

Medically intervening in newborns born at 22–24 weeks' gestation is a controversial area of obstetrics and neonatology and it is not possible to standardize the data available [4]. We see that every week in utero confers better survival as the risk of death is 2.5 times higher in infants born from 24 to 27 weeks compared to those who are born at 28 weeks and more than three times higher for the 22-week newborns [4]. However, morbidity in the survivors is high in the 22–28 week

PCA group and one report showed that 93 percent of these patients will have respiratory distress, 46 percent will have patent ductus arteriosis (PDA), 16 percent will have severe intraventricular hemorrhage (IVH), 11 percent will have necrotizing enterocolitis (NEC), and 36 percent will have late sepsis [4]. The most common issues for the smallest of patients are bronchopulmonary dysplasia (BPD) and infections [4]. All of these issues in and of themselves may require surgical attention or add to the anesthetic risk if the patient is taken to surgery. Other common problems that are seen in or result from preterm birth include: retinopathy of prematurity (ROP), hypoglycemia, and neurodevelopmental delay [1,4].

Pediatric anesthesiologists must be vigilant and thoughtful in the provision and planning of care for all of their patients. Preterm newborns who present for surgery are uniquely challenging due to the immaturity of all the organ systems, the complexity of their ongoing medical care, and the often emergent reasons for any surgical procedures. It is unlikely that the surgical issues these patients deal with today will change drastically over the coming years as there seems to be a current plateau in survival [4]. That being said, these patients are usually not cared for on a daily basis by pediatric anesthesiologists and this fact contributes to their challenging care.

## Neurologic Issues

Over the past few decades, anesthetic care for preterm newborns has improved as research has allowed us to understand their complex physiology. We have come to learn that fetuses at 20 weeks' gestation have the neural substrate to transmit impulses due to noxious stimuli. All newborns the pediatric anesthesiologist deals with will require either pain medications or anesthetics to minimize the detrimental stress responses related to surgical procedures [5]. Currently, there are concerns about the long-term neurologic sequelae of exposing

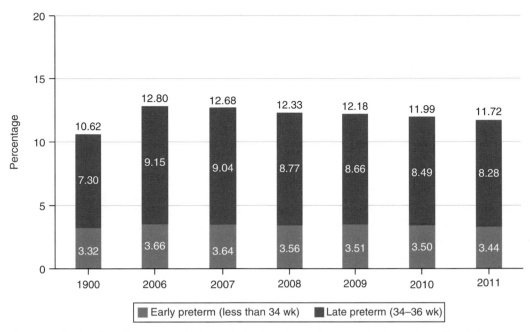

**Figure 2.1** Total, early, and late preterm birth rates in the United States. Reproduced with permission from: [2].

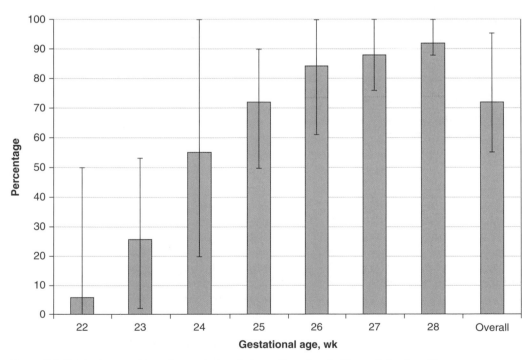

**Figure 2.2** Graph of neonatal mortality; survival to discharge. Reproduced with permission from [4].

the developing brain to anesthetics. This issue is far from resolved and clinical studies are underway that may add to our limited understanding of the effects of anesthetics on the developing CNS. Through vigilant observation and studies, practices are changing to optimize care. There has been recent change in NICU practice to avoid long-term midazolam administration to preterm newborns since this practice has led to the development of choreiform movements in these patients [1,5].

Preterm newborns are at risk for intraventricular hemorrhage (IVH), bleeding from the highly vascular periventricular germial matrix. IVH is multifactorial in nature, and almost 12 000 premature infants develop it every year [4,6]. Preterm newborns are at risk for neuronal injury, whether or not they require surgery, but changes in cerebral blood flow, possibly low or high blood pressure, swings in serum osmolalities, hypercarbia, thrombocytopenia, the presence of PDA, and restlessness are factors that may contribute to IVH [5,6]. The preterm brain lacks the ability to autoregulate blood flow on a consistent basis and this is a prevailing belief that predisposes them to neuronal injury [6]. Lower gestational age, lower birth weight, sicker, ventilated, and clinically unstable infants have been shown to autoregulate cerebral blood flow less well, and mortality is higher in these infants even without IVH [6]. Other types of brain injury are also commonly seen in preterm newborns; the "encephalopathy of prematurity" is a complex amalgam of destructive brain disease as well as maturational and growth dyscrasias affecting this population [7]. One of the most common manifestations is periventricular leukomalacia or disease of cerebral white matter, and its sequelae can be implicated in long-term cognitive and behavioral deficits found in up to 50 percent of formerly preterm newborns [7]. Neuronal damage can be caused by maternal infection, but also can be caused postnatally by sepsis, excitotoxicity, and inability to attenuate free radicals [7]. Also, ventilatory strategies may contribute to or protect infants from neuronal damage. Using pancuronium in intubated newborns to reduce asynchrony from the ventilator has been shown to eliminate fluctuations in cerebral blood flow and decrease risk for IVH [6]. Synchronized intermittent mandatory ventilation and assist control also reduce the fluctuation of cerebral blood flow in infants [6].

## Pulmonary Issues

Preterm newborns have a host of respiratory issues that the pediatric anesthesiologist has to deal with, due to maturation, neurologic, chemical, and structural factors.

Respiratory regulation in the preterm newborn can be drastically different from that of the term infant. Postconceptual age is more of a determinant for mature responses to hypoxemia than postnatal age [8]. Periodic breathing occurs in most preterm newborns during REM sleep. Respiration becomes more regular as the newborn matures [8]. The risk of apneic spells is up to 45 percent in infants younger than 48 weeks PCA and more common in younger children [5]. Apnea is defined as cessation of breathing for greater than 20 seconds or cessation of breathing accompanied with a heart rate below 100 bpm, cyanosis, or pallor [5,8]. Preterm newborns are at risk for cardiac arrest if the apnea is prolonged, thus they require close monitoring [8]. Sepsis, intracranial hemorrhage, metabolic acidosis, lack of normothermia, vagal reflexes and anesthetics all contribute to apnea [9]. Preterm newborns may also develop apnea after receiving opiates until around 55 weeks PCA. An additional risk factor for postoperative apnea is a hematocrit of less than 30 percent [1]. An oxygen-enriched environment will promote regular respirations in the preterm newborn and a hypoxic environment will increase apneic spells and respiratory variations [8], which is important with regards to post-anesthesia considerations for the preterm newborn. With vigilance and close monitoring, apnea may be treated with stimulation, bag-mask ventilation, and addition of caffeine or assisted ventilation with continuous positive airway pressure (CPAP) or endotracheal intubation [5]. Obstructive apnea may also occur postoperatively in the preterm newborn due to excessive relaxation [8]. For elective surgeries of the preterm newborn, it is recommended to wait until the newborn reaches almost 60 weeks PCA to decrease this risk of postoperative apnea [5].

Chemical factors also play a critical role in the preterm newborn's respiratory state. Surfactant, discovered by Dr. Mary Ellen Avery, is a substance that allows small alveoli to remain open in the presence of increased surface tension. Mature surfactant prevents the collapse of smaller alveoli into larger alveoli, thus maintaining functional residual capacity (FRC). Surfactant is made by pneumocytes after 24 weeks' gestation. The composition changes during gestation and it is not until about 36 weeks' gestation that there is sufficient mature, functional surfactant to prevent neonatal respiratory distress syndrome (RDS) [5,10]. Respiratory distress syndrome is due to a lack of surfactant, leading to decreased functional capacity [5]. Ninety percent of babies born at 26 weeks will experience RDS [5]. When requiring intubation and ventilation for surgery, these patients experience ventilation perfusion mismatch and may require additional support of PEEP [5]. Ventilation can be difficult and barotrauma and oxygen toxicity are risks of artificial ventilation in this age group; thus it is recommended to use the minimal concentration of oxygen necessary as well as to limit the peak inspiratory pressures used [5]. Because preterm newborns have decreased endogenous surfactant and will often develop respiratory distress, they may be treated with intratracheal surfactant ("surfed") in the NICU. Intratracheal surfactant has been shown to reduce air leaks, improve survival, and reduce the severity of chronic lung disease [9]. Despite the advantages of surfactant administration, the incidence of BPD in babies treated with surfactant has not been decreased and the use of surfactant in babies born at 28 weeks has decreased in recent years. Bronchopulmonary dysplasia is the requirement of supplemental oxygen at 28 days of life with a chest radiography demonstrating air trapping, atelectasis, and lung field opacification [9]. Assessment of the patient's respiratory status is important to drive decision-making and treatment plans about the use of surfactant. For example, if the patient is spontaneously breathing, requiring less than 0.4 $FiO_2$, then using a trial of nasal CPAP may be practiced in favor of intubating and instilling surfactant (Figure 2.3) [4,9].

Structural lung difference in the preterm newborn also contributes to their more delicate respiratory status. Preterm newborns have reduced lung volumes compared to term newborns. There is a four-fold increase in lung volume and alveolar surface area from 25 weeks to term. Preterm newborns also have a very compliant chest wall, which predisposes them to injury both via volutrauma (pneumothorax) and barotrauma (BPD) when positive pressure ventilation is used [1]. If intubated, NICU strategies are currently incorporating permissive hypercapnea, especially if PIPs are higher than 14–18 $cmH_2O$, and oxygenation goals are aiming for saturations in the upper eighties to decrease damage to the lungs [1]. A parameter of preterm newborn assisted ventilation is to prevent hypoxia, while at the same time avoiding hyperoxia, and it can be a delicate balance. A low range $SpO_2$ of 85–89 percent decreased retinopathy of prematurity, but increased mortality, in very low birth weight (VLBW) newborns on supplemental oxygen [9]. Hyperoxia plays a role in decreasing ciliary movement and adversely influencing bronchopulmonary development. The inspired oxygen concentration of oxygen seems to be the main factor, rather than the arterial

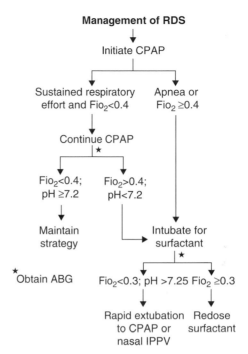

**Management of RDS**

Initiate CPAP

Sustained respiratory effort and $Fio_2 < 0.4$ / Apnea or $Fio_2 \geq 0.4$

Continue CPAP ★

$Fio_2 < 0.4$; pH $\geq 7.2$ / $Fio_2 > 0.4$; pH $< 7.2$

Maintain strategy / Intubate for surfactant ★

★ Obtain ABG

$Fio_2 < 0.3$; pH $> 7.25$ / $Fio_2 \geq 0.3$

Rapid extubation to CPAP or nasal IPPV / Redose surfactant

**Figure 2.3** CPAP surfactant. Source: [9].

concentration [9]. PEEP is often utilized in intubated preterm newborns, at around 5 $cmH_2O$, with the goal of keeping distal airways open to reduce shear stress from when they repeatedly close and reopen, improving oxygenation, and allowing down-titration of inspired oxygen [1,9]. Goal tidal volumes are often in the 6 ml $kg^{-1}$ range [1].

One must also consider the small size of the airway when choosing endotracheal tubes. The consideration of cuffed versus uncuffed tubes for risk of subglottic stenosis must be addressed. Also, if a patient is particularly small or requires sophisticated ventilation such as high-flow oscillatory ventilation, it may be beneficial to continue the NICU ventilator in the operating room in order to maintain clinical stability

## Cardiac Issues

The preterm newborn is at high risk for cardiovascular compromise when exposed to anesthetic agents and surgery. The physiology of the immature heart consists of poor diastolic function, fixed stroke volumes, and poor autoregulation of the systemic vasculature [5]. Patients administered potent inhalational anesthetics have impaired baroreceptor reflexes and compensate poorly, if at all, for blood loss and hypovolemia [5]. The pediatric anesthesiologist also must have an awareness of congenital anomalies of premature infants as they are 2.4 times more likely to have cardiovascular malformations than term newborns [11]. Preterm newborns are more likely than full-term babies to be born with pulmonary atresia with ventricular septal defect, complete atrioventricular septal defect, coarctation of the aorta, Tetralogy of Fallot, and pulmonary valve stenosis [11]. Also, a majority of preterm infants have a patent ductus arteriosus (PDA) that may require medical or surgical intervention [1,5]. In the term newborn, there is a rapid decrease in pulmonary vascular resistance due to a chemical response to increased $pO_2$, as well as a reduced $pCO_2$, and intrapulmonary cardiac and pulmonary pressure changes lead to a quick closure of the patent foramen ovale (PFO) and a PDA [8]. In preterm newborns there is a delay in the response to the increase of arterial oxygenation with extrauterine respirations. When preterm newborns become hypoxic, hypercarbic, or acidotic, they may revert back to a fetal circulation due to a relatively quick increase in pulmonary vascular resistance. This may result in right-to-left shunting via the PFO or opening of the PDA [8]. Monitoring of preductal (right upper extremity) and postductal (lower extremity) saturations is a common intraoperative practice of anesthesiologists that care for the preterm newborn. An open PDA with left-to-right shunting contributes to morbidity in the form of IVH, pulmonary edema and heart failure, NEC, renal insufficiency, or hemorrhage [1].

"Normal" blood pressures are difficult to define in the preterm newborns, but one may review recent blood pressures obtained to have a guide of what "normal" is for a particular patient. Intraoperative blood pressure measurement must use the same size non-invasive blood pressure (NIBP) cuff as was used prior to the trip to the operating room. Hypotension is found in up to 45 percent of premature infants, with hypertension being less common [6]. A common practice among pediatric anesthesiologists caring for patients in this group is to treat the blood pressure if the mean is lower than the GA plus 5 mmHg [5]. Blood pressure treatment can be with colloid, crystalloid, or vasopressors [5]. It is important to note that stroke volume is 1 ml kg⁻¹ and left ventricular end-diastolic volume is 2 ml kg⁻¹. Calcium supplementation may be helpful in augmenting blood pressure because preterm newborns have poor calcium reserves and their myocardial function is driven by extracellular calcium [1].

## Gastrointestinal Issues

The immature gastrointestinal tract of the preterm newborn requires consideration by the anesthesiologist. It is common for these patients to have reflux due to poor esophageal sphincter tone and impaired peristalsis [5]. Gastrointestinal reflux can contribute to aspiration, cough, laryngospasm, and other respiratory compromise that contribute to morbidity related to anesthetics [5]. Necrotizing enterocolitis can develop in the preterm newborn for many reasons and must be considered in these patients. Etiologic factors for the development of NEC are impaired intestinal blood flow, early and hyperosmolar feeds, and prematurity. Bowel perforation associated with NEC can lead to sepsis [5]. If the NEC does not respond to medical treatment, the patient may require an emergent exploratory laparotomy.

## Hematology Issues

Preterm newborns may present to the operating room relatively anemic and require transfusion after surgical blood loss. Anemia of prematurity is multifactorial and stems from delivery prior to placental transport of iron, incomplete fetal erythropoesis, recurrent phlebotomy of the hospitalized infant, low erythropoietin production, and rapid growth [9]. Preterm newborns, especially extremely low birth weight newborns, are likely to have received a transfusion if they have cardiopulmonary issues as the increased oxygen-carrying capacity of red blood cells will aid in patients with cardiorespiratory distress, though possibly increasing the risk of NEC [9]. The absolute blood volume of the smallest of patients is in the 100 ml kg⁻¹ range [5]. A few milliliters of blood loss during surgery may be a significant percent of total blood volume. The newborn born at less than 28 weeks will have hemoglobin levels of 13–15 g dl⁻¹, with 75 percent of it being fetal hemoglobin, which does not release oxygen as readily as adult hemoglobin [5]. Preterm newborns also have immature coagulation profiles with low platelet counts and vitamin K deficiency. All newborns should receive vitamin K if going for surgery [5]. Transfusion in these patients must be done after warming the blood, done in small volumes, and given slowly, with consideration of washing the blood to decrease the potassium load delivered over a short amount of time. A 10 ml syringe of packed red blood cells pushed quickly in a 1 kg weight baby via an IV increases the blood volume by 10 percent, which is analogous to pushing two units of packed red blood cells into an adult IV over less than one minute [1,5].

## Hepatic Issues

The immature liver of preterm newborns is not able to metabolize medications as well as a mature liver, does not synthesize certain proteins well, affecting drug metabolism, and does not have glycogen stores. Preterm newborns require the same glucose levels as term newborns, but because of their limited glycogen stores glucose must be supplemented when these babies are stressed or having feeds held in preparation for surgery [5]. Hypoglycemia is detrimental and may be difficult to recognize in these small patients, but hyperglycemia also carries an increased risk of intraventricular hemorrhage, dehydration, increased length of hospitalization, and death [5,9]. Infants most at risk for hyperglycemia, defined as >150 mg dl$^{-1}$ of glucose, are preterm newborns <1000 g, those receiving glucose infusions of >6 mg kg$^{-1}$ min$^{-1}$, those with illness, and those on glucocorticoid therapies [9]. Treatment of hyperglycemia can include decreasing glucose infusion rates, early amino acid administration to increase insulin release, and possibly instituting insulin infusions. Insulin infusions should be used with extreme caution, given the small doses involved and the significant morbidity associated with hypoglycemia, which may be difficult to recognize in the anesthetized patient [9].

## Renal Issues

The preterm newborn is at risk for hyponatremia since renal tubules do not have the ability to retain sodium until 32 weeks' gestation, the response of the distal tubules to aldosterone is low until 34 weeks' gestation and antidiuretic hormone levels are elevated [5]. Negative sodium balance is not uncommon in preterm infants of less than 35 weeks' gestation and this negative balance may last for up to three weeks after birth [9]. Hypernatremia may occur if there are insensible fluid losses not adequately replaced [1]. Newborn acid–base status is often on the acidotic side and in the first day of life they may show combined metabolic and respiratory acidosis. The renal tubules are not able to reabsorb bicarbonate well and there is normally mild metabolic acidosis seen in these patients [5]. For the first month they may have metabolic acidosis due to a net acid input from metabolism, protein intake, and bone mineralization with a decreased capacity for

acid excretion. This acidosis increases the risk of negative calcium balance and poor bone formation [9], which can impact cardiac function and fracture risk, respectively.

## Skin/Temperature Maintenance Issues

The epidermis of preterm newborns is very thin and requires the utmost of care and consideration. Preterm infants who are hypothermic on admission to the NICU after birth are at high risk for mortality [9]. There is a great amount of heat loss due to the large surface area to body size ratio, lack of adipose tissue, and thin skin. Infants less than 2 kg in weight are particularly efficient in transferring heat from the internal to external gradient [8,9]. Hypothermia leads to a decreased respiratory response to hypoxia. Infants born between 32 and 37 weeks will have an increase in ventilatory rate in response to hypoxia in a warm environment; this response is not seen in a cool environment [8]. Temperature monitoring and maintenance are very important in the preterm newborn. In environments of high temperature or when the environmental temperature fluctuates, these infants are at risk for apnea [9]. Their thin skin is also easily bruised and/or abraded by tape and monitors. These injuries are similar to partial thickness burns.

Total body water in these patients is 80 percent of body weight, and this amount decreases as the infant matures. This amount of fluid paired with the thin skin leads to evaporative fluid losses 15 times that of a full-term newborn in the first days of life. Newborns younger than 32 weeks are at the highest risk because they have the thinnest epidermal layer, but the skin does thicken over weeks of extrauterine life [1,5]. Also, preterm newborns rely on nonshivering thermogenesis, which includes utilization of their richly vascular and innervated brown fat, which has mitochondrial oxidative metabolism, to produce heat [9].

## Common Surgical Conditions of the Preterm Newborn

Common surgical conditions of preterm newborns include:

- Cut-downs for IV access
- Necrotizing enterocolitis exploratory laparotomy
- Patent ductus arteriosis ligation

## Inguinal Herniorrhaphy

The most common surgery performed in preterm newborns is inguinal herniorrhaphy. Thirty-eight percent of infants with a birth weight from 751 g to 1000 g will have an inguinal hernia, and since these hernias are larger than those seen in term newborns and infants, the risk for incarceration or strangulation is greater. The incidence of inguinal hernias is approximately 15 percent in infants born weighing 1001–1250 g [5]. Up to 49 percent of these babies are at risk for postoperative apnea [9].

## Preparation for Surgery

The pediatric anesthesiologist must review the patient's birth history, age at birth, current age in terms of PCA, and current weight. For all but the most minor procedures in relatively well preterm newborns, a complete blood count and coagulation profile should be obtained. Chest X-rays or echocardiograms should be reviewed to assess for significant cardiac or respiratory anomalies.

Guardians of preterm newborns presenting for surgery should be aware of the higher anesthetic risk. The anesthesiologist should review the possibility of difficulties in managing the airway, issues associated with intubation and having a breathing tube, the possibility of postoperative intubation, difficulties with vascular access, and the possibility of cardiorespiratory compromise and need for blood transfusion or blood products [5].

Premedication is not usually required as these small patients do not have perioperative anxiety or stranger awareness/anxiety. Atropine for prophylaxis against anesthesia-induced bradycardia is not as commonplace as in the past with current inhalational agents, but the correct dose of IV atropine should be immediately available [5].

The operating room thermostat should be kept very warm prior to arrival of the patient (27 °C/80 °F) and warm lights and hot air warming devices should be employed to maintain a neutral thermal environment for the patient [5]. Monitoring patient temperature must be done with care as esophageal or rectal probes may cause perforation even when placed gently [1,5]. Temperature should be maintained carefully so as to not cause hyperthermia [9]. Fluids and blood products should be warmed and given slowly.

Standard monitors should include pre- and postductal pulse oximeters. Noninvasive blood pressure cuffs should be appropriately sized as a large cuff may falsely read lower than the actual pressure, and placement should be careful as the bones are at risk for fracture [5]. The upper extremity blood pressure cuff may be a more reliable reading for mean arterial pressure, but may not be practical if lines are in place or if the extremity is part of the operative field. Invasive monitors are often extremely technically challenging and attempts to place them in very small patients may confer more harm than benefit, thus they may not be employed [1,5]. Some preterm newborns will present with umbilical lines in place and the arterial line can provide useful information or allow for easy lab draws; however, rapid flushing or drawing off of the line may cause morbidity and it should be used carefully [5]. The anesthesia machine used should be able to deliver reliably small volumes, PEEP, and limit pressure delivered to the patient to minimize barotrauma and optimize ventilation. If a patient is particularly small, a neonatal ventilator from the NICU may be required.

The patient may arrive already intubated, but the anesthesia team should be prepared if extubation occurs and have small face masks available, Miller 0 and 00 blades checked and ready to be used, a size 0 LMA available, and endotracheal tubes down to size 2.5 outer diameter with small stylets [1,5]. It is also important to have the proper size suction catheters available (a 5 French catheter for a 2.5 endotracheal tube, a 6–7 French catheter for a 3.0 endotracheal tube, and an 8 French catheter for a 3.5 endotracheal tube). The distance from vocal cords to carina in the trachea in preterm newborns may be less than 4 cm [5]; thus, care must be taken in tube placement and continuous assessment for extubation or mainstem intubation. A reference of tube length to guide for where to tape an oral endotracheal tube (OETT) at the gum of preterm newborns of various weights is to have the tip midtrachea; for newborns weighing 1, 2, 3, 4 kg the OETT should be taped at 7, 8, 9, 10 cm respectively [5]. A leak of the tube should be assessed. In order to minimize tracheal trauma and swelling, a leak should be audible between 10 and 30 cmH$_2$O [5,9]. These small endotracheal tubes are easily bent and kinked, and a small amount of secretions may block the tube. The anesthesiologist must be cognizant of these common complications. If a patient comes to the operating room already intubated, it is important to note the position of the tube, and it is not recommended to change out the endotracheal tube unless there is dislodgement, excessive leak, or occlusion due to secretions [9].

Inductions may be safely achieved with fentanyl and a neuromuscular blocking agent [1]. Propofol has been used to provide good intubating conditions in preterm neonates requiring intubation for surfactant administration, but it has been found to cause prolonged hypotension in this population and should be used with caution [12]. Preterm newborns born at 29–32 weeks who received 1 mg kg$^{-1}$ of propofol for intubation had a decrease in mean arterial pressure from 38 mmHg to 24 mmHg, ranging from 29–42 mmHg to 22–40 mmHg, respectively [12].

Maintenance of anesthesia should be done with moderate amounts of inhalational agents, such as sevoflurane, isoflurane, and desflurane. Halothane caused bradycardia and postoperative apnea in preterm newborns and is no longer is use [5]. Moderate amounts of inhalational agent should be dosed to avoid a decrease in systemic arterial pressures and to minimize increases in pulmonary vascular resistance [5]. Balanced anesthesia with fentanyl is commonly done as fentanyl provides cardiovascular stability while providing pain control, and is safe in patients at risk for, or with, pulmonary hypertension [5]. Many of the preterm newborns presenting for surgery will remain intubated and ventilated postoperatively, thus adequate dosing of fentanyl may be achieved. For the patients who will not remain intubated postoperatively, regional anesthesia with or without inhalational agents and acetaminophen will provide benefit [5]. A prospective study in 2006 showed that preterm newborns at less than 47 weeks PCA who presented for inguinal herniorrhaphy did not have postoperative apnea requiring airway intervention after an anesthetic with controlled ventilation with sevoflurane or desflurane, rectal acetaminophen 20 mg kg$^{-1}$ and a caudal block with 0.25 percent bupivacaine 1 ml kg$^{-1}$ [13]. Postoperative analgesia should be achieved with opiates only if the infant can be closely monitored, preferably in an ICU setting. Acetaminophen is the sole analgesic deemed safe for use in preterm newborns [5], as NSAIDs are not recommended for those under six months of age. Rectal acetaminophen is suggested for postoperative pain control after abdominal surgery in neonates, with a dose of 15 mg kg$^{-1}$ around the clock every 12 hours for newborns born at <32 weeks' gestation for four doses, or every eight hours for those patients born >32 weeks to 40 for six doses [9].

Once intubated, preterm neonates should not be exposed to high levels of oxygen. Oxygen toxicity to the lungs and developing retina is a concern in preterm neonates as high levels of oxygen administration contributes to morbidity and mortality [5,9]. It is recommended that after intubation is achieved, maintenance of inspired oxygen should be titrated to achieve oxygen saturations of 88–95 percent [5,9].

Regional anesthesia is safe in preterm neonates. Preterm neonates have a larger volume of cerebrospinal fluid compared to older children and they have an increased surface area around nerve roots, so medication dosing is higher and duration of block is shorter [5]. Blood pressure is well preserved when regional anesthesia is used, owing to the low vasomotor tone of preterm newborns and decreased vagal activity [5]. It is possible to place a spinal without IV access then secure lower extremity IV access once the spinal sets up. If a regional anesthetic is chosen for the preterm neonate, it should be noted that the procedure is technically more difficult than in term babies. One in seven attempts at spinal fails to find the intrathecal space, and one in three of these babies require additional anesthetic in addition to the spinal for adequate surgical conditions [5].

Intravenous fluids should be warm, free of air, and limited in volume delivered. Due to a high risk of hypoglycemia, dextrose-containing fluid given at maintenance should be part of the anesthesia care. This may mean glucose at a rate of 8–10 mg kg$^{-1}$ min$^{-1}$ or 10 percent dextrose at 110–120 ml kg$^{-1}$ day$^{-1}$ [1].

# References

1. Holzman R, Mancuso TJ, Polaner DM. *A Practical Approach to Pediatric Anesthesia.* Philadelphia, PA: Lippincott Williams & Wilkins; 2008. 601–8.

2. Hamilton BE, Hoyert DL, Martin JA, Strobino DM, Guyer B. Annual summary of vital statistics: 2010–2011. *Pediatrics.* 2013;131:548–58.

3. Costarino AT. Neonatology and premature birth outcome: a primer for pediatric anesthesiologists. Lecture presented at Society for Pediatric Anesthesia. October 11, 2013, San Francisco, CA.

4. Stoll BJ, Hansen NI, Bell EF, et al. Neonatal outcomes of extremely preterm infants from the NICHD neonatal research network. *Pediatrics.* 2010; 126(3):442–56.

5. Taneja B, Srivastava V, Saxena KN. Physiological and anesthetic considerations for the preterm neonate undergoing surgery. *J Neonat Surg.* 2012;1:14.

6. Ballabh P. Intraventricular hemorrhage in premature infants: mechanism of disease. *Pediatr Res*. 2010;67(1):1–8.

7. Volpe JJ. Brain injury in premature infants: a complex amalgam of destructive and developmental disturbances. *Lancet Neurol*. 2009.;8(1):110–24.

8. Cook DR, Marcy JH *Neonatal Anesthesia*. Pasadena, CA: Appleton Davies, Inc.; 1988.

9. Fanaroff AA, Fanaroff JM. *Klaus & Fanaroff's Care of the High-Risk Neonate*. 6th edn. New York: Elsevier Saunders; 2013.

10. MacDonald M, Mullet M, Seshia M. *Avery's Neonatology. Pathophysiology and Management of the Newborn*, 6th edn. New York: Lippincott Williams and Wilkins; 2005. 284–303.

11. Tanner K, Sabrine N, Wren C. Cardiovascular malformations among preterm infants. *Pediatrics*. 2005;116(6):e833–e838.

12. Welzing L, Kribs A, Eifinger F, et al. Propofol as an induction agent for endotracheal intubation can cause significant arterial hypotension in preterm neonates. *Pediatr Anes*. 2010;20(7):605–11.

13. Sale SM, Read JA, Stoddart PA, Wolf AR. Prospective comparison of sevoflurane and desflurane in formerly premature infants undergoing inguinal herniorrhaphy. *Br J Anaesth*. 2006;96:774–8.

Chapter

3

# Origin of the NICU

Amy Vinson

The Lion incubator was invented in 1891, but its approval for use in hospitals lagged behind. The first public use of an incubator for the care of an infant occurred in a side show of the Dreamland amusement park on Coney Island, NY and warmed a set of triplets born early to the owners of the show. Herein lies the birth of the specialized care of the premature infant in a world of modern medicine and technology [1]. A series of advancements, including portable incubators, ventilators, and antibiotics eventually led to the creation of the first official neonatal intensive care unit (NICU) at Vanderbilt University in 1961, when a ventilator was used (off-label) for the first time to help a struggling neonate.

While neonatology and pediatric anesthesia may not intuitively seem the closest of medical cousins, their developments have both relied heavily on technological advancements in order to care for ever sicker and more precarious neonates. The care of premature infants has continually fallen squarely into the hands of these two divisions, and an understanding of one another is paramount to the optimal care of patients in this unique population. The collaboration between the two groups is most notably recognized in the personage of Virginia Apgar (Figure 3.1), an anesthesiologist who developed the APGAR scoring system in 1952, to objectively assess the overall status of a newborn during the first moments of transition from fetal life [2].

## Population of the NICU

### Patients

The National Perinatal Information System collects data on admissions to special care nurseries. "Special care" nurseries (SCNs) are defined as either NICUs or neonatal intermediate care units (NINTs), and include data on children born at hospitals with these units on site as well as children transported into these units.

These data are prepared by the March of Dimes into a report titled "Special Care Nursery Admissions." The most salient statistics include the following regarding infants born during the study period (July 1, 2009 to June 30, 2010):

- 14.4 percent of all infants were admitted to an SCN;
- 49.1 percent of admissions were preterm (defined as <37 weeks gestational age [GA]);
- 70 percent of these premature infants were admitted to the NICU, not NINT;
- 23.6 percent of infants admitted to the SCN had a primary diagnosis of "prematurity";
- 11.9 percent of infants admitted to the SCN had a diagnosis of "respiratory distress syndrome";
- 90 percent of infants born less than 34 weeks GA were admitted to an SCN [3].

## Providers

As in other intensive care environments, the providers in the NICU are highly trained and varied in skillsets. The physician specialist associated with the NICU is the neonatologist (a pediatrician with subspecialty training in neonatology), though many NINTs are immediately staffed by pediatricians with neonatologist supervision. Other direct providers include neonatal nurse practitioners as well as neonatal clinical nurse specialists. In addition to these, and depending on the hospital environment, there may also be neonatology fellows and pediatric residents caring for the neonates. The success of an NICU depends on the collaboration of multiple providers working together as a team. Members of the team often include respiratory therapists, physical therapists, occupational therapists, speech therapists, registered dietitians, lactation consultants, pharmacists, and social workers.

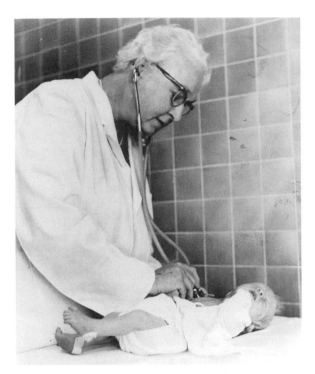

**Figure 3.1** Virginia Apgar, MD. Source: Library of Congress, public domain.

## Common Medical Issues in the NICU by Systems

The NICU population is unique in the medical system, and their problems and diagnoses are equally unusual. While other chapters in this book will look more exhaustively at each system described below, it is prudent in a discussion of the NICU to address the major conditions, abnormalities, and diagnoses found in the average NICU. We will address these conditions by systems.

## Neurologic

Neurodevelopment is a process that is ongoing throughout childhood and adolescence, but it is particularly dynamic in the neonate, and especially so in the preterm neonate. A more detailed review of neonatal response to pain, development, and drug toxicity can be found in other chapters of this book. Below, we briefly discuss the major neurologic conditions often uniquely found in the neonatal population: intraventricular hemorrhage (IVH), hypoxic-ischemic encephalopathy (HIE), retinopathy of prematurity (ROP), and the neonatal abstinence syndrome (NAS).

## Intraventricular Hemorrhage

The neonatal brain is a rapidly developing organ, with neuronal migration originating in the highly vascularized germinal matrix, which is a particularly delicate region, exquisitely sensitive to physiologic perturbations. With such changes, bleeding can develop within the germinal matrix; staging of IVH is based on the degree of blood spread into the periventricular parenchyma and adjacent lateral ventricles. Smaller infants are more susceptible to hemorrhage, especially within the first few days of life and since the presentation is often subtle, screening head ultrasounds have become routine for low birth weight neonates in most NICUs [4].

## Hypoxic-Ischemic Encephalopathy

While HIE remains a relatively rare occurrence in neonates (1–3 per 1000 live full-term births), the morbidity and mortality remains high. Fifteen to twenty percent of infants with HIE will die during the postnatal course and another 25 percent will develop significant and permanent neurologic sequelae, such as cerebral palsy, neurodevelopment impairment, and epilepsy. Currently there is much research into neuroprotective strategies that can be employed following a hypoxic insult. The only proven strategy is that of hypothermia (cooling the infant by 3–5 °C), although many other strategies (e.g., free radical scavengers and erythropoetin) are being investigated [5].

## Retinopathy of Prematurity

Premature infants are born with incompletely vascularized retinas. When subsequent vascularization does not proceed normally, ROP develops, which if left untreated could lead to retinal detachment and blindness. ROP generally occurs in two phases, with retardation in vessel growth occurring first at around 30–32 weeks post-GA and then a proliferative phase occurring at approximately 32–34 weeks post-GA. The most recognized risk factors are prematurity, low birth weight, and hyperoxygenation (including the use of unnecessary supplemental oxygen in the operating room), although infants exposed to very little supplemental oxygen have developed ROP. Improved screening, early diagnosis, and treatment (with bevacizumab [an angiogenesis inhibitor] or LASER treatment by an ophthalmologist) have improved the overall morbidity, despite the fact that the overall incidence of ROP has not declined [6].

## Neonatal Abstinence Syndrome

As the number of people dependent on opiates (both prescribed and illicit) and other psychotropic medications has increased in the last few decades, so has the incidence of intrauterine exposure and the number of infants born dependent on these same substances. The signs and symptoms displayed by neonates as they withdraw from these medications are collectively referred to as the "neonatal abstinence syndrome" or NAS. The timing of first symptoms is dependent on the type and dosage of the exposed medication, with heroin and oxycodone withdrawal occurring rapidly and methadone and buprenorphine withdrawal sometimes not occurring for several days. Treatment generally consists of the controlled replacement and weaning of opiate (usually morphine or methadone), with or without adjuncts such as phenobarbital or clonidine, while carefully monitoring for signs of withdrawal. Various scoring systems and weaning strategies are used, and are quite unit-specific. Many units are utilizing nonpharmacologic management techniques such as occupational and massage therapy [7].

## Cardiac

During fetal life, roughly 90 percent of combined ventricular output is directed toward the systemic circulation, with only 10 percent entering the pulmonary vasculature. This feat is accomplished mainly via two shunts: the intracardiac foramen ovale and the extracardiac ductus arteriosus; these two shunts close postnatally as the infant's pulmonary vascular resistance falls and the infant transitions away from the fetal circulation. Excluding congenital heart disease (CHD) and the hypotension associated with sepsis, the bulk of cardiac pathology in the NICU concerns an abnormal transition to postnatal circulation.

## Patent Ductus Arteriosus

The ductus arteriosus is a large conduit that links the fetal main pulmonary artery to the descending aorta, which usually closes early in postnatal life as oxygen tension increases and prostaglandin input decreases. Its closure is usually welcome, except in the case of so-called ductal-dependent cardiac lesions, but it often remains open in preterm neonates, leading to the unwanted shunting of blood. In fact, in infants born at <28 weeks GA, a majority (60–70 percent) will require either medical or surgical closure of a patent ductus arteriosus (PDA). There is considerable research into when a PDA is significant enough to warrant intervention, but two of the most important considerations are those of diastolic flow reversal and cerebral steal and pulmonary overcirculation. Once the decision has been made to intervene, a trial of medical closure is generally attempted, using cyclooxygenase inhibitors like indomethacin or ibuprofen. If medical treatment is unsuccessful or inappropriate, a surgical PDA ligation can be performed via a left thoracic approach [8].

## Persistent Pulmonary Hypertension of the Newborn

As its name implies, persistent pulmonary hypertension of the newborn (PPHN) occurs when the normal transition from fetal to postnatal circulation does not occur. Normally, shortly after birth, the systemic vascular resistance increases (due largely to the clamping of the umbilical cord), the pulmonary vascular resistance drops precipitously (due to multiple factors), and the major fetal shunts (the ductus arteriosus and foramen ovale) experience a functional followed by anatomical closure. When this drop in pulmonary vascular resistance does not occur, the closure of the shunts cannot occur, and the neonate will remain in a fetal circulation characterized by a circuit in parallel instead of a mature circuit in series. In other words, if a neonate has PPHN, shunting and variable systemic oxygen saturation and perfusion can result. The causes of PPHN are varied, but are generally due to abnormal parenchyma with resultant vasoconstriction (e.g., meconium aspiration syndrome, respiratory distress syndrome, pneumonia), abnormally deficient vasculature (e.g., pulmonary stenosis, lung hypoplasia), or are idiopathic. Treatment focuses on overall physiologic stability and efforts to decrease pulmonary vascular resistance through interventions such as inhaled nitric oxide, phosphodiesterase inhibitors, sedation, and methods to optimize oxygenation. When conventional therapies are unsuccessful, extra corporeal life support (ECLS) is offered to a select population [9].

## Congenital Heart Disease

An exhaustive discussion of CHD is beyond the scope of this section. We will instead focus on just

**Table 3.1** Ductal-dependent cardiac lesions

- Critical coarctation of the aorta (decreased systemic perfusion)
- Interrupted aortic arch (decreased systemic perfusion)
- Critical aortic stenosis (decreased systemic perfusion)
- Hypoplastic left heart syndrome (decreased systemic perfusion)
- Tricuspid atresia (decreased pulmonary perfusion)
- Pulmonary atresia (decreased pulmonary perfusion)
- Transposition of the great vessels (inability to deliver oxygenated blood to the systemic circulation) [10]

those conditions that will present within the first few hours or days of life. The immediate neonatal period is marked by a transition from fetal circulation to adult circulation and can often bring to light major congenital cardiac lesions. Certain lesions, such as total anomalous pulmonary venous return and critical pulmonary stenosis, are not even apparent on fetal surveys due to the significantly decreased pulmonary blood flow in the fetus. Other lesions, such as hypoplastic left heart syndrome and transposition of the great arteries, require a functional ductus arteriosus in order to supply oxygenated blood to the systemic circulation. In ductal-dependent cardiac lesions (see Table 3.1), an infusion of prostaglandin E1 can maintain patency of the ductus arteriosus and even open a functionally closed ductus arteriosus if anatomical closure has not occurred. Airway control is an important consideration when using prostaglandins, given associated apnea.

## Pulmonary

Lung immaturity is a predictable biochemical, physiologic, and anatomical phenomenon in premature infants, and this unique situation has led to the development of a different set of treatment and ventilation strategies than in adults and children.

The threshold of viability is accepted by many to occur at approximately 24 weeks GA, and this time corresponds with the embryological development of respiratory bronchioles and alveolar ducts and signifies the initiation of the ability to oxygenate and ventilate. At approximately 26 weeks GA, type II pneumocytes begin to populate the alveoli and begin the production of surfactant, which will ultimately prevent the collapse of alveoli with exhalation and dramatically improve pulmonary compliance [11].

Antenatal steroids are a mainstay in the treatment of women with preterm labor (less than 32–34 weeks GA) because of the known effect on fetal lung maturation and surfactant expression. The efficacy of antenatal steroids has been strongly validated, with multiple meta-analyses demonstrating a clear benefit [12].

One aspect of neonatal ventilation often not seen in older children is the relative immaturity of respiratory control that can lead to irregular breathing patterns and even life-threatening apnea. This is multifactorial, with causes ranging from altered response curves to hypoxia and hypercapnea, to immature brainstem and peripheral receptor networks. Furthermore, neonates do not seem to be able to handle an oxidant stress and are particularly vulnerable to oxygen toxicity. In fact, the 2010 American Heart Association Guidelines for neonatal resuscitation recommend initiating resuscitation for term infants with room air and blending in oxygen as needed to achieve an acceptable oxygen saturation [13].

## Respiratory Distress Syndrome

Respiratory distress syndrome (RDS), previously known as hyaline membrane disease, is best understood as difficulty ventilating due to the lack of surfactant and subsequent decrease in lung compliance and propensity for alveolar collapse. It is most commonly observed in premature neonates due to their natural surfactant-deficient state, but can be observed in full-term neonates whose surfactant, while present, might be inactivated by a variety of causes. Treatment depends on the degree of distress and prematurity and can include exogenous surfactant administration, noninvasive ventilatory support, and invasive ventilation [14].

## Chronic Lung Disease and Bronchopulmonary Dysplasia

Chronic lung disease (CLD) is a fairly generic term that refers to pulmonary disease that follows respiratory disorders of the neonate. Bronchopulmonary dysplasia (BPD) is a form of CLD with a specific definition: The need for supplemental oxygen at least 28 days after birth or the need for supplemental oxygen after 36 weeks corrected GA, depending on the definition being used. As one can imagine, this does not have a high predictive value for long-term respiratory dysfunction, as it does not take into account GA at birth or oxygen delivery method (e.g., nasal cannula versus endotracheal intubation). Bronchopulmonary dysplasia is a condition of prematurity, almost always occurring in infants born at less than 30 weeks GA and with low birth weight (under 1500 g). As improvements have been made to the treatment of RDS, fewer infants have developed BPD characterized by non-homogeneous parenchymal damage due to ventilator-associated trauma. Instead, as smaller and younger infants are now surviving, infants are now developing a more homogeneous BPD characterized by the reduced development of alveoli. Treatment is centered first on prevention. Frequent strategies employed may include the occasional use of diuretics to improve respiratory mechanics, optimizing nutrition, palivizumab for respiratory syncitial virus prophylaxis, short courses of steroids for exacerbations outside of the neonatal period, and inhaled bronchodilators for obstructive exacerbations [15,16].

## Transient Tachypnea of the Newborn

As discussed in the section on cardiac physiology of the neonate, the newborn infant must undergo a dramatic transition in order to move from a liquid environment reliant on maternal ventilation and oxygenation to one where ventilation and oxygenation are paramount to survival. The fetal lung is filled with fetal lung fluid up to a volume that is close to what will ultimately become the functional residual capacity. A small portion of this fluid is expelled due to external forces during labor, but the majority is reabsorbed by the lung epithelium once labor commences and levels of epinephrine increase. This is likely the reason that infants born via cesarean section without labor have a significantly increased incidence of transient tachypnea of the newborn (TTN) compared to those born by cesarean section after the beginning of labor [17]. When this fluid is not reabsorbed quickly enough, retained lung fluid will cause the infant to display symptoms of tachypnea, grunting, retractions, and variable hypoxia. This is usually a self-limited condition that resolves within 2–3 days [18].

## Ventilation Modes in the NICU

Given the physiologic challenge that incompletely developed neonatal lungs present, it is not surprising that neonatal ventilation strategies is an area of active research. There are multiple modes of noninvasive (i.e., without an endotracheal tube) as well as multiple modes of invasive ventilation utilizing endotracheal intubation. Because of the very small tidal volumes in the range of 4–6 ml kg$^{-1}$ (sometimes less than 5 ml in extremely low birth weight infants), the ventilators and circuitry have to operate in a precise manner with highly sensitive flow and pressure sensors [19].

In recent years, controversy has emerged regarding the use of cuffed versus uncuffed endotracheal tubes. In the past, the thought was to not use cuffed tubes in children younger than eight years because of the natural narrowing at the level of the cricoid cartilage, and because of the potential morbidity of subglottic trauma being caused by the cuff. With newer, lower profiled cuffs, this does not seem to be as much of an issue, and many practitioners are moving toward cuffed endotracheal tubes for neonates. The advantages of a cuffed tube include a good fit with fewer intubations, as well as a good seal with a minimized leak. Despite this movement, subglottic edema and remodeling continues to be a major concern of neonatologists and many units continue to use uncuffed endotracheal tubes as their standard of care [20].

### Noninvasive Modes

Nasal continuous positive airway pressure (NCPAP) has been well established as a method of noninvasive airway support in neonates, often used following extubation or in the attempt to prevent the need for endotracheal intubation. Recently, newer methods have developed using sensitive triggers and processors that can provide more advanced and timed support. Synchronized noninvasive positive pressure ventilation (SNIPPV) and non-synchronized noninvasive positive pressure ventilation (nsNIPPV) have also been studied. There is a Cochrane Database review showing a benefit of NIPPV over simple NCPAP for success in extubation when used as a bridge [21].

Finally, high-flow nasal cannula can deliver a small degree of CPAP and improvement in oxygenation, but the flow must always be humidified as this modality can quickly lead to significant mucosal drying and bleeding as well as a surprising degree of dehydration [22].

### Invasive Modes

Once the decision has been made to provide invasive ventilation utilizing endotracheal intubation, there are a wide variety of ventilation options that can be utilized, with the ultimate goal of preventing damage to premature, underdeveloped lungs when exposed to prolonged positive pressure ventilation. Generally, the first choice ventilation strategy is the use of conventional ventilation, but often this proves difficult due to either the need for high inspiratory pressures, hypoxemia, or both. When this modality is not adequate, the two main alternatives are high-frequency oscillatory ventilation (HFOV) and high-frequency jet ventilation (HFJV).

A recent meta-analysis in *Neonatology* investigated the use of conventional ventilation (CV) versus HFOV, specifically looking at short-term mortality, chronic lung disease, and other forms of morbidity. They found no change in short-term (~30-day) mortality. They found more pulmonary air leaks with HFOV as well as increased rates of significant IVH with certain modes of HFOV, although this particular finding was not consistent. There was, however, a decrease in the risk of ROP in the HFOV group [23].

### Conventional Ventilation

Conventional ventilation in neonates is not terribly different than CV in adults. Many of the same principles are utilized, such as lung-protective strategies and basic initial settings. One point that should be remembered is that lung-protective measures, such as low tidal volumes and peak inspiratory pressures, should be utilized on all premature neonates.

A recent meta-analysis suggests that using volume-targeted ventilation (as opposed to pressure-targeted ventilation) leads to decreased days on the ventilator, BPD, and significant IVH (grade 3 or 4) [24].

Time-cycled, pressure-limited ventilation (TCPL) is often utilized in neonates and is also known as intermittent positive pressure ventilation (IPPV). In this mode, the inspiratory and expiratory times are set, allowing many variables to affect the tidal volume with each breath, while providing a continuous background flow and limited pressure [20].

### High-Frequency Oscillatory Ventilation

Instead of utilizing conventional ventilation to provide close to physiologic tidal volumes using large pressure differences, HFOV relies on a completely different strategy. HFOV starts by providing a constant distending pressure (mean airway pressure, or MAP) about which a rapidly oscillating pressure difference, or amplitude, occurs. In fact, this occurs so rapidly that the oscillating pressure wave is attenuated and

the alveoli ultimately are exposed only to the MAP, or a very small pressure perturbation. This is thought to decrease the sheer stress, volutrauma, and barotrauma caused by large changes in pressure and distention experienced by alveoli during CV. Also, given the higher MAPs tolerated during HFOV, oxygenation is often vastly improved. Because the pressure difference is created by a piston driving an oscillating membrane back and forth to create the pressure change around the MAP, this is the only ventilation mode that utilizes an active expiratory phase.

With minimal changes in pressure seen by alveoli during HFOV, it is often not intuitive how gas exchange is accomplished. Gas exchange during HFOV seems to be accomplished via a variety of mechanisms, instead of the fairly simple bulk gas dispersion utilized by CV. A paper in *Critical Care Medicine* in 2005 sought to clarify these mechanisms, which include but are not limited to: molecular diffusion, turbulence, pendelluft, and laminar flow with Taylor dispersion [25].

The basic initial settings for HFOV involve setting a MAP, an amplitude (change in pressure around the MAP), a frequency (usually 8–15 Hz), and an $FiO_2$. Unlike in conventional ventilation, where oxygenation and ventilation are somewhat coupled, when utilizing HFOV, oxygenation and ventilation are mostly determined by different variables. The MAP and $FiO_2$ are the major determinants of oxygenation and the frequency and amplitude will largely determine the ventilation (with lower frequencies leading to increased ventilation and $CO_2$ elimination). It is important to appreciate a "wiggle," which is the subjective vibratory movement of the chest wall that occurs when there is an adequate pressure difference about the MAP. This is in fact how the amplitude is titrated to effect in neonatal HFOV. High-frequency oscillatory ventilation utilizes active exhalation, which means a negative pressure is applied to force volume out of the lungs.

### High-Frequency Jet Ventilation

High-frequency jet ventilation is another form of high-frequency ventilation, which uses a combination of conventional ventilation and high-frequency pulses. The general setup is to have a conventional ventilator deliver positive end-expiratory pressure (PEEP) as well as a low respiratory rate of physiologic tidal volumes referred to as "sigh breaths." Coupled to this is a jet injector that pulses short and rapid jets of gas into the trachea at a rate of 240–660 breaths per minute, although the usual operating range is more in the range of 320–450 breaths per minute. These jets entrain additional gas by creating an area of negative pressure, but do not employ active exhalation as seen in HFOV.

A Cochrane Database review looked at the elective use of HFJV versus CV in the population of preterm infants with RDS and found that those babies treated with HFJV had a lower incidence of chronic lung disease, but there was an unclear impact on the incidence of IVH [26].

## Gastrointestinal

The gastrointestinal system undergoes a complex developmental process to ready the fetus for enteral nutrition at birth. Despite this, a disproportionate amount of the oxygen delivery in a fetus is directed toward the head, leaving the gut vulnerable to ischemic insults in general. In addition to this, development does not always proceed perfectly and can lead to congenital defects noted at birth. For more in-depth and comprehensive information, please read the chapter on gastrointestinal disorders.

## Necrotizing Enterocolitis

Necrotizing enterocolitis (NEC) is bowel necrosis that occurs postnatally and is a significant source of morbidity for small and preterm infants, often carrying high mortality rates. NEC will classically present in a neonate with a variety of often subtle signs and symptoms, including feeding intolerance, apnea/bradycardia/desaturation events, abdominal distention, discoloration of the abdomen, peritonitis, and bloody stools. Abdominal radiographs may reveal pneumatosis intestinalis, free air, and portal venous gas in cases of severe or advanced NEC. The pathophysiology is not fully understood, but likely involves a combination of an immature gut with a delicate vascular supply, abnormal microbial colonization, immunoreactive mucosa, and a genetic predisposition. Treatment depends on the severity of illness and whether or not an intestinal perforation has occurred. The mainstay of treatment regardless of severity is a combination of bowel rest and intravenous antibiotics. For more severe cases a peritoneal drain may be placed at the bedside or an exploratory laparotomy with bowel resection may be performed, either at the bedside or in the operating room [27].

## Omphalocele and Gastroschisis

Omphalocele (Figure 3.2) and gastroschisis (Figure 3.3) are both congenital abdominal wall defects that must be addressed early in the neonatal course and are often diagnosed prenatally. Beyond the fact that significant evaporative losses can occur with both, the details most important to the anesthesiologist regarding these conditions are the associated comorbidities. Associated congenital abnormalities are far more common in patients with omphaloceles than those with gastroschisis. In fact, cardiac anomalies occur in 18–24 percent of infants with an omphalocele, making a preoperative (and often fetal) echocardiogram an essential part of the evaluation of an infant with an omphalocele. The bowel in gastroschisis, however, does not have the benefit of a protective sac, as in omphalocele, so patients with gastroschisis often have significant degrees of bowel inflammation and subsequent strictures. Depending on the size of the defects, they may require staged closures, allowing the abdominal cavity time to grow and accept the gut without significant diaphragmatic competition and respiratory compromise [28].

## Jaundice

Given the typical hematologic and hepatic state of the normal newborn, it is not surprising that neonatal jaundice occurs, to some degree, in every infant. Neonatal jaundice refers to an elevated level of indirect (or unconjugated) bilirubin that is manifest by the yellow discoloration of the skin in a level-dependent progression from the tip of the nose, down the body (the further caudad the spread, the higher the level). Left untreated, severe hyperbilirubinemia can lead to an acute bilirubin encephalopathy, also known as kernicterus. The factors leading to significant jaundice include the large erythrocyte volume, the faster turnover of erythrocytes, and the decreased activity of uridine diphosphate glucuronosyl transferase, which is responsible for the conjugation of bilirubin into a water-soluble form that can be excreted by the kidneys.

Often, phototherapy is utilized to provide conjugation via ultraviolet energy so that excess bilirubin can be conjugated and excreted (Figure 3.4). This condition is self-resolving once liver enzymes become upregulated and red cell turnover diminishes. ABO incompatibility (where maternal antibodies attack

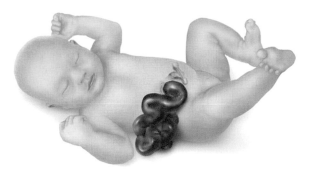

**Figure 3.2** Gastroschisis. Source: Centers for Disease Control and Prevention, National Center on Birth Defects and Developmental Disabilities, public domain.

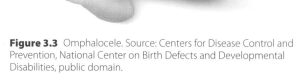

**Figure 3.3** Omphalocele. Source: Centers for Disease Control and Prevention, National Center on Birth Defects and Developmental Disabilities, public domain.

neonatal erythrocytes) is one of the more common situations leading to severe hemolysis and jaundice in the newborn. Routine screening and surveillance has significantly decreased the morbidity of this "setup" for jaundice [29].

## Fluid Management in the NICU

Perhaps the first thing a newcomer to the NICU will notice regarding fluid management is that it is reported as ml kg$^{-1}$ day$^{-1}$ and referred to as "total fluids" (TF). To the inexperienced, the selection of TF can seem random or arbitrary, but is based on a set of guiding principles.

Extremely premature infants are composed of almost entirely water, with a composition of water nearing 90 percent. These premature infants actually lose much more water transepidermally than their more mature counterparts, and this loss can quickly lead to dehydration. In fact, they can lose more water this way than through urine output. Many of the newer incubators incorporate variable humidification to counteract these losses in the first few days of life. Luckily, after birth, infants rapidly attain mature degrees of transepidermal losses and this is less of a concern with time.

The choices of TF as well as glucose and electrolyte additives must be managed carefully with frequent adjustments, at least on a daily basis. Smaller and earlier gestational age infants will require more fluids on a ml kg$^{-1}$ day$^{-1}$ basis, and this will often increase over the first few days of life. Modi suggests that a good starting point for an infant born at less than 1000 g is 100 ml kg$^{-1}$ day$^{-1}$, making adjustments based on strict inputs and outputs as well as weight and electrolyte measurements [30].

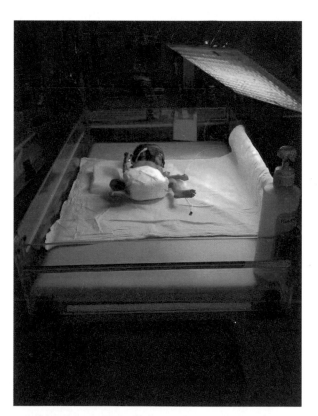

**Figure 3.4** A neonate with jaundice, receiving phototherapy. Source: Creative Commons Attribution-Share Alike 3.0 Unported license, by Vtbijoy.

As infants progress through their first few days of life, they have a natural diuresis as well as tremendous metabolic requirement needed for growth and their high basal metabolic rate. Because of this, infants will need more and more fluid as the days progress. O'Brien and Walker outlined general guidelines for low birth weight (LBW) (<2.5 kg), very low birth weight (VLBW) (<1.5 kg), and extremely low birth weight infants (ELBW) (<1 kg). They suggest starting with 50–60 ml kg$^{-1}$ day$^{-1}$ and 80–90 ml kg$^{-1}$ day$^{-1}$ for LBW and VLBW/ELBW infants, respectively, on day of life 0–1, and increasing progressively to 150–180 ml kg$^{-1}$ day$^{-1}$ by age five days, although many units stop at the lower end of this range [31].

Many NICUs will use mild fluid restriction as a strategy to decrease the incidence of PDA, NEC, BPD, and IVH. A Cochrane meta-analysis published in 2008 found a significant decrease in incidence of PDAs and NEC in premature infants and a trend toward a decreased incidence of BPD formation and IVH. There was, however, a greater weight loss in premature infants who were fluid restricted and many of these infants required higher-density caloric feeds in order to achieve adequate growth. In addition, many NICUs will also treat patients with BPD with diuretic therapy, which has been shown to be helpful in BPD exacerbations. Many of these infants will require electrolyte replacement, especially if they are treated with loop diuretics. Anesthetizing these infants is a challenge because of their relatively dehydrated state. Carefully crafting an anesthetic to minimize intraoperative hypotension in order to decrease the need for fluid boluses is helpful. Educating NICU providers about the cardiac depressant and hypotensive effects of most general anesthetics and the resultant need for fluid resuscitation is essential to avoid conflicts about the fluid management of these vulnerable patients in the operating room.

## Temperature Regulation

For the lay public, there is probably nothing more synonymous with premature infants than the incubator. As mentioned in the introduction, the invention of the neonatal incubator was the first step in the modern care of the neonate and in reality had a tremendous impact on neonatal mortality, especially in infants born at less than 1500 g. The neonate is accustomed to being in a warm intrauterine environment that is generally just a little warmer than the mother (a point often noted if a neonatal temperature is taken immediately after birth). Just like their adult counterparts, neonates attempt to maintain their core temperature within a narrow range, but they have far less ability to do so and have a massively increased potential for heat loss in comparison. However, unlike their older counterparts, neonates do not have the capability to shiver

in their attempt to increase their temperature – they instead rely solely on the metabolism of brown fat, which is present in the neonate as early as 25 weeks GA. This vulnerability to temperature applies also to hyperthermia. In short, neonates depend on a neutral thermal environment, which is the range of temperatures in which a neonate must expend minimal energy in order to maintain an acceptable core temperature.

Infants, and especially LBW infants, have a much higher surface area to volume ratio, and therefore can quickly lose heat to the environment via radiation, convection, and conduction. Immediately following birth, the most important mechanism of heat loss is via evaporation – the newborn emerges wet and must be quickly dried to prevent these losses. In addition to this, the skin of a premature neonate is thin, with very little subcutaneous fat, both of which decrease the neonate's insulating capacity. Small preterm infants are such poor insulators that simple measures such as placing the infant in a plastic bag or wrapping it in plastic wrap can greatly decrease heat loss.

As the infant's temperature falls below 36°C, active rewarming should be initiated to prevent further drops in temperature. However, when the temperature falls below 32°C, one may anticipate severe metabolic, cardiac, and neurologic derangements and corrective actions should be taken immediately [32].

## Neonatal Sepsis

Sepsis has been and continues to be a major source of morbidity and mortality for neonates, especially preterm neonates. Its presentation can be as overt or subtle as the presentation for NEC, and treatment must proceed immediately to prevent further insult or death. In fact, newborns will often react to bacteremia and sepsis with hypothermia, instead of pyrexia. Because neonatal sepsis can present in subtle ways and have devastating consequences, infants will often complete "rule-out sepsis" evaluations in which antibiotics are administered until surveillance body fluid cultures return negative at 48–72 hours. In addition, several biomarkers are gaining popularity to guide antibiotic treatment, including C-reactive protein and procalcitonin.

The organisms most commonly responsible for early-onset neonatal sepsis include, but are not limited to, group-B *Streptococcus* (GBS), *Escherichia coli*, *Listeria*, and *Enterococcus*. GBS infection was a significant pathogen in early neonatal sepsis that has been dramatically reduced with routine maternal GBS screening and treatment. GBS remains a concern in infants of inadequately treated mothers and later in infancy. Several neonatal sepsis evaluation algorithms exist, but most institutions in the United States utilize the guidelines distributed by the American Academy of Pediatrics in the Red Book [33].

## Common Surgical Procedures in the NICU

The major surgical interventions for neonates are covered in great detail throughout this book. In this section, however, we will focus only on those procedures commonly performed in the NICU at the bedside. The procedure location is highly hospital-dependent, with some institutions opting to perform the majority of procedures within the NICU and others opting to transport patients to the operating room for the majority of procedures.

## NEC Resection, Peritoneal Drain Placement

Exploratory laparotomies, intestinal resections, anastomosis, ostomy creations, and peritoneal drain placements are common in the NICU and, in fact, are the most common emergency surgical procedures performed on the neonatal population. It is more common among LBW and premature infants and presents in a myriad of subtle and overt ways. The choice of surgical procedure is highly dependent on the acuity of the infant, but it is well-recognized that infants requiring surgery of any kind have much higher morbidity and mortality [34].

## PDA Ligation

When medical closure of a PDA is unsuccessful or inappropriate, surgical closure is often indicated. In fact, in cases of hemodynamically significant PDAs, surgical ligation is often the initial approach since it has a much higher success rate than indomethacin (or other cyclooxygenase inhibitors). The approach is through a left thoracotomy or very rarely thoracoscopically in larger infants.

The only other option is an endovascular closure in the cardiac catheterization lab, but this is generally only feasible for larger patients and not the neonatal population. Smaller devices are being investigated in animal models, with the hope of providing a safer

and less expensive method of PDA closure than an operation [35].

A recent Cochrane review looked at the use of indomethacin for closure of a PDA versus a surgical closure and found no difference in any of the major morbidities queried, including mortality, NEC, sepsis, IVH, or CLD [36].

## Operating in the OR vs. the NICU

Certain procedures will almost always require a trip to the operating room due to the need for specialized equipment, personnel, or lighting, or the increased degree of sterility, but many procedures can be safely performed within the NICU. Any trip to and from the operating room carries with it inherent risks of airway dislodgment, invasive line dislodgment, thermal disruption, hemodynamic instability outside of a direct clinical area, and interruption in current ventilatory strategies. There are well-founded arguments for and against each option.

This is not a new controversy; in fact, a paper in 1993 lays out nicely the arguments on each side. They compared the procedures performed in the NICU to those performed in the operating room over a four-year period and found that overall the patients managed in the NICU were of lower GA, lower weight, increased severity of illness, and far more likely to be mechanically ventilated preoperatively. There was a higher mortality among the patients treated in the NICU compared to the group brought to the operating room – this was attributed to the severity of illness and not surgical complications. Of note, they found no difference in sepsis (culture-proven), length of surgery, or vital sign stability, except for hyperthermia, which was higher in the operating room group [37].

In 2012, Hall et al. published their ten-year experience with performing operations in the NICU over a wide range of procedures, including many laparotomies, repairs of congenital diaphragmatic hernias, tracheostomies, and the insertion of central venous lines. They argue that such operations are safe and especially suitable for unstable and ventilated infants in order to avoid the risks associated with transport [38].

More recently, a point–counterpoint was outlined in the journal *Pediatric Anesthesia*. To summarize, the group feeling that it is best to travel to the operating room seems to be working from the construct that whatever makes the surgical team more comfortable, safe, and efficient must be what is best for the infant.

They focus on issues such as resource familiarity and an aseptic environment. On the other hand, the group arguing for more operations occurring in the NICU seems to work from a construct of focusing on the neonate and minimizing transfers, interruptions in therapies, and physiologic perturbations. They feel that sick neonates should remain in place, and we, as providers, should be more flexible and accommodating in order to achieve this [39].

This controversy continues and does not appear to have an easy answer. Individual institutions will continue to have their preferences, but what is most important is to recognize when these preferences should be altered. For instance, in an institution where all neonatal surgery is performed in the operating room, there may be instances in which the transport is simply too precarious and an exception must be made. Conversely, in institutions frequently performing operations in the NICU, there may be circumstances in which it is more prudent to transport to the operating room. As in most areas of medicine, flexibility is vital in the care of our sickest, most vulnerable patients.

## Postoperative Care in the NICU

Prevailing thought regarding pain in the neonate has shifted drastically over the past century. Initially, many felt that the neonatal nervous system was not adequately mature to experience pain; while this may seem barbaric by today's standards, it certainly guided practice in the not too distant past. There is overwhelming evidence that even the smallest of neonates are capable of experiencing pain and discomfort, but what may be more important is newly emerging evidence that painful experiences may have consequences for years to come.

In 1987, Anand et al. published a study investigating the adjunctive use of fentanyl in neonates undergoing PDA ligation, in addition to the standard of care at the time, which was a mixture of oxygen and nitrous oxide. They observed significant physiologic changes in the non-fentanyl group in response to pain, including changes in cardiorespiratory, metabolic, and hormonal systems [40].

Later work has further clarified these acute physiologic alterations, which can in themselves have a significant impact on the neonate. In addition to these physiologic changes, infants will often display behavioral alterations in response to pain. Collectively, the behavioral and physiologic changes form the basis for neonatal pain scales.

Neonatal pain pathways are still in a state of development, so there is growing concern that painful stimuli, especially if repeated, could lead to desensitization and hyperalgesia. One of the more famous investigations centered on neonates who had received circumcisions without analgesia, and showed significantly altered behavior with subsequent vaccinations months later [41]. There is also evidence that surgery increases the degree of sensory processing dysfunction that occurs in children who have spent time in the NICU as premature neonates [42–44].

Pain control in the immediate postoperative period is of paramount importance and intraoperative strategies and observations should be communicated clearly with the NICU team in order to develop an appropriate postoperative analgesic regimen. Many units have created analgesic guidelines for common invasive procedures in the NICU, including the perioperative period.

## Ethics in the NICU

As in any critical care setting, ethical dilemmas are not infrequent, and the NICU is no exception. While it is clear that neonates lack the capacity to make decisions for themselves, there is no ethical basis for limiting their right to dignity, especially at the end of life. The tremendous improvements in neonatal care have allowed a survival rate approaching 80 percent for extremely premature infants. What this brings with it, though, are more complex ethical scenarios centering on quality of life and the rights of the newborn [45].

## Threshold of Viability

Within the past few decades, the mortality for extremely premature infants has fallen from ~80 percent to ~20 percent, but significant morbidities persist. We also lack consensus as to the definition of the "threshold of viability."

Certain seminal cases highlight the ethical dilemmas present when the subject is a patient who may or may not be a viable human being, depending on who one asks. In *Miller v. Hospital Corporation of America*, the Miller family sued the hospital organization for resuscitating their baby at less than 24 weeks GA despite their wishes to withhold resuscitation. This infant survived, but with profound neurologic deficits. The courts initially found in the family's favor, but they lost in appeals at the level of the Supreme Court of Texas on the grounds that parents cannot be fully informed as to the infant's prognosis until after birth, and could therefore not prenatally refuse resuscitation. This was further evaluated by Robertson in the 2004 Hastings Center Report, where the argument was made that parents could refuse life-saving treatment, but only if it was unlikely that the child could later interact symbolically [46,47].

A recent study looked at the guidelines for resuscitation at the threshold of viability in many countries. There was strong consensus that there is no chance for survival at less than 22 weeks GA, but at 25 weeks GA and above, resuscitation is generally offered except in cases of severe congenital abnormalities. Most countries consider the time between 23 and 24 weeks GA to be murkier, and these infants are approached on a more individual basis [48].

In the United States, the American Academy of Pediatrics published a clinical report addressing infants born between 22 and 25 weeks GA. They argue for full disclosure to the parents and a team approach to decision-making, including the parents. Furthermore, they recommend respecting the parents' wishes if found to be "within the limits of medical feasibility and appropriateness" [49].

## Conclusions

The NICU is a dynamic environment characterized by unique patients, comorbidities, treatment modalities, and technology. It is staffed by a highly trained team with exquisite attention to detail. The pediatric anesthesiologist and neonatologist arrive at their professions via somewhat different paths, but their understanding of one another's role and environment is critical to the optimal care of the neonate.

## References

1. McCullough E. *Good Old Coney Island: A Sentimental Journey Into the Past. The Most Rambunctious, Scandalous, Rapscallion, Splendiferous, Pugnacious, Spectacular, Illustrious, Prodigious, Frolicsome Island on Earth.* New York: Fordham University Press; 1957.

2. Apgar V. A proposal for a new method of evaluation of the newborn infant. *Curr Res Anesth Analg.* 1953;32:260–7.

3. National Perinatal Information System/Quality Analytic Services. Special care nursery admissions. www.npic.org. Prepared by March of Dimes Perinatal Data Center, 2011.

4. Ballabh P. Intraventricular hemorrhage in premature infants: mechanism of disease. *Pediatr Res.* 2010;67(1):1–8.

5. Lai MC, Yang SN. Perinatal hypoxic-ischemic encephalopathy. *J Biomed Biotechnol.* 2011;2011:609813.

6. Chen J, Stahl A, Hellstrom A, Smith LE. Current update on retinopathy of prematurity: screening and treatment. *Curr Opin Pediatr.* 2011;23(2):173–8.

7. Jansson LM, Velez M. Neonatal abstinence syndrome. *Curr Opin Pediatr.* 2012;24(2):252–8.

8. Hamrick SE, Hansmann G. Patent ductus arteriosus of the preterm infant. *Pediatrics.* 2010;125(5):1020–30.

9. Steinhorn RH. Neonatal pulmonary hypertension. *Pediatr Crit Care Med.* 2010;11(2 Suppl):S79–84.

10. Silberbach M, Hannon D. Presentation of congenital heart disease in the neonate and young infant. *Pediatr Rev.* 2007;28(4):123–31.

11. Moore KL, Persaud TVN (2002). *The Developing Human: Clinically Oriented Embryology*, 7th edn. Philadelphia, PA: Saunders.

12. Wapner R, Jobe AH. Controversy: antenatal steroids. *Clin Perinatol.* 2011;38(3):529–45.

13. Kattwinkel J, Perlman JM, Aziz K, et al. Neonatal resuscitation: 2010 American Heart Association guidelines for cardiopulmonary resuscitation and emergency cardiovascular care. *Pediatrics.* 2010;126(5):e1400–13.

14. Martin RJ, Fanaroff AA. The preterm lung and airway: past, present, and future. *Pediatr Neonatol.* 2013;54(4):228–34.

15. Baraldi E, Filippone M. Chronic lung disease after premature birth. *N Engl J Med.* 2007;357(19):1946–55.

16. Ehrenkranz RA, Walsh MC, Vohr BR, et al. Validation of the National Institutes of Health consensus definition of bronchopulmonary dysplasia. *Pediatrics.* 2005;116(6):1353–60.

17. Morrison JJ, Rennie JM, Milton PJ. Neonatal respiratory morbidity and mode of delivery at term: influence of timing of elective caesarean section. *Br J Obstet Gynaecol.* 1995;102(2):101–6.

18. Guglani L, Lakshminrusimha S, Ryan RM. Transient tachypnea of the newborn. *Pediatr Rev.* 2008;29(11):e59–65.

19. Brown MK, DiBlasi RM. Mechanical ventilation of the premature neonate. *Respir Care.* 2011;56(9):1298–311; discussion 1311–13.

20. Neumann RP, von Ungern-Sternberg BS. The neonatal lung: physiology and ventilation. *Paediatr Anaesth.* 2014;24(1):10–21.

21. Davis PG, Lemyre B, de Paoli AG. Nasal intermittent positive pressure ventilation (NIPPV) versus nasal continuous positive airway pressure (NCPAP) for preterm neonates after extubation. *Cochrane Database Syst Rev*. 2001;3:CD003212.

22. Roberts CT, Davis PG, Owen LS. Neonatal non-invasive respiratory support: synchronised NIPPV, non-synchronised NIPPV or bi-level CPAP: what is the evidence in 2013? *Neonatology*. 2013;104(3):203–9.

23. Soll RF. Elective high-frequency oscillatory ventilation versus conventional ventilation for acute pulmonary dysfunction in preterm infants. *Neonatology*. 2013;103(1):7–8; discussion 8–9.

24. Peng W, Zhu H, Shi H, Liu E. Volume-targeted ventilation is more suitable than pressure-limited ventilation for preterm infants: a systematic review and meta-analysis. *Arch Dis Child Fetal Neonatal Ed*. 2014;99(2):158–65.

25. Pillow JJ. High-frequency oscillatory ventilation: mechanisms of gas exchange and lung mechanics. *Crit Care Med*. 2005;33(3 Suppl.):S135–41.

26. Bhuta T, Henderson-Smart DJ. Elective high frequency jet ventilation versus conventional ventilation for respiratory distress syndrome in preterm infants. *Cochrane Database Syst Rev*. 2000;2:CD000328.

27. Neu J, Walker WA. Necrotizing enterocolitis. *N Engl J Med*. 2011;364(3):255–64.

28. Christison-Lagay ER, Kelleher CM, Langer JC. Neonatal abdominal wall defects. *Semin Fetal Neonatal Med*. 2011;16(3):164–72.

29. Maisels MJ. Neonatal jaundice. *Pediatr Rev*. 2006;27(12):443–54.

30. Modi N. Management of fluid balance in the very immature neonate. *Arch Dis Child Fetal Neonatal Ed*. 2004;89(2):F108–11.

31. O'Brien F, Walker IA. Fluid homeostasis in the neonate. *Paediatr Anaesth*. 2014;24(1):49–59.

32. Ringer SA. Core concepts: thermoregulation in the newborn part I – basic mechanisms. *Neoreviews*. 2013;14;e161–7.

33. Shah BA, Padbury JF. Neonatal sepsis: an old problem with new insights. *Virulence*. 2013;5(1):170–8.

34. Raval MV, Moss RL. Current concepts in the surgical approach to necrotizing enterocolitis. *Pathophysiology*. 2014; 21(1):105–10.

35. Bass JL, Wilson N. Transcatheter occlusion of the patent ductus arteriosus in infants: experimental testing of a new Amplatzer device. *Catheter Cardiovasc Interv*. 2014;83(2):250–5.

36. Malviya MN, Ohlsson A, Shah SS. Surgical versus medical treatment with cyclooxygenase inhibitors for symptomatic patent ductus arteriosus in preterm infants. *Cochrane Database Syst Rev*. 2013;28(3): CD003951.

37. Finer NN, Woo BC, Hayashi A, Hayes B. Neonatal surgery: intensive care unit versus operating room. *J Pediatr Surg*. 1993;28(5):645–9.

38. Hall NJ, Stanton MP, Kitteringham LJ, et al. Scope and feasibility of operating on the neonatal intensive care unit: 312 cases in 10 years. *Pediatr Surg Int*. 2012;28(10):1001–5.

39. Jenkins IA, Kelly Ugarte LR, Mancuso TJ. Where should we operate on the preterm neonate? *Paediatr Anaesth*. 2014;24(1):127–36.

40. Anand KJ, Sippell WG, Aynsley-Green A. Pain, anaesthesia, and babies. *Lancet*. 1987;2(8569):1210.

41. Taddio A, Katz J, Ilersich AL, Koren G. Effect of neonatal circumcision on pain response during subsequent routine vaccination. *Lancet*. 1997;349(9052):599–603.

42. Walker SM, Franck LS, Fitzgerald M, et al. Long-term impact of neonatal intensive care and surgery on somatosensory perception in children born extremely preterm. *Pain*. 2009;141(1–2):79–87.

43. Walker SM. Neonatal pain. *Paediatr Anaesth*. 2014;24(1):39–48.

44. Marlow N. Anesthesia and long-term outcomes after neonatal intensive care. *Paediatr Anaesth*. 2014;24(1):60–7.

45. Guimarães H, Rocha G, Bellieni C, Buonocore G. Rights of the newborn and end-of-life decisions. *J Matern Fetal Neonatal Med*. 2012;25(Suppl 1):76–8.

46. Lorenz JM. Ethical dilemmas in the care of the most premature infants: the waters are murkier than ever. *Curr Opin Pediatr*. 2005;17(2):186–90.

47. Robertson JA. Extreme prematurity and parental rights after Baby Doe. *Hastings Cent Rep*. 2004;34(4):32–9.

48. Pignotti MS, Donzelli G. Perinatal care at the threshold of viability: an international comparison of practical guidelines for the treatment of extremely preterm births. *Pediatrics*. 2008;121(1):e193–8.

49. MacDonald H, American Academy of Pediatrics, Committee on Fetus and Newborn. Perinatal care at the threshold of viability. *Pediatrics*. 2002;110(5):1024–7.

# Hemodynamics in the Infant

Viviane G. Nasr and James A. DiNardo

The physiologic changes that occur at birth and continue over the first few days and the first months of life are considerable and need to be appreciated in order to understand the hemodynamics of newborns.

## Fetal Circulation

Fetal circulatory channels shunt blood away from the lung, such that both ventricles, in parallel, contribute to systemic oxygen delivery by pumping blood to the systemic arterial system. This parallel circulation permits normal fetal growth and development even in fetuses with cardiac malformations.

Oxygenated blood from the placenta returns to the fetus via the umbilical vein, which enters the portal venous system. The ductus venosus connects the left portal vein to the left hepatic vein at its junction with the inferior vena cava (IVC). This allows approximately 50 percent of umbilical venous blood to bypass the hepatic sinuses. The remainder of the umbilical venous flow passes through the liver and enters the IVC via the hepatic veins. Fetal IVC blood is a combination of blood from the lower fetal body, umbilical vein, and hepatic veins. The stream of blood from the ductus venosus has a higher velocity in the IVC than the stream from the lower body and hepatic veins. This higher velocity facilitates delivery of this higher oxygen content blood across the foramen ovale (FO) into the left atrium (LA) [1] (Figure 4.1).

Inferior vena cava blood enters the right atrium (RA) and due to the position of the Eustachian valve, Chiari network, and FO enters the LA during 80 percent of the cardiac cycle. During the other 20 percent (atrial systole), IVC blood crosses the tricuspid valve and enters the right ventricle (RV). The overwhelming majority of superior vena cava (SVC) crosses the tricuspid valve and enters the RV as well. Blood from the RV is ejected into the pulmonary artery (PA). Approximately 10–15 percent of blood from the PA passes through the lungs to reach the LA and the rest

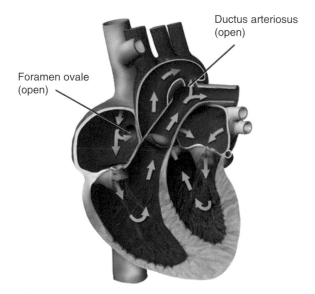

**Figure 4.1** Fetal circulation © Blausen Medical. Source: [1].

is shunted to the distal aorta via the ductus arteriosus (DA). As a result, two-thirds of total fetal cardiac output is provided by the RV with the remaining one-third provided via the LV.

The dynamics of shunting at the level of the ductus venosus, FO, and DA result in preferential delivery of the most highly oxygenated blood to the coronary and cerebral circulations. Obviously, this preferential delivery of oxygenated blood may be compromised in utero by cardiac lesions that prevent or reduce LV output. At birth, a series circulation is established in which each ventricle pumps into a specific vascular bed (RV to pulmonary artery; LV to aorta). The removal of the placenta and the initiation of alveolar ventilation at birth have the immediate effect of establishing this series circulation. To maintain the adult series circulation, the fetal channels must be closed (Table 4.1). Complex neurochemical and hormonal influences affect the closing of these fetal shunts. Acidosis, sepsis, hypothermia, hypoxia, and hypercarbia may cause

**Table 4.1** Fetal structures and their corresponding structure in adults

| Fetal structure | Adult structure |
| --- | --- |
| Foramen ovale | Fossa ovalis |
| Umbilical vein | Ligamentum teres |
| Ductus venosus | Ligamentum venosum |
| Umbilical arteries | Medial umbilical ligaments, superior vesicular artery |
| Ductus arteriosus | Ligamentum arteriosum |

reopening of the shunts and persistence of the fetal circulation (PFC).

# Closure of the Ductus Arteriosus

In the fetus, patency of the ductus arteriosus is maintained by high levels of prostaglandin ($PGI_2$ and $PGE_1$). There are two stages of ductal closure in the newborn: functional closure and permanent anatomic closure. Functional closure occurs by contraction of the smooth muscle of the ductal wall, usually within the first day of life. An increase in $PO_2$ and a decrease in prostaglandins contribute to functional closure. Oxygen is a dose-dependent ductal constrictor that acts by increasing the rate of oxidative phosphorylation within smooth muscle cells. In addition, the response to oxygen may be age-related; full-term neonates have a more dramatic response to oxygen than do immature newborns. Norepinephrine and epinephrine, by changing pulmonary and systemic vascular resistances, may secondarily contribute to ductal closure. Acetylcholine has a direct constrictor effect on ductal tissue. Permanent anatomic closure of the duct is usually accomplished by 2–3 weeks of life in the normal full-term neonate. The lumen is sealed by fibrous connective tissue, leaving the vestigial structure, known as the ligamentum arteriosum.

# Closure of the Foramen Ovale

In utero, the RA pressure is higher than the LA pressure. Inferior vena cava blood flows in such a manner as to keep the FO open. Cessation of umbilical vein flow causes a significant decrease in venous return to the right heart, causing a decrease in RA pressure. In addition, ventilation causes a marked increase in pulmonary arterial and venous blood flow, resulting in an increase in LA pressure. This elevation of LA relative to RA pressure causes the flap-like valve of the FO to functionally close. In instances in which RA pressure remains elevated, right-to-left shunting may persist. Functional closure usually progresses to anatomic closure. However, probe patency of the FO may persist in 30 percent of normal adults and 50 percent of children younger than five years of age.

# Closure of the Ductus Venosus

The umbilical vessels constrict strongly after mechanical stimulation and high oxygen tension facilitate this process. The resultant decrease in umbilical venous blood flow causes passive closure of the ductus venosus. The ductus venosus does not appear to be as sensitive as the ductus arteriosus to $PaO_2$, $PaCO_2$, or pH. The ductus venosus is functionally closed by one week of life and anatomically closed by three months. The remaining structure is the ligamentum venosum.

In addition to the establishment of the adult series circulation, dramatic alterations in pulmonary circulation, cardiac output and distribution, myocardial performance, and myocardial cell growth and hypertrophy continue to occur during the first weeks, months, and even years of life.

# Pulmonary Vascular Changes

The fetus has low pulmonary blood flow secondary to a high pulmonary vascular resistance. The minimal blood flow that reaches the pulmonary bed has a very low $PaO_2$, which may cause hypoxic pulmonary vasoconstriction and contributes to the elevated pulmonary resistance seen in the fetus. Morphologic examinations of the small arteries of the fetal and newborn lung show a thick medial smooth muscle layer. The fetal pulmonary vasculature is reactive to a number of stimulants. Vasoconstriction is induced by decreases in $PaO_2$, pH, and leukotrienes. Acetylcholine, histamine, bradykinin, $PGE_1$, $PGE_2$, $PGI_2$ (prostacyclin), and prostaglandin $D_2$ and beta-adrenergic catecholamines are patent vasodilators of fetal pulmonary vessels.

At birth, alveolar ventilation commences. This reduces the mechanical compression of small pulmonary vessels and increases $PaO_2$. The result is a dramatic reduction in pulmonary vascular resistance (PVR). During the following weeks and months, remodeling of the pulmonary vessels occurs; the most notable change is a thinning of the medial smooth muscle layer. By six months of life, this process results in reduction of PVR to near normal adult levels. The normal process of postnatal pulmonary maturation may be altered significantly by pathologic conditions, such as those associated with congenital heart disease.

# Myocardial Performance in the Neonate

In utero, the right ventricle (RV) has a cardiac output of approximately 330 ml kg$^{-1}$ min$^{-1}$ compared with the left ventricular (LV) output of 170 ml kg$^{-1}$ min$^{-1}$. Table 4.2 summarizes the percentage of combined CO at different gestational ages [2]. At birth, both RV and LV eject an output of approximately 350 ml kg$^{-1}$ min$^{-1}$. This requires minimal stroke volume increase for the RV but a considerable increase in stroke volume for the LV. The high-output state of the newborn effectively limits further increases in cardiac output. This high-output state decreases to about 150 ml kg$^{-1}$ min$^{-1}$ by 8–10 weeks of life.

# Hemodynamic Changes at Birth

Myocardial morphology and performance is notably different in the neonate. These differences are listed in Table 4.3 and summarized as follows.

**Afterload Mismatch.** The neonatal heart is more susceptible to afterload mismatch, and therefore stroke volume is poorly maintained in the face of increasing outflow resistance.

**Limited Preload Reserve.** The neonatal heart has limited preload reserve. Augmentation of stroke volume via the Frank–Starling mechanism is limited as compared with an adult.

**Reduced Contractile Capacity.** Neonatal cardiac cells contain more water and fewer contractile elements than mature myocardium. In addition, there are fewer mitochondria and sarcoplasmic reticulum (SR) and poorly formed T-tubule that make the myocardium more dependent on extracellular calcium. Development of the SR, T-tubular system, and calcium-handling proteins appear to be rapid and it has been suggested that they are relatively mature by three weeks in the neonatal heart [3].

**Reduced Ventricular Compliance.** The compliance of the neonatal myocardium is reduced because a deficiency of elastic elements parallels the deficiency of contractile elements.

**Increased Intraventricular Dependence.** Changes in ventricular pressure are transmitted to the opposite

**Table 4.2** Percentage of combined cardiac output at different gestational age

|  | 20 weeks | 30 weeks | 38 weeks |
| --- | --- | --- | --- |
| Combined CO | 210 ml min$^{-1}$ | 960 ml min$^{-1}$ | 1900 ml min$^{-1}$ |
| Left ventricle | 47 percent | 43 percent | 40 percent |
| Right ventricle | 53 percent | 57 percent | 60 percent |
| Data extrapolated from [2]. | | | |

**Table 4.3** Neonatal myocardial performance compared to the adult

Afterload mismatch

Limited preload reserve

Reduced contractile capacity

Reduced ventricular compliance

Increased intraventricular dependence

Incomplete autonomic sympathetic innervation and dominance of parasympathetic

Immature myocardial metabolism

ventricle via the ventricular septum more readily in the immature myocardium. Left ventricular diastolic filling is disproportionately impaired in the neonate by high RV end-diastolic pressure. This is due to a leftward shift of the intraventricular septum and a reduction in LV distensibility. Right ventricular diastolic filling is impaired to an equal extent by high LV end-diastolic pressure in neonates. This enhanced ventricular interaction is caused by reduced ventricular compliance and because, at birth, the LV and RV are of equal mass. The increased volume and pressure load experienced by the LV after birth produces relative LV hypertrophy. The normal adult LV to RV mass ratio of 2:1 is not seen until several months after birth.

**Incomplete Autonomic Innervation.** Sympathetic innervation, which is responsible for increasing heart rate and contractility, is incompletely developed at birth. As a result, local myocardial release of norepinephrine contributes less to increases in contractility than do increases in circulating catecholamine levels. For this reason, inotropic agents such as dopamine, the effects of which are partially mediated through release of norepinephrine from myocardial nerve endings, may have to be used in higher doses to be effective in younger patients. On the other hand, the parasympathetic system, which reflexly slows the heart, is fully functional at birth.

**Immature Myocardial Metabolism.** The neonatal myocardium is more dependent on anerobic metabolism than the adult heart using carbohydrates and lactate as primary energy sources. This may have a somewhat protective effect, making the neonatal myocardium more tolerant to the effects of hypoxia.

## Defining Hypotension

Defining hypotension in preterm and term neonates is problematic. As a consequence, there are multiple definitions of hypotension, incorporating both mean and systolic blood pressure, defined in the pediatric anesthesia and neonatology literature. The Pediatric Advanced Life Support definition of neonatal hypotension is a systolic blood pressure (SBP) less than 60 mmHg. A survey of members of the Society of Pediatric Anesthesia and the Association of Paediatric Anaesthetists identified an SBP of 45–50 mmHg as the threshold value for hypotension in neonates [4]. A mean arterial blood pressure (MAP) less than 20–30 percent of baseline is considered hypotension by many providers. In general, neonatologists define hypotension as blood pressure below the fifth or tenth percentile for gestational and postnatal age. A consensus statement addressing the lower limit of MAP by the Joint Working Group of the British Association of Perinatal Medicine and the Research Unit of the Royal College of Physicians recommended that MAP should not drop below the infant's gestational age in weeks, which also happens to be very close to the tenth percentile for age [5]. An absolute lower limit for mean blood pressure of 30 mmHg in infants <30 weeks' postmenstrual age has also been suggested because a MAP <30 mmHg is associated with lower cerebral blood flow and cerebral

injury [6]. Defining normal BP ranges in very low birth weight (VLBW, <1500 g) and extremely low birth weight (ELBW, <1000 g) preemies is even more complicated by the fact that ductal closure and transition from fetal circulation may be delayed. Nonetheless, BP ranges based on weight and gestational age have been defined [7–9] (Table 4.4; Figure 4.2)

In addition to the difficulty of defining normal blood pressure, anesthesiologists must consider the limitations of obtaining an accurate blood pressure in neonates (Chapter 20). In normal, healthy, awake neonates, there is a wide variation in blood pressures between limbs (>20 mmHg) as shown by Crossland et al. [10]. It is also important to note that treating hypotension with inotropic support is a challenge in neonates. The neonatal myocardium is vulnerable to

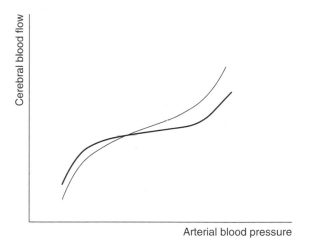

**Figure 4.2** The blood pressure increases over the first week of life and the slope of increase is similar irrespective of gestational age. Source: [9].

**Table 4.4** Blood pressure in premature infants: birth weight 600–1750 g with (2 × SD)

| Age(days) | Wt (g) | | | | | | | |
|---|---|---|---|---|---|---|---|---|
| | 600–999 | | 1000–1249 | | 1250–1499 | | 1500–1750 | |
| | sys | dia | sys | dia | sys | dia | sys | dia |
| 1 | 39(17) | 23(10) | 44(23) | 23(14) | 48(18) | 27(12) | 47(16) | 26(16) |
| 3 | 45(16) | 31(12) | 48(15) | 37(10) | 59(21) | 40(14) | 51(18) | 35(10) |
| 7 | 50(15) | 30(12) | 57(14) | 43(17) | 68(15) | 40(11) | 66(23) | 41(24) |
| 14 | 50(15) | 37(12) | 53(30) | | 64(21) | 36(24) | 76(35) | 42(20) |
| 28 | 61(24) | 46(27) | 57(30) | | 69(31) | 44(26) | 73(6) | 50(10) |

Data from Handbook of Anesthesiology, Department of Anesthesiology, Perioperative and Pain Medicine, Boston Children's Hospital.

the effects of catecholamines in terms of myocardial damage and depletion of energy substrates [11].

## Blood Pressure and Neurobehavioral Development

Blood pressure measurements during anesthesia are often used as a surrogate for organ perfusion. However, there are no clear data linking blood pressure measurements and neurocognitive outcomes, especially in preterm infants [12]. It is important to recognize that the level of hypotension, duration, and frequency of the hypotension are all important factors influencing neurobehavioral development [13]. It is also unclear if treating the hypotension with fluid and/or pressors is more harmful or helpful. In fact, overtreating may increase the risk of intraventricular hemorrhage in preterm infants [14,15].

## Cerebral Blood Flow and Autoregulation

Determining the lower BP limit of physiologic cerebral blood flow (CBF) in neonates is challenging and limited by the changing physiological conditions related to GA and postnatal development. Research efforts to make this determination are hampered by the fact that it is unethical to induce hypotension in a neonate in order to measure the lowest MAP below which the cerebral autoregulation is lost and that healthy neonates require sedation to obtain CBF measurements [16]. Cerebral autoregulation allows the maintenance of a CBF over a range of SBP, between 60 and 150 mmHg in adults [17]. Neonates may maintain autoregulation with respect to CBF within the MAP limits of 25–50 mmHg. The theoretical concept of autoregulation in the neonate may differ, as suggested by Greisen (Figure 4.3) [18].

The lower limits of cerebral autoregulation in neonates are not clearly defined, and there is likely a wide range of variability. A study in children younger than two years has shown that in infants less than six months of age, the lower limit of autoregulation occurred when MAP dropped by 20 percent, while in infants above six months of age, the lower limit occurred at a 40 percent drop [19,20]. Therefore, infants may be at a higher risk of inadequate perfusion following hypotension. Several studies have shown that the lower limit of cerebral autoregulation for some infants is indeed fairly close to the infant's age

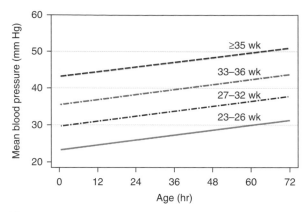

**Figure 4.3** Theoretical concept of autoregulation in the neonate. Source: [18].

in gestational weeks, which is consistent with the definition of hypotension. Other studies have shown that premature infants maintain cerebral autoregulation at a MAP level considerably lower than their gestational age in weeks [21,22]. However, in sick and preterm neonates, cerebral autoregulation may be lost [23].

Cerebral perfusion pressures vary directly with arterial blood pressures below and above the limits of cerebral autoregulation, provided that intracranial pressure is stable, which is almost always the case in neonates and infants with open fontanels. Acute increase in blood pressure can lead to rupture of the fragile vessels and bleeding, while hypotension can cause ischemia. Multiple additional factors interfere with CBF: (1) mechanical ventilation, (2) hypoxia, (3) hypercarbia, (4) hypoglycemia, (5) electrolyte imbalance, and (6) comorbidities such as congenital heart disease and sepsis.

As studies are not clear on the limits of autoregulation and lowest MAP, and given the effect of anesthetic agents on cerebral autoregulation, maintaining adequate BP and relying on noninvasive cerebral monitoring and trends is important when managing these critical patients in the operating room.

## References

1. Cote CJ, Lerman J, Anderson B. *A Practice of Anesthesia for Infants and Children*, 5th edn. Philadelphia, PA: Elsevier; 2013.

2. Rasanen J, Wood DC, Weiner S, Ludomirski A, Huhta JC. Role of the pulmonary circulation in the distribution of human fetal cardiac output during the second half of pregnancy. *Circulation.* 1996;94:1068–73.

3. Wiegerinck RF, Cojoc A, Zeidenweber CM et al. Force frequency relationship of the human ventricle increases during early post-natal development. *Pediatr Res*. 2009;65:414–19.

4. Nafiu OO, Voepel-Lewis T, Morris M, et al. How do pediatric anesthesiologists define intraoperative hypotension? *Pediatr Anesth*. 2009;19:1048–53.

5. Joint Working Group of the British Association of Perinatal Medicine and the Research Unit of the Royal College of Physicians. Development of audit measures and guidelines for good practice in the management of neonatal respiratory distress syndrome. Report of a Joint Working Group of the British Association of Perinatal Medicine and the Research Unit of the Royal College of Physicians. *Arch Dis Child*. 1992;67:1221–7.

6. Limperopoulos C, Bassan H, Kalish LA, et al. Current definitions of hypotension do not predict abnormal cranial ultrasound findings in preterm infants. *Pediatrics*. 2007;120:966–77.

7. Hegyi T, Anwar M, Carbone MT, et al. Blood pressure ranges in premature infants: II. The first week of life. *Pediatrics*. 1996;97(3):336–42.

8. Hegyi T, Carbone MT, Anwar M, et al. Blood pressure ranges in premature infants: I. The first hours of life. *J Pediatr*. 1994;124:627–33.

9. Nuntnarumit P, Yang W, Bada-Ellzey HS. Blood pressure measurements in the newborn. *Clin Perinatol*. 1999;26:981–96.

10. Crossland DS, Furness JC, Abu-Harb M, et al. Variability of four limb blood pressure in normal neonates. *Arch Dis Child Fetal Neonatal Ed*. 2004;89:F325–7.

11. Wolf AR, Humphry AT. Limitation and vulnerabilities of the neonatal cardiovascular system: considerations for anesthetic management. *Pediatr Anesth*. 2014;24:5–9.

12. McCann ME, Schouten ANJ. Beyond survival; influences of blood pressure, cerebral perfusion and anesthesia on neurodevelopment. *Pediatr Anesth*. 2014;24:68–73.

13. Logan JW, O'Shea TM, Allred EN, et al. Early postnatal hypotension is not associated with indicators of white matter damage or cerebral palsy in extremely low gestational age newborns. *J Perinatol*. 2011;31:524–34.

14. Fanaroff JM, Wilson-Costello DE, Newman NS, et al. Treated hypotension is associated with neonatal morbidity and hearing loss in extremely low birth weight infants. *Pediatrics*. 2006;117:1131–5.

15. Pellicer A, Bravo MC, Madero R, et al. Early systemic hypotension and vasopressor support in low birth weight infants: impact on neurodevelopment. *Pediatrics*. 2009;123:1369–76.

16. Vutskits L. Cerebral blood flow in the neonate. *Pediatr Anesth*. 2014;24:22–9.

17. Paulson OB, Strandgaard S, Edvinsson L. Cerebral autoregulation. *Cerebrovasc Brain Metab Rev*. 1990;2(2):161–92.

18. Greisen G. To autoregulate or not to autoregulate: that is no longer the question. *Semin Pediatr Neurol*. 2009;16(4):207–15.

19. Valvilala MS, Lee LA, Lam AM. The lower limit of cerebral autoregulation in children during sevoflurane anesthesia. *J Neurosurg Anesthesiol*. 2003;15:307–12.

20. Torvik A. The pathogenesis of watershed infarcts in the brain. *Stroke*. 1984;15:221–3.

21. Munro MJ, Walker AM, Barfield CP. Hypotensive extremely low birth weight infants have reduced cerebral blood flow. *Pediatrics*. 2004;114:1591–6.

22. Tyszczuk L, Meek J, Elwell C, et al. Cerebral blood flow is independent of mean arterial blood pressure in preterm infants undergoing intensive care. *Pediatrics*. 1998;102:337–41.

23. Boylan G, Young K, Panerai R, et al. Dynamic cerebral autoregulation in sick newborn infants. *Pediatr Res*. 2000;48:12–17.

**Chapter**

# 5

# Measures of Carbon Dioxide

Lawrence Rhein

Arterial carbon dioxide partial pressure ($PaCO_2$) is an essential indicator of ventilation and respiratory function. $PaCO_2$ represents the balance between production and elimination of carbon dioxide, and must be maintained within acceptable limits to ensure optimal acid–base homeostasis and health. This chapter reviews the basic physiology, interpretation, indications, and limitations of the two most common forms of noninvasive $CO_2$ monitoring – capnography and transcutaneous $CO_2$ monitoring – and will also review optimal $PaCO_2$ targets and the effect of hypocapnia on cerebral perfusion.

## Noninvasive Carbon Dioxide Monitoring

Arterial carbon dioxide partial pressure is an essential indicator of ventilation and respiratory function. Measurement of $PaCO_2$ through arterial blood gas (ABG) analysis is the gold standard for assessing ventilation. Unfortunately, measurement of $PaCO_2$ is invasive. Perhaps more importantly, $PaCO_2$ can be a dynamic and rapidly changing value. To overcome such problems, noninvasive monitors are used to provide a continuous estimate of $PaCO_2$. The two most primary noninvasive monitoring methods include capnography and transcutaneous monitors.

## Capnography

Capnography refers to the noninvasive measurement of the partial pressure of carbon dioxide in exhaled breath, expressed as the $CO_2$ concentration over time [1,2]. The relationship of $CO_2$ concentration to time can be represented graphically as a waveform or capnogram, or can be used to determine the maximum $CO_2$ concentration at the end of each tidal breath, or end-tidal $CO_2$ ($EtCO_2$). Capnography has been widely utilized in the United States since the 1980s, and has many clinical uses, including the assessment of disease

severity or response to therapy, or the confirmation of proper endotracheal tube (ETT) placement.

Capnography devices can be categorized based on their location for sampling, and therefore also on the types of patients for whom they are effective. Diverting capnometers are known as sidestream systems, and nondiverting capnometers are known as mainstream systems. Sidestream devices transport a sample of a patient's respired gases from the sampling site, through a sampling tube, to the sensor at a site distant from the sample site. Mainstream devices do not transport gas away from the sampling site, and therefore measure $CO_2$ at the actual sample site [3,4].

## Mechanism of $CO_2$ Detection: Capnography

Capnography uses infrared (IR) radiation and absorption to detect $CO_2$. Molecules of $CO_2$ absorb IR radiation at a very specific wavelength (4.26 μm). $CO_2$ monitors use lightweight IR sensors to emit IR light through adapter windows to a photodetector, which is sensitive to the IR band of $CO_2$. The detector is located on the other side of the airway adapter. The light that reaches the photodetector is used to measure $EtCO_2$. The IR radiation absorption is highly correlated with the $CO_2$ concentration present. Therefore, measurement of the IR radiation at the specific wavelength in a breath sample allows determination of $CO_2$ levels in that sample.

## Mainstream Versus Sidestream Capnographs

Mainstream devices measure $CO_2$ directly from the airway, with the sensor located on the airway adapter at the hub of the ETT, between the breathing circuit and the ETT. Mainstream capnography does not require gas sampling, as the measurement is made directly in the airway. Mainstream sensors are heated to slightly above body temperature to prevent condensation of water vapor, since this can cause falsely high $CO_2$ readings.

In mainstream capnography, a source emits IR that includes the absorption band for $CO_2$. The $CO_2$ within the exhaled gas in the circuit preferentially absorbs the radiation at its specific wavelength and passes other wavelengths. Photodetectors on the other side of the airway adapter measure the transmitted radiation. The detected signals are then amplified and transmitted via cable to a monitor where the partial pressure of the $CO_2$ is calculated and displayed.

In contrast, sidestream devices measure $CO_2$ via nasal or nasal–oral cannula by aspirating a small sample from the exhaled breath through cannula tubing to a sensor located inside the $CO_2$ monitor. This provides a unique advantage, allowing monitoring of non-intubated subjects, since sampling of the expiratory gases can be obtained from the nasal cavity. Gases can even be sampled from the nasal cavity during the administration of oxygen in patients receiving simultaneous oxygen administration using nasal cannula. Sidestream devices may require additional safeguards, including a gas scavenging system to collect anesthetics gases in the sample, and a water trap to collect condensation from humidified sample gas or patient secretions. Differences between mainstream and sidestream capnograms are summarized in Table 5.1.

Potential disadvantages of mainstream capnography include relative fragility of adapters, increased mechanical dead space, additional weight on the airway, and use limited to intubated patients. Sidestream capnography has different downsides. Measurement of $CO_2$ distant from the sampling site can potentially be affected by variation in humidity and temperature between the sampling and measurement sites, and pressure drops through the tubing [5,6]. In addition, using a remote location for measurement can result in a delay time of up to several seconds.

Sidestream gas analyzers continuously aspirate sample gas from the breathing circuit at variable sample flow rates. Low-flow sidestream systems usually utilize flow rates of approximately 50 ml min$^{-1}$ and are used for patients with low tidal volumes (i.e., neonates, infants, or patients of any age with low tidal-volume breathing). One advantage of such systems is that they have less dilution from supplemental oxygen compared to high-flow systems. High-flow systems utilize flow rates closer to 150 ml min$^{-1}$, but are less accurate in infants or patients with low tidal-volume breathing [7–9].

# Accuracy of $CO_2$ Detection by Capnography

Accurate assessment of $CO_2$ levels by capnography requires sampling of an accurate breath sample, reflective of a breath sample from the lower airways. In healthy lungs, there is limited anatomical or physiologic dead space, so the differences between EtCO$_2$ and PaCO$_2$ are relatively small. Patients with significant lung disease may have increased physiologic dead space and issues such as ventilation–perfusion mismatch, which may influence the correlation of the EtCO$_2$ with PaCO$_2$ [10,11]. For such patients, the EtCO$_2$ may only be useful for assessing trends in ventilatory status over time; isolated EtCO$_2$ values may or may not correlate with the PaCO$_2$.

**Table 5.1** Comparison of mainstream and sidestream carbon dioxide analyzers

|  | Mainstream | Sidestream |
|---|---|---|
| Location of infrared analysis unit | At airway connector | In the monitor |
| Use on extubated patients | No | Yes |
| Durability | Durable | Variable |
| Sample volume drawn | None | Low volume sample |
| Delay between sampling time and waveform display | None | Less than three seconds |
| Sensor 10–90 percent rise time | <70 milliseconds | >200 milliseconds |
| Waveform display | Crisp | Smooth appearance |
| Accuracy of waveform shape | Excellent | Variable |
| Changes in water vapor pressure | Not affected | Affected due to condensation and drying of sample |

## Indications for Capnography

Capnography has many potential clinical applications. The most common include:

(1) confirmation of ETT placement;
(2) assessment of trend of respiratory status (improvement versus maintenance versus deterioration) due to progression of clinical course or response to therapy;
(3) assessment of effectiveness of resuscitation in circulatory arrest.

### Endotracheal Tube Placement

Capnography has become a gold standard in the accurate determination of proper placement of an ETT (or any other advanced airway devices, like laryngeal mask airways) into the trachea [12–15]. Capnographic assessments may be quantitative, providing a numerical assessment of $EtCO_2$, or qualitative, which uses a colorimetric display to show a range of $EtCO_2$ values. Colorimetric capnography utilizes specially treated litmus paper that changes color when exposed to $CO_2$ [16,17]. Purple indicates $EtCO_2$ <3 mmHg, tan indicates $EtCO_2$ = 3 –15 mmHg, and yellow indicates $EtCO_2$>15 mmHg. Proper placement of an ETT in the trachea will therefore change the color of the litmus paper from purple to yellow. A monitor whose litmus paper remains purple has several possible explanations: (a) improper placement of the ETT into the esophagus; (b) proper tracheal placement with inadequate pulmonary blood flow; (c) obstruction of the ETT or airway just distal to the ETT; or (d) technical malfunction of the monitor or tubing.

Capnography has proven to be superior in sensitivity and specificity to other methods of ETT placement confirmation [12], including condensation in the tube [18], rise of the chest wall with breaths [19], and assessment of breath sounds [20]. Capnography may be slightly less sensitive in patients with circulatory failure, but remains highly accurate in determining ETT location. $EtCO_2$ should be the primary means to confirm tracheal placement of an ETT; the limitations of clinical methods indicates that these may be used adjunctively, but not primarily.

### Effectiveness of CPR

$EtCO_2$ reflects pulmonary blood flow during cardiac arrest, since alveolar ventilation and metabolism are otherwise constant. $EtCO_2$ can therefore be used as a noninvasive measure of cardiac output during cardiopulmonary resuscitation (CPR) [21]. Since effective CPR leads to improved cardiac output, the increase in perfusion will be reflected in a rise in the measured $EtCO_2$ [22].

## Transcutaneous Carbon Dioxide Monitoring

Transcutaneous $CO_2$ ($PtcCO_2$) devices provide another option for the continuous noninvasive estimation of $PaCO_2$. Rather than sample exhaled gas, $PtcCO_2$ monitoring uses skin sensors to calculate $CO_2$ through biochemical assessment of pH. This therefore provides an additional option for patients who are not intubated.

## Mechanism of $CO_2$ Detection: Transcutaneous Carbon Dioxide Monitoring

$PtcCO_2$ estimates the $PaCO_2$ through electrochemical measurements of $CO_2$ gas diffusing through body tissue and skin by a sensor at the skin surface by measuring the pH of an electrolyte solution that is separated from the skin by a permeable membrane [23,24]. The sensor is warmed to induce a local hyperemia, approximately 42–43 °C, which induces vasodilation of the dermal capillary bed below the sensor, increasing arterial blood flow. This vasodilation also facilitates diffusion of $CO_2$. $PtcCO_2$ is often slightly higher than the corresponding measured $PaCO_2$ value. This is likely due to two main factors. First, the elevated temperature alters the solubility of $CO_2$. Second, the hyperemia increases the metabolism of the skin cells, which contributes to $CO_2$ levels. The $PtcCO_2$ may therefore require a corrective algorithm to more closely align monitor values with the $PaCO_2$ [25,26].

Transcutaneous monitoring is considered a safe procedure; however, tissue injury may occur at the measuring site, including blisters, burns, and skin tears. Since the technology involves hyperemia where the probe is applied, continuous monitoring is generally avoided, since skin-related complications primarily occur when the $PtcCO_2$ is left in place for long periods of time. Some patients are not good candidates for $PtcCO_2$, including patients with poor skin integrity or adhesive allergy [27,28].

Besides the safety considerations, there are some clinical situations that may lead to an increased discrepancy between the $PtcCO_2$ and $PaCO_2$. These may include improper probe placement or application, factors associated with variable distance from probe to capillaries (such as body wall edema or thickness of the patient's skin or subcutaneous tissue), poor perfusion of the site of probe placement, or hyperoxia ($PaO_2$ > 100 torr) [24,27,28].

## Indications for Transcutaneous $CO_2$ Monitoring

Like capnography, $PtcCO_2$ assessment has many potential clinical applications. The most common include:

(1) assessment of trend of respiratory status (improvement versus maintenance versus deterioration) due to progression of clinical course or response to therapy;
(2) assessment of tissue perfusion;
(3) monitoring of acid–base status.

### Evaluation of Efficacy of Ventilation During Respiratory Failure

In some cohorts of patients, $PtcCO_2$ has been shown to be superior to capnography [27,28]. In particular, infants with congenital heart disease may have shunt or ventilation–perfusion mismatch that make $EtCO_2$ less accurate, but can benefit from $PtCO_2$ [29,30].

### Assessment of Tissue Perfusion

Several studies have looked at the use of $PtcCO_2$ to assess tissue perfusion in partial-thickness skin grafts for burn injury [31], and to evaluate changes in tissue perfusion during aortic cross-clamping for repair of coarctation of the aorta [32]. These studies suggest that $PtcCO_2$ may be useful in other clinical scenarios to noninvasively assess tissue perfusion.

### Monitoring of Acid–Base Status

Given the relationship of $PaCO_2$ to pH and serum bicarbonate, it is possible that changes in $PaCO_2$ can be used to reflect changes in pH. For example, in patients with diabetic ketoacidosis, $PtcCO_2$ may be utilized to follow the changes that occur during treatment and resolution of metabolic acidosis [33].

## Benefits and Limitations of $PtCO_2$ Compared to $EtCO_2$

Compared with $EtCO_2$ monitoring, $PtcCO_2$ monitoring requires a longer preparation time. Prior

to placement of the sensor, a calibration period of approximately 2–5 minutes is required. This is followed by another equilibration period of comparable duration after placement of the probe on the patient to allow for an equilibration between the $PtcCO_2$ and $PaCO_2$ values.

$PtcCO_2$ monitoring has been shown to be comparably accurate to capnography in patients with normal respiratory function and potentially more accurate in patients with congenital heart disease or ventilation–perfusion inequalities. $PtcCO_2$ monitoring also allows monitoring of $PaCO_2$ for patients on high-frequency oscillatory ventilation or non-intubated patients, for whom $EtCO_2$ is more challenging, and also allows monitoring metabolic status during treatment of acidosis.

In summary, both $PtcCO_2$ and capnography monitoring provide easily obtained, interpretable data that are within agreement of each other. Each method has unique advantages and limitations, but both provide important data that can assist in the optimal care of patients with a variety of pulmonary and metabolic diseases.

## Optimal Target $PaCO_2$

The optimal levels of $PaCO_2$ during anesthesia and controlled ventilation depends significantly on the underlying disease process and the potential risk of mechanical ventilation required to achieve optimal gas exchange.

The $PaCO_2$ is an indicator of $CO_2$ production and elimination: for a constant metabolic rate, the $PaCO_2$ is determined entirely by its elimination through ventilation. A normal value of $PaCO_2$ in a healthy patient is 35–45 mmHg.

In an otherwise healthy patient who requires ventilation assistance under anesthesia, the target $PaCO_2$ should therefore be in the normal physiologic range described above. There are a few clinical situations in which the risk of lung injury due to mechanical ventilation (to achieve normal $PaCO_2$) outweighs the benefit of normal $PaCO_2$. This ventilation approach is described as permissive hypercapnia.

The most common clinical scenarios in pediatrics that require a permissive hypercapnia ventilatory approach include most processes that involve lung hypoplasia. Premature infants, infants with congenital diaphragmatic hernia, and infants with primary or secondary lung hypoplasia fall into this category. Low tidal volume ventilation has been shown to improve important clinical outcomes in patients with such diseases, as they are particularly susceptible to permanent lung injury due to mechanical ventilation-induced volutrauma or barotrauma.

Other patient cohorts that may benefit from a low tidal volume ventilator strategy that results in permissive hypercapnia include those with acute respiratory distress syndrome. Finally, patients who have obstructive lung disease that does not allow complete exhalation, like severe asthma, may also benefit from permissive hypercapnia. Severe airway or bronchial obstruction increases the likelihood that inspiration will be initiated prior to the completion of expiration, creating intrinsic positive end-expiratory pressure (i.e., auto-PEEP). Ventilator strategies that allow complete exhalation, like decreasing tidal volume or inspiratory flow rate, necessarily may result in permissive hypercapnia.

The protective effects of hypercapnic acidosis may be a function of the acidosis or the hypercapnia *per se*, or a combination of both [34]. $PaCO_2$ in the range 50–80 mmHg, with pH between 7.20 and 7.30, reflect typical levels observed with institution of this technique.

## Hypocapnia

Hypocapnia can have potential significant health effects, specifically on cerebral perfusion. There are some clinical scenarios that can benefit from the physiologic changes induced by hypocapnia, but prolonged duration of hypocapnia can also have adverse neurologic consequences.

## Mechanism of Neurologic Effects of Hypocapnia

Systemic hypocapnia results in cerebrospinal fluid (CSF) alkalosis, which in turn decreases cerebral blood flow through potent vasoconstriction of cerebral vessels [35,36]. This can lower intracranial pressure, and be life-saving in situations in which intracranial pressure is severely elevated [37,38]. Cerebral vasoconstriction also has potential negative effects. Excessive vasoconstriction can cause reduced oxygen supply to the brain, and alkalosis can lead to reduced oxygen release from hemoglobin, resulting in cerebral ischemia [39]. Hypocapnia may also lead to increased neuronal excitability [40]. Over time, with buffering of CSF pH, the cerebral blood flow may return to normal. This may result in relative cerebral hyperemia and reperfusion injury to previously ischemic brain regions.

Hypocapnia can be particularly injurious to the developing brain, especially in premature infants. Relatively less well-perfused areas of the premature brain can be particularly susceptible to the ischemia resulting from severe cerebral vasoconstriction caused by severe or prolonged hypocapnia [41]. This results in a specific type of white matter brain injury, such as periventricular leukomalacia. Changes in cerebral blood flow due to swings in $PaCO_2$ can also result in intraventricular hemorrhage [42].

In summary, hypocapnia can have significant detrimental effects on cerebral perfusion, especially in premature infants. Close monitoring of ventilation, using blood gas measurements or noninvasive techniques, are critical to achieve optimal ventilation without negative pulmonary and neurodevelopmental effects.

## References

1.  Pfund AH, Gemmill CL. An infrared absorption method for the quantitative analysis of respiratory and other gases. *Bull Johns Hopkins Hosp*. 1940;67:61–5.

2.  Solomon, RJ. A reliable, accurate CO2 analyzer for medical use. *Hewlett-Packard Journal*. 1981;32:3–21.

3.  International Organization for Standardization. ISO 9918. Capnometers for use with humans: requirements, 1993.

4.  American Association for Respiratory Care. Clinical practice guideline: capnography/capnometry during mechanical ventilation. *Respir Care*. 1995;40(12):1321–4.

5.  Fletcher R, Werner O, Nordstrom L, Jonson B. Sources of error and their correction in the measurement of carbon dioxide elimination using the Siemens-Elema Co2 analyzer. *Br J Anaesth*. 1983;55(2):177–85.

6.  Williamson JA, Webb RK, Cockings J, Morgan C. The capnograph: applications and limitations: an analysis of 2000 incident reports. *Anaesth Intensive Care*. 1993;21(5):551–7.

7.  Friesen RH, Alswang M. End-tidal PCO2 monitoring via nasal cannulae in pediatric patients: accuracy and sources of error. *J Clin Monit*. 1996;12:155.

8.  Gravenstein N. Capnometry in infants should not be done at lower sampling flow rates. *J Clin Monit*. 1989;5:63.

9.  Sasse FJ. Can we trust end-tidal carbon dioxide measurements in infants? *J Clin Monit*. 1985;1:147.

10. Yamanaka MK, Sue DY. Comparison of arterial-end-tidal PCO2 difference and dead space/tidal volume ratio in respiratory failure. *Chest.* 1987;92:832.

11. Hardman JG, Aitkenhead AR. Estimating alveolar dead space from the arterial to end-tidal CO(2) gradient: a modeling analysis. *Anesth Analg.* 2003;97:1846.

12. Knapp S, Kofler J, Stoiser B, et al. The assessment of four different methods to verify tracheal tube placement in the critical care setting. *Anesth Analg.* 1999;88:766.

13. Ornato JP, Shipley JB, Racht EM, et al. Multicenter study of a portable, hand-size, colorimetric end-tidal carbon dioxide detection device. *Ann Emerg Med.* 1992;21:518.

14. Vukmir RB, Heller MB, Stein KL. Confirmation of endotracheal tube placement: a miniaturized infrared qualitative CO2 detector. *Ann Emerg Med.* 1991;20:726.

15. Grmec S, Mally S. Prehospital determination of tracheal tube placement in severe head injury. *Emerg Med J.* 2004;21:518.

16. Goldberg JS, Rawle PR, Zehnder JL, Sladen RN. Colorimetric end-tidal carbon dioxide monitoring for tracheal intubation. *Anesth Analg.* 1990;70:191.

17. MacLeod BA, Heller MB, Gerard J, et al. Verification of endotracheal tube placement with colorimetric end-tidal CO2 detection. *Ann Emerg Med.* 1991;20:267.

18. Kelly JJ, Eynon CA, Kaplan JL, et al. Use of tube condensation as an indicator of endotracheal tube placement. *Ann Emerg Med.* 1998;31:575.

19. Pollard BJ, Junius F. Accidental intubation of the oesophagus. *Anaesth Intensive Care.* 1980;8:183.

20. Birmingham PK, Cheney FW, Ward RJ. Esophageal intubation: a review of detection techniques. *Anesth Analg.* 1986;65:886.

21. Falk JL, Rackow EC, Weil MH. End-tidal carbon dioxide concentration during cardiopulmonary resuscitation. *N Engl J Med.* 1988;318:607.

22. Garnett AR, Ornato JP, Gonzalez ER, Johnson EB. End-tidal carbon dioxide monitoring during cardiopulmonary resuscitation. *JAMA.* 1987;257:512.

23. Monaco F, Nickerson BG, McQuitty JC. Continuous transcutaneous oxygen and carbon dioxide monitoring in the pediatric ICU. *Crit Care Med.* 1982;10:765–6.

24. Restrepo RD, Hirst KR, Wittnebel L, Wettstein R. AARC clinical practice guideline: transcutaneous monitoring of carbon dioxide and oxygen. *Respir Care.* 2012; 57:1955–62.

25. Severinghaus JW. Transcutaneous blood gas analysis. *Respir Care.* 1982;27:152–9.

26. Tremper KK, Shoemaker WC, Shippy CR et al. Transcutaneous PCO2 monitoring on adult patients in the ICU and the operating room. *Crit Care Med.* 1981;9:752–5.

27. Tobias JD. Transcutaneous carbon dioxide monitoring in infants and children. *Pediatr Anesth.* 2009, 19:434–44.

28. Tobias JD, Wilson WR, Meyer DJ. Transcutaneous monitoring of carbon dioxide tension after cardiothoracic surgery in infants and children. *Anesth Analg.* 1999;88:531–4.

29. Grenier B, Verchere E, Meslie A, et al. Capnography monitoring during neurosurgery: reliability in relation to various intraoperative positions. *Anesthesiology.* 1999;88:43–8.

30. Short JA, Paris ST, Booker BD, et al. Arterial to end-tidal carbon dioxide tension difference in children with congenital heart disease. *Br J Anaesth.* 2001;86:349–53.

31. Greenhalgh DG, Warden GD. Transcutaneous oxygen and carbon dioxide measurements for determination of skin graft "take." *J Burn Care Rehabil.* 1992;13:334–9.

32. Tobias JD, Russo P, Russo J. An evaluation of acid–base changes following aortic cross-clamping using transcutaneous carbon dioxide monitoring. *Pediatr Cardiol.* 2006;27:585–8.

33. McBride ME, Berkenbosch JW, Tobias JD. Transcutaneous carbon dioxide monitoring during diabetic ketoacidosis in children and adolescents. *Paediatr Anaesth.* 2004;14:167–71.

34. O'Croinin D, Chonghaile MN, Higgins B, Laffey JG. Bench-to-bedside review: permissive hypercapnia. *Crit Care.* 2005;9(1):51–9.

35. Kazemi H, Johnson, DC. Regulation of cerebrospinal fluid acid–base balance. *Physiol Rev.* 1986;66:953–1037.

36. Fortune JB, Feustel PJ, deLuna C, et al. Cerebral blood flow and blood volume in response to O2 and CO2 changes in normal humans. *J Trauma.* 1995;39:463–71.

37. Darby JM, Yonas H, Marion DW, Latchaw RE. Local "inverse steal" induced by hyperventilation in head injury. *Neurosurgery.* 1988;23:84–8.

38. Marion DW, Firlik A, McLaughlin MR. Hyperventilation therapy for severe traumatic brain injury. *New Horiz.* 1995;3:439–47.

39. Weckesser M, Posse S, Olthoff U, et al. Functional imaging of the visual cortex with bold-contrast MRI: hyperventilation decreases signal response. *Magn Reson Med.* 1999;41:213–16.

40. Vannucci RC, Brucklacher RM, Vannucci SJ. Effect of carbon dioxide on cerebral metabolism during hypoxia-ischemia in the immature rat. *Pediatr Res*. 1997;42:24–9.

41. De Reuck J. Cerebral angioarchitecture and perinatal brain lesions in premature and full-term infants. *Acta Neurol Scand*. 1984;70:391–5.

42. Gleason CA, Short BL, Jones MD Jr. Cerebral blood flow and metabolism during and after prolonged hypocapnia in newborn lambs. *J Pediatr*. 1989;115:309–14.

# Glucose Control

Monica Hoagland

## Glucose Homeostasis in Neonates

Under physiologic conditions, glucose levels are tightly controlled. Glucose loading stimulates insulin, which in turn stimulates peripheral glucose uptake, glycogen synthesis, and lipogenesis while also inhibiting processes that produce glucose. Fasting causes an increase in counter-regulatory hormones, including glucagon, catecholamines, cortisol, and growth hormone, which act to stimulate glucose production and decrease synthesis of glucose storage molecules. Early in a fast, euglycemia is maintained primarily by glycogenolysis. During a prolonged fast or in situations in which glycogen stores are limited, gluconeogenesis, lipolysis, and ketogenesis are more important. Amino acids from muscle catabolism and glycerol generated by lipolysis are substrates for gluconeogenesis. Lipolysis also produces free fatty acids, which are substrates for ketogenesis. Ketones can be used as an alternative fuel source by muscle to preserve adequate glucose for the brain and erythrocytes. Therefore, normal glucose homeostasis requires intact metabolic and endocrine pathways as well as adequate hepatic glycogen, muscle, and fat stores to drive endogenous energy production during times of fasting [1].

Neonates and small infants have a number of metabolic differences from older children and adults that affect glucose homeostasis. The fetus receives a continuous supply of glucose through placental blood flow. At birth, glucose levels abruptly decrease and subsequently increase over 1–2 hours due to increasing counter-regulatory hormones. Glucose levels stabilize as gluconeogenic and ketogenic pathways mature and oral glucose intake improves over the next 24 hours [2,3]. The endogenous glucose production rate in neonates is 4–6 mg kg$^{-1}$ min$^{-1}$, but is dependent on exhaustible glycogen, muscle, and fat stores [3]. Up to 80 percent of energy requirements are supplied by fat metabolism as glycogen stores fall [4]. Fetal weight doubles between 32 weeks gestational age and term,

mostly due to hepatic glycogen and adipose deposition [2]. Therefore, neonates that are premature or small for gestational age have significantly decreased metabolic reserve. Neonates also have higher energy requirements compared to adults. Glucose consumption in neonates is 6 mg kg$^{-1}$ min$^{-1}$ compared with 1–2 mg kg$^{-1}$ min$^{-1}$ in adults. This is primarily due to the increased brain-to-body size ratio and resulting increased cerebral glucose utilization in children [1,2].

The combination of increased metabolic rate and decreased energy reserves increases the risk of hypoglycemia in neonates. The presentation of hypoglycemia is nonspecific and includes autonomic symptoms (diaphoresis, tremor, and tachycardia) from increased catecholamine secretion and neuroglycopenic symptoms (altered mentation, lethargy, hypotension, and seizures) due to decreased cerebral glucose supply [1]. Multiple studies have shown an association between neonatal hypoglycemia and brain injury, as measured by structural abnormalities on radiologic studies and long-term neurodevelopmental abnormalities [1,5–7]. However, some studies have found no such correlation [8]. No study has determined a duration, severity or number of hypoglycemic episodes that is harmful to neonates and the contribution of hypoglycemia independent of other factors, such as hypoxia-ischemia, has not been proven [3]. Possible mechanisms for hypoglycemic cerebral injury include increased cerebral blood flow with decreased autoregulation due to the hormonal stress response and alterations in brain metabolism, neurotransmitters, and acid–base balance [9]. Glucose is the brain's primary fuel source. However, in contrast to adults, the neonatal brain also uses alternative energy sources, such as ketone bodies and lactate, under physiologic conditions. The presence of alternative fuels is therefore protective against hypoglycemic brain injury and their availability must be taken into account when assessing the severity of neonatal hypoglycemia. In patients with impaired metabolic responses, such as those with abnormal metabolic pathways, decreased substrate availability or insulin-driven hypoglycemia, mild hypoglycemia is more dangerous than in otherwise healthy patients [2,3,5,10]. This ability to use alternative fuels is a confounding factor in that it makes it difficult to define hypoglycemia in neonates.

Most studies use a threshold of 40–45 mg dl$^{-1}$ (2.2–2.6 mmol L$^{-1}$) to define neonatal hypoglycemia, though the threshold for intervention may be higher, especially in neonates with impaired metabolic responses [1–3]. However, glucose values in this range may occur normally in healthy, full-term neonates in the first 48–72 hours of life. Patients with increased risk for developing hypoglycemia include premature and small neonates, those with increased metabolic demands due to physiologic stressors, and patients with inappropriately elevated insulin levels or counter-regulatory hormone deficiency. Common physiologic stressors include sepsis, hypothermia, and hypoxia. Inappropriate insulin elevation can be iatrogenic, due to insulin administration or an abrupt discontinuation of glucose-containing fluids (including parenteral nutrition). Transient insulin elevation is also seen in neonates born to mothers with diabetes or those who received dextrose-containing fluids immediately prior to or during delivery. Sustained insulin elevations are seen in some endocrinopathies. Counter-regulatory hormone deficiency is seen in hypopituitarism, adrenal insufficiency, and patients receiving beta blockers [2,3,11].

Maintenance glucose administration in neonates is typically started at 4–7 mg kg$^{-1}$ min$^{-1}$ to match endogenous production. This is commonly supplied as 10 percent dextrose, requiring infusion rates of 60–100 ml kg$^{-1}$ day$^{-1}$ (2.5–4 ml kg$^{-1}$ h$^{-1}$). Patients with high volume requirements, such as extremely low birth weight infants, may require more dilute solutions to avoid hyperglycemia, while those who are fluid restricted may require more concentrated solutions to avoid hypoglycemia. Concentrations greater than 12.5 percent are rarely required, but should be given centrally to avoid sclerosis of peripheral veins or tissue damage from infiltration [3,12]. Neonates undergo a postnatal diuresis in the first few days of life that results in loss of 10–15 percent of body weight as water. This is a normal physiologic process and patients in whom this process is prevented by volume expansion have poor outcomes. Therefore, patients may require concentrated dextrose infusions

to meet nutritional requirements for the first few days of life [13,14]. Severe or symptomatic hypoglycemia requiring immediate intervention may be treated with a bolus of 3–5 ml kg$^{-1}$ of 10 percent dextrose (300–500 mg kg$^{-1}$) followed by an infusion [3].

Hyperglycemia is a common finding in critically ill patients that can also complicate the management of neonates. Physiologic stressors, such as acute illness, pain, or surgery disrupt normal glucose homeostasis by increasing counter-regulatory hormones and inducing insulin resistance. This results in inappropriate endogenous glucose production as well as decreased peripheral glucose uptake. Neonates that are premature or small for gestational age also have impaired glucose homeostasis at baseline. Iatrogenic factors, such as administration of dextrose-containing fluids (including parenteral nutrition and blood products), catecholamines, and corticosteroids, also contribute to hyperglycemia [1–3,15]. The detrimental effects of hyperglycemia and benefits of glucose control are established in some adult populations. Blood glucose abnormalities, including hypo- and hyperglycemia as well as glucose variability, have been associated with increased morbidity and mortality in a number of pediatric studies [16–18]. However, hyperglycemia is only a prognostic indicator in these studies. A directly causative effect of hyperglycemia on patient outcomes has not been proven [18] and the benefits of glucose control with insulin have not been established in pediatric patients due to increased risk of hypoglycemia [1,18].

Hyperglycemia is commonly defined as glucose greater than 126 mg dl$^{-1}$ (7 mmol L$^{-1}$), with treatment generally indicated above 180 mg dl$^{-1}$ (10 mmol L$^{-1}$) [1–3]. Hyperglycemia causes glycosuria and osmotic diuresis, which can result in significant volume depletion and electrolyte imbalances, especially in small infants [2,19,20]. Glycosuria may be present even with minimal hyperglycemia in preterm neonates who have a low renal threshold for glucose reabsorption [3,11,21]. There have been concerns that hyperglycemia can lead to significant fluid shifts with resultant cerebral pathology and neurodevelopmental effects, though there is no evidence that self-limited hyperglycemia below 360 mg dl$^{-1}$ (20 mmol L$^{-1}$) has significant effects in the absence of osmotic diuresis [3]. Hyperglycemia in the presence of hypoxia is associated with worsening of neurologic outcomes in adult and animal studies. This is due to anaerobic glycolysis of excess glucose with resultant intracerebral lactic acidosis and compromised cellular function [9,10]. In contrast, moderate hyperglycemia may not worsen, and actually may be protective from, ischemic damage in neonates due to differences in glucose and lactate metabolism in the neonatal brain [9–11,19,22]. Hyperglycemia in neonates is generally self-limited and related to iatrogenic factors or underlying medical comorbidities. Treatment involves limiting glucose administration and treating the underlying illness. Rarely, insulin is required and may be started at 0.03–0.05 units $kg^{-1} h^{-1}$ [3,12].

## Perioperative Glucose Management

Fasting, surgical stress, and anesthesia have significant effects on glucose homeostasis in the perioperative period. These effects are well-studied in pediatric patients, but studies including or focusing on neonates are limited. As noted in the previous section, neonates have significant metabolic differences from older children that may limit the applicability of pediatric studies to the neonatal population.

Hypoglycemia in healthy, fasting children presenting for surgery is rare (less than 2.5 percent) and the incidence has decreased as more liberal fasting guidelines, including intake of clear fluids until two hours preoperatively, have been implemented [18–21]. Most children who were hypoglycemic had very prolonged fasting times [19]. Children who underwent daytime fasting for afternoon procedures had lower glucose levels than children who fasted overnight for morning surgery, independent of the fast duration, due to diurnal variations in cortisol secretion [23]. In infants and young children, preoperative glucose levels did not correlate with age, weight, or duration of the fast [24]. Studies of fasting neonates have demonstrated that neonates under one week of age can maintain euglycemia without intraoperative glucose administration [4,25,26]. In one study, neonates of normal birth weight were able to maintain euglycemia for up to seven days without glucose administration due to increased fat mobilization [4]. However, hypoglycemia did occur in patients under 48 hours old or who were receiving preoperative glucose infusions that were stopped intraoperatively [25,26]. Preoperative oral and intravenous glucose loading raises insulin levels and can cause rebound hypoglycemia if glucose infusions are stopped intraoperatively [25].

Intraoperative increases in glucose due to surgical stress have been demonstrated in multiple pediatric studies [21]. Neonatal patients also mount an endocrine and metabolic stress response to surgical stimulation. Operative trauma in neonates results in an increase in oxygen consumption, energy expenditure, and blood glucose levels that persist until 12–24 hours postoperatively [4,27,28]. Glucose elevations are mediated by an early rise in catecholamines, followed by sustained cortisol and glucagon elevations. Insulin secretion remains low until 12–24 hours after surgery, with longer suppression in premature infants, who remain hyperglycemic longer in the postoperative period [27–29]. Increasing levels of surgical stress are associated with greater and more prolonged metabolic changes and worse outcomes [30]. In neonates, energy required for surgical trauma is diverted from energy used for growth. This avoids the overall increase in energy expenditure seen in adults, but does result in retarded neonatal growth during times of metabolic stress [27].

Anesthesia reduces the energy requirements of children up to 50 percent from their awake values [31,32]. The combination of reduced energy requirements and increased serum glucose due to impaired metabolism decreases the amount of glucose administration required intraoperatively [13]. However, the type of anesthetic also plays a role in determining intraoperative glucose requirements. In neonates and children, neuraxial anesthetics significantly decrease the hormone stress response compared to opioids [33,34] and volatile anesthetics [35,36]. Opioids, in turn, provide better suppression than volatile anesthetics [37]. Suppression of the surgical stress response blunts the normal intraoperative rise of glucose and places patients at risk for hypoglycemia. Consideration should be given to monitoring glucose levels in patients receiving neuraxial anesthetics [35].

The goals for intraoperative fluid management are to maintain adequate circulating volume to provide organ perfusion and oxygen delivery and to maintain electrolyte and glucose homeostasis [13]. Neonates are a particularly challenging group of patients in which to maintain these goals, as their volume, electrolyte, and glucose requirements are markedly different from older patients and change throughout the neonatal period. Maintenance volume requirements as determined by Holliday and Segar are approximately 4 ml $kg^{-1} h^{-1}$ in neonates [32]. Most neonates presenting for surgery from the NICU are well-resuscitated and receiving glucose-containing fluids. However, fasting neonates not receiving infusions will have a fluid deficit. In addition, surgical trauma requires additional fluid administration. Berry proposed administration of 15–20 ml kg$^{-1}$ of fluid over the first hour to correct volume deficits, followed by 6 ml kg$^{-1}$ h$^{-1}$ for maintenance fluids and an additional 2–6 ml kg$^{-1}$ h$^{-1}$ to cover surgical trauma [21]. Many studies employ fluid algorithms similar to that proposed by Berry. In some studies, glucose-containing solutions were administered at these high rates to cover maintenance requirements and replace fasting deficit and insensible loss without other crystalloid administration. It is therefore important to consider both the concentration of fluid administered and the rate at which it is given to determine the total glucose load in these studies.

Administration of 5 percent dextrose infusions to infants and young children causes hyperglycemia intra- and postoperatively. In most studies, the glucose rose intraoperatively whether or not dextrose was administered, and higher concentrations of dextrose were associated with increasing frequency of hyperglycemia. This has resulted in a trend toward using low glucose concentrations (1–2.5 percent dextrose) or avoiding glucose administration in these patients [15,19–21,38]. However, it should be noted that maintenance of euglycemia does not imply that patients have adequate glycogen stores for a prolonged intraoperative fast. In one study, infants under one year old not receiving glucose had an average increase in their glucose levels, but 40 percent of patients failed to increase or had a decrease in the glucose levels within normal limits. These patients required lipolysis to maintain euglycemia due to inadequate glycogen stores [39].

Studies assessing the need for intraoperative glucose administration in neonates are limited. Most neonates who did not receive intraoperative glucose were able to maintain euglycemia [25,26]. However, hypoglycemia was found in neonates less than 48 hours old or in whom preoperative glucose infusions were discontinued intraoperatively [25]. In addition, fat mobilization was required to maintain euglycemia in the fasting neonates due to limited glycogen stores [26]. Glucose administration at 100 mg kg$^{-1}$ h$^{-1}$ maintains euglycemia in neonates, though some patients did have declining glucose levels within the reference range [40]. Administration of 120–300 mg kg$^{-1}$ h$^{-1}$ of glucose is sufficient to prevent lipid mobilization and to allow glucose levels to rise without causing hyperglycemia in young infants [39] and neonates [26].

These rates are similar to the rates of endogenous glucose production in neonates (240–360 mg kg$^{-1}$ h$^{-1}$). However, hyperglycemia may still occur with these regimens during longer procedures. Higher rates of glucose administration resulted in hyperglycemia [25,41].

Given the risks of undetected hypoglycemia, intraoperative glucose administration is warranted in neonates. Neonates at particular risk include patients who are premature or small, less than 48 hours old, receiving glucose-containing solutions preoperatively, undergoing long procedures (2–3 hours), or who have a neuraxial block. Glucose can be supplied intraoperatively with D10% at a low infusion rate (1–3 ml kg$^{-1}$ h$^{-1}$) or with more dilute solutions close to normal maintenance rates. Separate, non-glucose-containing fluids should be used for boluses to replace the fasting deficit and intraoperative losses. Patients receiving glucose-containing fluids preoperatively require intraoperative glucose administration to prevent rebound hypoglycemia, though the rate can be decreased in anticipation of the surgical stress response. Glucose should be periodically monitored in neonates, especially for long procedures or if glucose-containing fluids are being withheld.

# References

1. Ulate K, Zimmerman J. Common endocrinopathies in the pediatric intensive care unit. In: Fuhrman B, Zimmerman J, Carcillo J, et al., editors. *Pediatric Critical Care*, 4th edn. Philadelphia, PA: Elsevier Health Sciences; 2011; 1105–23.

2. Jain V, Chen M, Menon R. Disorders of carbohydrate metabolism. In: Gleason C, Devaskar S, editors. *Avery's Diseases of the Newborn*, 9th edn. Philadelphia, PA: Elsevier Health Sciences; 2012; 1320–30.

3. Hawdon J, Cheetham T, Schenk D, et al. Metabolic and endocrine disorders. In: Rennie J, editor. *Rennie and Roberton's Textbook of Neonatology*, 5th edn. London: Churchill Livingstone; 2012; 850–67.

4. Elphick MC, Wilkinson AW. The effects of starvation and surgical injury on plasma levels of glucose, free fatty acids, and neutral lipids in newborn babies suffering from various congenital anomalies. *Pediatr Res*. 1981;15(4):313–18.

5. Burns CM, Rutherford MA, Boardman JP, et al. Patterns of cerebral injury and neurodevelopmental outcomes after symptomatic neonatal hypoglcyemia. *Pediatrics*. 2008;122(1):65–74.

6. Kinnala A, Rikalainen H, Lapinleimu H, et al. Cerebral magnetic resonance imaging and ultrasonography

findings after neonatal hypoglcyemia. *Pediatrics*. 1999;103(4):724–9.

7. Duvanel DB, Fawer C, Cotting J, et al. Long-term effects of neonatal hypoglycemia on brain growth and psychomotor development in small-for-gestational age and preterm infants. *J Pediatr*. 1999;134(4):492–8.

8. Boluyt N, van Kempen A, Offringa M. Neurodevelopment after neonatal hypoglcyemia: a systematic review and design of an optimal future study. *Pediatrics*. 2006;177(6):2231–43.

9. Sieber F, Traystman R. Special issues: glucose and the brain. *Crit Care Med*. 1992;20(1):104–14.

10. Vannucci RC, Vannucci SJ. Glucose metabolism in the developing brain. *Semin Perinatol*. 2000;24(2):107–15.

11. Murat I, Humblot A, Girault L, et al. Neonatal fluid management. *Best Pract Res Clin Anaesthesiol*. 2010;24(3):365–74.

12. Poindexter B, Denne S. Parenteral nutrition. In: Gleason C, Devaskar S, editors. *Avery's Diseases of the Newborn*, 9th edn. Philadelphia, PA: Elsevier Health Sciences; 2012; 963–72.

13. O'Brien F, Walker I. Fluid homeostasis in the neonate. *Paediatr Anaesth*. 2014;24(1):49–59.

14. Association of Paediatric Anaesthetists of Great Britain and Ireland. APA consensus guideline on perioperative fluid management in children, 2007. Available at: www.apagbi.org.uk/sites/default/files/Perioperative_Fluid_Management_2007.pdf.

15. Leelanukrom R, Cunliffe M. Intraoperative fluid and glucose management in children. *Paediatr Anaesth*. 2000;10(4):353–9.

16. Wintergest KU, Buckhingham B, Gandrud L, et al. Association of hypoglcyemia, hyperglcyemia, and glucose variability with morbidity and death in the pediatric intensive care unit. *Pediatrics*. 2006;118(1):173–9.

17. Hays SP, Smith EO, Sunehag AL. Hyperglcyemia is a risk factor for early death and morbidity in extremely low birth-weight infants. *Pediatrics*. 2006;118(5):1811–18.

18. Steven J, Nicolson S. Perioperative management of blood glucose during open heart surgery in infants and children. *Paediatr Anaesth*. 2011;21(5):530–7.

19. Paut O, Lacroix F. Recent developments in the perioperative fluid management for the paediatric patient. *Curr Opin Anaesthesiol*. 2006;19(3):268–77.

20. Murat I, Dubois M. Perioperative fluid therapy in pediatrics. *Paediatr Anaesth*. 2008;18(5):363–70.

21. Berleur MP, Dahan A, Murat I, et al. Perioperative infusions in paediatric patients: rationale for using Ringer-lactate solution with low dextrose concentration. *J Clin Pharm Ther*. 2003;28(1):31–40.

22. de Ferranti S, Gauvreau K, Hickey PR, et al. Intraoperative hyperglycemia during infant cardiac surgery is not associated with adverse neurodevelopmental outcomes at 1, 4 and 8 years. *Anesthesiology*. 2004;100(6):1345–52.

23. Redfern N, Addison GM, Meakin G. Blood glucose in anaesthetised children. Comparison of blood glucose concentrations in children fasted for morning and afternoon surgery. *Anaesthesia*. 1986;41(3):272–5.

24. Nilsson K, Larsson LE, Andreasson S, et al. Blood glucose concentrations during anaesthesia in children: effects of starvation and perioperative fluid therapy. *Br J Anaesth*. 1984;56(4):375–9.

25. Larsson LE, Nilsson K, Niklasson A, et al. Influence of fluid regimens on perioperative blood glucose concentrations in neonates. *Br J Anaesth*. 1990;64(4):419–24.

26. Sandstrom K, Nilsson K, Andreasson S, et al. Metabolic consequences of different perioperative fluid therapies in the neonatal period. *Acta Anaesthesiol Scand*. 1993;37(2):170–5.

27. Pierro A, Eaton S. Metabolism and nutrition in the surgical neonate. *Semin Pediatr Surg*. 2008;17(4):276–84.

28. Anand KJS, Brown MJ, Causon RC, et al. Can the human neonate mount an endocrine and metabolic response to surgery? *J Pediatr Surg*. 1985;20(1):41–8.

29. Srinivasan G, Jain R, Pildes RS, et al. Glucose homeostasis during anesthesia and surgery in infants. *J Pediatr Surg*. 1986;21(8):718–21.

30. Anand JS, Aynsley-Green A. Measuring the severity of surgical stress in newborn infants. *J Pediatr Surg*. 1988;23(4):297–305.

31. Lindahl S. Energy expenditure and fluid and electrolyte requirements in anesthetized infants and children. *Anesthesiology*. 1988;69(3):377–82.

32. Holliday MA, Segar WE. The maintenance need for water in parenteral fluid therapy. *Pediatrics*. 1957;19(5):823–32.

33. Wolf AR, Doyle E, Thomas E. Modifying infant stress responses to major surgery: spinal vs extradural vs opioid analgesia. *Paediatr Anaesth*. 1988;8(4):305–11.

34. Wolf AR, Eyres RL, Laussen PC, et al. Effect of extradural analgesia on stress responses to abdominal surgery in infants. *Br J Anaesth*. 1993;70(6):654–60.

35. Gouyet L, Dubois M, Murat I. Blood glucose and insulin level during epidural anaesthesia in children receiving dextrose-free solution. *Paediatr Anaesth*. 1994;4(5):307–11.

36. Nakamura T, Takasaki M. Metabolic and endocrine stress responses to surgery during caudal analgesia in children. *Can J Anaesth*. 1991;38(8):969–73.

37. Anand KJ, Sippell WG, Aynsley-Green A. Randomised trial of fentanyl anaesthesia in preterm babies undergoing surgery: effects on the stress response. *Lancet*. 1987;1(8524):62–6.

38. Bailey AG, McNaull PP, Jooste E, et al. Perioperative crystalloid and colloid fluid management in children: where are we and how did we get here? *Anesth Analg*. 2010;110(2):375–90.

39. Nishina K, Mikawa K, Maekawa N, et al. Effects of exogenous intravenous glucose on plasma glucose and lipid homeostasis in anesthetized infants. *Anesthesiology*. 1995;83(2):258–63.

40. Sumpelmann R, Mader T, Dennhardt N, et al. A novel isotonic balanced electrolyte solution with 1% glucose for intraoperative fluid therapy in neonates: results of a prospective multicentre observational postauthorisation safety study (PASS). *Paediatr Anaesth*. 2011;21(11):1114–18.

41. Fosel TH, Uth M, Wilhelm W, et al. Comparison of two solutions with different glucose concentrations for infusion therapy during laparotomies in infants. *Infusionsther Transfusionsmed*. 1996;23(2):80–4.

# Oxygen Management
## Concerns About Both Hyperoxia and Hypoxia in Neonates During Critical Care and Intraoperatively

Augusto Sola

## Introduction

Many therapies and interventions are not based on proven benefit, but on anecdotal evidence, expert opinion, and tradition. This is especially true for oxygen therapy, which is usually not questioned and has been used for more than 100 years. However, such a practice may be harmful when it is not truly necessary [1–5]; some of the available evidence will be provided in this chapter.

Oxygen is one of the most frequent drugs administered during critical care and during the pre-, intra-, and postoperative periods, and its administration and management has been fraught with problems, misunderstandings, and errors. We have all been taught about the many causes of hypoxemia and of the potential significant damage secondary to hypoxia. This is well taught in medical and nursing schools and throughout residency. Based on this education, no healthcare provider induces or tolerates hypoxemia in any patient. Regrettably, in many places there is still a lack of education about the potential damaging effects of hyperoxemia and hyperoxia. Additionally, and very differently from hypoxemia and hypoxia, the only reason that hyperoxemia can occur in a human being is us, the healthcare providers. We cause hyperoxemia and hyperoxia in the laudable effort to prevent or treat hypoxemia and when supplementary $O_2$ is provided unnecessarily. Even though we still do not know the perfect way to manage this potent drug, we have learned during the last decade that there are many things we should not continue to do as we have been doing [2–10].

This chapter reviews several aspects of oxygenation and oxygen management. The focus is more on hyperoxemia and hyperoxia, since hypoxia and hypoxemia are better known and well covered in many other places. With this in mind, this chapter describes the following in its different sections: (1) physiology of

oxygenation; (2) oxidative stress and oxidant injury; (3) oxygen as a health hazard; (4) assessment of oxygen in blood; and (5) targeting of $SpO_2$ and recommendations for clinical practice.

## Physiology of Oxygenation

Atmospheric pressure ($P_{atm}$) is about 765 mmHg at sea level. We all know that in room air the inspired fraction of $O_2$ ($FiO_2$) is 0.21; the rest (0.79) is nitrogen, regardless of the altitude above sea level. That is to say that 21 percent of the $P_{atm}$ is the partial pressure of inspired $O_2$ ($PiO_2$). If we are interested in knowing the $PiO_2$ of dry gas we have to subtract the estimated water vapor pressure ($P_{H2O}$), which is variable and frequently estimated at about 47–50 mmHg. Therefore, the $PiO_2$ in room air at sea level ($P_{atm}$ of about 765 mmHg) is about 150 mmHg ($P_{atm} - P_{H2O} \times 21 / 100$), varying also with ambient temperature. Of course, relative ambient humidity (water vapor pressure) is also variable. So the partial pressure of $O_2$ that reaches the upper and lower airway is about 150 mmHg, and this will reach the alveoli. Here there is another gas, $CO_2$, at an alveolar partial pressure ($PACO_2$) of about 40 mmHg. Therefore, "dry" alveolar $PO_2$ ($PAO_2$) in room air is about 110 mmHg ($PiO_2 - PACO_2$). This is in few and simple words the alveolar gas equation; the known formulae are given below.

$$PiO_2 = FiO_2 \times P_{atm} / 100 \qquad \text{Dry gas: } P_{atm} - P_{H2O}$$

$$PiO_2 \text{ in room air: } 21 \times (P_{atm} - P_{H2O}) / 100 \simeq 150 \text{ mmHg}$$

$$PiO_2 \text{ in pure oxygen: } 100 \times (P_{atm} - P_{H2O}) / 100 \simeq 710 \text{ mmHg}$$

$$PAO_2 = PiO_2 - PACO_2 \text{ (in room air about 100 mmHg; breathing pure oxygen about 670 mmHg)}$$

The $PAO_2$ then has to reach pulmonary capillaries and veins, left atrium, left ventricle, and systemic circulation. In normal healthy children and adults the $PaO_2$ is about 100 mmHg. In the neonatal period, due to intra- and extrapulmonary shunting, $PaO_2$ is usually 45–75 mmHg and rarely >80 mmHg.

Once in systemic circulation, oxygen has to be transported by hemoglobin (Hb) and circulated in the blood to reach tissues for adequate tissue oxygenation. However, tissue oxygenation is complex and multiple factors are related to achieving this process satisfactorily (Table 7.1).

Of all this, we frequently and easily measure $PaO_2$, but this is probably among the least important factors related to tissue oxygenation. Thus, there could be a low $PaO_2$ in blood (hypoxemia) with adequate tissue oxygenation (normoxia); furthermore, there could be normoxemia and even hyperoxemia but not sufficient oxygen in the tissue (hypoxia). A normal (or high) $PaO_2$ with tissue hypoxia generally occurs in one of several ways: (1) anemia; (2) altered affinity of hemoglobin for binding oxygen (for example in cases of methemoglobinemia or when the $Hb$–$O_2$ curve shifts markedly to the right); (3) poor perfusion (altered cardiac output and vascular resistance); (4) decreased oxygen delivery; or (5) altered microcirculation. In summary, to remain viable tissues require a certain amount of oxygen per minute, a need met by oxygen content ($CaO_2$) and delivery, and not oxygen pressure.

Oxygen has to be bound to Hb to be transported to the tissues; dissolved oxygen has extremely little participation in this process. In normal conditions, the normal Hb–O2 curve is sigmoid and maintains a predictable relation between $PaO_2$ and arterial saturation

**Table 7.1** Factors related to tissue oxygenation

| | |
|---|---|
| $PaO_2$ (mmHg) | Hematocrit (hyperviscosity) |
| Hb concentration (anemia) and quality | pH |
| | $CO_2$ local and systemic |
| (Hb F; Hb A; dyshemoglobins) | Temperature |
| Hb–$O_2$ relationship (saturation in percent) | Glycemia |
| | $O_2$ delivery |
| Oxygen content ($CaO_2$ in ml $O_2$/dl) | $O_2$ consumption |
| $[(SaO_2 \times Hb \times 1.34) +.003$ ml $O_2$/mmHg $PaO_2]$. | $PaO_2$ local (4–20 mmHg) |
| | Distance |
| Cardiac output | Microcirculation |
| (heart rate; stroke volume; minute volume) | |
| Peripheral vascular resistance and systemic blood flow | |
| Pulmonary vascular resistance and blood flow | |

($SaO_2$). One gram of Hb can carry about 1.34 ml of $O_2$ when fully saturated, a concept known as maximum oxygen carrying capacity. To make the necessary connection between $PaO_2$ and $O_2$ content requires applying the $CaO_2$ equation (described in Table 7.1). As shown, $SaO_2$ and Hb are key factors, while a very small quantity of oxygen is carried dissolved in plasma (0.003 ml $O_2$/mmHg $PaO_2$; which is to say only 0.3 ml $O_2$/dl plasma when $PaO_2$ is 100 mmHg). The following examples illustrate these concepts, using values of Hb that exist in neonates:

- With $SaO_2$ of 100 percent and Hb of 20 g dl$^{-1}$: $CaO_2$ is 26.8 ml dl$^{-1}$ (+0.003 ml $O_2$/mmHg $PaO_2$)
- With $SaO_2$ of 100 percent and Hb of 8 g dl$^{-1}$: $CaO_2$ is 10.72 ml dl$^{-1}$ (+0.003 ml $O_2$/mmHg $PaO_2$)

If desaturation occurs in the first case, $CaO_2$ is still usually much higher than in the second one:

- $SaO_2$ of 90 percent and Hb of 20 g dl$^{-1}$: $CaO_2$ is 24.12 ml dl$^{-1}$. Anemia, even with normal $SaO_2$, can therefore lead to hypoxia.

The most common method to try to clinically assess oxygenation is the noninvasive continuous measurement of arterial saturation by pulse oximetry ($SpO_2$), currently considered a "fifth vital sign." However, the pulse oximeter tells us very little about tissue oxygenation. In many clinical situations and practices, methods to determine cardiac output are infrequently available or not available at all. More so, in most situations peripheral vascular resistance, $O_2$ delivery and consumption, microcirculatory changes, and other factors cannot be assessed in critically ill infants and function of precapillary sphincters and of postcapillary venules is ignored in clinical care.

In summary, tissue oxygenation is a complex process involving many factors. Due to the issues discussed here and other factors, we need to handle $O_2$ administration with extreme care to preserve tissue oxygenation and prevent and treat hypoxia adequately, while at the same time always trying to avoid causing damage by inducing hyperoxemia, hyperoxia, oxidative stress, and oxidant damage.

## Oxidative Stress and Oxidant Injury

We all know that oxidation can be destructive. With iron and other metals $O_2$ creates a slow-burning process, which results in the brittle brown substance we call rust. The interaction between $O_2$ molecules and all the different substances they may contact can lead to oxidation. Chemically, oxidation is the loss of at least one electron when two or more substances interact.

Various environmental stresses lead to excessive production of reactive oxygen species (ROS), causing progressive oxidative damage and ultimately cell death. It is the imbalance between the systemic manifestation of ROS and a biological system's ability to readily detoxify the reactive intermediates or to repair the resulting oxidative damage. Thus, oxidative damage to the tissues depends on the delicate equilibrium between ROS production and their scavenging.

Mechanisms of DNA oxidation had been well described and summarized by the end of the previous century [11,12]. Every day there is about $10^{12}$ molecules of $O_2$ that enter each and every one of our cells, and there are an estimated 37.2 trillion cells in the adult human body! [13]. When 1/200 $O_2$ molecules are not balanced by antioxidants and act freely, our DNA starts to get affected; 1/100 affects our proteins [11,12]. In our daily lives, in normoxia, we are all subject to oxidant stress and oxidative damage. This is a well-known reason that our cells age in normoxia. The groups of genes that are more upregulated in aging are the response genes to oxidative stress and DNA damage. The repressor element 1-silencing transcription factor (REST) is a universal feature of normal aging in human cortical and hippocampal neurons. REST potently protects neurons from oxidative stress and amyloid beta-protein toxicity; conditional deletion of REST in the mouse brain leads to more oxidative stress and age-related neurodegeneration [14]. This obviously would not happen in hypoxia but, since we all know of the potentially serious side-effects of tissue hypoxia, we "tradeoff" accepting the perils of oxidant stress and live in normoxia. However, as care providers we must do everything possible to avoid inducing worse oxidative damage by producing and accepting hyperoxia when we care for patients.

Highly reactive ROS are produced by stepwise reduction of molecular oxygen ($O_2$) by high-energy exposure or electron-transfer reactions. Reactive oxygen species are summarized in Table 7.2. Some ROS are important as they act as cellular messengers in redox signaling, but excess or imbalance with antioxidants generates stress and disruptions in normal mechanisms of cellular signaling. Peroxides and free radicals can damage all components of the cell (proteins, lipids, and DNA).

The antioxidant system that protects against significant oxidative damage is well developed in adults,

**Table 7.2** Radical oxygen species

| Free radicals | Nonradical molecules |
|---|---|
| • Superoxide anion ($O_2^{\bullet-}$) <br> • Hydroxyl radical ($^{\bullet}OH$) <br>    $2\,O_2^{\bullet-} + 2H^+ \rightarrow H_2O_2 + O_2$ <br>    $2\,O_2^{\bullet-} + 2H^+ \rightarrow {}^{\bullet}OH + {}^{\bullet}OH$ | • Hydrogen peroxide ($H_2O_2$) <br> • Singlet oxygen ($^1O_2$) <br> • Others |

**Table 7.3** Summary of antioxidant defenses

| Enzymatic | Nonenzymic/dietary |
|---|---|
| Superoxide dismutase (SOD) | Ascorbate (AsA) |
| Catalase (CAT) | Glutathione (GSH) |
| Guaiacol peroxidase (GPX) | Carotenoids |
| Ascorbate-glutathione (AsA-GSH) | Tocopherols (vitamin E) |
| Ascorbate peroxidase (APX)]. | Coenzyme Q10 |
| Monodehydroascorbate <br>   reductase (MDHAR) | Vitamin C |
| Dehydroascorbate reductase <br>   (DHAR) | Phenolics |

but there is individual variability in its functioning. The best-known antioxidant defenses are summarized in Table 7.3. This system, however, is poorly developed or markedly impaired in newborns and infants, and is even more defective in preterm infants. This is one reason why hyperoxia and oxidative damage are more serious during development.

Acute oxygen therapy may have acute undesired effects such as an impact on respiratory control and on chemo- and baroreceptors, raised blood pressure and decreased cardiac index, heart rate, cardiac oxygen consumption, and blood flow in the cerebral and renal beds. It may also lower capillary density and redistribute blood in the microcirculation. Table 7.4 summarizes adverse conditions and damage associated with oxidant stress. Using excess oxygen for the treatment of nonhypoxemic patients is definitely a health hazard.

## Oxygen as a Health Hazard

A hazardous substance is one for which there is statistically significant evidence that danger to health, with acute or chronic health effects, may occur from exposure. OSHA's definition includes any substance, chemical, or agent that is, among other things, a carcinogen, damages the lungs and eyes, is combustible, explosive or flammable, oxidizes, and is unstable and reactive such that its use may produce or release other compounds that have any of the previously mentioned

**Table 7.4** Conditions associated to hyperoxia, oxidative stress, and damage

| | |
|---|---|
| Aging | Other |
| DNA impact – cancer | • Fragile X syndrome |
| Central nervous system | • Sickle cell disease |
| • Parkinson's disease | • Lichen planus |
| • Alzheimer's disease | • Vitiligo |
| • Neuronal degeneration | • Infection |
| • Autism | • Inflammation – fibrosis |
| • Altered blood flow | • Chronic fatigue syndrome |
| Cardiovascular | • Altered renal function |
| • Atherosclerosis | *Perinatal: Specific to mother, fetus, and neonate* |
| • Heart failure | • Placental defenses and genes |
| • Myocardial infarction | • ROP |
| • Decreased contractility | • BPD – lung injury |
| • Altered chemo- and baroreceptors | • Developing brain |
| Endocrine | • Increased PVR |
| • Insulin | • Abnormal response to iNO |
| • Glucagon | • Altered clock genes |
| Lung | • Altered ocular genes |
| • Atelectasis | • Thymus (T-cells) |
| • Alveolar collapse | |

ROP: retinopathy of prematurity; BPD: bronchopulmonary dysplasia; PVR: pulmonary vascular resistance; iNO: inhaled nitric oxide.

characteristics. Oxygen is a very potent drug that meets these criteria and has been used in inadequate ways in many healthcare settings. We must change the way we administer supplementary $O_2$ when a patient is not hypoxemic and stop using pure free-flowing oxygen, since 100 percent oxygen unleashes a cascade of dangerous chemicals [15]. More so, periods of fluctuating hypoxia–hyperoxia reperfusion are potentially very damaging [16–18].

Table 7.4 lists a summary of potential side-effects of $O_2$. Important conditions related to oxygen damage in adults are described, followed by several that may occur during the perinatal and infancy periods.

Most patients with acute myocardial infarction or acute coronary syndromes (ACS) receive $O_2$ therapy as part of their treatment, initiated most often before their first contact with a physician, but there is no evidence that this is beneficial. A survey among physicians found that 96 percent of their patients with ACS received oxygen therapy [19]. About 50 percent of all responders believed that $O_2$ decreases mortality, but this has never been shown. In fact, considerable data suggest that $O_2$ therapy may be detrimental in patients with both ACS and stable coronary disease when there is no hypoxia. $O_2$ administration may constrict the coronary vessels, lower myocardial oxygen delivery, and may actually worsen ischemia. Therefore, this

long-accepted but potentially harmful intervention needs to be revised, favoring use of $O_2$ only in hypoxemic patients, and titrating its administration to individual $PaO_2$ or $SpO_2$ [20].

The role played by oxidatively damaged DNA in carcinogenesis has been established. Oxygen free radicals' interaction with DNA can result in genetic changes which can lead to cancer [21]. Oxidative stress has been shown to contribute to the development of various cancer types and has recently been involved in the pathogenesis of pancreatic cancer [22]. Clinical studies on the effect of preventive antioxidants have shown surprisingly little or no effect on cancer incidence, and epidemiological trials, together with in vitro experiments, suggest that the optimal approach is not to increase intake of antioxidants but to reduce endogenous and exogenous sources of oxidative stress. One of the exogenous sources is clearly breathing supplemental $O_2$ when it is not needed. Additionally, a randomized study evaluating recovery post-anesthesia with 80 percent vs. 21 percent $O_2$ was interrupted by the safety review board as the incidence of infections was markedly higher in the $O_2$ group [23].

Both the mother and neonate are exposed to oxidative stress during birth. However, lipid peroxidation levels and antioxidant capacity in umbilical venous and arterial blood immediately after delivery at over 37 weeks' gestation are significantly different in patients delivered by planned Cesarean section (C-section) when compared to vaginal delivery [24]. The higher oxidative stress and alteration of the oxidant and antioxidant system during C-section must be added to the list of the many known risks associated with planned elective C-sections. Worse, if $O_2$ is used unnecessarily during C-sections and labor and delivery, the potential damage caused to mothers, placenta, and fetus increases markedly [25–32].

In a random prospective study [25], supplemental oxygen ($FiO_2$ 0.4) was compared to room air ($FiO_2$ 0.21) in elective C-sections under spinal anesthesia. Total antioxidant capacity, total oxidant status, and the oxidative stress index were measured in maternal pre- and postoperative blood and in umbilical artery blood samples. Fetal and maternal oxidative stress was significantly worse with $FiO_2$ 0.4 than with room air. The authors suggested a mandate to warn about the use of supplemental oxygen during this procedure and wrote that we must "handle the sword with care." A meta-analysis of the effect of inspired oxygen concentration and a Cochrane review, both from 2013, report significant differences in healthy pregnant women with supplemental $O_2$ during C-section with regional anesthesia compared with no supplemental $O_2$ [29,30]. $PaO_2$ in mother and neonate, and free $O_2$ radicals and ROS were all significantly higher with administration of supplemental $O_2$. Mean difference above the values found in room air for maternal $PaO_2$ was 141.8 mmHg, and for neonatal umbilical artery and vein $PO_2$ were 3.3 mmHg and 5.9 mmHg respectively ($p < 0.0001$). The levels of the $O_2$ free radicals malondialdehyde (MDA) and 8-isoprostane were also significantly higher (0.2 μmol $L^{-1}$ and 64.3 pg $ml^{-1}$, respectively, $p < 0.00001$).

The numerous functions of the placenta are astounding, but many are still not fully understood and the effects of hyperoxia have only recently started to be studied. Proteins of resistance to multiple drugs (glycoprotein-P) and of resistance to breast cancer (genes ABCB1 and ABCG2) are highly expressed in the placenta during the first trimester and they protect the fetus from maternally derived toxins and drugs, foreign chemical substances, and pollutants (i.e., xenobiotics). As $O_2$ is a regulator of the resistance to multiple drugs in various tissues, the effect of oxygen on multidrug resistance was studied in explants of villi of human placentas at different times during gestation. It was found that ABCG2 mRNA increases

after hours of hyperoxia. It is possible, therefore, that placental changes in $O_2$ tension and delivery may alter resistance to drug and toxin exposure during fetal life. In a different study, increased $PaO_2$ reduced the cellular pro-inflammatory response to *E. coli* and promoted an abnormal anti-inflammatory cytokine profile in the membranes. In addition, inflammatory pathways connect hyperoxic induced intra-amniotic inflammation with fetal and neonatal tissue damage. Even though the mechanisms and molecular pathways of acute lung injury in preterm fetuses and neonates are complex, tissue injury may occur as a result of injurious $O_2$ byproducts secondary to hyperoxia [31]. Finally, supplemental $O_2$ has been used for intrauterine resuscitation, but it is a practice of unproven benefit and potentially harmful due to increased free radical activity [32].

In summary, maternal $O_2$ supplementation during labor and in C-sections is potentially dangerous for mother and fetus, should be reserved only for documented maternal hypoxia, and should not be considered an indicated intervention for non-reassuring fetal status.

Neonatal and pediatric undesired effects of excess $O_2$ are listed in Table 7.4. Harper, studying 14 healthy children aged 8–15 with functional MRI, showed that only two minutes of 100 percent $O_2$ produces abnormal activation of the hippocampus, hypothalamus, and insula, areas that regulate blood pressure, heart rate, and response to stress [15]. Oxygen by itself also causes cell death in the developing brain [33,34], and worse long-term neurodevelopment outcomes have been associated with hyperoxia [9]. Oxygen toxicity has been identified as a contributing factor to the pathogenesis of cerebral palsy. In a large study of 1105 preterm infants [35], the risk of disabling cerebral palsy was double in those exposed to hyperoxia and eight-fold in the highest quintiles of oxygen exposure. The association of $O_2$ excess with retinopathy of prematurity (ROP) has been known since the 1940s and better characterized more recently [5,6,8,10,36–38]; the case is the same with bronchopulmonary dysplasia (BPD) [8,39] and other conditions in which the benefits of changing practice to try to maintain $SpO_2$ to decrease hyperoxia have been proven of benefit and are discussed later.

$O_2$ is a pulmonary vasodilator and hypoxia induces pulmonary vasoconstriction and increased pulmonary vascular resistance. However, pure $O_2$ produces oxidative stress in lungs and vessels, and alters pulmonary artery contractility. In animal models of persistent pulmonary hypertension of the newborn (PPHN), 100 percent $O_2$ increases ROS in the mitochondrial matrix prior to the cytosol and can produce significant changes in critical cellular signaling pathways. Additionally, 100 percent $O_2$ increases PDE5 activity, decreases NO-mediated cGMP-dependent vasorelaxation, and impairs the response to inhaled nitric oxide (iNO). Some of these alterations are prevented with the use of antioxidants such as superoxide dismutase and catalase, confirming the role of oxidative stress in these abnormal responses [40–42].

There has been growing interest in the impact of hyperoxia on gene alteration. Proteome changes are induced by oxidative stress in the developing brain [33,34], and two studies described a three-fold increase in the risk of leukemia and cancer in childhood with exposure to 100 percent $O_2$ in the delivery room for three minutes or more [43,44]. In experimental animals, a few minutes of hyperoxia at birth alter whole-genome expression in the newborn eye [45]. If this were to occur during induced hyperoxia after birth of preterm infants, predisposition for ROP could be markedly increased. Hyperoxic acute lung injury is characterized by inflammation and epithelial cell death. Circadian locomotor output cycles kaput (CLOCK) genes, master regulators of circadian rhythm, integrate various antioxidant and metabolic pathways. Circadian rhythm disruption is associated with many pathological conditions and is implicated in inflammation and lung diseases. Key circadian genes like Rev-erbα, Per, and Bmal modulate metabolism and inflammation. Hyperoxia-induced lung inflammation and injury can be promoted by dysregulation of circadian rhythm by alteration of CLOCK gene expression [46,47]. For example, Rev-erbα protein is degraded in hyperoxia and its disruption exacerbates hyperoxic lung injury, which is associated with decreased cell proliferation and distorted alveolar architecture. Stabilizing lung Rev-erbα protein prevents the loss of cell proliferation. Premature neonates are often exposed to hyperoxia and photo-oxidation with phototherapy in the NICU. In neonates <750 g birth weight, aggressive phototherapy was found to increase mortality. The potential cytotoxicity and disruption of circadian gene expression altering cell homeostasis as a combined effect of $O_2$ and phototherapy is concerning since preliminary data suggest that an alteration of circadian rhythm genes occurs in neonatal animals exposed to some hyperoxia associated with phototherapy. This cytotoxic effect can be partly reversed by stabilizing the Rev-erbα protein, which improves mitochondrial efficiency, conferring a survival advantage [47].

Oxygen should never be denied when necessary. Nonetheless, to avoid hypoxemia without inducing hyperoxemia is neither easy nor simple. Understanding oxygen toxicity provides us with new ways of interrupting pathologic sequences since the hazards described are "in our hands." We, the healthcare providers, are the only cause for a $PaO_2$ greater than normal in a human being of any age in a healthcare setting. We therefore have to assess $O_2$ levels and manage $O_2$ administration differently than we have been doing.

## Assessment of Oxygen in Blood

Cyanosis is the bluish discoloration of skin and mucous membranes due to an increased concentration of reduced (not saturated) Hb. As much as this sign is important, we must recognize its pitfalls. Human beings perceive color with variability. Furthermore, illumination, race, skin thickness, and total Hb concentration impact on this clinical assessment. We all have a "blind spot" for detecting cyanosis on the face of even significant Hb desaturation, more so in cases when total Hb concentration is low. In summary, some of the patients with what appears to be cyanosis do not need supplemental $O_2$, and in many more in whom we do not see cyanosis there is hypoxemia and a need for some evaluation and therapy. $SpO_2$ is currently the noninvasive way to assess hypoxemia.

Clinically we assess oxygen in blood by intermittent measurements of $PaO_2$ and/or $SaO_2$ in arterial or venous blood and by continuous noninvasive pulse oximetry ($SpO_2$) monitors. The pulse oximeter does not measure the same thing as arterial blood gas. $SpO_2$ monitors measure the Hb-$O_2$ saturation, while the arterial blood gas measures the pressure of oxygen gas dissolved in the blood (oxygen not bound to hemoglobin) and "calculates" oxygen saturation. The calculation or transformation of $PaO_2$ to $SaO_2$ by means of formulae or algorithms is of no value in hospitalized ill patients and in all newborns; therefore a $SaO_2$ derived from a blood gas should not be used for clinical management. Such calculation assumes a normal adult $O_2$ dissociation curve and $O_2$ affinity, with normal 2,3-DPG and Hb concentration, and a normal temperature, pH, and $PaCO_2$ for healthy adults. It also assumes that the patient has no dyshemoglobinemia and is without fetal hemoglobin (Hb F). These calculations are therefore correct only under standardized normal conditions that are usually not present in hospitalized pediatric patients with variable pH, $PaCO_2$, and temperature, and are never found in neonates in whom, in addition, a large and variable proportion of Hb is Hb F (not A), 2,3-DPG is low and Hb concentration is variable. Therefore, continuously monitored $SpO_2$ cannot be compared to a calculated $SaO_2$ derived from a $PaO_2$ from an arterial blood gas. To circumvent this problem, many healthcare settings customize the output of blood gas analyzers so they do not report $SaO_2$. Good and modern co-oximetry is the gold standard for $SaO_2$. Current models are called continuous wave spectrophotometers; these measure light absorbance at 100–130 μm wavelengths. However, co-oximeters are expensive, require blood sampling, and provide only intermittent, not continuous, monitoring. This is not ideal when one wants to closely monitor an unstable patient. Noninvasive pulse oximetry is used routinely to monitor $SpO_2$ continuously. They were created to aid in the diagnosis of desaturation, but they are of little to no value by themselves to tell us about hyperoxemia. The normal $SpO_2$ in room air ($FiO_2$ 0.21) is 95–100 percent. However, as shown in Figure 7.1, when a patient receives supplemental $FiO_2$ (i.e., >0.21) and the $SpO_2$ is >95 percent (i.e., "Normal"), there is a risk for the $PaO_2$ be above normal [48] because when we breathe supplemental

oxygen and the $SpO_2$ is >95 percent the $Hb–O_2$ relation is "lost" (Figure 7.1). When this happens it is impossible to predict $PaO_2$ from the $SpO_2$ digital readout. In the example in the figure, when $SpO_2$ is 86–93 percent, $PaO_2$ is 50–68 mmHg. However, when $SpO_2$ is 95–100 percent, the $PaO_2$ could be much higher than 85 mmHg. Following the concepts of the alveolar gas equation described earlier, the $PaO_2$ could actually be as high as 200–300 mmHg, or even higher if the lungs are normal, the $SpO_2$ is >95 percent, and the child is breathing pure oxygen ($FiO_2$ 1.0). In these cases, free dissolved $O_2$ will be circulating and ROS will increase (Figure 7.1). Therefore, in such situations, $FiO_2$ should be weaned.

The way these monitors function and their strengths and limitations are well-described [5], but they are beyond the scope of this chapter. In summary, $SpO_2$ monitors function by establishing the ratio between wavelength (red and IR) and displaying the ratio as $SpO_2$. $SpO_2$ monitors, just like any other medical equipment, are not perfect and all have an inherent bias (equipment error). In individuals under normal conditions this bias (or "standard deviation") could be as low as 2 percent in some monitors but as high as 5 percent in others. Therefore, it is nonsensical to argue about differences in $SpO_2$ values of 1–2 percent. Additionally, there are many $SpO_2$ monitors available in the market and there are more than 100 published studies that demonstrate that one monitor

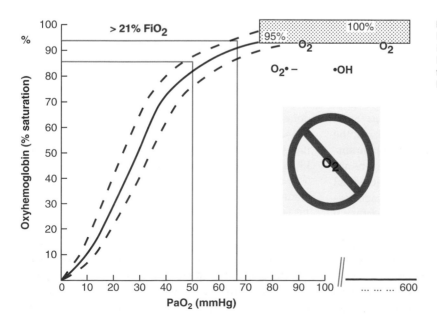

**Figure 7.1** $Hb–O_2$ relation when breathing supplemental $O_2$. When $SpO_2$ is 95–100 percent, $PaO_2$ could be much higher than 100 mmHg. In these cases, free dissolved $O_2$ will be circulating and ROS will increase.

is not the same as another monitor. The $SpO_2$ monitor with Signal Extraction Technology (SET®) has been demonstrated to be the one with better specificity and sensitivity, and to monitor the patient best when it is needed the most – during critical illness and periods of low perfusion and motion. Additionally, only one monitor on the market actually uses many wavelengths (not just two) and can measure Hb, methemoglobin, and carboxyhemoglobin in addition to $SpO_2$ (Rainbow, Masimo Corporation, Irvine, CA).

# Recommendations for Clinical Practice and Targeting of SpO$_2$

The $SpO_2$ in normal individuals in room air is 95–100 percent. However, if $SpO_2$ is >94 percent when breathing supplemental $O_2$, there is an abnormally elevated $PaO_2$ in 60 percent of arterial samples [48]. With the aim of avoiding hypoxemia and at the same time preventing hyperoxemic-induced oxidant stress, when a patient breaths supplemental $O_2$ we should target $SpO_2$ to avoid 96–100 percent and wean the $FiO_2$ in such cases. In all cases, $SpO_2$ alarms must be operative when a patient is receiving supplemental $O_2$; the low alarm should be about 1 percent below the lower limit chosen as acceptable according to the patient and diagnosis, and the high alarm 1 percent above the acceptable high limit of $SpO_2$. We include below clinical recommendations for cardiopulmonary resuscitation, apnea, surgery and anesthesia, PPHN, BPD, and during the first weeks of life in tiny preterm infants.

In all hospital settings, including operating rooms, pre- and post-anesthesia, and birthing centers, a heater humidifier (to provide adequately conditioned inhaled gas) and a blender (to accurately measure the dose of $O_2$) are mandatory. In addition, an adequate $SpO_2$ monitor that can rapidly measure $SpO_2$ even during poor perfusion is necessary to titrate the amount of $O_2$ administered. During cardiopulmonary resuscitation, particularly when the lungs are not affected, there is no need to provide any supplemental $O_2$, less so 100 percent $O_2$. Such a practice increases the risk of damage by hypoxia–hyperoxia reperfusion injury. Clear physiologic evidence that in many cases there is absolutely no need to provide excess $O_2$, with its associated risks, could be derived by the alveolar gas equation described earlier. The $FiO_2$ provided by mouth-to-mouth resuscitation is about 17 percent due to the exhaled $CO_2$ in the gas provided by the person providing resuscitation, and many human beings have been successfully resuscitated in this way with this $FiO_2$. A similar situation occurs in periods of apnea (spontaneous or medically induced), where the treatment is to ventilate the alveoli (breathe) and not to give supplemental $O_2$.

Newborns and children who require surgery are developing and many are critically ill, but the use of $O_2$ during neonatal and pediatric anesthesia has not been well studied. However, it has been over 45 years since Van Den Brenk and Jamieson [49] showed that, in mammals, there is potentiation by anesthetics of brain damage due to breathing high-pressure oxygen and that excess oxygenation during surgery of preterm infants is associated with ROP [50]. More recently there is concern about the negative impact of sedatives like midazolam [7] and ketamine, which alters NMDA receptors [51] and enhances human neural stem cell proliferation and induces neuronal apoptosis via ROS [52]. For these and other reasons the association of hyperoxia-induced oxidative stress and anesthetic drugs should be avoided and the practice of preoxygenation must be carefully evaluated. In addition, atelectasis can occur during and after anesthesia, and the rate at which absorption atelectasis occurs can be accurately predicted by known physiological principles: High $FiO_2$ worsens compliance and pure $O_2$ results in reabsorption atelectasis shortly after its application [50–58]. The alveolar to venous pressure gradient must be countered by the respiratory elastic recoil to keep alveoli open, but this gradient is too high with 100 percent $O_2$. With just three minutes of "preoxygenation," the higher the $FiO_2$, the greater the areas of atelectasis and the shorter the time required for collapse to occur, irrespective of the $FiO_2$ used after induction. Alveolar recruitment maneuvers to maintain functional residual capacity (FRC) and ventilation distribution are useful and more effective if done with positive end-expiratory pressure (PEEP) of 6 $cmH_2O$ with low $FiO_2$. When an $FiO_2$ of 1.0 is used, there is rapid recurrence of the atelectasis, decreased FRC, and alteration of ventilation homogeneity and lung units with low VA/Q ratios become more unstable when breathing $O_2$ [50–58]. Moreover, an $FiO_2$ of 1.0 before extubation increases the risk for postoperative atelectasis and more $O_2$ than necessary in the postoperative period can, paradoxically, aggravate central hypoventilation and apnea. Mental changes during oxygen therapy were described more than 65 years ago by Comroe [1]. Since then the body of knowledge showing potential adverse effects of providing unnecessary

$O_2$ has expanded exponentially, showing that excess $O_2$ should be avoided before, during, and after anesthesia.

In congenital diaphragmatic hernia (CDH) with PPHN, $SpO_2$ monitoring should be in the preductal territory (right hand). But if this is unavailable, in >80 percent of babies the left hand is preductal too. In the face of the abnormal vessel and alveolar development present in CDH, it is paramount to avoid any additional hypoxic pulmonary vasoconstriction; the challenge is to do this and at the same time avoid hyperoxic injury. Without any published solid evidence, this may be accomplished by aiming to maintain preductal $SpO_2$ between 91 and 96 percent, and weaning respiratory pressures and $FiO_2$ when $SpO_2$ ≥96 percent. The same is applicable to PPHN of other etiologies. Another challenging condition is chronic lung disease, where hypoxia leads to cor pulmonale, bronchoconstriction, and pulmonary vasoconstriction, but where $FiO_2$ should be titrated with the intention to maintain $SpO_2$ between 90 and 95 percent.

The ideal and best $SpO_2$ targets for preterm infants breathing $O_2$ during the first weeks of life has been a matter of controversy, but has been studied in detail [5,6,8–10,36–38]. For these infants a prudent approach is to avoid $SpO_2$ >94 percent, with an intention to treat with $SpO_2$ ranges of 87–94 percent and low and high $SpO_2$ alarms of 85 and 95 percent, respectively. When any dose of supplemental $O_2$ is given in these infants, monitoring with modern $SpO_2$ with SET technology to aim to avoid hyperoxemia and hypoxemic episodes followed by hyperoxia reperfusion is associated with decreased rates of severe ROP and does not increase mortality [5,10,38,59].

We have recently summarized what could be a safe oxygen saturation intention to treat and monitoring in preterm infants, with the aim to avoid hypoxia and hyperoxia [60,61]. In the last few years it has become clearer that oxidative stress is the unifying element in the process of perinatal programming of adult diseases. Oxidative stress may lead to cardiovascular and other diseases, but also to changes in neuro hormones and personality disorders [62,63]. Therefore, avoiding hyperoxia and induced oxidative stress can help prevent the neonatal origin of adult diseases. Regional anesthesia with supplemental oxygen is potentially harmful and unnecessary, as summarized in Cochrane reviews in 2016 [64].

In summary, cellular oxygenation is complex. Oxygen as a gas can be similar to the Janus god and Trojan Horse in Greek mythology. The former was a god of duality, two-faced and looking at opposing sides. The Trojan Horse was a present, perceived as likeable and innocuous but capable of generating serious consequences and igniting everything without anyone realizing until it was too late. Maybe our ability to clinically measure tissue oxygenation will improve in the future. In the meantime, we must do everything possible to avoid and treat hypoxemia, while at the same time be determined not to induce hyperoxemia, hyperoxia or oxidative injury.

## References

1. Comroe JH Jr., Bahnson ER, Coates EO Jr. Mental changes occurring in chronically anoxemic patients during oxygen therapy. *J Am Med Assoc.* 1950;143:1044–8.

2. Sola A, Rogido MR, Deulofeut R. Oxygen as a neonatal health hazard: call for detente in clinical practice. *Acta Paediatr.* 2007;96:801–2.

3. Saugstad OD. Take a breath: but do not add oxygen (if not needed). *Acta Paediatr.* 2007;96:798–800.

4. Vento M, Sastre J, Asensi MA, Vina J. Room-air resuscitation causes less damage to heart and kidney than 100% oxygen. *Am J Respir Crit Care Med.* 2005;172:1393–8.

5. Sola A, Golombek S, Montes Bueno MT, et al. Safe oxygen saturation targeting and monitoring in preterm infants: can we avoid hypoxia and hyperoxia? *Acta Paediatr.* 2014;103:164–80.

6. Chow LC, Wright KW, Sola A. Can changes in clinical practice decrease the incidence of severe retinopathy of prematurity in very low birth weight infants? *Pediatrics.* 2003;111:339–45.

7. Sola A. Oxygen in neonatal anesthesia: friend or foe? *Curr Opin Anaesthesiol.* 2008;21:332–9.

8. Sola A, Zuluaga C. Oxygen saturation targets and retinopathy of prematurity. *J AAPOS.* 2013;17:650–2.

9. Deulofeut R, Critz A, Adams-Chapman I, Sola A. Avoiding hyperoxia in infants ≤1250 g is associated with improved short- and long-term outcomes. *J Perinatol.* 2006;26:700–5.

10. Bizzarro MJ, Li FY, Katz K, et al. Temporal quantification of oxygen saturation ranges: an effort to reduce hyperoxia in the neonatal intensive care unit. *J Perinatol.* 2014;34:33–8.

11. Aust AA, Eveleigh F. Mechanisms of DNA oxidation. *Proc Soc Exp Biol Med.* 1999;222:246–52.

12. Acworth IN, Bailey B. *The Handbook of Oxidative Metabolism.* Chelmsford, MA: ESA; 1996).

13. Bianconi E, Piovesan A, Facchin F, et al. An estimation of the number of cells in the human body. *Ann Hum Biol.* 2013;40(6):463–71.

14. Lu T, Aron L, Zullo J, et al. REST and stress resistance in ageing and Alzheimer's disease. *Nature.* 2014;507(7493):448–54.

15. Macey PM, Woo MA, Harper RM. Hyperoxic brain effects are normalized by addition of CO2. *PLoS Med.* 2007;4(5):e173.

16. Levine RL. Ischemia: from acidosis to oxidation. *FASEB J.* 1993;7:1242–6.

17. Berkelhamer SK, Kim GA, Radder JE, et al. Developmental differences in hyperoxia-induced oxidative stress and cellular responses in the murine lung. *Free Radic Biol Med.* 2013;14:51–60.

18. Wollen EJ, Sejersted Y, Wright MS, et al. Transcriptome profiling of the newborn mouse brain after hypoxia-reoxygenation: hyperoxic reoxygenation induces inflammatory and energy failure responsive genes. *Pediatric Res.* 2014;75:517–26.

19. Meier P, Ebrahim S, Otto C, Casas JP. Oxygen therapy in acute myocardial infarction – good or bad? *Cochrane Database Syst Rev.* 2013;8:ED000065. dx.doi.org/10.1002/14651858.ED000065.

20. Kones R. Oxygen therapy for acute myocardial infarction: then and now. A century of uncertainty. *Am J Med.* 2011;124(11):1000–5.

21. Valko M, Izakovic M, Mazur M, Rhodes CJ, Telser J. Role of oxygen radicals in DNA damage and cancer incidence. *Mol Cell Biochem.* 2004:266:37–56.

22. Yu JH, Kim H. Oxidative stress and cytokines in the pathogenesis of pancreatic cancer. *J Cancer Prev.* 2014(2):97–102.

23. Pryor KO, Fahey TJ 3rd, Lien CA, Goldstein PA. Surgical site infection and the routine use of perioperative hyperoxia in a general surgical population: a randomized controlled trial. *JAMA.* 2004;291:79–87.

24. Noh EJ, Kim YH, Cho MK, et al. Comparison of oxidative stress markers in umbilical cord blood after vaginal and cesarean delivery. *Obstet Gynecol Sci.* 2014;57(2):109–14.

25. Yalcin S, Aydoğan H, Kucuk A, et al. Supplemental oxygen in elective cesarean section under spinal anesthesia: handle the sword with care. *Rev Bras Anesthesiol.* 2013;63(5):393–7.

26. Klimova NG, Hanna N, Peltier MR. Effect of oxygen tension on bacteria-stimulated cytokine production by fetal membranes. *J Perinat Med.* 2013;41(5):595–603.

27. Klimova NG, Hanna N, Peltier MR. Does carbon monoxide inhibit proinflammatory cytokine production by fetal membranes? *J Perinat Med.* 2013;41(6):683–90.

28. Lye P. Effect of oxygen on multidrug resistance in the first trimester human placentas. *Placenta.* 2013;34(9):817–23.

29. Klingel ML, Patel SV. Meta-analysis of the effect of inspired oxygen concentration on the incidence of surgical site infection following cesarean section *Int J Obstet Anesth.* 2013;22(2):104–12.

30. Chatmongkolchart S, Prathep S. Supplemental oxygen for caesarean section during regional anaesthesia. *Cochrane Database Syst Rev.* 2013;6:CD006161.

31. Iliodromiti Z, Zygouris D. Sifakis S, et al. Acute lung injury in preterm fetuses and neonates: mechanisms and molecular pathways. *J Matern Fetal Neonatal Med.* 2013;26(17):1696–704.

32. Hamel, MS, Anderson, BL, Rouse, DJ. Oxygen for intrauterine resuscitation: of unproved benefit and potentially harmful. *Am J Obstet Gynecol.* 2014;211(2):124–7.

33. Felderhoff-Mueser U, Bittigau P, Sifringer M, et al. Oxygen causes cell death in the developing brain. *Neurobiol Dis.* 2004;17:273–82.

34. Kaindl AM, Sifringer M, Zabel C, et al. Acute and long-term proteome changes induced by oxidative stress in the developing brain. *Cell Death Differ.* 2006;13:1097–109.

35. Collins MP, Lorentz JM, Jelton R, Paneth N. Hypocapnia and other ventilation related risk factors for cerebral palsy in low birth weight infants. *Pediatr Res.* 2001;50:712–19.

36. SUPPORT Study Group of the Eunice Kennedy Shriver NICHD Neonatal Research Network. Target ranges of oxygen saturation in extremely preterm infants. *N Engl J Med.* 2010;362:1959–69.

37. Stenson BJ, Tarnow-Mordi WO, Darlow BA, et al. Oxygen saturation and outcomes in preterm infants. *N Engl J Med.* 2013;368:2094–104.

38. Schmidt B, Whyte RK, Asztalos EV, et al. Effects of targeting higher vs lower arterial oxygen saturations on death or disability in extremely preterm infants: a randomized clinical trial. *JAMA.* 2013;309:2111–20.

39. Bhakta KY, Jiang W, Couroucli XI, et al. Regulation of cytochrome P4501A1 expression by hyperoxia in human lung cell lines: implications for hyperoxic lung injury. *Toxicol Appl Pharmacol.* 2008;233(2):169–78.

40. Lakshminrusimha S, Swartz DD, Gugino SF, et al. Oxygen concentration and pulmonary hemodynamics in newborn lambs with pulmonary hypertension. *Pediatr Res.* 2009;66(5):539–44.

41. Farrow KN, Lee KJ, Perez M, et al. Brief hyperoxia increases mitochondrial oxidation and increases

phosphodiesterase 5 activity in fetal pulmonary artery smooth muscle cells. *Antioxid Redox Signal.* 2012;17(3):460–70.

42. Lakshminrusimha S, Steinhorn RH, Wedgwood S, Savorgnan FJ. Pulmonary hemodynamics and vascular reactivity in asphyxiated term lambs resuscitated with 21 and 100% oxygen. *J Appl Physiol.* 2011;111(5):1441–7.

43. Naumburg E, Bellocco R, Cnattingius S, Jonzon A, Ekbom A. Supplementary oxygen and risk of childhood lymphatic leukaemia. *Acta Paediatr.* 2002;91(12):1328–33.

44. Spector LG. Childhood cancer following neonatal oxygen supplementation. *J Pediatrs.* 2005;147(1):27–31.

45. Wollen EJ, Kwinta P, Bik-Multanowski M, et al. Hypoxia-reoxygenation affects whole-genome expression in the newborn eye. *Invest Ophthalmol Vis Sci.* 2014;55(3):1393–401.

46. Lagishetty V, Parthasarathy PT, Phillips O, Fukumoto J, et al. Dysregulation of CLOCK gene expression in hyperoxia-induced lung injury. *Am J Physiol Cell Physiol.* 2014;306(11):C999–1007.

47. Sengupta S, Yang G, McCormack S, et al. Hyperoxia and phototherapy alter circadian gene expression: implications for cytotoxicity, metabolism and cellular homeostasis. Abstract 58, 2014, Pediatric Academic Societies Annual Meeting.

48. Castillo A, Sola A, Baquero H, et al. Pulse oximetry saturation levels and arterial oxygen tension values in newborns receiving oxygen therapy in the neonatal intensive care unit: is 85% to 93% an acceptable range? *Pediatrics.* 2008;121:882–9.

49. Van Den Brenk HA, Jamieson D. Potentiation by anaesthetics of brain damage due to breathing high-pressure oxygen in mammals. *Nature.* 1962;194:777–8.

50. Phibbs RH. Oxygen therapy: a continuing hazard to the premature infant. *Anesthesiology.* 1977;47:486–7.

51. Gressens P, Rogido M, Paindaveine B, Sola A. The impact of neonatal intensive care practices on the developing brain. *J Pediatr.* 2002;140:646–53.

52. Bai X, Yan Y, Canfield S, et al. Ketamine enhances human neural stem cell proliferation and induces neuronal apoptosis via reactive oxygen species-mediated mitochondrial pathway. *Anesth Analg.* 2013;116(4):869–80.

53. von Ungern-Sternberg BS, Regli A, Schibler A, et al. The impact of positive end-expiratory pressure on functional residual capacity and ventilation homogeneity impairment in anesthetized children exposed to high levels of inspired oxygen. *Anesth Analg.* 2007;104:1364–8.

54. Marcus RJ, van der Walt JH, Pettifer RJA. Pulmonary volume recruitment restores pulmonary compliance and resistance in anesthetized young children. *Paediatr Anaesth.* 2002;12:570–84.

55. Tusman G, Bohm SH, Tempra A, et al. Effects of recruitment maneuver on atelectasis in anesthetized children. *Anesthesiology.* 2003;98:14–22.

56. Edmark L, Kostova-Aherdan K, Enlund M, Hedenstierna G. Optimal oxygen concentration during induction of general anesthesia. *Anesthesiology.* 2003;98:28–33.

57. Halbertsma FJJ, van der Hioeven JG. Lung recruitment during mechanical positive pressure ventilation in the PICU: what can be learned from the literature? *Anaesthesia.* 2005;60:779–90.

58. Dantzker DR, Wagner PD, West JB. Instability of lung units with low VA/Q ratios during O2 breathing. *J Appl Physiol.* 1975;38:886–95.

59. Darlow BA, Marschner SL, Donoghoe M, et al. Benefits of oxygen saturation targeting: New Zealand (BOOST-NZ) Collaborative Group. *J Pediatr.* 2014;165:30–5.

60. Sola A. Oxygen saturation in the newborn and the importance of avoiding hyperoxia-induced damage. *Neoreviews.* 2015;16(7);e393 .

61. Sola A, Golombek S. Oxygen saturation monitoring in neonatal period. In: Buonocore G, et al. (eds.), *Neonatology.* New York: Springer; 2016.

62. Padmanabhan V, Cardoso RC, Puttabyatappa M. Developmental programming: a pathway to disease. *Endocrinology.* 2016;157(4):1328–40.

63. Verny T. The pre & perinatal origins of childhood and adult diseases and personality disorders. *J Prenat Perinat Psychol Health.* 2012;26(3).

64. Chatmongkolchart S, Prathep S. Comparing supplemental oxygen with room air for low-risk pregnant women undergoing an elective caesarean section under regional anaesthesia. *Cochrane Database Syst Rev.* 2016;3:CD006161.

**Chapter**

**8**

# Temperature Control

Benjamin Kloesel and Laura Downey

## Introduction

Thermoregulation refers to the ability of an organism to maintain a set body temperature by active and passive physiologic processes. Humans are able to maintain internal equilibrium within ±0.2 °C of a set point, usually 37 °C. This ability to maintain thermal stability despite changes in ambient temperature is an important part of homeostasis.

Compared with adults, neonates and infants are more susceptible to developing hypothermia. Prior studies demonstrated a clear relationship between poor temperature regulation in the preterm newborn and increased mortality [1]. Therefore, strategies to maintain normothermia are a critical part of perioperative care.

With a focus on neonates and infants, this chapter will discuss: the physiology and pathophysiology of temperature regulation; temperature monitoring devices; and strategies to maintain thermoregulation under general anesthesia.

## Normal Body Temperature

Body temperature varies with age, time of day, and level of activity, but is usually maintained within a narrow range with a mean of 37 °C (98.6 °F). When compared to older children and adults, infants and young children tend to have a higher core body temperature. In the neonatal period (0–28 days), temperatures as high as 37.5–38 °C are considered normal. These higher temperatures are attributed to the higher metabolic rates found in neonates and smaller children [2].

Hyperthermia, or fever, in neonates is defined by rectal temperature >38 °C (100.4 °F), while hypothermia is defined as core body temperature below 35 °C (95 °F). Mild hypothermia is defined as a core temperature 32–35 °C (90–95 °F); moderate hypothermia as 28–32 °C (82–90 °F); and severe hypothermia below 28 °C (82 °F) [3].

## Physiology of Temperature Regulation

Thermoregulation is the body's ability to maintain normothermia through a feedback system. The hypothalamus, which relies on afferent nerves to sense body temperature and efferent nerves to send signals to effector organs, is the central regulator that triggers actions to adjust body temperature [4].

The anterior hypothalamus receives afferent input from ascending spinal pathways via peripheral warm (via unmyelinated C-fibers) and cold (via thin myelinated Aδ fibers) receptors located in the skin, around great vessels, in the viscera, brain, and spinal cord. When the anterior hypothalamus detects deviations outside the normal temperature range, signals are sent to the posterior hypothalamus, which stimulates appropriate physiologic responses [4–6].

Input from receptors in the CNS and viscera control the majority of autonomic responses that regulate temperature. The main target organs are the blood vessels and muscles. When core temperature rises, vasodilation of blood vessels increases blood flow to the skin surface and excess heat is lost to the environment through radiation and conduction. Perspiration results in cooling through the evaporation of sweat from the skin. When core temperature falls, the body generates heat through voluntary muscle activity, called shivering. The body retains heat through vasoconstriction, which reduces blood flow to the skin and subsequently decreases heat loss to the environment [4,5].

Skin receptors only contribute about 20 percent of the input to the anterior hypothalamus. However, this input is the main driving force for behavioral responses seen in adults, who may put on/take off clothing or move to more/less warm environments. Neonates and children rely on their caregivers for behavioral modifications [6,7].

Although highly regulated mechanisms of thermoregulation are present in adults, these pathways are immature and inefficient in neonates/infants. Instead, neonates/infants have a unique method for maintaining thermoregulation – non-shivering thermogenesis.

# Neonatal Temperature Regulation: Non-Shivering Thermogenesis

Despite a lack of mature mechanisms to maintain normothermia, a drop in core body temperature, or cold stress, stimulates a sympathetic surge that initiates several downstream events to help neonates/infants maintain their core body temperature – non-shivering thermogenesis, increased metabolic rate, and augmented cardiac output.

Primarily, neonates generate heat through non-shivering thermogenesis. Its main source, brown adipose tissue, is highly vascular and located in the axilla, mediastinum, between scapulae, around the internal mammary vessels, blood vessels of the neck, and the adrenal glands. The large number of mitochondria and excess triglycerides make brown adipose tissue an excellent energy source for generating heat [8].

Non-shivering thermogenesis is activated through an increase in sympathetic activity initiated by hypothermia. The sympathetic surge releases norepinephrine and thyroid stimulating hormone (TSH) from the hypothalamic ventromedial nucleus. TSH stimulates release of thyroxine (T4), which is converted to triiodothyronine (T3). T3 upregulates thermogenin, a protein that uncouples oxidative phosphorylation in brown adipose tissue. When oxidative phosphorylation is uncoupled, heat is created instead of ATP. Since up to 25 percent of cardiac output is diverted through the brown adipose tissue, the generated heat is distributed throughout the body. Infants use this method of heat generation until the second year of life.

The circulating catecholamines released during a cold stress stimulate non-shivering thermogenesis to generate heat and augment the cardiac output to dissipate heat throughout the body. These adaptive mechanisms allow the infant to maintain body temperature for a few hours, but at the expense of an increased metabolic rate and exhaustion of thermogenic reserves of glycogen and brown fat. Since most brown adipose tissue is deposited during the third trimester of pregnancy, premature and low-birth weight infants have limited thermogenic capabilities and often fare worse than full-term infants.

# Mechanisms of Heat Exchange

Heat exchange with the environment occurs in humans via the skin and respiratory tract. Four different types of heat transfer are important for the anesthesiologist: radiation, evaporation, convection, and conduction. The primary source of heat loss in infants is radiation (39 percent), followed by convection (37 percent), evaporation (21 percent), and conduction (3 percent).

**Radiation** describes the emission of thermal energy away from the human body; it depends on the difference between skin temperature and the temperature of surrounding walls. **Convection** is thermal energy transfer from the body to its environment by movement of fluids. The driving force is the gradient between skin temperature and the temperature of ambient air and fluids. **Evaporation** is the transition of a molecule from a liquid at its surface into the gaseous phase. The energy required for this transition is drawn from thermal energy. Evaporation depends on the transepithelial/transepidermal water loss (TEWL). **Conduction** refers to thermal energy transfer between solid objects that are in contact. In patients, heat loss depends on the temperature difference between the patient's skin and the surface in contact with the skin. When the temperature of the surface in contact with the patient's skin is less than the skin temperature, heat loss occurs. Metallic surfaces have high thermal conductivity and facilitate rapid heat transfer. Table 8.1 discusses methods to avoid heat loss in neonates in the delivery room and the perioperative period [5].

# Hypothermia in Neonates/Infants

Several factors make neonates and infants more susceptible to hypothermia: immature thermoregulatory mechanisms, limited glycogen and brown fat stores, and physiologic factors that accelerate heat loss. During periods of cold stress, metabolic rates may rise by two- to three-fold, leading to further heat loss and other physiologic consequences that may increase morbidity and mortality during prolonged hypothermia (Table 8.2).

As discussed above, neonates/infants have immature thermoregulation mechanisms that impair their ability to maintain an appropriate core body temperature, while dramatically increasing their energy expenditure. Several anatomic and physiologic differences also contribute to their susceptibility to hypothermia. The reduced effectiveness of vasoconstriction

**Table 8.1** Mechanism of heat loss and preventive measures in neonates and children

| Type | Contribution of heat loss in infants | Definition | Prevention |
|------|--------------------------------------|------------|------------|
| Radiation | 39 percent | Heat transfer between objects of different temperature not in contact with each other | *Decrease the temperature gradient between patient and environment*<br>• warming the environment/operating room<br>• use of a radiant warmer<br>• covering patient with warm blankets |
| Convection | 37 percent | Heat transfer to moving molecules (air or fluids) | *Decrease the temperature gradient between the patient and ambient air*<br>• warming the environment/operating room |
| Evaporation | 21 percent | Heat transfer from transition of liquid to gaseous phase | *Minimize insensible losses*<br>• drying the infant<br>• covering the infant with polyethylene occlusive skin wraps or plastic bags<br>• using humidified inspired gases |
| Conduction | 3 percent | Heat transfer between two surfaces in direction contact | *Decrease temperature gradient between patient and operating room table/IV fluids*<br>• warming blanket/ pad on the operating table<br>• warming intravenous fluids and irrigation solutions |

**Table 8.2** Effects of hypothermia on neonates/children

Cardiovascular
• increased heart rate
• increased cardiac output
• increased vasoconstriction
• increased right-to-left shunting

Pulmonary
• increased pulmonary vascular resistance
• increased apnea/hypoventilation
• increased hypoxia/hypoventilation/hypocapnea

Endocrine/metabolic
• 2–3-fold increase in metabolic rate
• increased circulating catecholamines
• metabolism of brown fat
• metabolic acidosis
• increased ketone production

Renal
• osmotic diuresis

Hematologic
• increased PT/PTT
• inhibits normal coagulation pathways
• decreased platelet function

Immune
• impaired wound healing
• increased risk of infection
• impaired immune function

and decreased subcutaneous fat impair their ability to retain heat, while increasing radiant and conductive heat loss to the environment. Additionally, a large skin surface area-to-body-mass ratio and a high basal metabolic rate accelerate radiant and evaporative heat loss [5,9].

When faced with cold stress, the sympathetic surge initiates non-shivering thermogenesis and augments cardiac output to maintain thermoregulation. However, lipolysis of brown fat during non-shivering thermogenesis produces ketones, which results in metabolic acidosis and osmotic diuresis. The increase in cardiac output is coupled to an increase in cardiac oxygen consumption and workload, which may exhaust the reserves of brown fat and glycogen stores during prolonged hypothermia [9].

Hypothermia is a risk factor for hypoventilation and apnea, which results in hypercapnia, hypoxia and respiratory acidosis. In conjunction with the metabolic acidosis associated with non-shivering thermogenesis, the respiratory acidosis may further increase pulmonary vascular resistance (PVR). Increases in PVR can lead to persistent pulmonary hypertension of the newborn (PPHN), when blood shunts from right to left through fetal circulatory pathways. This may lead to severe hypoxemia that does not respond to normal measures [10,11]. Additionally, increases in PVR may worsen right-to-left shunting through a patent ductus arteriosus (PDA), a ductal-dependent cardiac lesion, or nonrestrictive anatomical shunt. In the setting of the preterm neonate, an increase in right-to-left shunting through a PDA may lead to systemic hypoperfusion, tissue hypoxia, and further metabolic acidosis [9].

Although somewhat impaired in neonates, hypothermia-induced vasoconstriction may reduce tissue oxygen partial pressure and impair wound healing. Furthermore, immune functions such as chemotaxis, migration, and phagocytosis are impaired and may increase infection rates. Hypothermia may inhibit normal coagulation pathways through prolonged prothrombin/partial thromboplastin time and impaired platelet function [9].

Hypothermia in neonates has detrimental effects on almost every body system, which contributes to increased morbidity and mortality in the perioperative period: cardiac (increased heart rate, cardiac output, vasoconstriction, right-to-left shunting); pulmonary (increased PVR, apnea/hypoventilation, hypoxia); metabolic and endocrine (increased metabolic rate, circulating catecholamines, metabolism of brown fat, metabolic acidosis); hematology (increased bleeding times, prolonged PT/PTT, inhibition of platelet function); and immune (impaired wound healing and immune function, increased infection rates) [5,9]. A notable exception is medically induced hypothermia, which has been found to minimize neural damage after hypoxia and ischemia in term infants.

## Thermoregulation During General Anesthesia

Operating rooms represent a specific hazard to thermoregulation in neonates/infants due to a combination of several factors: (1) anesthetic-induced inhibition of thermoregulatory mechanisms; (2) a reduction in metabolic rate under anesthesia; (3) redistribution of heat throughout the body; and (4) increased heat loss through environmental exposure and increased insensible losses [9].

Anesthetic agents significantly inhibit non-shivering thermogenesis and vasoconstriction, while decreasing metabolic rate. Opioids and propofol reduce the temperature threshold for vasoconstriction and shivering, while neuromuscular blockers completely abolish the shivering response. Although nitrous oxide has less inhibitory effect on vasoconstriction, halogenated volatile anesthetics cause vasodilation and inhibit thermoregulatory mechanisms

in a dose-dependent manner. Brismar et al. demonstrated almost a 30 percent reduction in metabolic rate in patients under general anesthesia [6,12].

Patients under general anesthesia show a characteristic temporal pattern of events that influences body temperature. Induction of general anesthesia leads to vasodilation and triggers phase 1, called **internal redistribution**. Within the first 30–45 minutes, the central core temperature drops by 0.5–1.5 °C. Importantly, the overall heat balance of the body only slightly decreases as the majority of energy is not lost to the environment but rather redistributed to the periphery and skin. In the first hour after induction, redistribution accounts for 81 percent of the temperature decrease. The second phase, termed **thermal imbalance**, lasts 2–3 hours and is characterized by a decrease in core body temperature of about 0.5–1.0 °C per hour. Thermal imbalance reflects a combination of reduced heat production (decreased metabolic rate, decreased muscle activity) and increased heat loss to the environment (radiation, evaporation, conduction, convection). During the third phase, **thermal steady state**, the decreased core body temperature causes a drop in the heat gradient between body and environment. At this point, the dissipation of heat equals heat production and the core temperature remains constant (usually between 34.5 and 35.5 °C) [9].

As a result of anesthetic-induced vasodilation and inhibited thermoregulatory mechanisms, neonates/infants are even more vulnerable to environmental heat loss in the operating room. Due to their high surface area-to-body-mass ratio, decreased subcutaneous fat, and high metabolic rate, rapid heat loss occurs through (1) radiant heat loss to the cold operating room; (2) conductive heat loss from cold intravenous fluids or blood products; and (3) evaporative heat loss from exposed viscera and mechanical ventilation. In an awake infant, heat loss to the environment is offset by a high metabolic rate. Since vasoconstriction, increases in metabolic rates, and non-shivering thermogenesis are the primary responses available to anesthetized infants, blunting of these responses can lead to profound hypothermia under general anesthesia [9].

Short procedures can lead to significant heat loss when the proper preventive steps are omitted, while lengthy surgeries can easily overwhelm the limited capabilities of newborns/infants to maintain adequate body temperature. Therefore, it is important for the anesthesiologist to take appropriate measures to reduce perioperative heat loss and maintain normothermia. Table 8.1 provides a summary of interventions to address perioperative heat loss. In brief, the following steps should be considered for every surgery: (1) warming of the operating room prior to patient arrival; (2) use of radiant warmers and heating pads/mattresses; (3) institution of closed-circuit anesthesia, with use of humidified/warmed gases; (4) warming of intravenous infusions/irrigation fluids; (5) use of forced-air warming blankets to cover body areas not involved in the surgical procedure; and (6) keeping the patient covered by blankets/clothes [5,13].

Anesthesiologists most often employ passive rewarming methods, which include forced-air warming devices and warm blankets. However, it is important to note that these techniques deactivate skin cold receptors and abolish the body's own thermoregulatory functions. This contributes to worsening hypothermia if passive surface rewarming is unable to maintain normothermia [9]. Forced-air warming devices have been associated with third degree thermal burns in infants. It is crucial that they be used according to manufacturers' recommendations, and caution should be used when using the highest temperature setting [14].

In summary, general anesthesia increases the risk of perioperative hypothermia in neonates and infants. Intraoperative hypothermia leads to several adverse effects in the perioperative period: (1) increased metabolic rate and oxygen consumption; (2) exhaustion of thermogenic reserves; (3) diminished metabolism of anesthetic agents resulting in prolonged opioid effects and neuromuscular blockade; (4) increased bleeding risk due to inhibition of normal coagulation pathways; (5) increased risk of wound infections. This underlines the importance of meticulous intraoperative temperature maintenance by addressing the various heat loss mechanisms [4].

## Temperature Measurement

Neonates and infants are at high risk for perioperative hypothermia; therefore, perioperative temperature monitoring and appropriate methods for maintaining normothermia are key aspects of intraoperative care (Table 8.3). The way by which those measurements are obtained should be reliable, reproducible, cost-effective, devoid of complications, and easy to implement. For a full discussion on various methods for monitoring intraoperative temperature, see Chapter 20 on monitors for neonates.

The most common thermometers used in the operating room are disposable. The decision on how to monitor temperature should be based on accuracy, safety, ease of placement, and operative considerations. The most accurate temperature monitors reflect core body temperatures, which measure central tissues that receive the majority of the blood flow. Common sites used in pediatric patients that reflect core body temperature include nasopharyngeal, esophageal, tympanic membrane, rectal, and, if placed properly, axillary artery temperatures. The procedure, improper placement of the monitor, and heating/cooling of the patient (such as during cardiopulmonary bypass) may affect the accuracy of the temperature readings.

Peripheral tissues are often cooler than the core compartment; the more peripheral the measurement site, the greater the discrepancy between obtained core and peripheral temperatures. The most common method using peripheral tissues is skin probes, which are easy to place but often correlate poorly with the core body temperature and are not recommended for use in neonates/infants undergoing general anesthesia [13].

## Temperature Regulation in Special Situations

Temperature control has been shown to be important in the setting of perinatal hypoxic-ischemic encephalopathy. Whole-body hypothermia (33.5 °C for 72 hours, initiated within six hours after birth) has beneficial outcomes in regards to the endpoints of death and severe disability, while temperature elevations during the first postnatal days were associated with an increased risk of death or worse neurological outcomes at age 6–7 years [15].

Hypothermia continues to be a key component for cerebral protection in patients on CPB. Hypothermia decreases metabolic rate and demand in the brain and other organ systems, which is important during the periods of low-flow or deep hypothermic circulatory arrest (DHCA) necessary to repair many neonatal congenital heart defects. Additionally, hypothermia reduces the inflammatory response from the CPB circuit, which is thought to be important for cerebral protection of the immature brain. Disadvantages of hypothermia include: prolonged CPB times, increased bleeding, and possible increased

**Table 8.3** Temperature monitoring methods

| Site | Advantages | Disadvantages | Sources of error |
|---|---|---|---|
| Pulmonary artery | • Gold standard<br>• Continuous reading | • Invasive | |
| Skin | • Easy placement | • Correlates poorly with core body temperature | • Variation in local skin perfusion<br>• Forced-air warmers, radiant warmer |
| Skin overlying temporal artery | • Easy placement<br>• Correlates with nasopharyngeal temperature | • Limited data available that support its use | • Variation in local skin perfusion<br>• Forced-air warmers, radiant warmer |
| Tympanic membrane | • Correlates with core body temperature | • Does not provide continuous measurements | • Technique |
| Nasopharynx | • Correlates with core body temperature<br>• Easy placement<br>• Continuous reading | • Contraindications: basilar skull fractures, major anatomic defects, coagulopathy<br>• Requires proper seating (posterior nasopharynx close to soft palate)<br>• Closest estimate of brain temperature | • High fresh-gas flows in setting of<br>  o mask anesthesia<br>  o uncuffed endotracheal tube |
| Esophagus | • Correlates with core body temperature<br>• Easy placement<br>• Continuous reading | • Requires proper seating (distal third of esophagus where heart sounds are loudest) | • High fresh-gas flows in setting of<br>  o omask anesthesia<br>  o ouncuffed endotracheal tube<br>• patient lacks insulating tissues between esophagus and tracheobronchial tree |
| Rectum | • Correlates with core body temperature<br>• Easy placement<br>• Continuous reading | • Requires proper seating (2–5 cm into rectum)<br>• Contraindications: neutropenia, thrombocytopenia, inflammatory bowel disease | • Insulation by feces, cold blood returning from the legs, bladder irrigation, open abdomen |
| Axilla | • Correlates with core body temperature<br>• Continuous reading | • Requires proper seating (above axillary artery with tight adduction of arm) | • Infusion of cold solutions through peripheral IV<br>• Proximity of forced-air warmer |
| Bladder | • Correlates with core body temperature<br>• Continuous reading<br>• Integrated in urinary catheter | • Requires bladder catheterization (invasive, infrequently needed) | • Oliguria/anuria |

risk of infection. While DHCA offers many advantages for congenital heart surgery, there continues to be controversy regarding the "safe" length of time for DHCA or low-flow CPB, and often this decision is institution-dependent [16].

Therapeutic hypothermia in the setting of extracorporeal membrane oxygenation (ECMO) support or traumatic brain injury has not resulted in improved clinical outcomes.

## Summary

In summary, perioperative temperature management in neonates and infants is of utmost importance, given their susceptibility to hypothermia due to anatomic (large skin surface-to-body mass ratio, reduced subcutaneous fat and skin keratin content, and limited glycogen and brown adipose tissue stores) and physiologic (increased metabolic rate, immature thermoregulatory mechanisms) factors. Hypothermia exerts detrimental effects on multiple organ systems and can lead to increased morbidity and mortality. As a result, the anesthesiologist caring for a neonate/infant needs to focus on meticulous temperature monitoring and targeted interventions addressing heat loss from radiation, convection, evaporation, and conduction to avoid perioperative hypothermia.

# References

1. Day RL, Caliguiri L, Kamenski C, Ehrlich F. Body temperature and survival of premature infants. *Pediatrics*. 1964;34:171–81.

2. Herzog LW, Coyne LJ. What is fever? Normal temperature in infants less than 3 months old. *Clin Pediatr (Phila)*. 1993;32:142–6.

3. Giesbrecht GG. Cold stress, near drowning and accidental hypothermia: a review. *Aviat Space Environ Med*. 2000;71:733–52.

4. Sessler DI. Temperature monitoring and perioperative thermoregulation. *Anesthesiology*. 2008;109:318–38.

5. Flick R. Clinical complications in pediatric anesthesia. In: Gregory GA, Andropoulos DB, e. *Gregory's Pediatric Anesthesia*, 5th edn. Chichester: Wiley-Blackwell; 2012; 1152–82.

6. Kurz A. Physiology of thermoregulation. *Best Pract Res Clin Anaesthesiol*. 2008;22:627–44.

7. Lenhardt R, Greif R, Sessler DI, et al. Relative contribution of skin and core temperatures to vasoconstriction and shivering thresholds during isoflurane anesthesia. *Anesthesiology*. 1999;91:422–9.

8. Himms-Hagen J. Brown adipose tissue metabolism and thermogenesis. *Annu Rev Nutr*. 1985;5:69–94.

9. Luginbuehl I, Bissonnette B, Davis PJ. Thermoregulation: physiology and perioperative disturbances. In: Davis PJ, Cladis FP, Motoyama EK, editors. *Smith's Anesthesia for Infants and Children*, 8th edn. Philadelphia, PA: Mosby; 2011; 157–78.

10. Murphy JD, Rabinovitch M, Goldstein JD, Reid LM. The structural basis of persistent pulmonary hypertension of the newborn infant. *J Pediatr*. 1981;98:962–7.

11. Walsh-Sukys MC, Tyson JE, Wright LL, et al. Persistent pulmonary hypertension of the newborn in the era before nitric oxide: practice variation and outcomes. *Pediatrics*. 2000;105:14–20.

12. Brismar B, Hedenstierna G, Lundh R, Tokics L. Oxygen uptake, plasma catecholamines and cardiac output during neurolept-nitrous oxide and halothane anaesthesias. *Acta Anaesthesiol Scand*. 1982;26:541–9.

13. Lyon AJ, Freer Y. Goals and options in keeping preterm babies warm. *Arch Dis Child Fetal Neonatal Ed*. 2011;96:F71–4.

14. Siddik-Sayyid SM, Abdallah FW, Dahrouj GB. Thermal burns in three neonates associated with intraoperative use of Bair Hugger warming devices. *Paediatr Anaesth*. 2008;18:337–9.

15. Shankaran S, Pappas A, McDonald SA, et al. Childhood outcomes after hypothermia for neonatal encephalopathy. *N Engl J Med*. 2012;366:2085–92.

16. Jonas R. Hypothermia, reduced flow, and circulatory arrest. In: Jonas R, editor. *Comprehensive Surgical Management of Congenital Heart Disease*. London: Hodder; 2004; 161–73.

**Chapter**

**9**

# Neonatal Resuscitation

Monica E. Kleinman

The transition from in utero fetal physiology to the immediate postnatal state involves rapid changes in cardiopulmonary function and metabolic regulation. Among the most significant events are (1) the initiation of spontaneous respiration to create a fluid–air interface for alveolar gas exchange; (2) the clearance of fetal lung fluid via the pulmonary lymphatic system; (3) the reduction in pulmonary vascular resistance and increase in pulmonary blood flow due to lung inflation and oxygen exposure; and (4) the increase in systemic vascular resistance from umbilical cord clamping, leading to closure of the foramen ovale and reduced flow across the ductus arteriosus, thus increasing systemic arterial oxygen saturations.

Resuscitation in the delivery room is unique because the primary goal is to support the process of cardiopulmonary transition. Interruption at any point can lead to critical consequences such as persistent pulmonary hypertension of the newborn, in which the pulmonary vascular resistance remains elevated and there is shunting of desaturated venous blood to the systemic circulation via the foramen ovale and ductus arteriosus. In most cases, the use of basic resuscitation measures such as stimulation, airway suctioning, and positive pressure ventilation are sufficient. Less frequently, the neonate requires tracheal intubation, chest compressions, or administration of intravascular fluids or medications.

There are multiple antenatal and intrapartum factors that increase the likelihood that neonatal resuscitation will be necessary, in addition to a number of congenital conditions that may compromise the neonate immediately after birth. Aziz et al. [1] developed a predictive model using a large database of deliveries and found that the elements listed in Table 9.1 were most highly associated with the need for positive pressure ventilation or tracheal intubation. The presence of major congenital malformations or hydrops fetalis was also significantly associated with the need for resuscitative measures.

**Table 9.1** Risk factors for neonatal resuscitation

| Antenatal risk factors | Intrapartum risk factors |
| --- | --- |
| Multiple pregnancy < 35 weeks | Prematurity <36 weeks |
| Maternal infection | Breech presentation |
| Hypertension | Meconium-stained amniotic fluid (MSAF) |
| Oligohydramnios | Non-reassuring fetal heart rate |
| | Emergency Cesarean section |
| | Shoulder dystocia |
| | Scalp pH <7.1 |

## Oxygen Therapy and Airway Management

Perhaps the most fundamental difference between delivery room resuscitation and resuscitation in other settings is the recommendation regarding the use of supplemental oxygen for term newborns. A landmark prospective controlled trial by Scandinavian investigators challenged the assumption that initial resuscitation of the newborn should be performed with 100 percent oxygen and, in fact, found that the use of room air for asphyxiated newborns with birthweight $\geq$1000 g decreased the time to first spontaneous breath [2]. Meta-analyses of several trials furthermore demonstrated decreased mortality for the groups resuscitated with room air [3,4]. Many areas of the world now initiate resuscitation with room air; current North American recommendations for initial resuscitation of both term and preterm infants is to use room air or a blended air/oxygen mixture titrated to achieve targeted oxygen saturations [5] (see Table 9.2). Preterm infants are more likely to require supplemental oxygen, based on studies demonstrating persistent hypoxemia in infants less than 32 weeks' gestation when using ventilation with room air [6–8].

69

**Table 9.2** The Neonatal Resuscitation Program's targets for oxygen saturations in the immediate newborn period

| Time after birth | Preductal SpO$_2$ |
| --- | --- |
| 1 min | 60–65 percent |
| 2 min | 65–70 percent |
| 3 min | 70–75 percent |
| 4 min | 75–80 percent |
| 5 min | 80–85 percent |
| 10 min | 85–95 percent |

Cyanosis is common immediately after birth as the fetal oxyhemoglobin saturation is around 60 percent. Preductal room air oxygen saturations in healthy term infants will typically reach 85–95 percent by ten minutes of life [9]. The Neonatal Resuscitation Program (American Academy of Pediatrics/American Heart Association) recommends targets for oxygen saturations in the immediate newborn period as shown in Table 9.2 [5].

If the newborn has respiratory effort but oxygen saturations fail to improve in the first few minutes of life, administer supplemental oxygen and consider CPAP. If the infant has absent of ineffective respiratory effort or becomes bradycardic, positive pressure ventilations with titrated concentrations of oxygen are indicated. For term newborns, initial inflating pressures of 30–40 cmH$_2$O may be required to recruit lung volume and establish an air–alveolar interface. Preterm infants are more prone to barotrauma and should be ventilated with enough inflating pressure to generate chest rise, usually ≤20 cmH$_2$O. In either population, ventilation pressures should be adjusted as lung compliance improves. The associated application of positive end-expiratory pressure (PEEP) in the delivery room supports the establishment of functional residual capacity (FRC) [10]. Neonates that remain cyanotic or bradycardic despite the use of effective positive pressure ventilations via facemask should undergo tracheal intubation and assisted ventilation. Laryngeal mask airways are an alternative if manual ventilations or tracheal intubation are not effective in infants ≥34 weeks' gestation and ≥2000 g [11]. Persistent bradycardia despite a secure airway and effective ventilations is an indication for chest compressions and ventilation with 100 percent oxygen (Figure 9.1).

## Emergency Vascular Access

The presence of patent umbilical vessels facilitates emergency vascular access in the delivery room. Indications for umbilical line placement include the need to administer volume expanders or medications. While several drugs can be delivered intratracheally (e.g., epinephrine), the intravenous route is always preferred. During resuscitation the placement of an umbilical venous catheter (UVC) provides rapid access to the central circulation for fluids, blood products, or medications. In the delivery room setting it is appropriate to place a "low" UVC in which the catheter is advanced only a few centimeters until blood return is achieved. Further advancement of the catheter requires X-ray confirmation of placement to ensure the line traverses the ductus venosus and is not positioned in the portal vein or a hepatic vein. If umbilical venous catheterization is not possible, alternatives include peripheral intravenous access or intraosseous infusion. Cannulation of the umbilical artery is typically reserved for neonates requiring continuous arterial blood pressure monitoring or frequent laboratory sampling in the intensive care unit. If volume expansion is indicated based on poor perfusion or a history of blood loss, isotonic crystalloid or packed red blood cells (PRBCs) can be administered in aliquots of 10 ml kg$^{-1}$ followed by reassessment.

## Resuscitation Medications

While it is rare to require medication administration during neonatal resuscitation, dosing accuracy is critical, especially with low birth weight infants. Other than volume expansion for suspected hypovolemia, the only other medication that is routinely used in the delivery room is epinephrine. Epinephrine is indicated when, despite effective ventilations with 100 percent oxygen and chest compressions, the newborn remains bradycardic (heart rate <60 min$^{-1}$) [5]. Although epinephrine can be administered intratracheally, the intravenous route is strongly preferred. The recommended dose of intravenous epinephrine is 0.01–0.03 mg kg$^{-1}$ of 1:10,000 (0.1 mg mL$^{-1}$) epinephrine. The use of high-dose (0.1 mg kg$^{-1}$) intravenous epinephrine is not recommended, although doses of 0.05–0.1 mg kg$^{-1}$ may be given via the endotracheal tube if intravenous access cannot be established [5].

Of note, the use of naloxone for newborns with respiratory depression in the delivery room is not recommended; instead, the patient's cardiorespiratory status should be supported with ventilation and oxygenation. Other medications such as sodium bicarbonate, glucose, or vasopressors are typically initiated

## Neonatal Resuscitation Algorithm—2015 Update

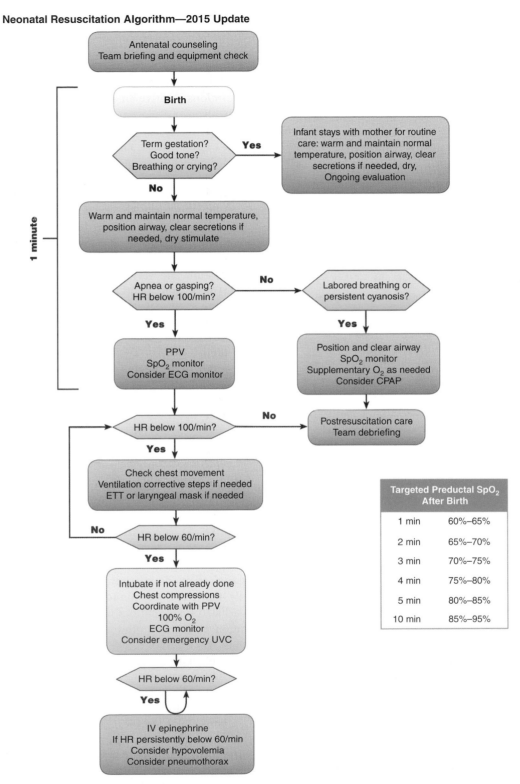

**Figure 9.1** The Neonatal Resuscitation Program (American Academy of Pediatrics/American Heart Association) algorithm illustrates the progressive escalation of measures for delivery room resuscitation. Source: [5].

once the neonate is in the intensive care unit with additional laboratory and monitoring capabilities.

## Special Circumstances

### Meconium-Stained Amniotic Fluid

In utero passage of meconium occurs in both normal pregnancies and those characterized by fetal distress during labor. Meconium-stained amniotic fluid (MSAF) is seen more commonly in post-date newborns and those who are small for gestational age (SGA). Meconium-stained amniotic fluid is a major risk factor for development of meconium aspiration syndrome (MAS), a potentially life-threatening respiratory disorder. Tracheal suctioning prior to initiation of respirations was widely used in the past to prevent MAS; however, management of MSAF has changed significantly over the past two decades due to findings from large studies demonstrating no benefit of tracheal suctioning for vigorous neonates [12]. Even for infants who are depressed at birth, current recommendations are to initiate the usual steps of resuscitation, including clearance of the mouth and nose, to avoid harm related to delay in ventilation [13].

### Prematurity

Prematurity carries a unique set of considerations for resuscitation, including regulation of temperature, pulmonary immaturity, and risk of oxygen toxicity. Outcome for preterm infants is related to both gestational age and birth weight, and is also influenced by gender and singleton vs. multiple births. The use of antenatal corticosteroids to accelerate fetal lung development is also associated with lower mortality and morbidity [14]. The National Institute of Child Health and Human Development (NICHD) maintains a Neonatal Research Network that provides extremely preterm birth outcome data for gestational ages between 22 and 25 weeks [15].

Preterm infants are more likely to require advanced respiratory management in the delivery room due to surfactant deficiency associated with pulmonary immaturity. Surfactant, a phospholipid produced by type II pneumocytes, reduces alveolar surface tension and facilitates elastic recoil and maintenance of lung volume at end-expiration. Pulmonary surfactant production begins at 23–24 weeks' gestation, and can be stimulated by the use of

antenatal corticosteroids [14]. Surfactant deficiency results in neonatal respiratory distress syndrome (RDS) characterized by atelectasis, hypoxemia, and decreased lung compliance. The initial treatment for RDS includes supplemental oxygen and application of continuous positive airway pressure (CPAP) to maintain alveolar inflation. Despite the use of noninvasive ventilation, the premature newborn is at high risk of respiratory failure due to unfavorable pulmonary mechanics and immature control of respiration.

For infants requiring assisted ventilation, surfactant replacement therapy with synthetic or animal-derived exogenous surfactant reduces neonatal mortality and the risk of acute and chronic lung disease. Prophylactic surfactant administration (i.e., tracheal intubation and surfactant instillation prior to development of signs of RDS) is no longer used routinely with the widespread adoption of early nasal CPAP [16]. However, the use of early, selective surfactant administration for preterm infants with respiratory failure is favored over delayed administration in the setting of worsening RDS [17]. A recent multicenter study showed no difference in the composite outcome of death or bronchopulmonary dysplasia (BPD) for extremely preterm infants (24–27 weeks' gestation) receiving nasal CPAP versus tracheal intubation and surfactant administration in the first hour of life [18].

Exogenous surfactant is administered intratracheally in a volume based on weight, using a small feeding tube to provide 2–4 aliquots while adjusting the infant's position. During surfactant administration the neonate may experience desaturation and bradycardia that typically responds to assisted ventilation. Following surfactant administration, lung compliance may rapidly improve; close monitoring of chest excursion and exhaled tidal volumes is critical to prevent overdistention and pneumothorax, especially if the infant is to be transported.

Exposure to high concentrations of supplemental oxygen is potentially toxic to the immature lung and the developing retina. Although BPD is multifactorial, oxidative stress and inflammation from oxygen exposure are major contributors. Oxygen saturation goals for preterm infants represent a balance between avoiding oxygen toxicity and providing adequate oxygen delivery to developing organs. The SUPPORT study (Surfactant, Positive Pressure, and Oxygenation Randomized Trial) was a large randomized trial that compared two saturation targets, 85–89 percent vs. 90–95 percent, in preterm infants of less than 28 weeks' gestational age [19]. The higher oxygen saturation target was associated with lower rates of necrotizing enterocolitis (NEC) and higher survival rates, despite an increased incidence of retinopathy of prematurity (ROP).

Based on similar findings from studies in the United Kingdom, Australia, and New Zealand, current recommendations for preterm infants after initial resuscitation are for titration of oxygen concentration to achieve saturation goals of 90–95 percent [20]. In terms of ventilation targets, hypocarbia is to be avoided as it is associated with a higher incidence of BDP and periventricular leukomalacia [21]. Likewise, hypercarbia is associated with worse outcomes when combining death with serious intraventicular hemorrhage, bronchopulmonary dysplasia, and neurodevelopmental impairment [22].

Preterm neonates are vulnerable to hypothermia due to their lack of subcutaneous fat, thin skin, and high body surface area-to-mass ratio. Deleterious effects of hypothermia include hypoglycemia, metabolic acidosis, and RDS, and hypothermia is associated with increased mortality [23]. The neutral thermal environment (ambient temperature at which heat is neither gained or lost) depends on the gestational age and weight. Extremely low birth weight (<1000 g) or very low birth weight (<1500 g) neonates require active warming in addition to measures to prevent heat loss, such as head covering and occlusive wrap to the skin. The use of a servo-controlled radiant warmer is preferred to a conventional incubator immediately after birth [24]. Other measures to combat hypothermia include increasing the room temperature, use of an insulated transwarmer mattress, and warming inspired gases [25,26].

## Congenital Anomalies

Advances in prenatal imaging and genetic testing have afforded the opportunity to anticipate resuscitation needs for neonates with specific prenatally diagnosed conditions. The fetus with congenital diaphragmatic hernia (CDH), for example, is often referred for delivery in a perinatal center with the capability of extracorporeal membrane oxygenation (ECMO), but the initial steps of resuscitation are adjusted due to the anatomic considerations. Newborns with a prenatal diagnosis of CDH should undergo prompt tracheal intubation, avoiding the use of positive-pressure

ventilation by mask to prevent gaseous distention of the stomach and intestines. Immediately following tracheal intubation, placement of a sump-type naso- or orogastric tube is essential to remove any swallowed air using continuous suction. Since the stomach and/or intestines may be in an intrathoracic location, failure to decompress gastric air can lead to further cardiopulmonary compromise. As the presence of CDH is associated with significant pulmonary hypoplasia and pulmonary hypertension, these patients may remain desaturated, with evidence of ductal-level right-to-left shunting based on pre- and postductal oxygen saturation differences. It is important to recognize that the ipsilateral lung in CDH patients is also abnormal, and a high rate, low tidal volume mechanical ventilation strategy is recommended. In the immediate post-delivery period, ventilate with 100 percent oxygen to achieve a preductal oxygen saturation goal of >85 percent using a peak inspiratory pressure $\leq 25$ cmH$_2$O while transferring to the intensive care unit.

The EXIT procedure (ex utero intrapartum therapy) has been attempted for infants with severe pulmonary hypoplasia who are unlikely to survive without immediate use of ECMO. In the EXIT to ECMO approach the infant is partially delivered via C-section and cannulation of the neck vessels is performed while maintaining uteroplacental circulation. Although results are limited to retrospective reviews, the use of peripartum ECMO has not been shown to improve outcome for this specific patient population [27]. In other conditions the EXIT procedure has been used successfully to allow for immediate surgical intervention for critical high airway obstruction syndrome (CHAOS) or life-threatening neck or lung masses [28].

## Hydrops Fetalis

Hydrops fetalis is a life-threatening complication for the fetus characterized by diffuse body wall edema and effusions in pleural, pericardial, and peritoneal spaces.

The etiologies of hydrops fetalis are diverse and include "non-immune" causes such as chromosomal abnormalities, congenital infections, congenital heart disease, and in utero cardiac rhythm disturbances (complete heart block, supraventricular tachycardia). Immune causes such as hemolytic diseases are less common with the use of maternal therapy to prevent

Rh-isoimmunization in mothers with Rh-negative blood types.

Hydrops fetalis has a high rate of premature birth and postnatal morbidity and mortality, depending on the underlying cause. Delivery room resuscitation may be complicated by poor lung and chest wall compliance, requiring urgent pleural drainage to facilitate ventilation. In the setting of longstanding fetal hydrothorax pulmonary hypoplasia may be significant and there is high risk of pneumothorax during attempted resuscitation.

## Post-Resuscitation Care

The most significant recent advance in neonatal resuscitation has been the use of therapeutic hypothermia to improve outcome for newborns with hypoxic-ischemic encephalopathy related to perinatal asphyxia. The use of moderate hypothermia (core temperature 33.5–34.5 °C) for depressed newborns ≥36 weeks reduces mortality and neurodevelopmental disability as found in several randomized clinical trials [29–31]. Clinical criteria for induced hypothermia typically include a combination of Apgar scores, umbilical cord or patient pH or base deficit, duration of resuscitation, and exam consistent with moderate or severe encephalopathy. Some centers also include the results of amplitude-integrated encephalography (aEEG). Hypothermia is typically provided using a similar approach to the published clinical trials, with initiation within six hours of age and continuation for 72 hours, followed by gradual return to normothermia.

Therapeutic hypothermia is typically provided in tertiary care centers with neonatal expertise. Timely identification of eligible newborns delivered in the community is essential due to the time-sensitive nature of initiating therapy. Passive cooling with careful temperature monitoring may be recommended prior to transfer, with caution to avoid excessive hypothermia [32]. Alternatively, a servo-controlled device can be used to provide controlled active cooling [33].

## References

1. Aziz K, Chadwick M, Baker M, Andrews W. Ante- and intra-partum factors that predict increased need for neonatal resuscitation. *Resuscitation*. 2008;79:444–52.

2. Saugsted OD, Rootwelt T, Aalen O. Resuscitation of asphyxiated newborn infants with room air or oxygen: an international controlled trial – the Resair 2 study. *Pediatrics*. 1998;102:e1.

3. Davis PG, Tan A, O'Donnell CP, Schulze A. Resuscitation of newborn infants with 100% oxygen or air: a systematic review and meta-analysis. *Lancet*. 2004;364:1329–33.

4. Rabi Y, Rabi D, Yee W. Room air resuscitation of the depressed newborn: a systematic review and meta-analysis. *Resuscitation*. 2007;72:353–63.

5. Wyckoff MH, Aziz K, Escobedo MB, et al. Part 13: Neonatal resuscitation: 2015 American Heart Association guidelines update for cardiopulmonary resuscitation and emergency cardiovascular care. *Circulation*. 2015;132:S543–60.

6. Wang CL, Anderson C, Leone TA, et al. Resuscitation of preterm neonates by room air or 100% oxygen. *Pediatrics*. 2008;121:1083–9.

7. Rabi Y, Singhal N, Nettel-Aguirre A. Room-air versus oxygen administration for resuscitation of preterm infants: the ROAR study. *Pediatrics*. 2011;128:e374.

8. Escrig R, Arruza L, Izquierdo I, et al. Achievement of targeted saturation values in extremely low gestational age neonates resuscitated with low or high oxygen concentrations: a prospective randomized trial. *Pediatrics*. 2008;121:875–81.

9. Rabi Y, Yee W, Chen SY, Singhal N. Oxygen saturation trends immediately after birth. *J Pediatr*. 2006;148:590–4.

10. Hooper SB, Siew ML, Kitchen JM, te Pas AB. Establishing functional residual capacity in the non-breathing infant. *Semin Fetal Neonatal Med*. 2013;18:336–43.

11. Schmolzer GM, Agarwal M, Kamlin CO, Davis PG. Supraglottic airway devices during neonatal resuscitation: an historical perspective, systematic review and meta-analysis of available clinical trials. *Resuscitation*. 2013;84:722–30.

12. Wisell TE, Gannon CM, Jacob J, et al. Delivery room management of the apparently vigorous meconium-stained neonate: results of the multicenter, international collaborative trial. *Pediatrics*. 2000;105:1–7.

13. Chettri S, Adhisivam B, Bhat BV. Endotracheal suction for nonvigorous neonates born through meconium stained amniotic fluid: a randomized controlled trial. *J Pediatr*. 2015;166:1208–13.

14. Roberts D, Dalziel SR. Antenatal corticosteroids for accelerating fetal lung maturation for women at risk of preterm birth. *Cochrane Database Syst Rev*. 2006;19(3):CD004454.

15. www.nichd.nih.gov/about/org/der/branches/ppb/programs/epbo/pages/epbo_case.aspx.

16. Rojas-Reyes MX, Morley CJ, Soll R. Prophylactic versus selective use of surfactant in preventing morbidity and mortality in preterm infants. *Cochrane Database Syst Rev*. 2012;14:CD000510.

17. Bahadue FL, Soll R. Early versus delayed selective surfactant treatment for neonatal respiratory distress syndrome. *Cochrane Database Syst Rev*. 2012;11:CD001456.

18. SUPPORT Study Group of the Eunice Kennedy Shriver NICHD Neonatal Research Network, Finer NN, Carlo WA, et al. Early CPAP versus surfactant in extremely preterm infants. *New Engl J Med*. 2010;362:1970–9.

19. SUPPORT Study Group of the Eunice Kennedy Shriver NICHD Neonatal Research Network, Carlo WA, Finer NN, et al. Target ranges of oxygen saturation in extremely preterm infants. *N Engl J Med*. 2010;362:1959–69.

20. The BOOST II United Kingdom, Australia, and New Zealand collaborative groups. Oxygen saturation and outcomes in preterm infants. *N Engl J Med*. 2013;368:2094–104.

21. Erickson SJ, Grauaug A, Gurrin L, et al. Hypocarbia in the ventilated preterm infant and its effect on intraventricular hemorrhage and bronchopulmonary dysplasia. *J Paediatr Child Health*. 2002;38:560–2.

22. Ambalayanan N, Carlo WA, Wrage LA, et al. PaCO2 in surfactant, positive pressure, and oxygen randomised trial (SUPPORT). *Arch Dis Child Fetal Neonatal Ed*. 2014;100:F145–9.

23. Laptook AR, Salhab W, Ghaskar B. Admission temperature of low birth weight infants: predictors and associated morbidities. *Pediatrics*. 2007;119:e643.

24. Sinclair JC. Servo-control for maintaining abdominal skin temperature at 36°C in low birth weight infants. *Cochrane Database Syst Rev*. 2002;1:CD001074.

25. McCall EM, Alderdice F, Halliday HL, Jenkins JG, Vohra S. Interventions to prevent hypothermia at birth in preterm and/or low birthweight infants. *Cochrane Database Syst Rev*. 2010;3:CD004210.

26. te Pas AB, Lopriore E, Dito I, Morley CJ, Walther FJ. Humidified and heated air during stabilization at birth improves temperature in preterm infants. *Pediatrics*. 2010;125:e1427–32.

27. Stoffan AP, Wilson JM, Jennings RW, Wilkins-Haug LE, Buchmiller TL. Does the ex utero intrapartum treatment to extracorporeal membrane oxygenation procedure change outcomes for high-risk patients with congenital diaphragmatic hernia? *J Pediatr Surg*. 2012;47:1053–7.

28. Moldenhauer JS. Ex Utero Intrapartum Therapy. *Semin Pediatr Surg*. 2013;22:44–9.

29. Gluckman PD, Wyatt JS, Azzopardi D, et al. Selective head cooling with mild systemic hypothermia after neonatal encephalopathy: multicentre randomised trial. *Lancet*. 2005;365:663–70.

30. Shankaran S, Laptook AR, Ehrenkranz RA, et al. Whole-body hypothermia for neonates with hypoxic-ischemic encephalopathy. *N Engl J Med*. 2005;353:1574–84.

31. Azzopardi DV, Strohm B, Edwards AD, et al. Moderate hypothermia to treat perinatal asphyxial encephalopathy. *N Engl J Med*. 2009;361:1349–58.

32. Committee on Fetus and Newborn, American Academy of Pediatrics. Hypothermia and neonatal encephalopathy. *Pediatrics*. 2014;133:1146–50.

33. Chaudhary R, Farrer K, Broster S, McRitchie L, Austin T. Active versus passive cooling during neonatal transport. *Pediatrics*. 2013;132:841–6.

## Chapter 10

# Congenital Abnormalities and Syndromes

Katherine R. Gentry and Anne M. Lynn

This chapter is dedicated to presenting an approach to evaluating neonates with congenital anomalies and a review of commonly presenting syndromes seen in the nursery. There is likely to be significant overlap with other chapters in this book and cross-referencing is recommended. Following a discussion of some of the more common syndromes seen in neonates, we have included a table of additional syndromes not covered in the text, with particular emphasis on features of the airway and/or the presence of congenital cardiac disease (see Table 10.1).

## Chromosomal and Genetic Abnormalities

**Trisomy 21 (T21, Down Syndrome).** A genetic syndrome resulting from an extra copy of chromosome 21, either through maternal nondisjunction in meiosis I (>90 percent of cases), chromosomal translocation, or abnormal mitosis resulting in mosaicism.

*Incidence:* T21 is the most common chromosomal abnormality, with an incidence of about 1:700 live births [1].

*Diagnosis:* Prenatal diagnosis can be made via cell-free DNA screening for fetal aneuploidy, chorionic villus sampling, or amniocentesis. After birth, diagnosis is based upon clinical features and karyotyping.

*Clinical features:* Features found in the neonate include a flat facial profile, slanted palpebral fissures, anomalous ears, hypotonia, poor Moro reflex, midphalangeal dysplasia of the fifth finger, a transverse palmar crease, excessive skin at nape of neck, hyperflexibility of joints, and dysplasia of the pelvis [2]. Features involving the airway include: protruding tongue (appears large relative to the hypoplastic midface), subglottic stenosis and narrow tracheal diameter, and obstructive sleep apnea [3,4]. Greater than 40 percent of children with Trisomy 21 have a cardiac defect; atrioventricular canal defects, patent ductus arteriosus, and Tetralogy of Fallot (ToF) are the most

common. Patients have immune deficiency and an increased risk of leukemia, including congenital leukemia, which develops within the first three years of life. The skin can be dry and coarse.

*Anesthetic considerations:* Careful assessment of respiratory and cardiac status is vital. Prepare for a potentially difficult airway due to relative macroglossia, small hypopharynx, and precautions in the case of an unstable cervical spine. A smaller-sized endotracheal tube (ETT) than predicted by age may be indicated due to the risk of subglottic stenosis [3]. Similar considerations apply when planning a nasal tube, as the nasal passages may be smaller. IV access may be difficult, and sterile technique for placement is recommended due to immune suppression. Anesthetic management will be dictated by the presence and status of cardiac disease [1].

*Pharmacologic and other considerations:* Atropine may cause pronounced mydriasis and tachycardia. High concentrations of sevoflurane, i.e., during inhalational induction, may precipitate bradycardia [5].

**22q11 Deletions.** The 22q11.2 deletions include a spectrum of features including congenital heart disease, hypocalcemia, immune deficiency, palate abnormalities, and abnormal facies. DiGeorge syndrome will be described as a representative example.

DiGeorge is a genetic syndrome with varied phenotypes, most commonly including cardiac outflow tract obstruction, hypoparathyroidism with hypocalcemia, and immune defects due to thymic hypoplasia.

*Incidence:* 22q11 deletions occur in 1:3000–1:5000 live births. DiGeorge syndrome involves a monoallelic microdeletion at 22q11.2 (DiGeorge syndrome critical region [DGCR]). It is the most frequent gene deletion and, after trisomy 21, the second most common genetic cause of congenital heart disease. Males and females are equally affected [6].

*Diagnosis:* Thymic aplasia may be noted during cardiac surgery. This, plus clinical findings (described

**Table 10.1** Syndromes, include those not covered by this chapter, with features of the airway and/or the presence of congenital cardiac disease

| Syndrome | Airway/respiratory concerns | Cardiac disease (incidence, if known) | Other features of note |
|---|---|---|---|
| **Chromosomal** | | | |
| Trisomy 21 | Large tongue, small trachea, C-spine instability | AV canal, ASD, VSD (50 percent) ToF (8 percent) | See text |
| Trisomy 13 (Patau syndrome) | Cleft lip and palate, choanal atresia Facemask ventilation may be impossible | 90 percent: ASD, VSD, coarctation, bicuspid aortic valve, dextroversion | Associated with midline defects High mortality in first six months of life |
| Trisomy 18 (Edwards syndrome) | Microstomia, micrognathia, high arched palate | ASD, VSD, PDA, PS, coarctation | High mortality in first year of life |
| 3 p duplication | Large mouth, cleft lip and palate, choanal atresia | ToF, VSD, hypoplastic heart, TGA | >50 percent die in first two years of life |
| 4 p duplication (trisomy 4p) | Cleft lip and palate, macroglossia, microglossia | Congenital heart disease often present: ASD, VSD | Recurrent pulmonary aspiration → chronic respiratory disease Life expectancy approxlmately two years |
| Trisomy 8 mosaicism | Short neck, microretrognathia, difficult mask fit | Cardiac septal defects and great vessel abnormalities | Mental deficiency, seizures, Factor VIII deficiency |
| Trisomy 9 | Short neck, ankyloglossia, microretrognathia | ASD, VSD, PDA, valve abnormalities, DORV | Severe mental deficiency Death in infancy or early childhood IV access difficult |
| 5p Cri du Chat | Microcephaly, occasional micrognathia, long epiglottis, difficult DL | CHD in 33 percent: PDA, ASD, VSD, or PS | Developmental delay, aspiration risk Life expectancy early childhood |
| 22q11.2 deletion DiGeorge | Midface hypoplasia, microretrognathia, high arched palate, tracheal anomalies | IAA (30–56 percent), ToF (20–30 percent), truncus arteriosus (13–30 percent), right aortic arch (14–26 percent), VSD (8–25 percent), DORV, TGA, PS, R infundibular stenosis | Hypocalcemia (hypoplasia of parathyroid), immunodeficiency (thymic aplasia) |
| 22q11.2 deletion velocardiofacial | Prominent nose, retrognathia, high arched palate (mandibular abnormalities appearing like Robin Sequence) | R aortic arch (50 percent), VSD (75 percent), ToF (20 percent), abnormal carotid and L subclavian arteries | Hypothyroidism, hypocalcemia, T-cell immunodeficiency, thymic hypoplasia |
| 22q11 conotruncal anomaly face (variant of DiGeorge) | Cleft lip/palate microglossia | ToF, PA, DORV, TA, aortic arch abnormalities | Thymic and parathyroid hypoplasia, with immunodeficiency and neonatal hypocalcemia, anal atresia, abdominal hernias |
| CHARGE | Midface hypoplasia, micrognathia, anterior larynx, microstomia, choanal atresia, laryngomalacia, subglottic stenosis | Cardiac defects in 80 percent: ASD, VSD, AV canal, conotruncal malformations, HLHS, PS, coarctation | Cranial nerve dysfunction increases aspiration risk; TEF/EA in 20 percent, see text. |

*(continued)*

**Table 10.1** (continued)

| Syndrome | Airway/respiratory concerns | Cardiac disease (incidence, if known) | Other features of note |
|---|---|---|---|
| Noonan | Micrognathia, dental malocclusion, short webbed neck<br>Can have atlantoaxial instability | Cardiac defects in 50 percent: PS, hypertrophic cardiomyopathy, ASD, ToF, AV canal, coarctation | Coagulopathy: Factor XI deficiency, thrombocytopenia, other factor deficiencies |
| Prader–Willi (Neonatal) | None in infancy | None in infancy | Hypotonia, possible history of aspiration, pneumonia |
| Tuberous sclerosis (TSC-1: chrom 9) (TSC-2: chrom 16) | Oral and laryngeal tumors possible | Cardiac rhabdomyosarcoma | Neurodegenerative<br>Skin: adenoma sebaceum, angiofibromas<br>Neurologic: seizures, obstructive hydrocephalus |
| Turner syndrome | Short webbed neck, micrognathia | Coarctation of the aorta, dissecting aortic aneurysm, VSD, ASD, dextrocardia, bicuspid AV, HLHS | Infantile presentation: lymphedema |
| Williams Beuren syndrome | Mandibular hypoplasia | Supravalvar aortic stenosis can lead to sudden death on induction<br>Other cardiac anomalies also possible (see text) | Infantile hypercalcemia<br>Mild mental retardation but normal language development |
| **Mucopolysaccharidoses** | Coarse facies make mask fit difficult<br>Thick tongue and stiff neck complicate DL and intubation | Valve thickening, systolic and diastolic dysfunction, arteriosclerosis | Features develop over time as GAGs accumulate (see text) |
| **Endocrine** | | | |
| Beckwith–Wiedemann | Large tongue, maxillary hypoplasia, large size | Cardiomyopathy, cardiac hamartomas, or other congenital heart disease has been described | Severe hypoglycemia in newborn period (see text) |
| Congenital adrenal hyperplasia syndromes | None | None | Impaired synthesis of cortisol or aldosterone from cholesterol, due to enzymatic defects<br>21-hydroxylase deficiency responsible for 90 percent of cases<br>Phenotype includes virilization (ambiguous genitalia) ± salt wasting |
| **Immunologic** | | | |
| DiGeorge (see above) | | | |
| Neonatal lupus erythematosus | None | Congenital heart disease in ~50 percent (10 percent both cutaneous and cardiac manifestations)<br>Complete heart block, PDA, VSD, TGA, ASD coarctation, ToF<br>Pacemaker required in ~ 1/3 of infants with neonatal lupus | Skin lesions in ~50 percent, ("raccoon eyes" generalized, non-scaling, erythematous) disappear at ~6 months of age<br>Occurs in infants of mothers with SLE, resulting from placental transfer of autoantibodies |

**Table 10.1** (*continued*)

| Syndrome | Airway/respiratory concerns | Cardiac disease (incidence, if known) | Other features of note |
|---|---|---|---|
| **Metabolic** | | | |
| Mitochondrial DNA deletion syndromes:<br>• Pearson<br>• Kearns–Sayre (KSS)<br>• Leigh (LS) | Risk of postoperative respiratory failure due to neuromuscular weakness (LS, KSS) | Heart block and/or cardiomyopathy can occur (KS) | Pearson: infantile disease with sideroblastic anemia and dysfunction of the exocrine pancreas (→ steatorrhea) – often fatal<br>LS: psychomotor delay or regression presenting in infancy<br>KS: presents in childhood<br>*Avoid lactated Ringer's and large doses of propofol. Maintain normothermia, normocarbia, and euglycemia. Minimal fasting period, give IV dextrose |
| Smith Lemli Opitz | Micrognathia, difficult DL | Heart defects in >40 percent: AV canal, TGA, anomalous pulmonary drainage, ToF, VSD | Pulmonary hypoplasia, aspiration risk, hypotonia<br>Multi-organ failure in first week of life due to defective cholesterol production |
| **Skin, muscle, connective tissue** | | | |
| Epidermolysis bullosa | Precautions to minimize mucosal and skin trauma | None | See text |
| Ehlers–Danlos: encompasses a number of inherited connective tissue disorders | Risk of airway trauma/bruising with any invasive technique. Risk of TMJ dislocation, C-spine subluxation | Valvular insufficiency, conduction system defects | Risk of excessive bleeding: have adequate venous access, blood products available |
| Marfan syndrome (early-onset form presents in infancy) | Micrognathia, potential TMJ dislocation | Severe cardiac valve insufficiency (MV prolapse common), aortic root dilatation | Multiple systems affected including: eyes, skin, skeletal system, cardiovascular system |
| Central core myopathy | Occasional mandibular hypoplasia<br>Avoid succinylcholine for intubation | Evaluate for cardiomyopathy and valvular pathology | High susceptibility to MH |
| King Denborough syndrome | High arched or cleft palate, micrognathia, webbed neck, crowded teeth | Cardiac disease unusual, but should be investigated. | Noonan-like features in infancy, high MH susceptibility |
| Myotonia congenita<br>• Becker disease<br>• Thompsen disease | No airway anomalies | No cardiac involvement | Thompsen disease presents in infancy to early childhood: see inability to relax muscles, blepharospasm, diffuse muscular hypertrophy<br>Possible MH risk<br>Do not use succinylcholine to avoid fasciculation-induced myotonia<br>Response to nondepolarizing agents normal<br>Pain with propofol can also precipitate myotonia |

(*continued*)

**Table 10.1**  (*continued*)

| Syndrome | Airway/respiratory concerns | Cardiac disease (incidence, if known) | Other features of note |
|---|---|---|---|
| Myotonic dystrophy •Types I, II | Aspiration risk due to dysphagia, gastric distention<br>Muscle weakness may cause postoperative respiratory failure | Cardiac conduction defects in 90 percent, cardiomyopathy or valvular pathology possible<br>Degree of cardiac disease does not correlate with severity of muscle disease | Pain and shivering can incite a myotonic reaction<br>No succinylcholine<br>Normal response to nondepolarizing agents<br>Temperature maintenance important |
| Spinal muscular atrophy I (Werndig Hoffman) | Postoperative respiratory failure serious risk, aspiration risk | – | Presents before three months |
| SMA II | As above | – | Presents between 3–18 months |
| **Skeletal/musculoskeletal** | | | |
| Arthrogryposis | Difficult DL if TMJ or C-spine involved | Rare | Difficult IV access (see text) |
| Freeman Sheldon | Small puckered mouth, high arched palate, small mandible | Not typical | Arthrogryposis type IIA<br>Thought to involve fibrous replacement of muscle fibers → possible myopathy<br>Masseter spasm, hyperpyrexia, and tachycardia reported after GA |
| Multiple pterygium | Diff DL if oral, head, neck involvement; LMA has been successful | Rare | Restrictive lung disease |
| Klippel Feil | Difficult DL with C-spine limited motion | CHD, usually VSD | See text |
| VACTERL | TE fistula | CHD common | See text |
| Osteogenesis imperfecta | Fragile teeth, risk for mandibular fracture so gentle DL | Rare aortic root dilation, MV prolapse | Four types – type 1 most common: blue sclerae, fragile bones, teeth, hearing loss<br>Hyperthermia with anesthesia, not thought to be MH |
| Jeune syndrome | Small larynx, reduce ETT size | Possible pulmonary hypertension from restrictive lung disease | Hypoplastic lungs, stiff chest wall so low ventilator press<br>Renal cysts – check renal function<br>Postoperative ventilation possible |
| Robinow syndrome | Possible micrognathia, with difficult DL | CHD – RV outflow obstruction | "Fetal Face S" |
| Thrombocytopenia with absent radius | Avoid nasal ETT/NG due to low platelet counts | CHD, usually ToF or ASD | Absent radii, decreased platelet count (decreased megakaryocytes) |

**Table 10.1** (*continued*)

| Syndrome | Airway/respiratory concerns | Cardiac disease (incidence, if known) | Other features of note |
|---|---|---|---|
| **Craniosynostosis** | | | |
| Antley–Bixler | Choanal atresia, possible need for tracheostomy | Rare | Trapezoidocephaly, eye protection important |
| Apert | Difficult DL, abnormal trachea | CHD 10 percent – PS, VSD, overriding aorta | Syndactyly – possible difficult IV (see text) |
| Carpenter | High arch palate, hypoplastic mandible – difficult DL | CHD 50 percent – ASD, VSD, PDA, ToF, TGA | Possible ICP elevation (see text) |
| Crouzon | Hypoplastic midface | | See text |
| Saethre Chotzen | Occasional C-spine fusion – difficult DL | | Possible increased ICP |
| Kleeblattschaedal | – | – | Cloverleaf skull Eye care important Possible risk for ICP |
| **Other craniofacial** | | | |
| Robin Sequence | Micrognathia, cleft palate, glossoptosis. Obstructive apnea, possible difficult facemask and laryngoscopy Must plan ahead for airway management. | Not typical | May be seen with other syndromes, such as Stickler, Cornelia de Lange, Hallerman-Streiff, or femoral hypoplasia syndromes |
| Treacher Collins | Malar and mandibular hypoplasia, cleft palate, wide mouth | Cardiac defects possible | |
| Goldenhar | Facial asymmetry, mandibular hypoplasia, unilateral hypoplasia of palate and tongue Possible C1–C2 subluxation | Frequently associated: VSD, ASD, PDA, ToF, coarctation of the aorta | Arnold–Chiari malformation, encephalocele, spina bifida, hydrocephalus |
| Nager syndrome | Malar hypoplasia, maxiallary and mandibular hypoplasia, posteriorly displaced tongue, cleft lip and palate, laryngeal hypoplasia, absent epiglottis | Not typical | Upper limb malformation always present: hypoplastic or aplastic thumb, to absent radius. Cervical spine deformities frequent |
| **Other anatomical** | | | |
| Bladder exstrophy | None | Not typical, but ductus arteriosus may still be open during first stage repair if performed in first few days of life | Midline structures in lower abdomen fail to fuse Ranges from simple epispadias to cloacal exstrophy exposing bladder and rectum |
| Pentalogy of Cantrell | None | ASD, VSD, ToF | (1) Midline supraumbilical abdominal defect, (2) Sternal defect (3) Diaphragmatic pericardium deficiency (4) Anterior diaphragm deficiency (5) Congenital cardiac disease |

(continued)

**Table 10.1** *(continued)*

| Syndrome | Airway/respiratory concerns | Cardiac disease (incidence, if known) | Other features of note |
|---|---|---|---|
| Prune Belly syndrome | No difficult airway association Lack of abdominal muscles may complicate respiratory function pre- and postoperatively | 10 percent incidence of heart disease: PDA, ASD, VSD, ToF | (1) Abdominal wall muscular deficiency<br>(2) Urinary tract dilatation<br>(3) Cryptorchidism |
| Sturge Weber | Facial deformation may make facemask fit difficult. Possible hemangioma of oro- or posterior pharynx Avoid nasotracheal intubation due to increased vascularity | Cardiac malformations possible including coarctation of the aorta | Neurologic: seizures, intracranial calcifications, arachnoid hemangiomas<br>Skin: hemangiomas (port-wine stain) on the face<br>Eyes: coloboma, glaucoma, enlarged globe with choroidal calcification |
| PHACES | Possible hemangioma in airway Large "plaque-like" facial hemangioma, usually unilateral, in V1 distribution | Cardiac disease in ~1/3 of patients: coarctation of the aorta most common, PDA, ASD, VSD, aberrancies of subclavian artery takeoff | **P**osterior fossa brain malformations<br>**H**emangiomas of face<br>**A**rterial abnormalities<br>**C**ardiac anomalies<br>**E**ye abnormalities<br>**S**ternal clefting or **s**upraumbilical raphe |

**Cardiac malformations**: ASD, atrial septal defect; AV canal, atrioventricular canal; DORV, double outlet right ventricle.; HLHS, hypoplastic left heart syndrome; IAA, interrupted aortic arch; PDA, patent ductus arteriosus; PS, pulmonary stenosis; TA, tricuspid atresia; TGA, transposition of the great arteries; ToF, Tetralogy of Fallot; VSD, ventricular septal defect.
**Other**: DL, direct laryngoscopy; EA, esophageal atresia; ETT, endotracheal tube; GAGs, glycosaminoglycans; ICP, intracranial pressure; NG, nasogastric; TEF, tracheoesophageal fistula; TMJ, temporomandibular joint.

below), make the diagnosis. CD4+ counts, karyotyping, and fluorescent in situ hybridization (FISH) using probes from within the deletion segment are confirmatory. Abnormal migration of neural crest cells in the fourth week of gestation affects the development of the third and fourth pharyngeal pouches, leading to cardiac defects, abnormal or absent thymus, and hypoparathyroidism [6].

*Clinical features:* Neonatal hypocalcemia, cardiac defects, and recurrent infections are the hallmarks of neonatal disease. Hypocalcemia results from parathyroid hypoplasia, and may present as tetany or seizures. Associated cardiac malformations include ToF, type B interrupted aortic arch, truncus arteriosus, double outlet right ventricle, transposition of the great arteries, and ventriculo-septal defects, among others. Immune dysfunction begins in the first six months of life. In up to 60 percent of patients, craniofacial anomalies are present. These include small dysplastic ears, hypertelorism, downward-slanted palpebral fissures, a cupid-bow mouth, cleft palate, midface hypoplasia, micrognathia, and retrognathia. Anomalies of the airway and

esophagus can be associated, such as tracheoesophageal fistula, and laryngo-, tracheo-, or bronchomalacia. Hydronephrosis or nephrocalcinosis can be seen [1,6].

*Anesthetic considerations:* Assess cardiac anatomy and function with echocardiography. Anticipate possible difficult intubation. Check CBC including lymphocyte count, and electrolytes with kidney function; monitor calcium levels throughout the case. Use sterile technique due to immune compromise. If giving blood products, only use CMV-negative, irradiated products (Graft Versus Host Disease [GVHD] can result from donor T-lymphocytes attacking the host's cells; irradiation reduces this risk) [1].

*Pharmacologic and other considerations:* Exercise caution using drugs with renal excretion in the setting of kidney disease; avoid cardio-depressive medications; consider antibiotic prophylaxis needs.

*Further reference:* GeneReviews® – www.ncbi.nlm.nih.gov/books/NBK1523.

**Williams-Beuren Syndrome (WBS; 7q11.23 deletion).** Growth retardation, cardiovascular anomalies, with characteristic facial appearance and personality are features of this hemizygous continuous gene deletion syndrome.

*Incidence:* The incidence of WBS has been estimated at 1:20 000–1:50 000 live births [7,8]. Prevalence estimates range from 1:7500–1:20 000 [9].

*Diagnosis:* A contiguous deletion within the Williams Beuren syndrome critical region (WBSCR), which includes the elastin gene, is present in 99 percent of individuals with the diagnosis. FISH or deletion/duplication testing can detect this deletion.

*Clinical features:* Distinctive facial features, cardiovascular disease, connective tissue abnormalities, endocrine disorders, and intellectual disability (mild) are hallmarks of the disease. The characteristic "elfin facies" includes a broad forehead, short nose with a broad tip, a wide mouth with full lips, and large cheeks. Mandibular hypoplasia and dental abnormalities may be present. Elastin arteriopathy underlies cardiovascular disease; supravalvular aortic stenosis (SVAS), peripheral pulmonary stenosis, coronary disease, mitral valve prolapse, coarctation of the aorta, and patent ductus arteriosus have been reported. Intracardiac lesions such as ToF and ventricular septal defects also occur. Connective tissue abnormalities that might be present in the neonate include hoarse voice/cry, inguinal and umbilical hernias, plus joint and skin laxity. Hypercalcemia is common in the neonate, which can lead to nephrocalcinosis [10].

*Anesthetic considerations:* Patients with WBS have an increased risk of cardiac arrest and sudden death under anesthesia. The incidence of sudden death in WBS (due to all causes), has been estimated at 1/1000 patient-years [11]. It has also been noted that such arrests tend to be refractory to resuscitation [12]. Obtain an ECG and ECHO prior to providing an anesthetic. However, it appears that the severity of SVAS is not a predictor of sudden death [13]. Check for hypercalcemia and manage if present. The anesthetic plan should anticipate a possible difficult airway due to dental abnormalities and mandibular hypoplasia [1].

*Other:* The WBSCR is near the gene for the L-type voltage gated calcium channel alpha-2/delta subunit 7q11.23-q21.1 that has been implicated in some forms of malignant hyperthermia (MH) susceptibility. There is one case report of a child developing masseter spasm with halothane without progression to MH, and another report of a child developing an elevated temperature and creatinine phosphokinase (CPK) after general anesthetic with sevoflurane, $N_2O$, and oxygen, that resolved 12 hours after the anesthetic. It is probably best to avoid succinylcholine and be alert to signs of MH if using volatile agents [1].

*Further reference:* GeneReviews® – www.ncbi.nlm.nih.gov/books/NBK1249.

**CHARGE:** A syndrome with multiple features due to a mutation in CHD7, at locus 8q12, with autosomal dominant inheritance.

*Incidence:* 1:13 000–1:15 000 live births [1].

*Diagnosis:* The definitive diagnosis of CHARGE syndrome requires having all four major features or three major and three minor features (see below).

*Clinical features:* CHARGE is an acronym for **c**oloboma, **h**eart defects, choanal **a**tresia, **r**etarded growth and development, **g**enital abnormalities, **e**ar anomalies.

Major features: coloboma, choanal atresia or stenosis, cranial nerve dysfunction or anomaly (CN I and VIII particularly frequent), and characteristic ear.

Minor features: genital hypoplasia, developmental delay, cardiovascular malformation (present in 75–85 percent), growth deficiency, orofacial cleft, tracheoesophageal fistula (15–20 percent), distinctive facial features.

Cardiac malformations include atrioventricular canal defects, conotruncal defects (e.g., ToF), aortic arch anomalies, hypoplastic left heart syndrome, and patent ductus arteriosus. Facial features include square face with broad forehead, prominent nasal bridge, flat midface, midface hypoplasia, and micrognathia. Tracheomalacia and subglottic stenosis are occasionally seen.

*Anesthetic considerations:* Choanal atresia is bilateral in 50 percent of cases and these neonates, as obligate nasal breathers, may present to the operating room for stent placement. Define cardiac anatomy with echocardiography. Anticipate possible difficult mask ventilation and intubation due to micrognathia, midface hypoplasia, and cleft lip and palate. A smaller ETT may be required if subglottic stenosis is present. Patients with CHARGE are at high risk for aspiration due to CN IX and X anomalies ± presence of tracheoesophageal fistulae. The risk of a difficult airway must be weighed against the possibility of aspiration for each patient.

*Other:* If a difficult airway is expected, only give muscle relaxants once the airway is secured. Check if subacute bacterial endocarditis prophylaxis is indicated.

*Further reference:* GeneReviews® – www.ncbi.nlm.nih.gov/books/NBK1117 and http://ghr.nlm.nih.gov/condition/charge-syndrome.

**Noonan syndrome:** A genetic syndrome characterized by short stature, congenital heart defects, and developmental delay. Several genes are implicated: *PTPN11*, *SOS1*, *RAF1*, and *KRAS* to name the most common.

*Incidence:* 1:1000–1:2500 live births. Females and males are equally affected [1].

*Diagnosis:* The clinical diagnosis is based on the presence of key features. A variety of single gene mutations have been reported in affected individuals, the most common being a mutation in *PTPN11* in 50 percent of cases. It has been called "Turner-like syndrome" though the karyotype in Noonan's syndrome is normal [14].

*Clinical features:* Short stature, congenital heart defects, and developmental delay are characteristic. Other important features include broad/webbed neck, abnormal chest shape with pectus carinatum and excavatum, low-set nipples, cryptorchidism in males, characteristic facies (most apparent in newborns and children) include low-set posteriorly rotated ears, vivid blue/green irises, wide-set eyes, epicanthal folds, thick eyelids. Coagulation defects may also be present. The most common cardiac anomalies include pulmonary stenosis, hypertrophic cardiomyopathy, atrial septal defect, ToF, atrioventricular canal defects, and coarctation of the aorta [1]. It has been reported that many patients with Noonan syndrome have a history of abnormal bruising or bleeding. A recent case series of patients with *PTPN11* mutations, however, suggests that the rates of actual coagulopathy are lower than initially thought [15].

*Anesthetic considerations:* Carefully evaluate for the potentially difficult airway, cervical spine instability, and cardiac abnormalities. A history of abnormal bleeding should be sought and first-line coagulation studies should be obtained.

*Other:* There are reports that isoflurane can cause tachycardia. Noonan-like features in infancy are seen in King Denborough syndrome (an MH-susceptible disorder) [1].

*Further reference:* GeneReviews® – www.ncbi.nlm.nih.gov/books/NBK1124.

# Congenital Endocrine Disorders

**Beckwith-Wiedemann Syndrome.** A syndrome of macroglossia, hypoglycemia, and gigantism due to hyperinsulinemia.

*Incidence:* 1.5:100 000 live births in most of the world. 1:13 700 live births in the West Indies [1].

*Diagnosis:* Molecular genetic testing is used to identify genomic and epigenetic changes at chromosome 11p15. Clinical features are often used to make a provisional diagnosis (see below). Major findings are common in BWS and uncommon in the general population, while minor findings are found in both BWS and the general population.

*Clinical features:* Major findings (selection): macrosomia (height and weight >97th percentile); macroglossia (98 percent); anterior linear ear lobe crease/posterior ear pits; omphalocele/umbilical hernia; visceromegaly involving one or more organs including liver, spleen, kidneys, adrenal glands, and pancreas; embryonal tumor (e.g., Wilms tumor, hepatoblastoma, neuroblastoma, rhabdomyosarcoma); hemihyperplasia (asymmetric growth of one or more body regions); cytomegaly of the fetal adrenal cortex; renal abnormalities; and cardiomegaly.

*Minor findings:* Pregnancy-related findings (polyhydramnios, prematurity), neonatal hypoglycemia, facial nevus flammeus, characteristic facies, and structural cardiac anomalies [16].

*Anesthetic considerations:* Check for hypoglycemia and correct if present, continue to monitor glucose throughout perioperative period. Anticipate possible difficult intubation due to large tongue and maxillary hypoplasia; have fiberoptic bronchoscope available. Echocardiography if concerns about heart disease [1].

*Further reference*: GeneReviews® – www.ncbi.nlm.nih.gov/books/NBK1394.

# Inborn Errors of Metabolism

**Mitochondrial Disorders.** Please refer to the table and separate chapter by Hsieh and Morgan on mitochondrial diseases (Chapter 11).

**Mucopolysaccharidoses (MPS).** The mucopolysaccharidoses are a heterogeneous group of disorders in which defects in lysosomal enzyme activity lead to accumulation of glycosaminoglycans (GAGs) – long unbranched polysaccharides. The phenotypes vary based upon the specific enzyme affected and the tissues in which GAGs are deposited.

*Incidence:* There are seven distinct forms of MPS resulting from 11 known enzymatic deficiencies, with an overall incidence of >1/25 000 live births. In the United States it is estimated that about 200 babies are born with a form of MPS each year [17].

*Diagnosis:* While clinical features (below) are suggestive, MPS diagnosis requires laboratory testing. MPS is commonly diagnosed using dye spectrometric tests of urine samples to detect partially degraded GAGs or oligosaccharides, with subsequent assays for particular enzyme activity in serum, white blood cells, or skin fibroblasts. Genetic inheritance is autosomal recessive except for MPS-II Hunter syndrome, which is transmitted in an X-linked fashion [18]. Prenatal diagnosis is also possible via amniocentesis or chorionic villus sampling.

*Clinical features:* Clinical features vary by specific form. General features include: coarse facial features, macrocephaly, premature closure of saggital and metopic sutures, wide mouth, protuberant tongue, short neck, stiff rib cage with pectus deformity, joint contractures and stiffness, possible atlantoaxial instability, gibbus deformity of the spine, arteriosclerosis, valve thickening, hepatosplenomegaly, recurrent pulmonary infections, early and accelerated growth followed by growth failure, and mental retardation [1].

Infants typically appear normal at birth. In severe MPS-1, nonspecific symptoms such as umbilical hernia and frequent upper respiratory tract infections may be seen in the first year of life. In general, signs and symptoms develop after age one year [19].

The advent of enzyme replacement therapy and hematopoetic stem cell transplantation (HSCT) is altering the course of the MPS syndromes. Benefits of enzyme replacement therapy may include improved physical functioning, while HSCT may improve neurocognitive status. These therapies remain under investigation [20].

*Anesthetic considerations:* Oral secretions may warrant premedication with glycopyrrolate. Mask ventilation may be difficult due to poor fit (facial features), obstruction from the large tongue, and limited neck range of motion. Anticipate difficult laryngoscopy for the same reasons. Of note, nasal airways may be difficult to place due to narrowing of the choanae due to GAG accumulation, while oral airway placement may also be difficult to place and cause downward displacement of the epiglottis. Have a laryngeal mask airway and a fiberoptic bronchoscope available. A stiff chest wall may render ventilation difficult.

While poor gag reflexes increase risk of aspiration, a careful inhalational induction maintaining spontaneous ventilation ± fiberoptic intubation is probably safest. Intellectual disability and behavioral problems may render patients uncooperative. Use caution with premedication as it may precipitate airway obstruction. If cardiac disease is present, tailor anesthetic accordingly [1].

*Further reference:* GeneReviews® – www.ncbi.nlm .nih.gov/books/NBK1162.

*Names for MPS:*

**MPS I:** Classically considered to have one of three forms: Hurler, Hurler–Scheie, or Schie syndrome. However, since no biochemical differences have been found among them, the recommended classification is as Severe MPS I and Attenuated MPS I [19].

**MPS II:** Hunter syndrome

**MPS III:** San Fillipo syndrome

**MPS IV:** Morquio syndrome

**MPS VI:** Marioteaux–Lamy syndrome

**MPS VII:** Sly syndrome

**MPS VIII:** (no eponym)

# Disorders of Skin, Muscle, and Connective Tissue

**Epidermolysis Bullosa (EB).** A genetic disorder resulting in blistering of the skin and mucosal surfaces following minor trauma. Three primary subtypes are **junctional EB, EB simplex, and dystrophic EB.**

*Incidence:* Varies by country and subtype. Highest rates are in the United States (1:12 500) and United Kingdom (1:17 000), while much less common in Canada (1:300 000) [1].

*Diagnosis:* Initially made upon clinical features of blistering ± scarring following minor skin or mucosal trauma. A skin biopsy is necessary to distinguish among subtypes. In addition, molecular genetic testing is available.

*Clinical features:* Extremely sensitive skin, particularly to friction and shearing forces, results in blistering. "Pseudosyndactyly" can occur from scarring and joint contractures are seen. Damage to the oral and nasal mucosae can cause narrowing of these passages, and esophageal strictures may develop. Eyelid retraction can lead to corneal abrasions.

**Junctional EB, Herlitz-Type.** This is the most common form of junctional EB and can be life-threatening in young children. Skin infections can lead to sepsis, respiratory infections and distress can occur and death can result before the age of two.

**EB Simplex, Downing-Mara Type.** This has a wide range of clinical symptoms. Early neonatal death can be seen in the severe form. Blisters may be hemorrhagic. Oral and laryngeal involvement affects respiration and feeding.

**EB Simplex.** This can occur with **extracutaneous manifestations**, including pyloric atresia or muscular dystrophy [1].

*Anesthetic considerations:* Preoperative evaluation should include a complete blood count to look for anemia, and renal function if there is concern for kidney involvement (dystrophic EB). Careful airway evaluation and planning for IV access is important. Most importantly, management is with a "no-touch" technique as much as possible to reduce blistering. Use monitors without adhesive and place Vaseline gauze between skin and the BP cuff. Vaseline on the facemask, a lubricated laryngoscope and ETT, and an ETT securing system that avoids adhesive are recommended precautions. The IV cannula should also be secured with Vaseline gauze padding and a light dressing. Anticipate possible difficult airway and realize that traumatic intubations may lead to blistering in the airway. A half-size smaller ETT than usual may be warranted. LMAs can be used if well-lubricated. Regional anesthesia may be safe if the skin at the injection site is unaffected. Sterile technique is mandatory due to increased risk of skin infections. Surgical preparation should be performed with a spray technique rather than rubbing.

*Other*: There are reports of sensitivity to nondepolarizing neuromuscular blockers. If muscular dystrophy present, avoid succinylcholine. Consider an anticholinergic to reduce oral secretions [1].

*Further reference:* GeneReviews®:

EB simplex www.ncbi.nlm.nih.gov/books/NBK1369;
junctional EB www.ncbi.nlm.nih.gov/books/
    NBK1125;
dystrophic EB www.ncbi.nlm.nih.gov/books/
    NBK1304;
EB with pyloric atresia www.ncbi.nlm.nih.gov/books/
    NBK1157.

**Central Core Disease (CCD).** A congenital myopathy with high susceptibility to malignant hyperthermia

*Incidence:* The incidence of all congenital myopathies is 6/100 000 live births, and CCD is probably the most common myopathy (estimated at ~ 15 percent) [1,21].

*Diagnosis:* Muscle biopsy reveals a central core of low staining for enzyme activity within a transverse section of muscle fiber. MH susceptibility is determined by halothane–caffeine contraction testing.

*Clinical features:* In infancy, CCD presents with hypotonia and delayed achievement of motor milestones. There may even have been reports of decreased fetal movement in utero. In other cases, it presents as a progressive limb-girdle syndrome in adolescence. Associated skeletal abnormalities may include hip and patellar dislocation, kyphoscoliosis, and abnormalities of the feet. Mandibular hypoplasia has been reported.

*Anesthetic considerations:* Evaluate for cardiac dysfunction (mitral valve prolapse, systolic or diastolic dysfunction), and respiratory function. Blood work should include electrolytes and CPK. Because of MH susceptibility, these patients should receive a non-triggering anesthetic. Refer to your institution's guidelines and MHAUS for MH precautions. Regional anesthesia, if appropriate, is a good option. Nitrous oxide can be safely used to help facilitate IV placement. Evaluate for possible difficult airway if mandibular hypoplasia present and position carefully if joint contractures are present [1].

*Other:* Avoid succinylcholine and volatile anesthetics. Consider if subacute bacterial endocarditis (SBE) prophylaxis if indicated.

# Skeletal/Musculoskeletal

**Arthrogryposis.** Arthrogryposis describes the condition of having multiple congenital contractures affecting two or more parts of the body.

*Incidence:* Arthrogryposis is a feature of several disorders. The incidence is estimated at 1 in 3000 live births [22].

*Diagnosis:* Clinical features present at birth suggest the diagnosis. Differentiation among the different types of the disorder may begin with assessment of neurological status. In those with normal neurological function, amyoplasia, distal arthrogryposis, a connective tissue disorder, or fetal crowding may be the cause. Abnormal neurological function suggests a primary neuromuscular cause [22].

*Clinical features:* **Amyoplasia:** internally rotated shoulders, elbows extended, wrists flexed, stiff fingers, dislocated hips, extended knees, and equinovarus contractures of the feet. Midfacial hemangioma in many patients. Intelligence normal. Around 10 percent may have gastrointestinal anomalies such as gastroschisis or intestinal atresia. **Distal arthrogryposes (DA):** hands and feet are primarily affected. In DA type 2, aka Freeman Sheldon syndrome, patients have a very small mouth, puckered lips, scoliosis, in addition to distal contractures. Among forms of arthrogryposis associated with **abnormal neurological function**, there are some associated with myopathies and muscular dystrophies [22].

*Anesthetic considerations:* Anesthetic management can be very challenging due to a potentially difficult airway (small mouth, micrognathia, limited temporomandibular joint (TMJ) motion, atlanto-occipital instability) and difficult venous access. Assess cardiac and respiratory function. In infants, a scalp IV may be a possibility. Have a laryngeal mask and a fiberoptic bronchoscope available [1].

*Other:* There is weak evidence suggesting a link between arthrogryposis and MH: two case reports of hypermetabolism and hyperpyrexia in children with arthrogryposis exist, but of the two the patient that went on to have contracture testing tested negative. It has been suggested that succinylcholine be avoided due to this potential risk of MH and the risk of hyperkalemia in patients with limited mobility [23].

**Klippel Feil.** Congenital fusion of any two cervical vertebrae leading to short neck with limited range of motion and a low hairline. Congenital heart defects and hearing loss are other features.

*Incidence:* Estimated to occur in 1:40 000–1:42 000 births worldwide. Slight female predominance, 65 percent.

*Diagnosis:* Physical exam features and neck radiography determine preliminary diagnosis. Some patients have a mutation in *GDF6* or *GDF3* genes. Genetic locus is 8q22.2.

*Clinical features:* Classically, the triad of short neck, limited range of motion, and low posterior hair line is described. Additional features include other skeletal anomalies (e.g., scoliosis, sacral agenesis), spinal canal stenosis, webbed neck, Sprengel deformity of the scapula, renal and genitourinary anomalies, congenital heart disease (15 percent, particularly ventricular septal defect), and deafness. Cleft palate, malformed laryngeal cartilage, and vocal cord paresis are also common [1].

*Anesthetic considerations:* Careful assessment of the cervical spine and airway is imperative. Document any preexisting neurological abnormalities. Evaluate for cardiac and renal disease. Due to the high risk of spinal cord injury during standard laryngoscopy and intubation, alternatives to general anesthesia necessitating intubation should be considered, if possible. Nasal fiberoptic intubation is the technique of choice, but may be quite challenging in an infant. Consider use of an intubating LMA to provide guidance for a small fiberoptic scope. Neck positioning must be done with extreme care, particularly if the surgery requires turning the patient prone. Extubate fully awake with neck stabilization [1].

*Other:* Consider the use of an antisialagogue prior to induction. Avoid neuromuscular blockade until the airway is secured.

**VACTERL. V**ertebral anomalies, **a**nal atresia, **c**ardiac defects, **t**rach**e**oesophageal fistula (TEF), **r**enal and **l**imb anomalies

*Incidence:* 1:3500–1.6:10 000 live births.

*Diagnosis:* Association of the classic clinical features either on prenatal ultrasound or in the neonatal period.

*Clinical features:* In addition to the most common features listed above, several other defects can be present. These include deformities of the head (e.g., micrognathia), respiratory tract and lung abnormalities (e.g., laryngeal stenosis and lung hypoplasia). The most common cardiac anomalies are ventricular septal defects, patent ductus arteriosus, ToF, transposition of the great arteries. Limb anomalies include humeral hypoplasia, radial aplasia, and polydactyly. Scoliosis and other vertebral anomalies can be seen [1].

*Anesthetic considerations:* Anesthetic implications depend on the surgical procedure and whether a TEF and/or cardiac anomaly is present. Airway management in the presence of TEF should avoid positive pressure mask ventilation due to risk of gastric distention and aspiration. Careful placement of the ETT is mandatory and may involve auscultation over the stomach and bilateral lung fields as well as chest radiography. Bronchoscopy is sometimes done to confirm the site of TEF relative to the carina for endotracheal tube positioning. Anesthetic management and monitoring will also depend on the cardiac anomaly present. Neuraxial anesthesia is generally contraindicated in the presence of vertebral anomalies, unless imaging confirms normal segments and/or position of the conus medullaris (for caudal anesthesia) [24].

*Other:* Consider if SBE prophylaxis is indicated. Manage fluid carefully if renal disease present.

# Craniofacial Disorders

**Craniosynostosis.** Non-syndromic craniosynostosis: 50 percent of cases [1]. Major classes of syndromic craniosynostosis are due to mutations in the Fibroblast Growth Factor Receptor gene:

**FGFR1-related:** Pfeiffer 1,2,3

**FGFR2-related:** Apert, Beare-Stevenson, Crouzon, FGFR2-related isolated coronal synostosis, Jackson-Weiss syndrome.

**FGFR3-related:** Crouzon with aganthosis nigricans, FGFR3-related isolated coronal synostosis (Muenke syndrome)

*Incidence:* Overall 1:2000–1:2500 live births.

*Crouzon* 1:25 000

*Apert* 1:100 000

*Pfeiffer (combined)* 1:100 000 [25].

*Diagnosis:* 6/8 FGFR-related synostosis syndromes can be diagnosed based on clinical findings alone. Muenke syndrome (FGFR3) and FGFR2-related isolated coronal synostosis are diagnosed using molecular genetic tests for disease-causing mutations [26].

*Clinical features:* Characteristic facial features shared by the FGFR-related syndromes (except Muenke and FGFR2-related isolated coronal synostosis) include midface hypoplasia, small nose, hypertelorism, proptosis, and prognathism. In the neonatal period, airway obstruction may result from midface hypoplasia. Patients may have noncommunicating hydrocephalus; the risk of high intracranial pressure (ICP) is greatest in Crouzon syndrome. A Chiari malformation may be congenital or acquired. Even when treated promptly, developmental delay may occur.

Features of Apert syndrome include cervical spine fusion, polysyndactyly of the hands and feet, occasional cardiac and GI malformations, and the highest risk of intellectual disability among the FGFR-related syndromes.

*Anesthetic considerations:* Identify the syndrome (if present) and comorbidities. Evaluate for increased intracranial pressure and tailor anesthetic plan accordingly. Check complete blood count, electrolytes, and coagulation studies prior to craniosynostosis repair.

Type and cross for blood and plasma (adult units). Anticipate difficult airway management, have alternative devices available. Place corneal protectors on eyes. These procedures entail massive blood loss, thus good IV access is essential along with intra-arterial blood pressure monitoring. There are risks of venous air embolism (VAE) throughout many stages of the procedure. Precordial Doppler can facilitate air embolism detection.

*Other:* Consider pre- and intraoperative use of tranexamic acid to reduce operative blood loss [27,28]. Consider dexamethasome to reduce airway and facial edema. Given the risk of VAE, N2O is not recommended. Use caution with neuromuscular blockade until airway is secured.

*Further reference:* GeneReviews® – www.ncbi.nlm .nih.gov/books/NBK1455.

**Robin Sequence.** Micrognathia, glossoptosis, and cleft palate.

*Incidence:* Isolated Robin sequence affects 1:8500–1:14 000 people. Both sexes are equally affected except in an X-linked form [1].

*Diagnosis:* The triad of micrognathia, glossoptosis, and airway obstruction make the diagnosis. Cleft palate may be present. It is termed a sequence because it is thought that mandibular hypoplasia leads to posterior displacement of the tongue, preventing closure of the palate. Robin sequence may have a partial genetic basis with multiple genes contributing to the phenotype. Investigation into causative genes is ongoing [29].

*Clinical features:* The classic triad listed above has implications for other organ systems. Most importantly, these patients are at high risk for airway obstruction and obstructive sleep apnea. This may be managed with prone positioning, a nasopharyngeal airway, mandibular distraction osteogenesis, or tracheostomy. Vagal hyperactivity and dysfunctional neurologic control of breathing may also be present [1].

*Anesthetic considerations:* Robin sequence represents a classic example of the difficult pediatric airway. Obtaining a view with direct laryngoscopy can be quite challenging due to the small chin and posteriorly displaced tongue. Successful techniques described include awake fiberoptic intubation (FOI), FOI through an LMA, video laryngoscopy, and standard direct laryngoscopy, typically with a straight blade [30,31]. Ease of intubation tends to improve as patients get older. It is crucial to establish whether mask ventilation is adequate prior to giving neuromuscular blockers or respiratory depressants. Evaluate for comorbid conditions such as cardiac dysfunction, respiratory infections, and reflux disease. If the patient has had prior anesthetics, these records warrant careful review.

*Other:* Robin sequence occurs as part of a number of other syndromes. Two of note include campomelic dysplasia and Stickler syndrome.

**Treacher Collins Syndrome (TCS).** Treacher Collins syndrome involves craniofacial anomalies including mandibular and zygomatic hypoplasia, large mouth, microtia, downward slanting eyes, and coloboma of the lid.

*Incidence:* 1:10 000 live births [1].

*Diagnosis:* Clinical and radiographic findings suggest the diagnosis. See below for major and minor clinical features. Radiography can demonstrate zygomatic hypoplasia or aplasia, malar hypoplasia, and mandibular retrognathia. Three mutations have been associated with TCS, *TCOF1*, *POLR1D*, *POLR1C*, and can be detected with molecular genetic testing. Individuals with physical signs of TCS may not have mutations in any of these genes, however.

*Clinical features:*

Major features: Hypoplasia of the zygoma and mandible, external ear abnormalities (microtia), lower eyelid abnormalities, family history consistent with autosomal dominant inheritance.

Minor features: External ear abnormalities (stenosis or atresia of external auditory canals), conductive hearing loss, defects of the eye, cleft palate.

The most common manifestations in infants are airway and feeding issues. Other features that may be present include cardiac defects, cervical spine abnormalities, kidney defects, choanal atresia, sleep apnea, early failure to thrive, and cryptorchidism [32].

*Anesthetic considerations:* Infants are at risk for airway obstruction due to choanal atresia or stenosis and micrognathia with glossoptosis. The primary concern is difficult airway management. Fiberoptic intubation and avoidance of neuromuscular blocking agents is recommended until the airway is secured. In contrast to Robin sequence, intubation may become more difficult as patients get older. A tracheostomy may be necessary [1].

*Further reference:* GeneReviews® – www.ncbi.nlm.nih.gov/books/NBK1532.

# References

1. Bissonette B, Luginbuehl I, Marciniak B, Dalens B, editors. *Syndromes: Rapid Recognition and Perioperative Implications.* New York: McGraw-Hill; 2006.

2. Ostermaier K. *Down Syndrome: Clinical Features and Diagnosis.* UpToDate®; 2013.

3. Shott SR. Down syndrome: analysis of airway size and a guide for appropriate intubation. *Laryngoscope.* 2000;110(4):585–92.

4. Shott SR. Down syndrome: common otolaryngologic manifestations. *Am J Med Genet C Semin Med Genet.* 2006;142C(3):131–40.

5. Kraemer FW, Stricker PA, Gurnaney HG, et al. Bradycardia during induction of anesthesia with sevoflurane in children with Down syndrome. *Anesth Analg.* 2010;111(5):1259–63.

6. McDonald-McGinn D, Emanuel B, Zackai E. 22q11.2 deletion syndrome. GeneReviews® 1999, updated 2013.

7. Tassabehji M. Williams–Beuren syndrome: a challenge for genotype–phenotype correlations. *Hum Mol Genet.* 2003;2:R229–37.

8. Schubert C. The genomic basis of the Williams–Beuren syndrome. *Cell Mol Life Sci.* 2009;66(7):1178–97.

9. Strømme P, Bjørnstad PG, Ramstad K. Prevalence estimation of Williams syndrome. *J Child Neurol.* 2002;17(4):269–71.

10. Morris C. Williams Syndrome. GeneReviews®, 1999, updated 2013.

11. Wessel A, Gravenhorst V, Buchhorn R, et al. Risk of sudden death in the Williams–Beuren syndrome. *Am J Med Genet A.* 2004;127A(3):234–7.

12. Gupta P, Tobias JD, Goyal S, et al. Sudden cardiac death under anesthesia in pediatric patient with Williams syndrome: a case report and review of literature. *Ann Card Anaesth.* 2010;13(1):44–8.

13. Bird LM, Billman GF, Lacro RV, et al. Sudden death in Williams syndrome: report of ten cases. *J Pediatr.* 1996;129(6):926–31.

14. Allanson J, Roberts A. Noonan syndrome. GeneReviews®, 2001, updated 2011.

15. Derbent M, Öncel Y, Tokel K, et al. Clinical and hematologic findings in Noonan syndrome patients with PTPN11 gene mutations. *Am J Med Genet A.* 2010;152A(11):2768–74.

16. Shuman C, Beckwith J, Smith A, et al. Beckwith–Wiedemann syndrome. GeneReviews®, 2001, updated 2010.

17. Tomatsu S, Fujii T, Fukushi M, et al. Newborn screening and diagnosis of mucopolysaccharidoses. *Mol Genet Metab.* 2013;110(1–2):42–53.

18. Wraith JE. Mucopolysaccharidoses and mucolipidoses. *Handb Clin Neurol.* 2013;113:1723–9.

19. Clarke L, Heppner J. Mucopolysaccharidosis type I. GeneReviews®, 2002, updated 2011.

20. Valayannopoulos V, Wijburg FA. Therapy for the mucopolysaccharidoses. *Rheumatology (Oxford).* 2011;50(Suppl. 5):v49–59.

21. Jungbluth H. Central core disease. *Orphanet J Rare Dis.* 2007;2:25.

22. Bamshad M, Van Heest AE, Pleasure D. Arthrogryposis: a review and update. *J Bone Joint Surg Am.* 2009;91(Suppl 4):40–6.

23. Benca J, Hogan K. Malignant hyperthermia, coexisting disorders, and enzymopathies: risks and management options. *Anesth Analg.* 2009;109(4):1049–53.

24. Willschke H, Bosenberg A, Marhofer P, et al. Epidural catheter placement in neonates: sonoanatomy and feasibility of ultrasonographic guidance in term and preterm neonates. *Reg Anesth Pain Med.* 2007;32(1):34–40.

25. Derderian C, Seaward J. Syndromic craniosynostosis. *Semin Plast Surg.* 2012;26(2):64–75.

26. Robin N, Falk M, Haldeman-Englert C. FGFR-related craniosynostosis syndromes. GeneReviews®, 1998, updated 2011.

27. Goobie SM, Meier PM, Pereira LM, et al. Efficacy of tranexamic acid in pediatric craniosynostosis surgery: a double-blind, placebo-controlled trial. *Anesthesiology.* 2011;114(4):862–71.

28. Goobie S. The case for the use of tranexamic acid. *Paediatr Anaesth.* 2013;23(3):281–4.

29. Jakobsen LP, Knudsen MA, Lespinasse J, et al. The genetic basis of the Pierre Robin sequence. *Cleft Palate Craniofac J.* 2006;43(2):155–9.

30. Fiadjoe JE, Stricker PA. The air-Q intubating laryngeal airway in neonates with difficult airways. *Paediatr Anaesth.* 2011;21(6):702–3.

31. Marston AP, Lander TA, Tibesar RJ, Sidman JD. Airway management for intubation in newborns with Pierre Robin sequence. *Laryngoscope.* 2012;122(6):1401–4.

32. Katsanis S, Jabs E. Treacher Collins syndrome. GeneReviews®, 2004, updated 2012.

# Myopathies of the Newborn

Vincent Hsieh and Phil G. Morgan

## Introduction

The differential diagnosis of hypotonia in newborns and infants is significantly different from that of older pediatric patients. Core myopathies (central core disease and multiminicore disease), which are considered highly susceptible to malignant hyperthermia (MH), for example, are the most common causes of congenital myopathy, but not of myopathy in older children [1]. Congenital hypotonia may be caused by primary muscle disorders as well as motor neuron disorders, myasthenia gravis, and mitochondrial defects. Pediatric anesthesiologists will require a working understanding of the causes of hypotonia in newborns and infants in order to avoid potentially disastrous consequences and provide the safest possible care [2].

Primary muscle disorders in neonates consist of a heterogeneous group of diseases that can be broadly divided into congenital muscular dystrophies and congenital myopathies [3]. Research in the last two decades has led to identification of hundreds of genetic loci responsible for the molecular basis of neuromuscular disorders [4–6]. While the identification of specific defective proteins has added to our understanding of the pathophysiology of muscle development and the neuromuscular junction, the landscape of muscle disorders in neonates is confusing since there are numerous naming conventions in widespread use. The aim of this chapter is to provide an overview of primary muscle disorders in newborns and infants, as well as the other major causes of hypotonia in this age group. The final part of the chapter summarizes the approach to the anesthetic management of the hypotonic patient.

## Primary Muscle Disorders

Primary muscle disorders presenting in the neonatal period are broadly divided into congenital muscular dystrophies (CMDs) and congenital myopathies (CMs) [3]. In general, the CMDs are characterized by severe disruption of muscle architecture on tissue biopsy, whereas CMs show a relative preservation of muscle cell structure and fiber type proportion.

## Congenital Muscular Dystrophies

Congenital muscular dystrophies are a heterogeneous group of conditions that result from disruption of the structural connection between the contractile elements of the muscle cell (the actin–myosin filaments) and extracellular matrix. These connections are crucial for transducing the contractile force of actin–myosin filaments to the surrounding connective tissue. Loss of this transduction results in muscle weakness, disruption of related elements of the muscle cell, and progressive deterioration of the muscle fiber. CMDs should be considered multi-organ system diseases and often present with significant central nervous system (CNS) involvement. While Duchenne and Becker muscular dystrophies are well-known to most anesthesiologists, the CMDs may seem unfamiliar by comparison.

CMDs are classified by their genetic mutations and resultant biochemical defects. The most well-known are the dystroglycanopathies caused by defects in connective tissue glycoproteins which form the contractile element–extracellular matrix connection described above. Of these, the most familiar is caused by defects in the LAMA2 extracellular matrix protein (primary merosin deficiency) often with profound loss of motor function and some CNS white matter deterioration. Patients with primary merosin deficiency are usually symptomatic at birth with generalized hypotonia, weak cry, respiratory insufficiency, seizures, and sometimes multiple congenital joint contractures (arthrogryposis) [7,8].

Mutations in the POMT1, POMT2, and FCMD glycoproteins are also common (Walker–Warburg syndrome [WWS], Muscle–Eye–Brain [MEB] disease, and Fukuyama CMD, respectively). Walker–Warburg

Syndrome and the less severe MEB disease typically present at birth with hypotonia, lissencephaly, hydrocephalus, cerebellar and retinal dysplasia, arthrogryposis, respiratory insufficiency, and sometimes cleft lip and palate [9]. Patients with WWS rarely live beyond one year. Fukuyama CMD presents with hypotonia and respiratory insufficiency in early infancy along with cerebral and cerebellar dysplasia, hydrocephalus, and seizures. Cardiomyopathy occurs in patients that survive into the second decade of life [10]. An increasingly large group of other genetic defects can cause rare forms of CMD, most of which require similar perioperative considerations as those listed above [3].

The final common form of CMD is myotonic dystrophy type 1 (DM1), which results from an unstable trinucleotide expansion in the DMPK gene on chromosome 19. While there is rough correlation between the number of triplets and earlier age of onset when CTG repeats are less than 400, the congenital phenotype is often characterized by more than 1500 CTG repeats. Prenatal findings often include polyhydramnios and decreased fetal movements. Postnatally, hypotonia and immobility are apparent, as are clubfoot deformities and arthrogryposis. Weakness in the head and neck results in a weak cry, impaired swallowing, and a characteristic triangular open mouth. Respiratory muscle weakness is common and mechanical ventilation is often required for the first weeks of life. Cardiovascular problems are not common in the newborn period, but cardiomyopathy and pulmonary hypertension have been reported [11]. Although DM1 is an autosominal dominant trait, the mother is the transmitting parent in 94 percent of cases because the female locus is more unstable than the male locus [12]. In most cases the mother is unaware of being affected, but detailed examination reveals mild facial weakness and grip myotonia.

Muscular dystrophies associated with older pediatric patients have also been reported in patients younger than one year of age. In particular, limb-girdle muscular dystrophy and Emery–Dreifuss muscular dystrophy have been described in the newborn period, presenting with reduced fetal movements and severe hypotonia at birth [13,14].

# Congenital Myopathies

Congenital myopathies are primary muscle disorders that are typically nonprogressive and characterized

by "nondystrophic" changes on muscle biopsy, i.e., no degeneration of the muscle. Traditionally, CMs are classified by histopathologic staining patterns.

## Nemaline Myopathies

Nemaline (from Greek *nema*, thread) myopathies first took their name from the threadlike structures seen on muscle biopsy specimens. Two forms are seen when the disease presents in the newborn period: classical and severe. In the classical form, infants show generalized weakness involving facial and axial muscles as well as bulbar and feeding difficulties often requiring frequent suctioning and tube feeding. The severe phenotype is characterized by a history of polyhydramnios, severe weakness, arthrogryposis, severe feeding difficulties, and respiratory failure [15]. Serum CPK levels are normal or mildly elevated. No susceptibility to MH is documented in nemaline myopathies. However, as is the case with all myopathies, depolarizing muscle relaxants should be avoided due to the potential for hyperkalemia.

## Central Core Disease

Central core disease (CCD) is one of the most common CMs [1]. With histochemical staining, distinct cores of absent oxidative activity are seen running the length of Type 1 muscle fibers. There is a wide variation in the clinical presentation of CCD, and while weakness may become clinically apparent for most affected individuals during infancy and early childhood, contractures are frequently present at birth (hip dislocation, equinovarus foot deformities). For the majority of patients, there is no bulbar or diaphragmatic weakness. Severely affected patients, however, may present in the neonatal period with scoliosis, arthrogryposis, and facial, bulbar, and respiratory insufficiency [16]. Serum CK levels are normal or mildly elevated [17]. Central core disease is usually inherited in an autosomal dominant fashion and is associated with at least 22 different mutations in the skeletal muscle ryanodine receptor (RyR1). Sporadic mutations and even recessive pedigrees have also been reported [18]. The RyR1 mutations seen in CCD are associated with susceptibility to MH in older patients; however, MH-like responses have not been reported in neonates.

## Multiminicore Disease

Multiminicore Disease (MmD) is a rare autosomal recessively inherited CM. In contrast to CCD, the cores are multiple and indistinct and do not extend the length of the muscle fiber. Four clinical phenotypes have been described: a classical form with predominantly axial muscle weakness progressing to scoliosis; a moderate form with generalized muscle weakness affecting the pelvic girdle and hand involvement; a classical form with external ophthalmoplegia; and an antenatal onset form with arthrogryposis. Both the moderate and external ophthalmoplegia forms are associated with an RyR1 mutation, whereas other forms are associated with mutations in SEPN1 and ACTA1. Malignant hyperthermia has been reported only in MmD with RyR1 mutations, unlike with the other forms of MmD; nonetheless, some authors have advised caution in using volatile anesthetics in all patients with the disease [17,19].

### Centronuclear Myopathy

Histochemical staining in centronuclear (myotubular) myopathy demonstrates a characteristic pattern of numerous centrally placed nuclei with a surrounding zone of absent oxidative enzyme activity. Like other CMs, there is a high degree of variability in clinical phenotype. The most severe neonatal form follows an X-linked mode of inheritance and presents with marked hypotonia, respiratory failure, dysphagia and undescended testes, whereas the autosomal recessive forms are more variable, ranging from significant weakness and inability to walk to milder phenotype with presentation in later childhood. Centronuclear myopathy is not associated with MH [20].

## Motor Neuron Disorders

## Spinal Muscular Atrophy

Spinal muscular atrophy (SMA) is a relatively common autosomal recessive progressive degenerative disease affecting motor neurons of the anterior spine and brainstem. SMA is the result of mutations in the protein survival motor neuron 1 (SMN1). The function of SMN1 is unclear, although it is thought to have an anti-apoptotic role specifically in motor neurons. The classification of SMA is based on age of onset and severity of symptoms. Type 1 SMA, also known as Werdnig–Hoffman disease, presents at birth to six months of age with sudden-onset axial and proximal limb weakness without facial weakness. Intercostal muscles are severely affected, but the diaphragm is spared. As a result, the chest assumes a characteristic

bell-shaped appearance, but overt respiratory failure usually does not occur in infancy. Bulbar weakness is a classic feature, which results in difficulty swallowing and pooling of secretions in the hypopharynx. Infants with SMA are prone to recurrent respiratory infections and are rarely expected to survive beyond two years of age without tracheostomy placement. Type 2 SMA presents at 6–18 months of age and is less severe than Type 1. Type 3 presents in later childhood and has the slowest progression of disease. Cardiac malformations such as hypoplastic left heart and atrial and ventricular septal defects have been reported in babies with SMA Type 1. Pulmonary complications are the leading cause of anesthetic mortality and morbidity in SMA Types 1 and 2. In addition to the classical SMA Types 1–3, a more profound form of the disease has been more recently described. Type 0 SMA presents prenatally and requires mechanical ventilation immediately at birth [21,22]. The anesthetic approach to these patients must be individualized depending on the severity of the disease, although succinylcholine should be avoided to prevent hyperkalemia [23].

## Diaphragmatic Spinal Muscular Atrophy

Diaphragmatic SMA, also known as spinal muscular atrophy with respiratory distress (SMARD), has features in common with SMA but with additional diaphragmatic weakness. SMARD therefore presents in infancy with life-threatening respiratory failure. Unlike with SMA, the distal rather than proximal muscles tend to be affected in SMARD. Mutations in the gene encoding immunoglobulin-binding protein 2 are responsible for the disease.

## Pontocerebellar Hypoplasia

Pontocerebellar hypoplasia is a progressive degenerative disease of motor neurons as well as neurons of the brainstem and cerebellum. Like SMA, respiratory and feeding difficulties may be present at birth or in early infancy.

## Myasthenia Gravis

## Transient Neonatal Myasthenia

Transient neonatal myasthenia is a phenomenon occurring in 20 percent of infants born to mothers with myasthenia gravis and is the result of placental transfer of acetylcholinesterase receptor antibody. The severity of maternal myasthenia gravis does not correlate to severity of neonatal signs and symptoms, and the disease is sometimes seen in babies born to undiagnosed mothers with subclinical myasthenia. Transient neonatal myasthenia presents at birth or within the first three days of life with generalized hypotonia and weakness including facial involvement. The diagnosis is confirmed by administration of anticholinesterase. Ventilatory and nutritional support may be needed until spontaneous recovery occurs by 2–4 months. Symptomatic infants may be given scheduled pyridostigmine until symptoms resolve [24].

Rarely, other forms of neonatal myasthenia present and are the result of genetic defects in neuromuscular transmission (e.g., decreased or dysfunctional acetylcholine receptors, defective acetylcholine recycling, abnormalities in synapse formation). These forms of disease are difficult to treat and may present with arthrogryposis and profound weakness in all muscle groups.

## Glycogen Storage Diseases

Glycogen storage diseases are generally thought to appear later in childhood; however, the severe forms listed below can present during the neonatal period and even prenatally.

## Infantile Glycogen Storage Disease Type II (GSD II, Pompe Disease)

Pompe disease (also known as infantile acid maltase deficiency) can manifest in the first weeks or months of life with diffuse hypotonia and weakness, giving these infants an extremely hypotonic appearance (floppy baby or rag doll syndrome) [25]. The early onset of the infantile form compared to forms appearing later in childhood is likely due to less residual enzyme activity. Cardiomegaly is often pronounced and there is progression of respiratory insufficiency due to hypotonia. Of importance, there is a neurogenic component to the weakness with motor neuron involvement. Apparent muscle bulk may be increased, however, and macroglossia, along with pharyngeal muscle weakness, predisposes the patient to upper airway obstruction. Fortunately, the prognosis for this disease has greatly improved in the last decade with enzyme replacement therapy.

## Glycogen Storage Disease Type IV (GSD IV, Branching Enzyme Deficiency, Andersen Disease)

This defect can also present in infancy and is termed fatal infantile GSD IV (a fetal version also occurs and is a more severe form than the infantile version) [25]. The infantile version is characterized by hypotonia, muscle and neuronal involvement, cardiomyopathy and, often, early death. However, occasional patients survive into childhood and may be seen by the anesthesiologist. At present, there is no effective therapy for this defect.

## Mitochondrial Myopathies

Mitochondrial myopathies are (as their name implies) caused by abnormalities in mitochondrial function. Mitochondria are the principal source of energy metabolism within cells and have critical effects on anesthetic management [26]. Within mitochondria reside the enzymes responsible for the Krebs cycle, fatty acid β-oxidation, and, most importantly, oxidative phosphorylation. Since mitochondria are important for supplying ATP in most tissues (most importantly nerve and muscle), the symptoms usually include myopathy and cardiomyopathy, and in the nervous system encephalopathy, seizures, and developmental delay. Mitochondria are also important in triggering cell death, or apoptosis, thus mitochondrial diseases may also lead to other organ dysfunction via this mechanism as well.

Cells are also able to use glucose to generate ATP by use of glycolysis without involvement of the mitochondria. Restriction of energy production to glycolysis is an anaerobic process and postnatally often leads to lactic acidosis. However, in utero, in the presence of low oxygen tension, most ATP is normally generated by glycolysis, which explains why many infants with severe mitochondrial defects do well until birth. The resulting lactate is then removed by the maternal circulation. In fact, fetal demise is not noted as a common component of mitochondrial disease in multiple reviews of neonatal disease. Other than glycolysis, all other energy-producing substrates (further oxidation of the glucose product pyruvate, fatty acids, amino acids) require the mitochondrion for their effective use. Inhibition of any of these metabolic pathways will lead to chemical derangements, often with profound effects. In general, mitochondrial defects can be recognized by increases in lactate or pyruvate, increases in systemic acylcarnitines, or altered amounts of amino acids. Generally, a metabolic abnormality in a patient with a myopathy or encephalopathy should raise the possibility of a mitochondrial defect. Great care must be taken to account for these defects when caring for these patients in the operative or perioperative period since the abnormal metabolite may be partially causative for the disease symptoms (e.g., acidosis).

The more commonly seen neonatal mitochondrial syndromes are *Leigh disease, Kearns–Sayre syndrome,* and *Leber hereditary optic neuropathy.* Much has been written about the presentation of mitochondrial disease in children and adults; however, little has been presented about mitochondrial disease prenatally or in the neonate. Prenatal presentations were discussed in 2003 by von Kleist-Retzow et al. [27]. Generally the authors noted intrauterine growth retardation and a variety of developmental abnormalities. A recent review reported on the neonatal presentation of 32 infants with mitochondrial disease, diagnosed as Leigh-like syndrome (encephalopathy with brainstem involvement), mitochondrial cytopathy, or lethal infantile mitochondrial disease [28]. The most common symptoms were poor feeding, recurrent vomiting, and failure to thrive with a lactic acidosis. Common clinical signs including encephalomyopathy, hepatopathy, intestinal dysmotility and cardiomyopathy were accompanied by an extremely high mortality regardless of presentation [28,29]. Twenty-seven of the neonates with documented disease had defects in the electron transport chain, while the others had various other enzymatic deficiencies. The most common of the other deficiencies was a defect in the DNA polymerase, POLG, which was associated with a hepatopathy.

Complex I is the largest component of the electron transport chain, consisting of at least 45 protein subunits, and represents the most common type of mitochondrial defect in the neonatal period [30]. Distelmaier et al. found the clinical presentation of newborns with complex I disease to include profound hypotonia, respiratory failure, seizures, and neurologic regression (consistent with early-onset Leigh disease) and notable in that there was generally no prenatal disease [31]. Similarly, defects in Coenzyme Q synthesis may cause multisystemic disease in the neonatal period, often accompanied by nephrosis [32,33]. Defects in other complexes can also cause

neonatal disease, but the presentations are similar to those for complex I defects.

It is a common mistake to regard all mitochondrial diseases as a singular entity. Even family members carrying the identical mitochondrial gene mutation may present with dramatically different symptomatology. Because of this variability, it is dangerous to imply that, because an anesthetic technique was successful in a few patients with mitochondrial disease, it is safe for all patients with mitochondrial dysfunction. Since motor neurons may be affected, a hyperkalemic response to succinylcholine may be seen. Lastly, although MH is occasionally reported to be associated with some forms of mitochondrial myopathies, at present there is no documentation of a causal relationship [34,35].

## Anesthetic Considerations

The anesthetic management of newborns and infants with congenital myopathy begins with the usual considerations for hypotonic patients in this age group. Nondepolarizing muscle relaxants should be omitted or used sparingly, and elective use of succinylcholine should be avoided entirely. Some additional specific points should also be raised. The first is that many of these children will have metabolic abnormalities that result in increased dependence on normal intravascular volume and on normal serum glucose levels. Fluids should therefore be managed closely by minimizing NPO times and providing continuous dextrose-containing IV fluids intraoperatively. Monitoring of serum glucose intra- and postoperatively is encouraged.

For a review of other perioperative considerations for the infant or child with undiagnosed muscle disease, the reader is referred to the practical approach discussed by Brandom and Veyckemans [36]. In particular, these authors (and others) emphasize the importance of evaluating these patients preoperatively to determine if their hypotonia is more consistent with a primary muscle disorder versus a mitochondrial myopathy. Elevated CK values are most consistent with a dystrophic disease and make the use of volatile agents less desirable. If, on the other hand, lactate, pyruvate, or acylcarnitines are elevated, a mitochondrial disease is more likely and a propofol-based anesthetic is less favored. At the present time, there is no evidence that a brief induction with a volatile agent is contraindicated, even in cases more likely to have a dystrophic pathology. Given the uncertainty of choice between non-triggering agents and volatile anesthetics, intraoperative monitoring for acidosis is also recommended.

Compared to myopathies in older children, there is an increased likelihood of MH-associated myopathies in neonates and infants. However, this is coupled with a paucity of reports of MH in infants, particularly under two months of age. Given the lack of case reports in this age group, neonates and infants under two months of age may have an inherently lower susceptibility to MH. As a result, we really do not know at what developmental point a neonate becomes susceptible to MH. If one is relatively certain that a neonate has a core myopathy, then it seems prudent to avoid volatile agents to the extent possible. On the other hand, most physicians who treat patients with mitochondrial disorders tend to avoid propofol, and such an approach would seem wise if that diagnosis is more likely. Narcotics, regional analgesia, dexmedetomidine, and ketamine have all been used successfully in both groups and are excellent primary anesthetics or additions when appropriate [26].

# References

1. Amburgey K, McNamara N, Bennett LR, et al. Prevalence of congenital myopathies in a representative pediatric United States population. *Ann Neurol*. 2011;70(4):662–5.

2. Kinder Ross A. Muscular dystrophy versus mitochondrial myopathy: the dilemma of the undiagnosed hypotonic child. *Paediatr Anaesth*. 2007;17:1–6.

3. Bonnemann CG, Wang CH, Quijano-Roy S, et al. Diagnostic approach to the congenital muscular dystrophies. *Neuromuscul Disord*. 2014;24(4):289–311.

4. Bharucha-Goebel DX, Santi M, Medne L, et al. Severe congenital RYR1-associated myopathy: the expanding clinicopathologic and genetic spectrum. *Neurology*. 2013;80(17):1584–9.

5. Shieh PB. Muscular dystrophies and other genetic myopathies. *Neurol Clin*. 2013;31(4):1009–29.

6. Laing NG. Genetics of neuromuscular disorders. *Crit Rev Clin Lab Sci*. 2012;49(2):33–48.

7. Scrivener TA, Ross SM, Street NE, Webster RI, De Lima JC. A case series of general anesthesia in children with laminin alpha2 (merosin)-deficient congenital muscular dystrophy. *Paediatr Anaesth*. 2014;24(4):464–5.

8. Online Mendelian Inheritance in Man. Muscular dystrophy, congenital merosin-deficient, 1A, 2003 Available at: www.omim.org/entry/607855.

9. Online Mendelian Inheritance in Man. Muscular dystrophy-dystroglycanopathy (congenital with brain and eye anomalies), Type A, 1, 1986 Available at: www.omim.org/entry/236670.

10. Online Mendelian Inheritance in Man. Muscular dystrophy-dystroglycanopathy (congenital with brain and eye anomalies), Type A, 4, 1986. Available at: www.omim.org/entry/253800.

11. Schara U, Schoser BG. Myotonic dystrophies type 1 and 2: a summary on current aspects. *Semin Pediatr Neurol*. 2006;13(2):71–9.

12. Mulley JC, Staples A, Donnelly A, et al. Explanation for exclusive maternal origin for congenital form of myotonic dystrophy. *Lancet*. 1993;341(8839):236–7.

13. Quijano-Roy S, Mbieleu B, Bonnemann CG, et al. De novo LMNA mutations cause a new form of congenital muscular dystrophy. *Ann Neurol*. 2008;64(2):177–86.

14. Mercuri E, Poppe M, Quinlivan R, et al. Extreme variability of phenotype in patients with an identical missense mutation in the lamin A/C gene: from congenital onset with severe phenotype to milder classic Emery–Dreifuss variant. *Arch Neurol*. 2004;61(5):690–4.

15. North KN, Laing NG, Wallgren-Pettersson C. Nemaline myopathy: current concepts. The ENMC International Consortium and Nemaline Myopathy. *J Med Genet*. 1997;34(9):705–13.

16. Jungbluth H, Sewry CA, Muntoni F. Core myopathies. *Semin Pediatr Neurol*. 2011;18(4):239–49.

17. Klingler W, Rueffert H, Lehmann-Horn F, Girard T, Hopkins PM. Core myopathies and risk of malignant hyperthermia. *Anesth Analg*. 2009;109(4):1167–73.

18. Jungbluth H, Muller CR, Halliger-Keller B, et al. Autosomal recessive inheritance of RYR1 mutations in a congenital myopathy with cores. *Neurology*. 2002;59(2):284–7.

19. Brislin RP, Theroux MC. Core myopathies and malignant hyperthermia susceptibility: a review. *Paediatr Anaesth*. 2013;23(9):834–41.

20. Jungbluth H, Wallgren-Pettersson C, Laporte J. Centronuclear (myotubular) myopathy. *Orphanet J Rare Dis*. 2008;3:26.

21. MacLeod MJ, Taylor JE, Lunt PW, Mathew CG, Robb SA. Prenatal onset spinal muscular atrophy. *Eur J Paediatr Neurol*. 1999;3(2):65–72.

22. D'Amico A, Mercuri E, Tiziano FD, Bertini E. Spinal muscular atrophy. *Orphanet J Rare Dis*. 2011;6:71.

23. Islander G. Anesthesia and spinal muscle atrophy. *Paediatr Anaesth*. 2013;23(9):804–16.

24. Papazian O. Transient neonatal myasthenia gravis. *J Child Neurol.* 1992;7(2):135–41.

25. Dimauro S, Garone C. Metabolic disorders of fetal life: glycogenoses and mitochondrial defects of the mitochondrial respiratory chain. *Semin Fetal Neonatal Med.* 2011;16(4):181–9.

26. Niezgoda J, Morgan PG. Anesthetic considerations in patients with mitochondrial defects. *Paediatr Anaesth.* 2013;23(9):785–93.

27. von Kleist-Retzow JC, Cormier-Daire V, Viot G, et al. Antenatal manifestations of mitochondrial respiratory chain deficiency. *J Pediatr.* 2003;143(2):208–12.

28. Gibson K, Halliday JL, Kirby DM, et al. Mitochondrial oxidative phosphorylation disorders presenting in neonates: clinical manifestations and enzymatic and molecular diagnoses. *Pediatrics.* 2008;122(5):1003–8.

29. Uziel G, Ghezzi D, Zeviani M. Infantile mitochondrial encephalopathy. *Semin Fetal Neonatal Med.* 2011;16(4):205–15.

30. Fassone E, Rahman, S. Complex I deficiency: clinical features, biochemistry and molecular genetics. *J Med Genet.* 2014;49:578–90.

31. Distelmaier F, Koopman WJ, van den Heuvel LP, et al. Mitochondrial complex I deficiency: from organelle dysfunction to clinical disease. *Brain.* 2009;132(Pt 4):833–42.

32. Jakobs BS, van den Heuvel LP, Smeets RJ, et al. A novel mutation in COQ2 leading to fatal infantile multisystem disease. *J Neurol Sci.* 2013;326(1–2):24–8.

33. Falk MJ, Polyak E, Zhang Z, et al. Probucol ameliorates renal and metabolic sequelae of primary CoQ deficiency in Pdss2 mutant mice. *EMBO Mol Med.* 2011;3(7):410–27.

34. Fricker RM, Raffelsberger T, Rauch-Shorny S, et al. Positive malignant hyperthermia susceptibility in vitro test in a patient with mitochondrial myopathy and myoadenylate deaminase deficiency. *Anesthesiol.* 2002;97(6):1635–7.

35. Keyes MA, Van de Wiele BV, Stead SW. Mitochondrial myopathies: an unusual cause of hypotonia in infants and children. *Paediatr Anaesth.* 1996;6(4):329–35.

36. Brandom BW, Veyckemans F. Neuromuscular diseases in children: a practical approach. *Paediatr Anaesth.* 2013;23(9):765–9.

Chapter

**12**

# Preoperative Preparation

Lynne R. Ferrari

## Preoperative Evaluation

The objective of the preoperative evaluation of the pediatric surgical patient is to assess current clinical status and alleviate fear and anxiety of the child and family. The process of anesthetizing an infant or child and the associated risks must be demystified during the preoperative visit since parents often have more anxiety about their child undergoing anesthesia than they do for themselves. The preoperative visit is an opportunity for the anesthesiologist to evaluate the child's psychological status and family interactions. It has been demonstrated that parental anxiety surrounding anesthesia is highest when surgery is scheduled for infants less than one year of age and is the child's first surgical experience [1].

## Psychosocial Preparations of the Family

Anesthesiologists and other healthcare professionals who treat children face the unique challenge of caring for two patients at once. As a result of the child's dependence, the child and parent become the patient–parent dyad. The psychological differences between children and adults are well known, and in recent years it has also been well documented that differences are seen in the emotional and cognitive development of the child as compared to that of an adult. Since reasoning skills have not yet matured in children, the understanding of and response to illness is affected. Communication skills are not highly developed either, therefore the medical practitioner is required to anticipate the child's needs and concerns and be able to interpret nonverbal expressions and actions [2].

The anesthesiologist must offer advice, support, and reassurance on two levels and must not only be aware and sensitive to the child's needs, but must also be able to support the parent's need for information that will enable them to remain a strong advocate for their child throughout the medical system. For most parents, the prospect of their child's impending hospitalization is more frightening than almost anything else. Perioperative anxiety is greatest for parents of infants between the ages of 0–6 months. Factors that influence parental anxiety include the age of the child, previous surgery in the patient or a sibling, parental gender, highest level of education obtained by the parent and preoperative discussion. Interestingly, these factors were more significant for mothers when parents were assessed by gender [3].

As infants begin to differentiate their primary caregivers from others, they develop a previously absent wariness of strangers. This change begins to occur at approximately eight months of age, whereas infants younger than this will usually separate easily from their primary caregiver. A discussion of the infant's behavior and the presence of stranger anxiety should be included in the preoperative interview so that the anesthesiologist may obtain a sense of how easily the infant will separate from the parent and how anxious the parent is. Prior to the onset of stranger anxiety in an infant, parental presence is not required or advisable during the induction of anesthesia; therefore parents of young infants should not be invited into the operating room. An explanation of what will occur after the infant is taken from the parents is usually sufficient. If stranger anxiety is already present in an older infant, then a parent may be invited into the operating room until the child is unaware of his or her presence if the anesthesiologist feels it would be safe. An explanation of the induction process should occur, including what the parent will observe, the operating room configuration, and the personnel that will be present. They should also be instructed on when they will be asked to leave and how they will be escorted from the operating room to avoid any distress regarding leaving their child with the operating room team.

## Premedication

Infants under one year of age have varying degrees of separation anxiety. Stranger anxiety develops slowly; it does not just appear suddenly. As cognitive skills in a child develop and improve, typically around 12 months of age, their stranger anxiety can become more intense. The nature of anxiety in children is dependent on many factors, including age, temperament, past experience, and family background. Parental presence, distraction, and premedication have all been used successfully, but no single strategy is effective for all children [4]. When the need for premedication arises, the standard agent of choice has been midazolam, which has been shown to be effective in infants not only for premedication but to decrease anxiety during interventional procedures performed without general anesthesia [5]. The recent introduction of dexmedetomidine as an intranasal as well as oral agent for premedication has provided an alternative choice [6]. The most recent meta-analysis demonstrated that dexmedetomidine premedication is superior to midazolam with respect to satisfactory separation from parents and mask acceptance, and has an additional clinical advantage of reducing the requirement for rescue analgesia during the postoperative period. There are, however, increased risks of decreased heart rate and blood pressure compared to midazolam when dexmedetomidine is used for premedication [7]. Ketamine has been a longstanding choice for premedication in older infants, but it should be noted that children premedicated with ketamine require close observation in a quiet environment where resuscitation equipment is readily available. Studies have shown midazolam to be a more effective and safer premedication than ketamine [8].

## Informed Consent About Short- and Long-Term Morbidity

The process of informed consent for anesthesia is carried out during the preoperative discussion. An assessment of risk that is specific to each patient with regard to the planned procedure and each patient's current state of health as compared to the usual state of health should be discussed. The overall incidence of cardiac arrest during anesthesia in children under 18 years of age has been reported to be 2.9–4.95/10 000 and 18.28/10 000 below one year of age, making cardiac arrest in infants 3–6 times more common than in older children. The greatest risk occurs in patients

with an American Society of Anesthesiologists risk stratification of III and IV, as well as those undergoing emergency surgery [9].

The most common surgical procedures associated with highest risk of cardiac arrest in children include airway procedures, followed by abdominal, thoracic, and cardiovascular procedures. The vast majority of neonatal cardiac arrest occurs in patients who have congenital heart disease [10]. The most frequent noncardiac causes of anesthesia-related cardiac arrests are medication and airway related [11,12]. Any medical comorbidities that exist which increase anesthetic risk should be described in detail and the measures that the anesthesia team will take to safely care for patients with regard to these risks should be explained. An explanation of the monitoring equipment in place in each operating room and the specific physiologic parameter that it measures is useful information to parents. In addition, a description of the number of personnel in the operating room as well as those available in case of an emergency is a reassuring piece of information for parents.

## Ambulatory Surgery

The greatest risk for infants undergoing ambulatory surgery is post-anesthetic apnea. There is controversy regarding the lowest age at which both full-term babies and former premature babies may be discharged home after surgery. Former preterm infants born prior to 37 weeks' gestational age as well as full-term infants less than 28 days of life are at increased risk for respiratory depression and apnea after general anesthesia. It is therefore recommended that the period of postoperative respiratory monitoring be extended for these patients. In former preterm infants without additional comorbidities, six hours of post-anesthesia respiratory monitoring is satisfactory since the first apneic episode usually occurs within the first four hours postoperatively [13]. In the presence of additional risk factors, including chronic lung disease, anemia (as defined by hematocrit <30 percent), recurrent apnea at home, or neurologic disease, the period of observation should be extended to 12 hours [14,15]. Whenever possible, elective surgery should be postponed until a postconceptual age of 60 weeks has been achieved.

Within the pediatric population, perioperative cardiac arrest under general anesthesia is more frequent in infants than in older children and beyond the first year of life age does not noticeably affect incidence of cardiac arrest [16,17]. Most cardiac arrests in the operating room are not a direct result of the anesthetic, and intraoperative cardiac arrests occur more frequently in children with congenital cardiac disease. Although there are no data to support discouraging elective ambulatory anesthesia in children less than one year of age, many institutions do not discharge children to home after general anesthesia until they are older than six months of age.

## Smoking in the House

Exposure to environmental tobacco smoke is associated with detrimental effects on pulmonary function in infants and children. There is a strong association between passive inhalation of tobacco smoke and airway complications in children receiving general anesthesia. Interestingly, studies indicate that this relationship is greatest for girls and for those whose mothers have a lower level of education. Significant physiologic effects may be documented as a result of passive tobacco smoke exposure. Cotinine is an alkaloid found in tobacco and is also a measurable metabolite of nicotine. The level of cotinine in the blood is proportionate to the amount of exposure to tobacco smoke, thus it is a valuable indicator of tobacco smoke exposure, including secondary (passive) smoke. In recent reports, perioperative airway complications occurred in 42 percent of patients with urinary concentrations of cotinine >40 ng ml$^{-1}$, in 33 percent of patients with concentrations of cotinine between 10.0 and 39.9 ng ml$^{-1}$, and in 24 percent of patients with concentrations of cotinine <10 ng ml$^{-1}$ (the three groups) [18]. The presence of a smoking caregiver is a significant independent risk factor for upper respiratory infection during the first three years of life. An increased risk of lower respiratory infections of two-fold or more occurs in infants and children from four months of age to three years. The risk of wheezing as a result of lower respiratory infections in the presence of a smoking caregiver was more than three-fold in this patient age group [19]. The exposure of infants to passive tobacco smoke should be investigated and, if present, minimized to decrease the risk of adverse respiratory events during the perioperative period.

## Fasting Requirements

It is no longer advisable or safe to restrict children to "NPO after midnight" [20]. This severe restriction routinely increases each child's chance of undergoing the induction of anesthesia when dehydrated, hypoglycemic, and irritable, all of which lead to increased risk under anesthesia. The risk of pulmonary aspiration of gastric contents in healthy children undergoing elective surgery is only 0.04 percent [21]. The American Society of Anesthesiologists (ASA) has proposed practice guidelines that may be followed when determining the NPO restrictions in children [22]. The ASA and others recommend fasting from clear fluids for two hours prior to anesthesia. Clear liquids consist of water, non-particulate juices (apple, white grape, etc.), Pedialyte®, and Popsicles®. Fasting from breast milk for four hours and formula for six hours is recommended. The composition of human milk varies among mothers and is dependent on the mother's diet, but in general is composed of 50 percent lipids, 40 percent carbohydrate in the form of lactose, and 10 percent protein divided into casein and whey [23]. Breast milk may cause significant pulmonary injury if aspirated due to a high fat content as determined by the maternal diet. The suggested fasting period for solid food is six hours for regular meals and eight hours for fat-containing meals; however, a large survey of pediatric institutions recommends fasting from all solids for at least eight hours in all children [24]. It is best to check with each surgical facility for specific practice guidelines.

## Immunization

There is no direct evidence of any major interaction between immunization and commonly used anesthetic agents and techniques in children, but it is possible that immunosuppression caused by anesthesia and surgery may lead to decreased vaccine effectiveness. In addition, diagnostic difficulty may arise if a recently immunized child suffers from postoperative temperature elevation or malaise [25]. From a risk management perspective, a review of the available evidence suggests that it would be prudent to adopt a cautious approach where the timing of elective surgery is discretionary. It is therefore recommended that elective surgery and anesthesia should be postponed for one week after inactive vaccination and three weeks after live attenuated vaccination in children.

Anesthesia and surgery exert immunomodulatory effects and some authors argue that they may exert additive or synergistic influences on vaccine efficacy and safety. Alternatively, inflammatory responses and fever elicited by vaccines may interfere with the postoperative course. There is a lack of consensus approach among anesthesiologists regarding the theoretical risk of anesthesia and vaccination. The immunomodulatory influence of anesthesia during elective surgery is both minor and transient (around 48 hours) and the current evidence does not provide any contraindication to the immunization of healthy children scheduled for elective surgery. Respecting a minimal delay of two days for inactivated vaccines or 14–21 days for live attenuated viral vaccines between immunization and anesthesia may be useful to avoid the risk of misinterpretation of vaccine-driven adverse events as postoperative complications [26].

# Prematurity

Preterm births as defined by completion of 37 weeks' gestation or 260 postmenstrual days are estimated to occur in 12.7 percent of live births [27,28]. This group of infants has a unique subset of perioperative comorbidities that the anesthesiologist should be alert to and investigate preoperatively to avoid any unexpected untoward events related to the anesthesia or perioperative episode of care.

Thorough preoperative assessment of the former preterm infant is essential and allows time for optimization of medical conditions. These infants present for a variety of surgical procedures and some, like hernia repair, may seem minor, but the anesthetic management remains challenging. Two major areas of concern for professionals and family alike are the extent of chronic lung disease and the possibility for postoperative apnea. Concise delineation of other coexisting conditions is also extremely important to anesthesiologists.

Infants born prematurely may range from having no residual lung disease to significant bronchopulmonary dysplasia (BPD). The latter condition is extremely variable in its manifestations from mild radiographic changes in an asymptomatic patient to pulmonary fibrosis, emphysema, reactive airway disease, chronic hypoxemia and hypercarbia, tracheomalacia or bronchomalacia, and increased pulmonary vascular resistance with cor pulmonale. If pulmonary hypertension and cor pulmonale are suspected, a pre-anesthetic echocardiogram is useful not only to confirm the diagnosis, but also to guide optimization of medical therapy. Diuretics, bronchodilators, and corticosteroids are medications that many of these patients require to optimize the child's respiratory

function, and should be continued up to and including the day of surgery. Measurement of serum electrolytes to evaluate the degree of hypokalemia and compensatory metabolic alkalosis may be valuable, especially if therapy has recently been altered. Consideration of pharmacological "stress" doses of steroids should be considered in infants receiving steroid treatment.

Postoperative apnea has been reported following anesthesia in former preterm and term infants alike. The incidence of post-anesthetic apnea is inversely related to the postconceptual age and gestational age. Infants younger than 56 weeks postconceptual are at greatest risk since the risk of post-anesthetic apnea does not fall to less than 1 percent until 55 weeks postconceptual age. This risk is present in full-term infants under 28 days of life. The concurrent presence of anemia is a confounding factor that further increases the risk of post-anesthetic apnea. Hematocrit should be targeted at a minimum of 30 percent in this patient population [29–31]. There is no consensus about the patient profile of at-risk infants. Reports are not consistent in identifying the postconceptional age or gestational age of at-risk patients, the methods used to detect apnea or periodic breathing, the surgical procedure, other confounding medical conditions, or even the definition of apnea [14].

A combined analysis of eight prospective studies investigated postoperative apnea in former preterm infants following inguinal herniorrhaphy. A uniform definition of apnea was cessation of breathing or no detection of air flow for ≥15 seconds or ≤15 seconds with bradycardia defined as heart rate <80 bpm. Examination of the data revealed that hematocrit <30 percent, apnea at home, postconceptional age, and gestational age are all important risk factors for postoperative apnea [32]. This supports claims that the risk of postoperative apnea is inversely related to postconceptional age and that infants as old as 60 weeks postconceptional age may be susceptible. Also, some authors suggest that infants with a prior history of apnea and bradycardia, respiratory distress, intubation, and mechanical ventilation may be at further increased risk [33–35]. Any child considered to be at risk for postoperative apnea should have arrangements made for overnight observation and monitoring. The former preterm infant should also have a recent hematocrit available since a value of <30 percent is associated with an increased incidence of post-anesthesia apnea irrespective of postconceptional age [36,37].

Intraventricular hemorrhage is a frequent finding in premature infants and is categorized as Grade 1–4 depending on the extent of hemorrhage beyond the germinal matrix, into the ventricular system, and finally penetration into the brain parenchyma. Grade 1 hemorrhage will usually not result in significant concern for the anesthesiologist, however more extensive blood pressure control is warranted for higher grade hemorrhage.

Retinopathy of prematurity is inversely related to gestational age. It occurs in up to 50 percent of premature infants [38,39]. The presence of retinopathy of prematurity should be noted in the preoperative review since the goal of the anesthetic plan should be to maintain oxygen saturation between 90 and 95 percent with the minimal concentration inspired oxygen [40].

The incidence of hypoglycemia, defined as less than 45 mg dl$^{-1}$, is three-fold higher in preterm infants as a result of decreased glycogen stores and feeding challenges. It is essential that this be identified so that a perioperative plan for glucose supplementation be made. Sepsis as a result of perinatal or postnatal acquired organisms is not an uncommon finding in the premature infant. A treatment plan for the infection as well as for hemodynamic support if the surgical procedure cannot be postponed should be identified. Because of their relatively smaller size, preterm infants are susceptible to periods of hypothermia and cold stress. Physiologic immaturity of thermoregulation, the lack of brown adipose tissue, and the lack of non-shivering thermogenesis predispose to the inability to generate heat in the same way that full-term and older infants do. A perioperative plan for temperature regulation and heat conservation is essential during the preoperative period.

## Review of Systems

### Cardiovascular

Effective cardiorespiratory function is represented by a respiratory rate under 60 breaths/minute, oxygen saturation above 95 percent by the first several hours of life, and the absence of respiratory distress, nasal flaring, grunting, or chest wall retractions [41]. When confronted with a neonate with respiratory abnormalities, important diagnostic considerations include: complex structural cardiac lesions, diaphragmatic hernia, persistent pulmonary hypertension, meconium aspiration syndrome, especially in infants greater than 40 weeks' gestational age, spontaneous pneumothorax, transient tachypnea of the newborn, or pneumonia [42,43].

The etiology of a new murmur or abnormality in the cardiovascular system must be fully investigated prior to the planning and induction of general anesthesia. The timing, location, intensity, radiation, quality, and pitch are characteristics of heart murmurs that can distinguish physiologic from pathologic murmurs. Physiologic murmurs detected during the first 48 hours of life are usually attributed to flow across the ductus arteriosis as it closes or across the pulmonic valve as pulmonary vascular resistance changes. These murmurs are transient, soft ejection murmurs, usually Grade 1 or 2. Pathologic murmurs detected in the first few hours of life are caused by outflow tract obstruction as occurs in aortic or pulmonic stenosis, as well as subaortic stenosis associated with hypertrophic cardiomyopathy. These Grade 2 or 3 murmurs are characteristically crescendo–decrescendo in nature. Defects that produce left-to-right shunting appear within the first few days of life when the pulmonary vascular resistance has dropped. Pan-systolic murmurs early after birth are most commonly caused by AV value insufficiency. Shunting through a ventricular septal defect produces a pan-systolic murmur that appears after several days of life. A continuous murmur heard in an infant most often represents an extra thoracic arteriovenous communication. Referral to a cardiologist should be made during the preoperative assessment if cardiac disease is suspected.

### Respiratory

The child with a recent upper respiratory infection (URI) poses a clinical dilemma for the anesthesiologist. Because most young children can have up to six URIs per year, this is a common problem for which no absolute rules exist. Most children have clear breath sounds during quiet respirations. Cough is a sign of lower respiratory involvement and should be evaluated for origin (upper or lower airway) and quality (wet or dry). Several potential risks are encountered in the perioperative period in the child who has an active cold or is recovering from a recent one.

Adverse perioperative events occur more frequently in infants with URIs. These include atelectasis, oxygen desaturation, bronchospasm, croup, and laryngospasm [44,45]. Decisions to cancel or postpone surgery should be made in conjunction with the surgeon and should be based on the type of procedure, the urgency of the procedure, and the child's overall medical condition. Bronchial hyper-reactivity may exist for up to seven weeks after the resolution of URI symptoms, and delaying surgery for this length of time is often impractical. Most practitioners would agree that surgery may be scheduled after the acute symptoms have resolved and no sooner than two weeks after the initial evaluation.

Infants with an anterior mediastinal mass are at significant risk for airway compromise during sedation due to compression of the intrathoracic larynx. Although lymphomas constitute the largest group of masses that arise in the anterior mediastinum in infants and children, other masses that may present in this location include teratomas, cystic hygromas, thymomas, hemangiomas, sarcomas, desmoid tumors, pericardial cysts, and diaphragmatic hernias of the Morgagni type. Patients with anterior mediastinal masses may present with varied signs and symptoms referable to both the cardiovascular and respiratory systems and are directly related to the location and size of the mass, as well as the degree of compression of surrounding structures. The most commonly observed respiratory symptom is cough, especially in the supine position, which results from anterior compression of the trachea. Infants less than two years of age are more likely to experience wheezing as a sign of tracheal compression. Other respiratory symptoms include tachypnea, dyspnea, stridor, retractions, decreased breath sounds, and cyanosis on crying, all of which should alert the practitioner to some degree of airway compromise that may worsen when positive intrathoracic pressure is generated. Preoperative computerized axial tomography may be beneficial in determining the degree of compromise and anesthetic plan.

Choanal atresia may be found as part of a constellation of congenital abnormalities, including those associated with CHARGE syndrome: **c**oloboma, **h**eart disease, **a**tresia choanae, **r**etarded growth, **g**enital abnormalities, and **e**ar abnormalities. Infants with choanal atresia are unable to change to oral breathing during periods of nasal obstruction, which may result in cyanosis at rest, which resolves with crying or placement of an oral airway. The incidence is approximately 1 in 8000 births [46]. Respiratory distress during the newborn period may be a result of obstruction at the level of the larynx – maybe due to laryngeal web, subglottic stenosis, or vascular ring. This should be clarified prior to induction of general anesthesia to avoid airway complications.

Infants born with congenital diaphragmatic hernia may present with severe respiratory distress as a result of lung hypoplasia and inadequate pulmonary gas exchange. Tachycardia, tachypnea, and cyanosis along with a scaphoid abdomen should suggest this diagnosis, which may be confirmed by radiographic evidence of a mediastinal shift and bowel loops in the chest.

## Gastric

Congenital obstruction of the gastrointestinal tract may result in vomiting, abdominal distention, aspiration with or without pneumonia, dehydration, hypovolemia, and electrolyte abnormalities. Correction of these abnormalities during the preoperative period is essential for safe preparation for general anesthesia. Associated anomalies of other organs are found in more than 50 percent of cases of children with gastroesophageal abnormalities. Often there is a combination of vertebral, anal, cardiac, tracheal, esophageal, renal, and limb anomalies (VACTERL). Cardiac anomalies are found in 15–40 percent of cases. Esophageal malformations can occur in several forms: tracheoesophageal fistula, isolated esophageal atresia with or without tracheal communication, or double fistulae. The incidence is estimated at 1 in 4000 live births. Prenatal diagnosis can be made with ultrasonography. Signs noted soon after birth include drooling due to excessive secretions, regurgitation with subsequent aspiration, choking spells, abdominal distention, and inability to pass a gastric tube beyond the atretic esophagus. Contrast radiographic studies are often conclusive. The clinical course can be complicated by the consequences of prematurity, pulmonary aspiration, and abdominal distention.

## Neurologic

The incidence of myelomeningocele is 1/1000 live births and although 75 percent of lesions occur in the lumbosacral region, affected children may present with a defect anywhere along the neuraxis. Dysfunction of the skeletal system, skin, genitourinary tract, and peripheral and central nervous system may also be present, so these organ systems should be fully evaluated during the preoperative visit. These children are frequent visitors to the operating room and need careful attention to their perioperative needs to avoid trauma that would make future encounters more difficult. There is high incidence of sensitivity to latex-containing products, so an attempt to limit exposure to latex should be made. This caution should be noted during the preoperative visit and "Latex Sensitivity" should be posted clearly on the front of the patient chart.

Seizures are a frequently encountered component of many early childhood illnesses and occur in 4–6/1000 children. Seizures are a symptom of an underlying central nervous system disorder that must be fully investigated and understood. The history should provide a detailed description of the seizure, including the type, frequency, and severity of symptoms, as well as the characteristics of the postictal state so that it may easily be recognized by the OR team should it occur during the perioperative period. All anticonvulsant therapy should be recorded and serum drug levels should be checked. All anticonvulsants should be taken up to and including the morning of surgery. If the infant has seizures despite adequate therapy, this should be noted.

Infants with significant trauma as well as infants who have a variety of congenital abnormalities are at risk for cervical spine instability. Infants younger than three months are unable to adequately support their head and are at heightened risk for cervical cord injuries, which can result from excessive forces during delivery or in the first few months of life. Altered mucopolysaccharide metabolism may predispose children to deformities of the odontoid process, resulting in cervical spine instability. Atlantoaxial instability and superior migration of the odontoid process may occur in children with rheumatoid arthritis and skeletal dysplasia. Children with trisomy 21 have laxity of the transverse ligament and abnormal development of the odontoid process, which results in cervical spine instability in 15 percent of cases. Symptoms include clinical manifestations of cord compression which usually are not manifested until after five years of age. The American Academy of Pediatrics' guidelines suggest that parents be aware of the importance of cervical spine-positioning precautions to avoid excessive extension or flexion to protect the cervical spine during any anesthetic, surgical, or radiographic procedure. In infants in which cervical abnormalities are noted,

intubation of the trachea should be undertaken in a neutral head position or with somatosensory evoked potential (SSEP) monitoring of the upper extremities [47].

## Physical Examination

A full physical examination of the neonate and infant is an essential component of the preoperative review. As assessment of gestation age as well as chronologic age should be made. The examination should begin with an observation of the infant in an undisturbed state, since a great deal may be learned about relevant physical findings without touching the child. The entire skin surface should be inspected for temperature, moisture, elasticity, and fragility. The color of the skin and the presence of pallor, cyanosis, rash, jaundice, unusual markings, birthmarks, and scars from previous operations should be noted. When examining a newborn, the head should be examined by inspection and palpation to determine if there is any bruising as a result of delivery, as well as the fullness of the fontanels to determine alterations in intracranial pressure. Abnormal facies might be an indication of a syndrome or constellation of congenital abnormalities. One congenital anomaly is often associated with others.

Inspection of the oral cavity may reveal normal variants such as small cysts, Epstein's pearls, Bohn's nodules, and dental lamina cysts. These are of no consequence and should not cause difficulty with laryngoscopy or endotracheal intubation. A gloved finger may be inserted into the oral cavity to determine the shape and integrity as well as to identify any abnormalities such as cleft palate. The neck should be observed for range of motion to detect spine abnormalities such as Klippel–Feil syndrome, congenital torticollis, and any anterior midline abnormalities such as branchial cleft or thyroglossal duct cyst. Short or webbed neck may be an indication of chromosomal abnormalities such as Down or Turner syndrome.

The shape of the chest and mechanics of respiration should be observed even before the lungs are auscultated. A normal infant is observed to be centrally acyanotic, resting comfortably, breathing easily with clear breath sounds when the lungs are auscultated. The color, viscosity, and quantity of nasal discharge should be documented. Respiratory rate may be irregular and pauses up to 20 seconds are normal in the infant. Common causes of mild respiratory distress in the newborn include transient tachypnea of the newborn due to retained fetal lung fluid, spontaneous pneumothorax, neonatal sepsis, pneumonia, meconium aspiration, or congenital heart disease. The respiratory system should be evaluated by noting the rate and quality of respirations, the presence of noisy breathing, coughing, purulent nasal discharge, stridor, and wheezing. Retractions, nasal flaring, grunting, and paradoxical respiration may be signs of increased work of breathing and respiratory distress in the infant. Noisy or labored breathing may indicate nasal or upper respiratory obstruction. If the child is coughing, the origin of the cough (upper versus lower airway) and the quality (dry or wet) can be evaluated even before auscultation of the lungs. Signs of an acute upper respiratory infection should be documented if present. The ease of mouth opening should be determined and the airway should be evaluated for ease of intubation. If the child will not open his or her mouth, a manual estimation of the thyrohyoid distance should be made. Children with micrognathia, as in Pierre Robin syndrome or Goldenhar's syndrome, may be especially difficult to intubate.

The goal of the cardiovascular examination in the infant is two-fold; to assess the status of the circulatory system and to detect congenital heart disease. The rate, rhythm, volume, and character of the pulses in all four extremities should be evaluated. The resting heart rate of the healthy newborn averages 120–130 bpm. The precordium is examined by inspection, palpation, and auscultation. Clicks, murmurs, or other abnormal heart sounds should be sought. If a heart murmur is detected on the cardiovascular examination, there are specific concerns that must be addressed. An innocent murmur may be due to turbulent blood flow, whereas a pathological murmur is usually due to a structural abnormality; this distinction must be made. Lesions in which bacterial endocarditis prophylaxis or protection from paradoxical air embolism are required must be documented so that the anesthesia team is made aware. The child with a heart murmur or a history of a murmur warrants special consideration. The determination of an innocent versus pathologic murmur as well as the presence of hemodynamic compromise should be made. Innocent or non-pathologic heart murmurs can be identified by four characteristics: the murmur is early systolic to mid-systolic; it is softer than grade 3 of 4; the pitch is low to medium; and the sound has a musical, not harsh, quality. The infant should be evaluated for risk of paradoxical air embolus and evaluated for the need for prophylaxis for subacute bacterial endocarditis [48].

The abdomen should be observed for configuration, fullness, and movement with respiration. Major abdominal wall abnormalities such as gastroschisis, omphalocele, prune belly, or bladder extrophy will be obvious on inspection. A scaphoid abdomen may be an indication of abdominal contents that are displaced into the chest, as occurs in diaphragmatic hernia. A distended abdomen may be a sign of intestinal obstruction, ascites, or an abdominal mass. Palpation of the abdomen should include examination of the liver, and bowel sounds should be present on auscultation. Risk for aspiration of gastric contents should be determined.

The physical examination should include an evaluation of the level of consciousness, ability to swallow, intactness of the gag reflex, and an adequate cervical spine range of motion, hypotonia, spasticity, or flaccidity. General muscle tone and the presence of signs of an increase in intracranial pressure should also be noted.

## Laboratory Testing

It is important to remember that phlebotomy is often traumatic for infants and their families, and an event that is not easily forgotten. For this reason, it is best to limit the number of invasive tests performed. The diagnostic studies should be selected based on the general medical health and the procedure being performed. In general, measurement of hematocrit in a healthy older infant undergoing elective surgery is unnecessary [49]. A hematocrit *should* be measured if significant blood loss is anticipated, if the child is less than six months of age or was born prematurely. Neither the routine measurement of the coagulation profile nor a history of "easy bruising" is reliable in predicting surgical bleeding [50]. The presence of prior hematoma, bleeding from circumcision or large bruises should prompt an investigation; however, a negative history for bruising in an otherwise healthy child would require no further testing. Routine preoperative urinalysis is not indicated in children, and serum chemistries should only be performed when an abnormality is suspected. Infants who are treated with anticonvulsants should have these medication levels checked and an electrocardiogram or chest radiograph should only be ordered if the general medical condition warrants.

# References

1.  McCann ME, Schouten AN. Beyond survival: influences of blood pressure, cerebral perfusion and anesthesia on neurodevelopment. *Paediatr Anaesth.* 2014;24:68–73.

2.  Moynihan R, Kurker C. The perioperative environment and the pediatric patient. In: Ferrari LR, editor. *Anesthesia and Pain MAnagement for the Pediatrician.* Baltimore, MD: Johns Hopkins University Press;1999; 67–89.

3.  Litman RS, Berger AA, Chhibber A. An evaluation of preoperative anxiety in a population of parents of infants and children undergoing ambulatory surgery. *Paediatr Anaesth.* 1996;6:443–7.

4.  Banchs RJ, Lerman J. Preoperative anxiety management, emergence delirium, and postoperative behavior. *Anesthesiol Clin.* 2014;32:1–23.

5.  Weiser G, Cohen D, Krauss B, Galbraith R, Shavit I. Premedication with midazolam for urethral catheterization of febrile infants. *Eur J Emerg Med.* 2013;21(4):314–18.

6.  Wang SS, Zhang MZ, Sun Y, et al. The sedative effects and the attenuation of cardiovascular and arousal responses during anesthesia induction and intubation in pediatric patients: a randomized comparison between two different doses of preoperative intranasal dexmedetomidine. *Paediatr Anaesth.* 2014;24:275–81.

7.  Sun Y, Lu Y, Huang Y, Jiang H. Is dexmedetomidine superior to midazolam as a premedication in children? A meta-analysis of randomized controlled trials. *Paediatr Anaesth.* 2014;24(8):863–74.

8.  Khatavkar SS, Bakhshi RG. Comparison of nasal midazolam with ketamine versus nasal midazolam as a premedication in children. *Saudi J Anaesth.* 2014;8:17–21.

9.  Ahmed A, Ali M, Khan M, Khan F. Perioperative cardiac arrests in children at a university teaching hospital of a developing country over 15 years. *Paediatr Anaesth.* 2009;19:581–6.

10. Flick RP, Sprung J, Harrison TE, et al. Perioperative cardiac arrests in children between 1988 and 2005 at a tertiary referral center: a study of 92,881 patients. *Anesthesiology.* 2007;106:226–37; quiz 413–14.

11. Bhananker SM, Ramamoorthy C, Geiduschek JM, et al. Anesthesia-related cardiac arrest in children: update from the Pediatric Perioperative Cardiac Arrest Registry. *Anesth Analg.* 2007;105:344–50.

12. Jimenez N, Posner KL, Cheney FW, et al. An update on pediatric anesthesia liability: a closed claims analysis. *Anesth Analg.* 2007;104:147–53.

13. Allen GD, Ward RJ, Green HD, Perrin EB. Reversal of apnea following artificial ventilation under anesthesia. *Anesth Analg.* 1967;46:690–7.

14. Cote CJ, Zaslavsky A, Downes JJ, et al. Postoperative apnea in former preterm infants after inguinal herniorrhaphy: a combined analysis. *Anesthesiology.* 1995;82:809–22.

15. Walther-Larsen S, Rasmussen LS. The former preterm infant and risk of post-operative apnoea: recommendations for management. *Acta Anaesthesiol Scand.* 2006;50:888–93.

16. Morray JP, Posner K. Pediatric perioperative cardiac arrest: in search of definition(s). *Anesthesiology.* 2007;106:207–8.

17. Flick RP, Sprung J, Harrison TE, et al. Perioperative cardiac arrests in children between 1988 and 2005 at a tertiary referral center: a study of 92,881 patients. *Anesthesiology.* 2007;106:226.

18. Skolnick ET, Vomvolakis MA, Buck KA, Mannino SF, Sun LS. Exposure to environmental tobacco smoke and the risk of adverse respiratory events in children receiving general anesthesia. *Anesthesiology.* 1998;88:1144–53.

19. Holberg CJ, Wright AL, Martinez FD, Morgan WJ, Taussig LM. Child day care, smoking by caregivers, and lower respiratory tract illness in the first 3 years of life: Group Health Medical Associates. *Pediatrics.* 1993;91:885–92.

20. Cote CJ. NPO after midnight for children: a reappraisal. *Anesthesiology.* 1990;72:589–92.

21. Warner MA, Warner ME, Warner DO, Warner LO, Warner EJ. Perioperative pulmonary aspiration in infants and children. *Anesthesiology.* 1999;90:66–71.

22. ASA ATFoPF. Practice guidelines for preoperative fasting and the use of pharmacologic agents to reduce the risk of pulmonary aspiration: application to healthy patients undergoing elective procedures. *Anesthesiology.* 1999;90:896–905.

23. Picciano MF. Nutrient composition of human milk. *Pediatr Clin North Am.* 2001;48:53–67.

24. Ferrari LR, Rockoff MA. Preoperative fasting practices in pediatrics. *Anesthesiology.* 1999;90:978–80.

25. Short JA, van der Walt JH, Zoanetti DC. Immunization and anesthesia: an international survey. *Paediatr Anaesth.* 2006;16:514–22.

26. Siebert JN, Posfay-Barbe KM, Habre W, Siegrist CA. Influence of anesthesia on immune responses and its effect on vaccination in children: review of evidence. *Paediatr Anaesth.* 2007;17:410–20.

27. Raju TN. Epidemiology of late preterm (near-term) births. *Clin Perinatol.* 2006;33:751–63; abstract vii.

28. Raju TN. The problem of late-preterm (near-term) births: a workshop summary. *Pediatr Res.* 2006;60:775–6.

29. Tetzlaff JE, Annand DW, Pudimat MA, Nicodemus HF. Postoperative apnea in a full-term infant. *Anesthesiology.* 1988;69:426–8.

30. Cote CJ, Kelly DH. Postoperative apnea in a full-term infant with a demonstrable respiratory pattern abnormality. *Anesthesiology.* 1990;72:559–61.

31. Noseworthy J, Duran C, Khine HH. Postoperative apnea in a full-term infant. *Anesthesiology.* 1989;70:879–80.

32. Kurth CD, Spitzer AR, Broennle AM, Downes JJ. Postoperative apnea in preterm infants. *Anesthesiology.* 1987;66:483–8.

33. Steward DJ. Preterm infants are more prone to complications following minor surgery than are term infants. *Anesthesiology.* 1982;56:304–6.

34. Liu LM, Cote CJ, Goudsouzian NG, et al. Life-threatening apnea in infants recovering from anesthesia. *Anesthesiology.* 1983;59:506–10.

35. Welborn LG, Ramirez N, Oh TH, et al. Postanesthetic apnea and periodic breathing in infants. *Anesthesiology.* 1986;65:658–61.

36. Kurth CD, LeBard SE. Association of postoperative apnea, airway obstruction, and hypoxemia in former premature infants. *Anesthesiology.* 1991;75:22–6.

37. Welborn LG, Hannallah RS, Luban NL, Fink R, Ruttimann UE. Anemia and postoperative apnea in former preterm infants. *Anesthesiology.* 1991;74:1003–6.

38. Lermann VL, Fortes Filho JB, Procianoy RS. The prevalence of retinopathy of prematurity in very low birth weight newborn infants. *J Pediatr (Rio J).* 2006;82:27–32.

39. Sapieha P, Joyal JS, Rivera JC, et al. Retinopathy of prematurity: understanding ischemic retinal vasculopathies at an extreme of life. *J Clin Invest.* 2010;120:3022–32.

40. Askie LM, Henderson-Smart DJ, Ko H. Restricted versus liberal oxygen exposure for preventing morbidity and mortality in preterm or low birth weight infants. *Cochrane Database Syst Rev.* 2009;21:CD001077.

41. Levesque BM, Pollack P, Griffin BE, Nielsen HC. Pulse oximetry: what's normal in the newborn nursery? *Pediatr Pulmonol.* 2000;30:406–12.

42. Konduri GG, Kim UO. Advances in the diagnosis and management of persistent pulmonary hypertension of the newborn. *Pediatr Clin North Am.* 2009;56:579–600.

43. Guglani L, Lakshminrusimha S, Ryan RM. Transient tachypnea of the newborn. *Pediatr Rev.* 2008;29:e59–65.

44. Rolf N, Cote CJ. Frequency and severity of desaturation events during general anesthesia in children with and without upper respiratory infections. *J Clin Anesth.* 1992;4:200–3.

45. Tait AR, Malviya S, Voepel-Lewis T, et al. Risk factors for perioperative adverse respiratory events in children with upper respiratory tract infections. *Anesthesiology.* 2001;95:299–306.

46. Rodenstein DO, Perlmutter N, Stanescu DC. Infants are not obligatory nasal breathers. *Am Rev Respir Dis.* 1985;131:343–7.

47. Cunningham MJ, Ferrari LR, Kearse LA, McPeck K. Intraoperative somatosensory evoked potential monitoring in achondroplasia. *Paediatr Anaesth.* 1994;4:129–32.

48. Wilson W, Taubert KA, Gewitz M, et al. Prevention of infective endocarditis: guidelines from the American Heart Association – a guideline from the American Heart Association Rheumatic Fever, Endocarditis, and Kawasaki Disease Committee, Council on Cardiovascular Disease in the Young, and the Council on Clinical Cardiology, Council on Cardiovascular Surgery and Anesthesia, and the Quality of Care and Outcomes Research Interdisciplinary Working Group. *Circulation.* 2007;116:1736–54.

49. Steward DJ. Screening tests before surgery in children. *Can J Anaesth.* 1991;38:693–5.

50. Burk CD, Miller L, Handler SD, Cohen AR. Preoperative history and coagulation screening in children undergoing tonsillectomy. *Pediatrics.* 1992;89:691–5.

**Chapter**

# 13

# Developmental Pharmacology
## The Neonate

Cynthia Tung and Robert S. Holzman

## Neonatal and Pediatric Pharmacology: The Evolution of Scaled Modeling

In 1950, Terry et al. boldly stated what practicing pediatricians had known clinically for so long – neither age nor weight were satisfactory metrics for drug calculations in children. They therefore proposed scaling drug dosages according to body surface area, and were able to support this hypothesis with empirical evidence [1]. This scaling calculation was extended to water, electrolytes, and calories, preceding Holliday and Segar's guidance for parenteral fluid therapy according to basal metabolic rate by seven years [2]. Allometric (nonlinear, growth-based) scaling entered the mainstream of dosing concepts at that time, but was embraced by relatively few, and rather simplistic pharmacology models persisted for decades (Figure 13.1).

Pediatric *pharmacokinetic* parameters are now understood with increasing precision. Age-adjusted volume of distribution is important for the loading dose and of crucial importance in anesthetic practice because of the need to rapidly achieve a target effect. Clearance determines the maintenance dose rate. Together, clearance and volume of distribution determine the shape of the concentration–time curve [3]. *Pharmacodynamic* parameters, particularly for children and more so for neonates, are a far different story. Almost all neonatal organ systems are still developing; some enzymes are present, some are absent, some are increasing in activity, some are decreasing. Hematocrit affects drug delivery, as does the concentration of proteins (and the types of proteins) in the blood. Many organ systems have a relatively larger mass within a neonates body – does that mean they function as hypercellular systems, or are those systems less mature despite the increase in mass? Effective drug delivery to the receptor/effector sites depends on blood flow, tissue volume, tissue

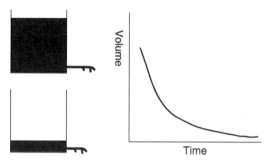

**Figure 13.1** A simplistic – and common – concept map of dosing and elimination.

solubility coefficients, and protein binding. Babies are different in almost all of these respects than children and adults.

## Effective Modeling: *Why* are Children Different?

### Volume of Distribution

Because a child's job is growth and development, he or she is obligated to a ravenous early life of oxygen consumption, acquisition of calories, and production of heat. In order to survive as homeotherms – without burning up – they must have a way to exquisitely balance heat generation and heat loss, which led to the proposal of the Surface Law (homeotherms maintain their temperature homeostasis in proportion to their body surface area, i.e., heat production = heat loss) [4]. This turned out to be *almost* right. When oxygen consumption is measured directly or indirectly, it is actually more proportional to body mass $(kg)^{3/4}$ (Figure 13.2), whereas body surface area is calculated as $(kg)^{2/3}$ [5]. It turns out that thermal homeostasis is proportional to the vascular branching necessary to deliver heat to the skin surface, rather than the skin surface itself. The capacitance of this branched system,

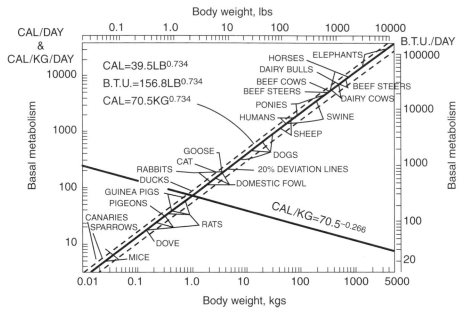

**Figure 13.2** A log-linear plot of basal metabolism of mature animals of different species, with an almost uniform slope of 0.75 – the ¾ power, if expressed exponentially. The slope of the line is the exponent of the function. When the exponent = 1, there is isometry (isometric growth), meaning there is no change in shape during growth. Source: [5].

influenced by the scaling concept, formed the basis for Holliday and Segar's fluid recommendations [2].

Accurate anticipation of differences in the volume of distribution is of crucial importance in anesthesiology in order to rapidly achieve a target effect. With a naturally larger volume of distribution because of allometric scaling as well as a larger "effective" volume of distribution because of a decrease in plasma proteins, a larger (apparent) volume of distribution is the result. This may explain the rather ironic requirement for a larger initial drug dose in infants and small children in order to achieve target concentration parity with adults and even older children (Figure 13.3).

## Clearance

Scalar "per kilogram" models of clearance under-predict, while surface area models over-predict clearance, leading to errors in calculating clearance with decreasing weight. Scalar modeling, for example, will lead to the false conclusion that children possess an enhanced capacity to metabolize drugs due to proportionally larger livers and kidneys (more "cellularity" per kilogram of body weight) than in adults [7]. As a better alternative, allometry is a good method of scaling clearance when only size differences exist [3]; however, it will overestimate clearance in children

when metabolic clearance pathways are developmentally immature (e.g., activity of the enzyme per unit volume of tissue is lower). This method should only be used alone when the patient's clearance for age reaches similar activity (>2 years) to that of adults [8]. A maturation model is required to describe clearance in neonates and infants (<2 years) to account for changes independent of size.

## Cardiac Output

One consequence of the allometrically scaled increased cardiac output and organ size in infants (i.e., the brain receives 30 percent compared to 15 percent of this proportion-adjusted cardiac output) is that more drug reaches target receptors more rapidly in vessel-rich organ groups (brain, kidney, intestinal viscera, especially the liver).

## Renal Clearance

Excretion may be reduced compared with older children and adults because glomerular *and* tubular renal function are reduced in newborns. Using an allometrically scaled postmenstrual age (gestational age + chronological age = PMA) model, Rhodin et al. reported adult GFR as 121.2 ml min$^{-1}$ per 70 kg, with half of the adult value reached at 47.7 postmenstrual weeks.

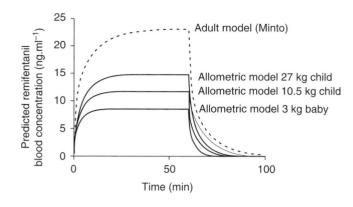

**Figure 13.3** Enhanced clearance and a larger central compartment volume results in reduced blood concentrations compared with adults. Smaller children require higher infusion rates (weight-based) than larger children or adults to achieve equivalent blood concentrations. Source: [6].

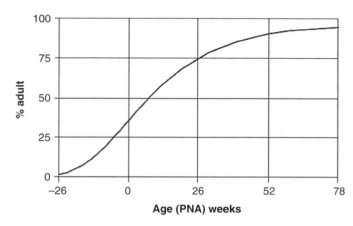

**Figure 13.4** Maturation of GFR showing the predictions of the sigmoid hyperbolic function. The abscissa is expressed as weeks of postnatal age so that 0 would be a full-term infant with a postmenstrual age (PMA) of 40 weeks. Source: [9].

At one-year postnatal age, the GFR is predicted to be 90 percent of the adult GFR [9] (Figure 13.4)

## Hepatic Biotransformation

Hepatic biotransformation is unrelated to body weight and scaled growth. Some cytochrome P450 (CYP) enzymes are present at birth (CYP3A7, uridine 5′-diphospho-glucuronosyltransferase [UGT]), while others are not (CYP2E1, CYP2D6, CYP3A4, CYP2C9). Some achieve adult activity in a few days (UGT2B7), while some require months to years to mature (UGT1A6) [10] (Figure 13.5). Hepatic activity cannot be anticipated by weight, body surface area (BSA), nor allometric scaling [11].

The CYP system is immature at birth and does not reach adult functionality until the first or second month (Figure 13.6). This immaturity may explain the prolonged clearance or elimination of some drugs in the first few days to weeks of life, as well as the inability of the liver to convert a precursor into its active form. The CYP450 system can be induced by a variety of drugs (e.g., phenobarbital). The age from birth – not

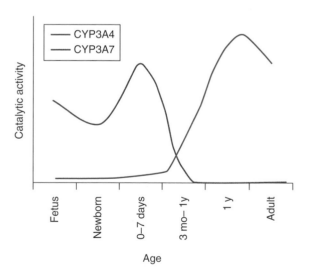

**Figure 13.5** Development and regression of cytochrome P450 (CYP) 3A4 and 3A7 as activity measured using isoform-specific probes in human liver microsomes. Source: [10].

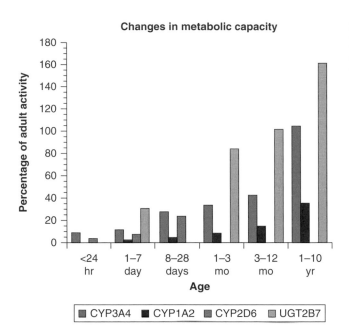

**Changes in metabolic capacity**

**Figure 13.6** The activity of many cytochrome P450 (CYP) isoforms and a single glucuronosyltransferase (UGT) isoform is diminished during the first two months of life. The achievement of adult activity over time is enzyme- and isoform-specific. Source: [12].

the gestational age – determines how premature or full-term infants metabolize drugs.

Elimination may be further affected by abnormal or decreased liver blood flow as a result of illness or surgery. Certain neonatal conditions may increase intra-abdominal pressure, and also decrease liver blood flow (e.g., closure of an omphalocele or gastroschisis, reopening of a ductus venosus, positive pressure ventilation).

## Binding

Opioids, amide local anesthetics, and muscle relaxants, for example, bind to albumin and alpha-1 acid glycoprotein. The unbound (free) drug is available to cross biological membranes, bind to receptors, and achieve a therapeutic concentration. Lower concentrations of albumin and alpha-1 acid glycoprotein result in more unbound drug availability to target receptors.

## Organ Function

Pharmacodynamics are affected in a substantial way by anesthetic and critical care interventions. For example, positive pressure ventilation may be associated with reduced clearance. This effect may be attributable to reduced hepatic blood flow with a drug that has perfusion-limited clearance (e.g., propofol, morphine) [3].

# Pharmacodynamics: Developing Organ Systems and Drug Targeting

Most investigations center on pharmacokinetics (PK), but dosing predictions as well as monitoring for therapeutic and adverse effects also requires a better understanding of pharmacodynamics. The challenge in caring for infants is that receptors themselves are in a state of development and may therefore express themselves with much greater variability quantitatively and qualitatively [7]. For example, neuroplasticity is characteristic of the developing nervous system centrally and peripherally, and there is no reason to think that it is not integral to developmental nociception. Maturation considerations for neurochemistry and neuroanatomy may alter drug efficacy in the neonate. While anatomic and neurotransmitter mechanisms are present at birth for the processing of painful stimuli, these systems evolve through the fetal and newborn period and into adult life, and it is not likely that they function in an identical manner during these lifecycle changes. Glutamine and substance P (SP) are colocalized in C fiber terminals in the dorsal horn and facilitate pain transmission in part by activating N-methyl-D-aspartate (NMDA) receptors. In the adult rat, NMDA receptor binding is restricted to the substantia gelatinosa (SG), but at postnatal day 7 (P7) in rat models it is distributed throughout the spinal cord;

A: Development

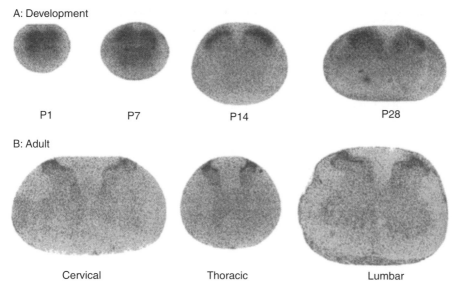

P1          P7          P14          P28

B: Adult

Cervical          Thoracic          Lumbar

**Figure 13.7** Mu receptor binding sites at P1, P7, P14, and P28 and at different levels of the adult rat spinal cord. In human terms, these ages are approximately 1.5 m, 19 m, 3.3 y, and 7 y. Source: [13].

the more mature and discretely distributed pattern is not achieved until P28 and parallels SP and other neuropeptides (Figure 13.7). In the rat, SP receptors move from a diffuse, nonspecific distribution in the neonate to discrete and concentrated loci in the mature SG. These developmental considerations in the expression of SP as well as other neurotransmitter systems make the neonatal SG substantially different than that found in adults, notwithstanding the achievement of calculated adequate drug levels systemically or for regional anesthetics.

Cardiac effects of many anesthetic drugs are not the same in neonates because the neonatal heart is different than the adult heart, or even the heart of an older child. Neonates have a cardiac output 2–3 times that of adults, about 180–240 ml kg$^{-1}$ min$^{-1}$. Cardiac muscle mass is smaller in newborns and infants than in older children and adults, the ventricles are less compliant, and in addition, there is a higher resting tone at end-diastole, with a lower peak pressure achieved during systole. There is also a developmental basis for differences in excitation–contraction coupling. Tension development in the myocardium is activated by the influx of Ca$^{2+}$ across the sarcolemma. As the myocardium matures, intracellular Ca$^{2+}$ uptake and re-release by the sarcoplasmic reticulum plays an increasingly important role in tension development [14]. Calculations for drug dosing in neonates must

take into account that neonatal myocardial depression may be more than just a dosing effect, but rather an adverse effect in the context of a substantially dissimilar myocardium.

## Population Pharmacokinetics and Neonatal Variability

Classical pharmacokinetic studies involve administering single or multiple doses of a drug to a small group of subjects and then obtaining multiple samples to describe the concentration and time profile of the drug. The highly charged ethical and practical issues of conducting such studies in children, especially neonates, are obvious. A preferable approach in most pediatric situations is the population pharmacokinetics (PPK) approach, combining fewer samples of individual data with blood sampling from a large target population at varying times.

Population pharmacokinetics is focused on absorption, distribution, metabolism, and excretion, using mathematical and statistical modeling, typically nonlinear mixed effects modeling (NONMEM). For example, using PPK and NONMEM modeling, Anderson et al. have shown that size explains 49.8 percent, age 18.2 percent, and renal function 14.1 percent of clearance variability of vancomycin in neonates [7].

## Better Prediction Through Better Modeling?

In an attempt to incorporate the many aspects of pharmacokinetic pharmacodynamic modeling, particularly with regard to infants and small children, Simcyp® software (Simcyp Limited, Blades Enterprise Center, John Street, Sheffield S2 4SU, UK) integrates demographic, genetic, physiological, and pathological information on adults with in vitro data on human drug metabolism and transport to predict population distributions of drug clearance (CL) and the extent of metabolic drug–drug interactions (Figure 13.8). The algorithms have now been extended to pediatric populations by incorporating information on developmental physiology and the development/maturation of specific cytochrome P450s [15]. Simcyp® algorithms have been reported to provide reasonable estimates of the in vivo drug clearance of 11 drugs commonly used in neonates, infants, and children [16].

## Inhalation Anesthetics

The effects of chloroform are more quickly produced and also subside more quickly in children than adults, owing no doubt to the quicker breathing and circulation [17].

So observed John Snow about inhaled anesthetics in children, providing early insight into fundamental differences and paving the way for pediatric anesthesiologists to be leaders in pediatric pharmacology.

Most of the PK differences are due to allometrically scaled parameters. Scaled branching and volume of the circulation is directly related to metabolic activity, since heat delivery from the core to the periphery has to be exquisitely balanced to maintain the homeothermic state. Developmental blood chemistry

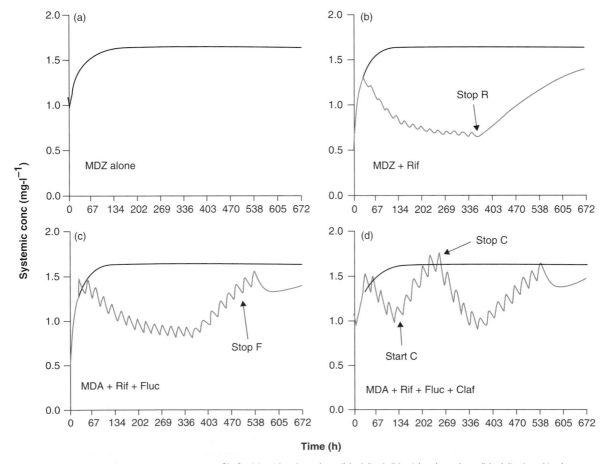

**Figure 13.8** Simulated concentration–time profile for (a) midazolam alone (black line); (b) midazolam alone (black line) and in the presence of rifampicin (gray line); (c) midazolam alone (black line) and in the presence of rifampicin and fluconazole (gray line); and (d) midazolam alone (black line) and in the presence of rifampicin, fluconazole, and clarithromycin (gray line). Source: [15].

**Table 13.1** Key differences in pharmacokinetic effects

|  | Children | Adults | Implication |
|---|---|---|---|
| Alveolar ventilation: FRC ratio | 5:1 | 1.5:1 | Enhanced wash-in |
| Cardiac output | 20 dl min$^{-1}$ (2 dl kg$^{-1}$ min$^{-1}$) | 50 dl min$^{-1}$ (0.75 dl kg$^{-1}$ min$^{-1}$) | Shorter time to equilibrium and enhanced speed of induction |
| Tissue:blood solubility |  |  | Neonates have lower levels of total protein, albumin, and cholesterol, and higher levels of total body water |
| Total protein | 50 g L$^{-1}$ | 70 g L$^{-1}$ | Less protein available for binding therefore increased free fraction |
| Albumin | 30 g L$^{-1}$ | 37 g L$^{-1}$ | Less protein available for binding therefore increased free fraction |
| Cholesterol | 1.3 g L$^{-1}$ | 2.09 g L$^{-1}$ | Lower cholesterol, lower solubility, and increased free fraction |
| Total body water | 689 g kg$^{-1}$ | 605 g kg$^{-1}$ | Greater dilution |

balance (differences in total proteins, albumin, cholesterol, and total body water) also affects tissue/blood solubility such that lower solubility is characteristic of neonates. These differences add to enhancing the speed of induction and the rapidity of therapeutic as well as adverse effects in children. These PK effects are outlined in Table 13.1.

In addition to the differences in PK outlined above, anesthetic potency also influences the ability to rapidly adjust an inhaled anesthetic, whether during induction or any other phase. The minimum alveolar concentration (MAC) has been the standard used to express anesthetic potency, and in general the lower the MAC the more potent the anesthetic. Lipid solubility of the specific agent is inversely related to the MAC of that agent; in addition, MAC has long been recognized to be different for different age groups (Figure 13.9).

Carbon monoxide (CO) can be produced in subclinical concentrations by all of the current methyl ethyl ethers (desflurane > isoflurane > halothane and sevoflurane) in the presence of desiccated soda lime or baralyme. Newer $CO_2$ absorbents (those that contain a lithium-based catalyst) do not have the typical strong bases (KOH, NaOH) and do not result in carbon monoxide or Compound A production. Furthermore, they are not significantly exothermic. Mitigating effects in infants and children include a lower total minute $CO_2$ production despite a higher per kilogram per minute value due to increased oxygen consumption.

Post-anesthesia delirium has been associated with all of the currently utilized inhalation agents, and there seem to be numerous cofactors that make it all the more difficult to discriminate a single etiology [19]. Again, this is a difficult assessment in the neonate and infant.

Specific adverse effects of inhalation agents more prominent in the neonatal and infant age group include:

- **Myocardial effects.** Cardiac muscle mass is smaller in newborns and infants than in older children and adults, the ventricles are less compliant, and in addition there is a higher resting tone at end-diastole, with a lower peak pressure achieved during systole [20]. Conduction delays are almost uniformly predictable with halothane but are variable with the newer ethers.

- **Baroreceptor effects**. Baroreception, like myocardial performance, "matures" postnatally. The sensitivity of carotid baroreceptors is reset as arterial pressure increases throughout the last third of gestation and the first postnatal month. Postnatally, baroreflex sensitivity increases from birth to six weeks of age with the most rapid changes occurring after two weeks of age [21–23]. Inhalation anesthetics may aggravate the relative insensitivity of the baroreceptor response in neonates [24,25].

- **Respiratory effects.** All potent volatile agents depress minute ventilation and shift the $CO_2$ response curve "up and to the left" in infants, more so than in older children and adults.

**115**

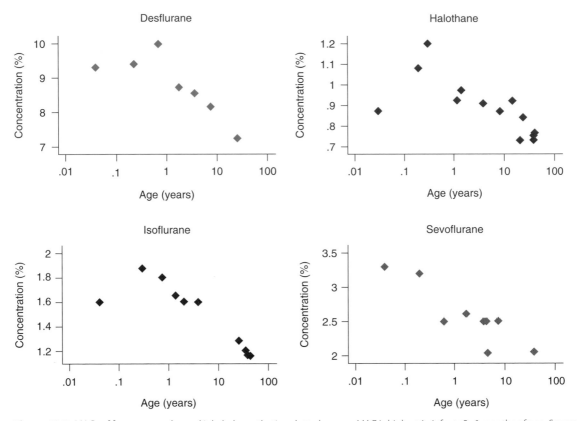

**Figure 13.9** MACs of four commonly used inhaled anesthetics plotted vs. age. MAC is highest in infants 3–6 months of age. Source: [18].

Comorbidities such as the Chiara II malformation commonly associated with spina bifida worsen this finding.

## Sevoflurane

Sevoflurane has become the most popular inhalation anesthetic for children because of its ease of acceptance, non-pungency, and relative forgiveness with regard to adverse cardiovascular effects in comparison with the previous generation's gold standard, halothane [26]. After passing through soda lime or baralyme, sevoflurane is degraded into five compounds (Compounds A–E). Only Compound A accumulates significantly in the circuit when the following conditions are met: increased temperature, low water content, high concentration of sevoflurane, the use of baralyme rather than soda lime, or the use of new soda lime.

Sevoflurane has half the potency of isoflurane and one-third that of halothane. Interestingly, sevoflurane MAC does not increase with decreasing age,

in contrast to the other inhaled agents. For unclear reasons, the additive effect of nitrous oxide is not as prominent with sevoflurane as it is with other agents.

There seem to be some unique electroencephalographic effects of sevoflurane, specifically epileptiform-like patterns, as well as rare facial or limb twitching during light levels that seem to disappear in deeper planes. The significance of these findings is also unclear and no adverse outcomes have been linked to these findings.

## Desflurane

Desflurane is isoflurane with replacement of the chlorine with a fluorine – but what a difference pharmacologically! The blood–gas and tissue–blood solubilities are dramatically decreased and consequently the uptake and distribution as well as the washout of desflurane is the most rapid of any of the potent inhaled anesthetics. Unfortunately, the pungency and airway irritability of desflurane make it a poor clinical choice for inhalation inductions in children, but maintenance and emergence are not problematic following an intravenous induction or an inhalation induction with a less pungent (i.e., sevoflurane) anesthetic.

Emergence, as expected, is quite rapid because of the rapid washout, and therefore a plan for preemptive postoperative analgesia should be coupled with the use of desflurane as the principal anesthetic. There would appear to be little need for utilizing desflurane clinically in neonates and infants for the sake of facilitating rapid emergence or even rapid intraoperative adjustments in anesthetic depth because of their relatively small tissue stores and rapidity of equilibration with changes in the inspired agent concentration.

## Isoflurane

The wash-in and wash-out of isoflurane is slower than desflurane or sevoflurane. Like desflurane, it has a pungent odor, making it less favorable for mask induction in children; maintenance and emergence do not present significant clinical issues, the pungency notwithstanding. Infants anesthetized with isoflurane do not exhibit the same degree of reduction in heart rate that results from halothane use.

## Nitrous Oxide

Nitrous oxide has a long history of use in infants and small children. Its low blood–gas partition coefficient and low potency have two very appealing features for use in infants – it works rapidly and because of its lower potency may actually provide a greater margin of safety for infants. As a carrier gas it has featured prominently throughout the history of pediatric anesthesia because of the second gas effect.

Caution must be applied with regard to its tendency to occupy air-filled spaces due to its blood–gas partition coefficient being 34-fold greater than nitrogen. Inasmuch as bowel obstruction is one of the more common newborn surgical emergencies, clinicians must be circumspect about the use of nitrous oxide. More subtle considerations include its effect on the inhibition of methionine synthetase, an important consideration for infants with their developing bone marrow and nervous systems.

## Intravenous Induction Agents

Barbiturates have long been the standard intravenous induction agent for all age groups. Special pediatric considerations over the years have been recognized – for example, prolongation of sleep times of newborns (presumably due to greater blood–brain barrier permeability), impaired biotransformation due to glucuronic acid conjugation immaturity in the first several weeks of life, and an increased dosing requirement in the newborn period and especially for the first six months of life.

**Thiopental** is a highly lipid-soluble ultra-short-acting barbiturate that results in rapid unconsciousness. Plasma protein binding is reduced in the neonate, resulting in a doubling of the plasma-free fraction in comparison to children and adults. In addition, clearance is substantially reduced in infants (less than half that of adults). Because its effect is primarily terminated by redistribution, recovery in infants nevertheless is on par with older children and adults. Thiopental has not been available in the United States since 2011.

**Methohexital**, a more potent barbiturate than thiopental, has not commonly been used by the intravenous route in children. It has mainly been used rectally, and a body of literature has described blood levels and reliability as an induction agent in infants and older children, but not in neonates.

Virtually all intravenous inductions, when chosen, are currently accomplished with **propofol**. Its short duration of action because of rapid redistribution and biotransformation permit its use by bolus as well as continuous infusion. Glucuronidation is the major route of elimination. Uridine 5-diphosphate-glucuronosyltransferases (UGTs) occur at varying times during early infancy, and some UGTs are present at birth while others develop during early infancy. A decrease in total requirements may be due to a net immaturity of neonatal enzyme systems while a decrease in induction dose requirements probably has more to do with a greater tendency toward hypotension and bradycardia in infants [27]. Propofol may also limit its own biotransformation by virtue of its effect on cardiac output and hepatic blood flow in neonates and infants, although few studies exist describing neonatal propofol pharmacology. Other features noted in patients who can self-report them – pain on injection, antiemetic effects – may occur in infants as well, but are probably more difficult to detect.

**Ketamine** remains a significantly utilized alternative to propofol because it preserves cardiovascular stability and rapidly results in unconsciousness.

Infants typically require a much larger dose to produce lack of movement with induction than older children. In infants younger than three months, the volume of distribution is similar to older infants, but the elimination half-life is prolonged. Clearance is reduced in younger infants with reduced metabolism; slower renal excretion is the likely cause. While respiratory efforts tend to be preserved in children and adults, respiratory depression and apnea may be the result of higher doses required in infants. Muscular (extensor) spasm may also occur, as well as elevations in pulmonary artery pressure in infants with an underlying elevation in baseline pulmonary artery pressure (congenital heart disease).

# Sedatives

## Benzodiazepines

Benzodiazepines are commonly used in pediatric patients to provide sedation, anxiolysis, anterograde amnesia, as well as anticonvulsant therapy. Benzodiazepines bind to gamma amino butyric acid (GABA) receptors, which are distributed throughout the frontal cortex and cerebellum in varying densities during the fetal through neonatal period [28]. Metabolism occurs in the liver by cytochrome P450 enzymes with excretion in the urine. The clearance of these drugs varies depending on clearance of the parent drug and its metabolites, as well as the intrinsic physiology of neonates and their comorbidities.

**Midazolam** is lipid-soluble at physiological pH and therefore has a rapid onset compared to other benzodiazepines. It also has a shorter half-life compared to diazepam and lorazepam. Absorption via the gastrointestinal tract is slower in premature neonates, full-term neonates, and young infants secondary to delayed gastric emptying [12,29]. Rectally administered midazolam may have faster absorption, but the bioavailability may vary.

Midazolam is converted to the active metabolite 1-hydroxymidazolam (1-OH-midazolam) by cytochrome P450 enzymes CYP3A4, CYP3A5, and, to a lesser extent, CYP3A7 [30,31]. 1-OH-midazolam has a shorter half-life compared to other benzodiazepine metabolites, yet in neonates the half-life can be anywhere from four to six hours, compared to two hours in adults [30,31]. CYP3A4 and CYP3A5 are activated during the first week of life [29] and, therefore, the formation of 1-OH-midazolam is decreased and

clearance of midazolam is slower in preterm and full-term neonates [31,32].

**Diazepam** is a longer-acting benzodiazepine commonly administered via oral, intravenous, or rectal routes. It is also metabolized by cytochrome P450 enzymes into desmethyldiazepam, which has a longer half-life in premature and term neonates compared to older children [28]. While highly bound to plasma proteins, the amount of unbound drug in newborns is double that of adults, so there is a potential for accumulation and a prolonged drug effect. The adult ratio of bound:unbound drug is reached by the first week of life.

**Lorazepam** is usually administered intravenously to the neonatal population. While some PK data exist for intramuscular and submucosal routes in the healthy adult population [33], there is still a lack of data in neonates and infants. It is a long-acting benzodiazepine, with half-life ranging from 18 to 73 hours in neonates, compared with 10–12 hours in older children and adults [34]. While also metabolized by cytochrome P450 enzymes, its metabolite is inactive. Lorazepam is about 75 percent plasma protein bound and also excreted in urine.

Any comorbidities that cause changes in hemodynamic, renal, or hepatic function or concomitant medication administration may also alter metabolism and excretion of benzodiazepines, leading to accumulation and prolonged sedation. Burtin et al. showed decreased clearance by 30 percent in neonates receiving sympathomimetic drugs, which the authors attributed to compromised cardiac output in critically ill neonates [32]. De Wildt et al. showed newborns exposed to indomethacin for treatment of patent ductus arteriosus (PDA) had higher clearance of midazolam compared to those who were not exposed; however, a decrease in renal function with the use of medications such as indomethacin and NSAIDs should also be considered in the neonate receiving benzodiazepines [31].

Interindividual variability in expression and activity of the CYP enzymes may also account for the interindividual variability in the clearance of benzodiazepines in neonates [28,29,30,32]. Exact neonatal dosing for a target concentration is difficult. Moreover, drugs like midazolam, which is considered short-acting in adults, may not have the same clinical profile in neonates. Benzodiazepines should therefore be administered and titrated to clinical effect, with the potential for accumulation in mind.

# Dexmedetomidine

**Dexmedetomidine** is a selective α2-agonist increasingly used in pediatric anesthesia for sedation or as an adjunct [35–39]. It has an α2:α1 activity of 1620:1, compared to clonidine's 200:1, and acts on the locus ceruleus to provide sedation and analgesia. Dexmedetomidine is metabolized in the liver by glucuronidation, hydroxylation, and N-methylation. It is about 90 percent protein-bound to albumin, and is eliminated primarily in the urine. In adults, dexmedetomidine has a half-life of about two hours, compared to clonidine's half-life of 12–24 hours. In newborns, the half-life is about 7.6 hours in preterm neonates and 3.2 hours in term neonates [40]. Using PPK, Potts et al. found clearance in neonates in the ICU to be about one-third that of adults. Clearance reaches about 87 percent of adult values by one year of age [41]. All of these findings are attributed to immature metabolic and elimination pathways in the neonate.

The hemodynamic profile of dexmedetomidine has also been widely studied in adults and children [42–46]. Its known effects on heart rate, and blood pressure, have also been seen in neonates [39,47]. While its safety profile continues to be studied and its use generally accepted among the pediatric population, it's PK profile in the neonate may warrant lower dosages to avoid unwanted effects [40].

# Opioids

Opioids are commonly used in neonates for analgesia and sedation. Similar to benzodiazepines, several studies have shown age to be the most important variable that affects metabolite formation, morphine clearance, and plasma concentration [48,49]. In neonates and infants, the beta elimination half-life of opioids is prolonged compared to adults and older children, so respiratory depression may also be prolonged. Opioids are primarily metabolized in the liver via oxidation, except morphine which undergoes glucuronidation and remifentanil which clears via ester hydrolysis [50]. Most opioids are also protein-bound to albumin and α1-acid glycoprotein, both of which are decreased in the neonate and, therefore, cause increased concentrations of unbound drug. Excretion is mainly via the kidneys.

**Morphine** is metabolized into morphine-3-glucoronide (M3G), which has no analgesic properties, and morphine-6-glucoronide (M6G), the active metabolite. The plasma concentration ratio of M6G:morphine is higher after oral administration than after intravenous administration due to the first-pass mechanism [50]. Among neonates and infants, the M3G metabolite also predominates [49]. Since there is less of the active metabolite, M6G, there may be a need for a higher concentration for an analgesic effect compared to older children and adults. As a result, there may also be more undesirable effects of the opioid, such as hypotension, bradycardia, hypercarbia, and seizures. Using a PPK approach, Bouwmeester et al. found that higher morphine infusion rates were necessary for infants and young children to achieve a target plasma concentration of 10 ng mL$^{-1}$, with the highest rate required at one year of age. Total body clearance of morphine reached 80 percent that of adults by age six months [49]. Once M3G and M6G metabolites are formed, they are excreted via the kidneys. Excretion then becomes a function of GFR. Because neonates have decreased glomerular and tubular function, the rate of elimination will also be slower and lead to accumulation of active metabolites.

**Fentanyl** is highly lipid-soluble and 50–100 times more potent than morphine, with rapid onset and shorter duration. It is also known to be relatively cardiac-stable and used widely in cardiac anesthesia as well as for sedation in the NICU. Fentanyl is metabolized in the liver by CYP3A4 enzymes via N-dealkylation and hydrozylation into inactive metabolites, and excreted in the urine. It is mostly bound to albumin, and less so to α1-acid glycoprotein. In adults, metabolism of fentanyl is not significantly altered with liver cirrhosis, but may be altered with impaired hepatic blood flow [50]. Transmucosal and transdermal routes of administration have been used and studied in older children [48,49], but their use and pharmacokinetic profile has not been delineated in neonates.

**Remifentanil** is a synthetic opioid with a potency similar to that of fentanyl. It is fast-acting and has a very short half-life. In adults, the beta elimination half-life is 9.5 min, while studies in neonates show it to be 3.4–5.7 min [51,52]. It is unique compared to other opioids because it undergoes ester hydrolysis in the plasma. The clearance rate in neonates is about twice as long as adults; however, liver disease, kidney disease, or the use of cardiopulmonary bypass do not appear to affect the clearance of remifentanil [51,53].

**Sufentanil** is also a highly lipid-soluble, synthetic opioid 5–10 times more potent than fentanyl. Like fentanyl, it has been shown to be appropriate for use in pediatric cardiac patients because it maintains relative hemodynamic stability. Sufentanil is metabolized by N-dealkylation into inactive metabolites and excreted in the urine [50]. It is mostly bound to α1-acid glycoprotein [54,55]; thus, more active, unbound drug can be found in the plasma of neonates. Moreover, protein binding is affected by plasma pH such that alkalosis would decrease and acidosis increase binding [55].

**Alfentanil** is another fast-acting opioid with a short half-life (5–10 min). It is one-third less potent than fentanyl and bound mainly to α1-acid glycoprotein. Unlike sufentanil, plasma pH does not affect its protein binding [50]. Alfentanil is metabolized by CYP3A4 and excreted in the urine. Like fentanyl, muscle rigidity has been found to occur in neonates receiving alfentanil infusions [56].

# Acetaminophen

**Acetaminophen** is a commonly used over-the-counter drug to treat fever and pain. It is water-soluble and therefore has potentially a lower peak concentration in neonates, given their higher volume of distribution. This would lead to less effectiveness and the need for a higher loading dose. While maturation may account for about one-third of the variability in absorption, other factors that can contribute to slower absorption in the neonate include their slower gastric emptying, and concomitant administration of food or other medications [57]. Absorption after rectal administration is much faster compared to oral administration, but the bioavailability of the drug may also have interindividual variability, depending on where in the rectum it is delivered. Although metabolism is by glucuronidation in a mature system, acetaminophen undergoes primarily sulfate conjugation and renal excretion in the neonate. Thus, one can expect slower clearance and the potential for accumulation and toxicity. Adult clearance is usually reached by 12 years of age [58].

# Muscle Relaxants

Neuromuscular blockers (NMBs) are used intraoperatively and postoperatively for endotracheal intubation, immobilization and decreasing barotrauma, oxygen consumption, and anesthetic or sedative requirements. While some data exist in neonates and infants, the only current consensus guidelines for use of NMBs in the pediatric population comes from the United Kingdom [59]. However, this consensus only addresses use in critically ill children, and does not include neonates.

Categorized into depolarizing and nondepolarizing agents, NMBs essentially bind directly or competitively to acetylcholine receptors (AChRs) on the neuromuscular junction (NMJ) and block transmission of the electrical impulse that causes muscle contraction. A higher volume of distribution generally means a higher concentration of drug needed to reach motor endplates; however, the number and type of AChRs present change throughout development. In neonates, maturation of the NMJ occurs during the first two months of life [60]. Mature AChRs are produced only in the junctional area, but an immature type of receptor is also formed during development and in cases of denervation. These immature AChRs are located in areas outside of the junctional area, have a greater affinity for succinylcholine than nondepolarizing agents, and have sodium channels that are more easily depolarized and open for a longer period of time [61]. Clinically, this may result in variability and unpredictability of results after administration of NMBs. Older children have a higher muscle mass:fat ratio compared to infants, so will have more AChRs and require a higher drug concentration for a desired effect [60].

**Succinylcholine** is the only nondepolarizing agent used clinically and it is well established that larger doses are required in neonates and infants because of their increased volume of distribution [62]. Recommended doses are 2–3 mg kg$^{-1}$ in neonates and infants, 1 mg kg$^{-1}$ in older children, and 4 mg kg$^{-1}$ for intramuscular administration. Succinylcholine is hydrolyzed by plasma cholinesterases into succinic acid and choline, so conditions like liver disease and atypical plasma cholinesterase may prolong its metabolism. Acute denervation injuries, crush injuries, and burns can result in a hypersensitivity to succinylcholine and lead to hyperkalemia, hyperkalemic dysrhythmias, or cardiac arrest. Children with undiagnosed myopathies, such as Duchenne muscular dystrophy, are at risk for malignant hyperthermia after succinylcholine administration. These and other known serious side-effects have led to the black box warning that recommends limiting use of succinylcholine to rapid sequence intubation and emergent securing of an airway in children [63].

The nondepolarizing muscle relaxants can be categorized into long-, intermediate-, and short-acting

**Table 13.2** The comparative effective dose to produce 95 percent depression of twitch height (ED95)

| | ED95 (mcg/kg) | | | Onset (min) | | | Duration (min) | | | Recovery (min) | | |
|---|---|---|---|---|---|---|---|---|---|---|---|---|
| | Infant | Child | Adult | Infant | Child | Adult | Infant | Child | Adult | Infant | Child | Adult |
| Pancuronium | 66 | 93 | 67 | 2–5 | 2–4 | 3–5 | – | 24 | 22 | – | 33 | 37 |
| Cisatracurium | – | 41 | 48 | – | 1–3 | 2–4 | – | 25 | 25 | – | 40 | 45 |
| Vecuronium | 47 | 81 | 43 | – | 1–3 | 2–3 | – | 22 | 26 | 73 | 35 | 53 |
| Rocuronium | 255 | 402 | 350 | – | 0.8–1.5 | 1–2 | – | 27 | 42 | – | 42 | 69 |
| Succinylcholine | 650 | 400 | 300 | 0.5 | 0.6 | 1 | 4.6 | 5.8 | 6.0 | 7.4 | 9.7 | 10 |

Source: adapted from [60].

groups. With the exception of cisatracurium, they are primarily metabolized by the liver, with biliary and renal excretion. The comparative effective dose to produce 95 percent depression of twitch height (ED95) for commonly used NMBs is listed in Table 13.2.

**Pancuronium** is a bisquaternary aminosteroid, long-acting, nondepolarizing muscle relaxant. It is favored in critically ill pediatric patients because of its known sympathomimetic effects resulting in tachycardia, hypertension, and increased cardiac output. There are sparse data on neonates. Some have shown the ED50 of children to be greater than that of adults overall, [64] and the ED95 to be greater in children compared to neonates, likely due to the difference in volume of distribution and protein binding.

**Vecuronium** is a monotertiary, monoquaternary aminosteroid derivative of pancuronium that is an intermediate-acting NMB. It does not have the same hemodynamic effects as pancuronium. Meretoja et al. found that neonates and infants less than one year had a lower ED95 compared to children aged 2–13 years, which the authors again attribute to the difference in volume of distribution and protein binding between age groups [65]. These differences also account for the prolonged effect of vecuronium in infants compared to older children [66].

**Rocuronium** is a monoquaternary aminosteroid, intermediate-acting NMB, that is six times less potent and has faster onset than vecuronium and pancuronium [67]. Its ED95 also appears to be age-dependent and it does not cause histamine release or hemodynamic changes [67,68].

**Cisatracurium** is the cis–cis isomer of atracurium, a bisquaternary ammonium benzylisoquinolinium that primarily undergoes Hoffman elimination. It is organ-independent for clearance and desirable for use in neonates and children with renal impairment. Inasmuch as Hoffman elimination depends on pH and temperature, lower pH and lower temperature will increase time to elimination. This should be considered when cisatracurium is used in patients with a metabolic acidosis. Cisatracurium is 3–4 times more potent than atracurium and does not cause significant histamine release [59]. Few studies exist for cisatracurium in infants and neonates. Some suggest that in neonates with congenital cardiac repairs, recovery from cisatracurium infusion is faster than from vecuronium infusion, but there was no difference in general patient outcomes.

# References

1. Crawford J, Terry M, Rourke G. Simplification of drug dosage calculation by application of the surface area principle. *Pediatrics.* 1950;5:783–90.

2. Holliday M, Segar W. The maintenance need for water in parenteral fluid therapy. *Pediatrics.* 1957;19:823–32.

3. Anderson B, Holford N. Tips and traps analyzing pediatric PK data. *Pediatric Anesthesia.* 2011;21:222–37.

4. Robiquet T. Rapport sur un memoire adresse a l'Academie royale de medecine par MM Sarrus et Rameaux. *Bull Acad R Med.* 1839;3:1094.

5. Brody S: *Bioenergetics and Growth: With Special Reference to the Efficiency Complex.* New York: Reinhold Publishing Corporation; 1945.

6. Rigby-Jones AE, Sneyd, JR. Pharmacokinetics and pharmacodynamics-is there anything new? *Anesthesia.* 2012;67:1–11.

7. Anderson B, Allegaert K, Holford N. Population clinical pharmacology of children: modelling covariate effects. *Eur J Pediatr.* 2006;165:819–29.

8. Edginton A. Knowledge-driven approaches for the guidance of first-in-children dosing. *Pediatric Anesthesia.* 2011;21:206–13.

9. Rhodin M, Anderson B, Peters A, et al. Human renal function maturation: a quantitative description

using weight and postmenstrual age. *Pediatr Nephrol.* 2009;24:67–76.

10. de Wildt S, Kearns G, Leeder J, van den Anker J. Cytochrome P450 3A: ontogeny and drug disposition. *Clin Pharmacokinet.* 1999;37:485–505.

11. Cella M, Knibbe C, Danhof M, Pascua, OD. What is the right dose for children? *Br J Clin Pharmacol.* 2010;70:597–603.

12. Kearns G, Abdel-Rahman S, Alander S, et al. Developmental pharmacology: drug disposition, action, and therapy in infants and children. *N Engl J Med.* 2003;349:1157–67.

13. Marsh D, Hatch D, Fitzgerald M, et al. Opioid systems and the newborn. *Br J Anaes.* 1997;79:787–95.

14. Klitzner T, Friedman W. A diminished role for the sarcoplasmic reticulum in newborn myocardial contraction: effects of ryanodine. *Ped Res.* 1989;26:98–101.

15. Johnson T, Rostami-Hodjegan A. Resurgence in the use of physiologically based pharmacokinetic models in pediatric clinical pharmacology: parallel shift in incorporating the knowledge of biological elements and increased applicability to drug development and clinical practice. *Paediatr Anesth.* 2011;21:291–301.

16. Johnson T, Rostami-Hodjegan A, Tucker G. Prediction of the clearance of eleven drugs and associated variability in neonates, infants and children. *Clin Pharmacokinet.* 2006;45:931–56.

17. Keys T. *The History of Surgical Anesthesia.* New York: Dover Publications; 1963.

18. Coté CJ. Pediatric anesthesia. In: Miller RD, Eriksson LI, Fleisher LA, et al., editors. *Miller's Anesthesia,* 7th edn. Philadelphia, PA: Churchill Livingstone; 2010.

19. Vlajkovic G, Sindjelic R. Emergence delirium in children: many questions, few answers. *Anesth Analg.* 2007;4:84–91.

20. Friedman W. The intrinsic physiologic properties of the developing heart. *Prog Cardiovasc Dis.* 1972;15:87–111.

21. Blanco C, Dawes G, Hanson M. Carotid baroreceptors in fetal and newborn sheep. *Ped Res.* 1988;24:342–6.

22. Friedman W, George B. Treatment of congestive heart failure by altering loading conditions of the heart. *J Ped.* 1985;106:697–706.

23. Holden K, Morgan J, Krauss A. Incomplete baroreceptor responses in newborn infants. *Amer J Perinat.* 1985;2:31–4.

24. Gournay V, Drouin E, Rozé J. Development of baroreflex control of heart rate in preterm and full term infants. *Arch Dis Child Fetal Neonatal Ed.* 2002;86: F151–4.

25. Patton D, Hanna B. Postnatal maturation of baroreflex heart rate control in neonatal swine. *Can J Cardiol.* 1994;10:233–8.

26. Holzman R, van der Velde M, Kaus S, et al. Sevoflurane depresses myocardial contractility less than halothane during induction of anesthesia in children. *Anesthesiology.* 1996;85:1260–7.

27. Steur R, Perez R, De Lange J. Dosage scheme for propofol in children under 3 years of age. *Paediatr Anaesth.* 2004;14:462–7.

28. Jacqz-Aigrain E, Burtin P. Clinical pharmacokinetics of sedatives in neonates. *Clin Pharmacokinet.* 1996;31:423–43.

29. Anderson B, Allegaert K. The pharmacology of anaesthetics in the neonate. *Best Pract Res Clin Anaesth.* 2010;24:419–31.

30. Pacifici G. Clinical pharmacology of midazolam in neonates and children: effect of disease – a review. *Int J Pediatr.,* 2014. doi: 10.1155/2014/309342.

31. de Wildt S, Kearns G, Hop W, et al. Pharmacokinetics and metabolism of intravenous midazolam in preterm infants. *Clin Pharmacol Ther.* 2001;70:525–31.

32. Burtin P, Jacqz-Aigrain E, Girard P, et al. Population pharmacokinetics of midazolam in neonates. *Clin Pharmacol Ther.* 1994;56:615–25.

33. Wermeling D, Miller J, Archer S, Manaligod J, Rudy A. Bioavailability and pharmacokinetics of lorazaepam after intranasal, intravenous and intramuscular administration. *J Clin Pharmacol.* 2001;41:1225–31.

34. McDermott C, Kowalczyk A, Schnitzler E, et al. Pharmacokinetics of lorazepam in critically ill neonates with seizures. *J Pediatr.* 1992;120:479–83.

35. Chrysostomou C, Zeballos T. Use of dexmedetomidine in a pediatric heart transplant patient. *Pediatr Cardiol.* 2005;26:651–4.

36. Finkel J, Johnson Y, Quezado Z. The use of dexmedetomidine to facilitate acute discontinuation of opioids after cardiac transplantation in children. *Crit Care Med.* 2005;33:2110–12.

37. Ard J, Doyle W, Bekker A. Awake craniotomy with dexmedetomidine in pediatric patients. *J Neurosurg Anesth.* 2003;15:263–6.

38. Tobias J, Berkenbosch J. Sedation during mechanical ventilation in infants and children: dexmedetomidine versus midazolam. *J Neurosurg Anesthesiol.* 2003;15:263–6.

39. Berkenbosch J, Tobias J. Development of bradycardia during sedation with dexmedetomidine in an infant concurrently receiving digoxin. *Pediatr Crit Care Med.* 2003;4:203–5.

40. Chrysostomou C, Schulman S, Castellanos M, et al. A phase II/III, multicenter, safety, efficacy,

and pharmacokinetic study of dexmedetomidine in preterm and term neonates. *J Pediatr*. 2014;164:276–82.

41. Potts A, Warman G, Anderson B. Dexmedetomidine disposition in children: a population analysis. *Ped Anaesth*. 2008;18:722–30.

42. Talke P, Richardson C, Scheinin M, Fisher D. Postoperative pharmacokinetics and sympatholytic effects of dexmedetomidine. *Anesth Analg*. 1997;85:1136–42.

43. Talke P, Chen R, Thomas B, et al. The hemodynamic and adrenergic effects of perioperative dexmedetomidine infusion after vascular surgery. *Anesth Analg*. 2000;90:834–9.

44. Hsu Y, Cortinez L, Robertson K, et al. Dexmedetomidine pharmacodynamics: part I. *Anesthesiology*. 2004;101:1066–76.

45. Cortinez L, Hsu Y, Sum-Ping S, et al. Dexmedetomidine pharmacodynamics: part II. *Anesthesiology*. 2004;101:1077–83.

46. Petroz G, Sikich N, James M, et al. A phase I, two-center study of the pharmacokinetics and pharmacodynamics of dexmedetomidine in children. *Anesthesiology*. 2006;105:1098–110.

47. Berkenbosch J, Wankum P, Tobias J. Prospective evaluation of dexmedetomidine for noninvasive procedural sedation in children. *Pedatr Crit Care Med*. 2005;6:435–9.

48. Bouwmeester N, van den Anker J, Hop W, Anand K, Tibboel D. Age- and therapy-related effects on morphine requirements and plasma concentrations of morphine and its metabolites in postoperative infants. *Br J Anaesth*. 2003;90:642–52.

49. Bouwmeester N, Anderson B, Tibboel D, Holford N. Developmental pharmacokinetics of morphine and its metabolites in neonates, infants and young children. *Br J Anaesth*. 2004;92:208–17.

50. Tegeder I, Lotsch J, Geisslinger G. Pharmacokinetics of opioids in liver disease. *Clin Pharmacokinetics*. 1999;37:17–40.

51. Davis P, Wilson A, Siewers R. The effects of cardiopulmonary bypass on remifentanil kinetics in children undergoing atrial septal defect repair. *Anesth Analg*. 1999;89:904–8.

52. Ross A, Davis P, Dear G, et al. Pharmacokinetics of remifentanil in anesthetized pediatric patients undergoing elective surgery or diagnostic procedures. *Anesth Analg*. 2001;93:1393–401.

53. Welzing L, Roth B. Experience with remifentanil in neonates and infants. *Drugs*. 2006;66:1339–50.

54. Greeley W, de Bruijn N, Davis D. Sufentanil pharmacokinetics in pediatric cardiovascular patients. *Anesth Analg*. 1987;66:1067–72.

55. Lundeberg S, Roelofse J. Aspects of pharmacokinetics and pharmacodynamics of sufentanil in pediatric practice. *Paediatr Anaesth*. 2011;21:274–9.

56. Pokela M, Ryhanen P, Koivisto M, Olkkola K, Saukkonen A. Alfentanil-induced rigidity in newborn infants. *Anesth Analg*. 1992;75:252–7.

57. Anderson B, van Lingen R, Hansen T, Lin Y, Holford N. Acetaminophen developmental pharmacokinetics in premature neonates and infants: a pooled population analysis. *Anesthesiology*. 2002;96:1336–45.

58. Allegaert K, Naulaers G, Vanhaesebrouck S, Anderson B. The paracetamol concentration-effect relation in neonates. *Pediatric Anesthesia*. 2013;23:45–50.

59. Playfor S, Jenkins I, Boyles C, et al. Consensus guidelines for sustained neuromuscular blockade in critically ill children. *Pediatr Anesth*. 2007;17:881–7.

60. Martin L, Bratton S, O'Rourke P. Clinical uses and controversies of neuromuscular blocking agents in infants and children. *Crit Care Med.*. 1999;27:1358–68.

61. Martyn J, White D, Gronert G, Jaffe R, Ward J. Up-and-down regulation of skeletal muscle acetylcholine receptors. *Anesthesiology*. 1992;76:822–43.

62. Meakin G, McKiernan E, Morris P, Baker R. Dose–reponse curves for suxamethonium in neonates, infants and children. *Br J Anaesth*. 1989;62:655–8.

63. Hospira Inc. Succinylcholine chloride IV injection [Package insert]. Lake Forest, IL, Hospira, Inc, 2005

64. Goudsouzian N, Ryan J, Savarese J. The neuromuscular effects of pancuronium in infants and children. *Anesthesiology*. 1974;41:95–8.

65. Meretoja O, Wirtavuori K, Neuvonen P. Age-dependence of the dose–response curve of vecuronium in pediatric patients during balanced anesthesia. *Anesth Analg*. 1988;67:21–6.

66. Fisher D, Castagnoli K, Miller R. Vecuronium kinetics and dynamics in anesthetized infants and children. *Clin Pharmacol Ther*. 1985;37:402–6.

67. Foldes F, Nagashima H, Nguyen H, et al. The neuromuscular effects of ORG9426 in patients receiving balanced anesthesia. *Anesthesiology*. 1991;75:191–6.

68. Woelfel S, Brandom B, Cook D, Sarner J. Effects of bolus administration of ORG-9426 in children during nitrous oxide–halothane anesthesia. *Anesthesiology*. 1992;76:939–42.

# The Newborn Airway

Shivani S. Patel and Narasimhan Jagannathan

Airway management poses a challenge due to the newborn's small size, unique anatomy, and physiology. Thus, the approach to newborn airway management differs from that for older children and adults. This chapter provides an overview of a spectrum of topics important in newborn airway management, including airway anatomy and physiology, tips for adequate ventilation and intubation, one-lung ventilation techniques, management of mediastinal masses, difficult airway management, and airway management in infants undergoing mandibular distraction and tongue–lip adhesion.

## Infant Airway Anatomy and Physiology

The infant respiratory system is not simply a miniaturized version of the adult system. In addition to anatomical differences (Table 14.1), significant differences in respiratory physiology exist. The newborn's smaller airway radius creates greater resistance to air flow that in turn increases the work of breathing and offers added pressure on the lumen of the airway. Any amount of airway narrowing caused by edema, and congenital malformations, can have serious consequences on the overall work of breathing and respiratory function [1]. Combined with the infant's higher chest wall compliance, the narrow airway also increases the incidence of airway obstruction [2]. The reduced outward recoil of the highly compliant chest wall produces low transpulmonary pressures and causes small peripheral airways to collapse during tidal breathing, predisposing to ventilation/perfusion mismatch (V/Q) [2,3] and oxygen desaturation.

The lungs of newborns are very compliant, contributing to low functional residual capacity (FRC) and dynamic airway collapse [3]. Combined with their higher oxygen consumption, this may lead to rapid oxygen desaturation during apneic periods [4,5]. Infants also have increased carbon dioxide production when compared with adults. Therefore, infants require a higher respiratory rate to achieve a relatively higher minute ventilation needed to eliminate carbon dioxide [15].

## Practical Tips to Adequately Ventilate and Intubate Young Infants

### Bag-Mask Ventilation

Bag-mask ventilation (BMV) is a critical component of airway management as it provides oxygenation and ventilation prior to placement of a definitive airway [16,17]. Selection of an appropriate-sized mask is essential to obtain an adequate seal. The mask should fit over the bridge of the nose, seal on the sides of the nasolabial folds, and fit between the lower lip and chin.

### BMV Technique

The facemask should be held tightly to the patient's face with the thumb and forefinger of the anesthesia providers' left hand while the other fingers lift the mandible toward the facemask. Care should be taken to avoid excessive pressure on the submandibular soft tissue as this may cause airway obstruction. The pharyngeal space can be opened via displacement of the mandible, chin lift, jaw thrust, and atlanto-occipital joint extension, leading to greater patency of the airway [18]. While the left hand seals the mask, the right hand is used to compress the reservoir bag on the anesthesia breathing circuit to generate positive pressure. Peak inspiratory pressure should be kept below 20 cmH$_2$O to avoid gastric insufflation of air. If a one-handed approach is insufficient, additional help may be recruited to attempt a two-handed technique in which the initial provider either maintains the same position while the secondary provider performs a jaw thrust, or uses both hands to secure the facemask while the secondary provider squeezes the reservoir

**Table 14.1** Unique infant airway anatomy compared to adults, and its clinical significance

| Infant airway anatomy | Clinical significance in airway management |
|---|---|
| Larger occiput | Supine positioning on a flat surface causes neck flexion that may lead to airway obstruction; consider use of a shoulder roll |
| Shorter and narrow hypopharynx, higher larynx | Barrier to aligning oral, laryngeal, and tracheal axes for laryngoscopy |
| Relative macroglossia, shorter mandible | Reduced upper airway space to displace tongue into the submandibular space |
| Vocal cords angled more cephalad rather than at 90 degrees | Vocal cords appear more anterior, potentially more traumatic tracheal tube insertion |
| U-shaped, long, floppy epiglottis | Use of semi-straight laryngoscope blade is preferable |
| Cartilaginous larynx and trachea (not yet calcified) | Extra compliance increases incidence of airway obstruction with positive-pressure ventilation |
| Funnel-shaped airway with cricoid cartilage as the functionally narrowest point; elliptical-shaped cricoid ring with larger anterior–posterior diameter | Affects the airway seal of both cuffed and uncuffed tracheal tubes |

Data from: [4,5,6,7,8–14].

bag. Additionally, use of an oral or nasal airway may help overcome difficulties in mask ventilation.

## Tracheal Intubation Technique

Endotracheal intubation via direct laryngoscopy is normally chosen unless specific indications require a different approach. When intubating an infant, placing a rolled towel under the supine patient's neck or shoulders helps improve airway patency. A laryngoscope can then be inserted to the right of the tongue to facilitate visualization. Because the infant's epiglottis is U-shaped, long, and floppy, and less in line with the trachea, a straight laryngoscope blade is preferable to a curved blade since it directly displaces the epiglottis out of view rather than using the vallecula's ligamentous connection with the epiglottis [6]. If the vocal cords cannot be visualized, gentle downward pressure at the level of the thyroid or cricoid cartilage may be helpful.

The tracheal tube (TT) should be introduced from the right side of the patient's mouth with the natural curve of the tube directed anteriorly. Insertion from the right is necessary to maintain visualization of the glottic opening. The TT should be advanced so that its distal end is midway between the vocal cords and carina. It is imperative to confirm position of the TT after securing it and anytime thereafter when there is a change in position because the infant's short trachea allows the TT to easily advance into the right mainstem bronchus [19]. Diminished breath sounds in the left lung may indicate right endobronchial intubation.

Use of a straight blade via a retromolar approach may allow better glottic visualization in infants with large tongues or small mandibles. A straight blade is inserted into the right side of the mouth, while the head is rotated to the left. This technique allows the tongue to be completely bypassed. The tip of the laryngoscope blade is then used to lift the epiglottis when it comes into view.

## One-Lung Ventilation, Video Assisted Thoracoscopy

Video assisted thoracoscopic surgery (VATS) is a less invasive approach to thoracoscopic surgery, making it advantageous to use in patients. Successful VATS requires proper one-lung ventilation (OLV), with efforts to promote a quiet surgical field, avoid contamination of the normal lung, prevent hypoxemia, and minimize respiratory insults inherent in the ventilation technique [20].

### Physiology of OLV

One-lung ventilation decreases functional residual capacity and tidal volume, predisposing to higher incidence of V/Q mismatch and oxygen desaturations. Hypoxic pulmonary vasoconstriction (HPV) diverts blood away from atelectatic lung tissue, normally minimizing V/Q mismatch. However, inhalational anesthetic agents in conjunction with high or low fractions of inspired oxygen reduce the HPV response [21,22].

Patients are placed in lateral decubitus position during VATS to allow for optimal access of the affected lung. However, this positioning has an unfavorable effect on respiratory physiology due to infants' compliant lungs, underdeveloped rib cage, and low functional residual capacity [3]. When the healthy lung is ventilated in the dependent position, it will have a decrease in compliance, potentially increasing the incidence of airway closure [23]. In adults, the lateral decubitus position increases the hydrostatic pressure gradient between the dependent and nondependent lungs, favorably increasing perfusion in the healthy lung while decreasing perfusion in the diseased lung. This results in relatively even distribution of ventilation and perfusion. In infants, however, this hydrostatic pressure gradient when in the same position results in uneven distribution of ventilation and perfusion as a result of their smaller size [24]. Therefore, infants may be at risk for hypoxia during OLV in the lateral decubitus position.

## OLV Techniques

The repertoire of devices suitable for OLV of the infant airway is limited. Currently, OLV in infants can be performed with a single-lumen TT or bronchial blocker, including the Fogarty® embolectomy catheter and Arndt Endobronchial Blocker® (Cook, WEB, Critical Care, Bloomington, IN, USA), because they are available in sizes suitable for the infant airway [25–27]. For neonates, these options may be more limited because of sizing availabilities in the small neonate or ex-preemie. In these patients, the surgeon may find retraction of the operative lung suitable while intermittently ventilating this lung during periods of oxygen desaturations.

A single-lumen TT can be advanced to isolate the bronchi after intubation. However, intubating the left main bronchus may be challenging. Suggested techniques to facilitate blind intubation of the left bronchus include use of a stylet to curve the distal end of the tube [28] or use of a distally curved rubber bougie which can be inserted blindly into the left main bronchus, followed by insertion of the TT over the bougie [29]. It should be noted that the right upper lobe bronchus may be obstructed when intubating the right main bronchus, causing hypoxia. Also, a single-lumen TT may not adequately seal the bronchus, risking contamination of the healthy lung and preventing collapse of the pathologic lung [25,30].

The bronchial blocker (BB) may also be used to achieve OLV in infants. An advantage of a BB versus a TT in sealing the bronchus is that the former provides a tighter seal. The Fogarty embolectomy catheter and Arndt Endobronchial Blocker have been successfully used for lung isolation in infants [31]. Proper placement of the Fogarty catheter is facilitated by bending the tip of its stylet toward the bronchus on the operative side. Positioning can be directed and confirmed with fiberoptic bronchoscopy (FOB) or fluoroscopy. Infants may require parallel insertion of the Fogarty catheter alongside the TT [32]. One such method for parallel insertion involves intubating the bronchus on the operative side with an TT, advancing a guide wire through the TT and into the bronchus, then removing the TT, and finally advancing the blocker over the guidewire into the bronchus [32]. It should be noted that since embolectomy catheters have low compliance and high pressure properties, the balloon should be inflated with incremental volumes of air until the airway is sealed. This will prevent overdistention, which can damage or rupture the airway [27,33].

More recently, the Arndt Endobronchial Blocker has been successfully used for OLV in small infants [31,34]. An advantage of the Endobronchial Blocker is that a central channel is present to allow for complete lung deflation. This feature is not present in the Fogarty catheter, so complete lung deflation may not be possible when using this device. The Arndt Endobronchial Blocker has a flexible wire loop and a three-part swivel adaptor. This adaptor allows for insertion of an FOB and balloon-tipped BB in two ports, and use of the third port as a ventilation circuit. The balloon is high-volume, low-pressure, and comes in two shapes to allow for optimal fit into the two mainstem bronchi: spherical for the right main stem bronchus and elliptical for the left main stem bronchus. Additionally, it is available in 1.0 cm length, corresponding to the length of the right main stem bronchus in the average child of two years of age. This enables it to fit entirely within the shorter right main stem bronchus, preventing obstruction of the upper lobe bronchus [35]. While coaxial insertion of the blocker and use of FOB can be accommodated in the relatively larger airway of older children, infants require a 5 French size Arndt Endobronchial Blocker and parallel insertion of the blocker due to the small diameter of their airway [27,36]. Additionally, passage of an FOB in an indwelling TT may be restricted in infants, in which case fluoroscopy may be used to guide insertion [36].

## Pre- and Intraoperative Management of Mediastinal Masses

Mediastinal masses encompass a diverse group of benign and malignant tumors that may be classified based on their location in the mediastinum [37]. These tumors have respiratory and hemodynamic consequences. In general, tumors of the anterior mediastinum comprise 46 percent of mediastinal masses in infants and children [38–41]. These tumors cause the most severe complications relating to compression of the airway and vasculature. It should be noted, however, that pediatric patients have an increased incidence of neurogenic tumors compared to adults [38–41], and these masses complicate airway management [42]. Although mediastinal tumors are rare in neonates, case reports have described mediastinal teratomas and cystic hygromas as important causes of respiratory distress in this population [43,44]. Cystic hygromas may be localized to the mediastinum or arise in the neck and extend down into the mediastinum, causing airway obstruction [43,45].

Tumors on the extreme end of the disease spectrum pose the greatest difficulty to management in the perioperative period, leading to severe cardiorespiratory complications and even death in children [46,47]. These problems can be exacerbated by general anesthesia [48,49]. As management of mediastinal masses in pediatric patients typically involves surgical biopsy or resection under general anesthesia with tracheal intubation, an understanding of risk factors for complications under anesthesia, preoperative testing, and intraoperative techniques to manage these tumors is necessary.

Mediastinal masses may lead to several forms of intrathoracic compromise, including one or a combination of compression of the tracheobronchial tree, compression of the pulmonary artery and heart, and superior vena cava syndrome [50,51]. Pulmonary symptoms such as dyspnea at rest, postural dyspnea, and stridor are strong risk factors for intraoperative airway complications [50,52], and symptoms such as syncope, arrhythmias, head and neck edema, and cyanosis predict cardiovascular complications in pediatric patients [50,52]. The absence of such symptoms, though, does not exclude the possibility

of airway or circulatory collapse under anesthesia [53,54]. Moreover, symptoms that are described may be worse in the postoperative period due to the effects to general anesthesia [47].

Careful preoperative testing can help gauge the severity of a patient's respiratory compromise and estimate the risk of adverse events under anesthesia. Computed tomography (CT) scanning is routinely used and provides the greatest amount of information concerning size of the mass, its location, and incursion on surrounding structures. Pulmonary function testing may reveal limited expiratory flow predictive of airway collapse under anesthesia [46], while echocardiography is useful in characterizing masses that may not compress the airway or cardiovascular systems but which will cause airway obstruction and cardiovascular collapse after induction of general anesthesia [55]. Additional tests may be used to enhance anesthetic management for specific tumors. A thyroid scan may be helpful when a thyroid mass is suspected, but should be performed first if iodinated contrast is used in the CT scan. Magnetic resonance imaging (MRI) may elucidate information on a neurogenic tumor, and positron emission tomography can be used for follow-up of germ cell tumors after treatment.

Intraoperatively, the anesthesiologist may employ a variety of techniques to manage mediastinal masses. Inhalational induction with maintenance of spontaneous respiration is recommended for infants with anterior mediastinal masses [56]. As functional residual capacity may be reduced under anesthesia, continuous positive airway pressure may also be helpful [46]. Elevation of the head of the bed mitigates undesirable effects of the supine position such as reduction of thoracic volume due to cephalad displacement of the diaphragm [47], and airway patency can also be maintained by placing the patient in partial or full lateral decubitus position [46].

When performing tracheal intubation, the clinician should consider placing an armored endotracheal tube without the assistance of neuromuscular blocking agents, as their administration may increase the risk of severe airway compression [57,58]. Alternatively, a supraglottic airway may provide sufficient ventilation [59]. If tracheal or bronchial collapse occurs, rigid bronchoscopy may be a useful option [46]. In general, when a compressed or distorted airway is a concern during anesthesia, a helium–oxygen gas mixture may be used as it allows for laminar air flow and minimizes resistance to gas flow in the airways [59,60].

127

If patients are at high risk of intraoperative airway obstruction, presurgical treatment of the mediastinal mass with steroids, chemotherapy, and/or radiotherapy may be helpful [52]. However, this approach may lessen the accuracy of diagnoses drawn from biopsies. Therefore, many clinicians recommend that, except in extreme circumstances, tissue diagnoses should be obtained prior to treatment, even if general anesthesia is required [61]. In patients with severe airway narrowing and pulmonary artery involvement, cardiopulmonary bypass may facilitate intraoperative gas exchange.

## Management of the Recognized and Unrecognized Difficult Airway

The difficult airway is typically defined by the inability to provide adequate mask ventilation and/or difficulty with tracheal intubation when using a traditional laryngoscope. The incidence of difficult airways is common in infants, particularly under the age of one year [62]. Therefore, it is prudent to have preplanned protocols in place to approach both the recognized and unrecognized difficult airway situations.

### The Anticipated Difficult Airway

The anticipated difficult airway scenario commonly arises in patients with craniofacial syndromes. Thus, it is imperative to perform a thorough preoperative assessment to pinpoint the area of obstruction and help gauge the success of various strategies to achieve adequate oxygenation. A useful approach to predict areas of obstruction is to group syndromes according to the associated functional abnormality [63]. Table 14.2 lists several encountered syndromes with abnormal airways grouped as such, and suggests airway management strategies.

Management of tracheal intubation poses a problem in infants and children as it is often impractical to perform awake intubations due to lack of cooperation [7]. Therefore, the clinician must consider whether or not intubation is safe to perform after induction of general anesthesia. Additionally, the feasibility of direct laryngoscopy is important to consider so that alternative devices can be readily available. Generally, direct laryngoscopy is difficult in these populations, particularly in patients with limited mouth opening [83]. If intubation is deemed unsafe to perform, alternative methods of achieving adequate oxygenation such as mask ventilation or use of a supraglottic airway (SGA) should be considered. It should be noted, however, that functional airway obstructions increase difficulty of mask ventilation [84] due to poor mask seal or supraglottic obstruction [83]. Supraglottic airways can often overcome these difficulties [83]. However, awake intubation may be the safest option in the case of difficult mask ventilation, severe upper airway obstruction, or risk of regurgitation and aspiration of gastric contents. It has been shown that placement of SGAs in the awake state may be useful in infants with craniofacial syndromes that exhibit upper airway obstructions [85,86].

Neuromuscular blocking drugs (NMBDs) help support tracheal intubation and also mitigate the risk of adverse events such as reflex airway activation [84]. They are not appropriate for every intubation scenario [65,87], and their use should be guided by the underlying airway pathology, expected ability to perform mask ventilation, and whether or not native muscle tone is needed to keep the airway patent (i.e., anterior mediastinal mass) [83]. Additionally, evidence is unclear on the use of NMBDs versus maintenance of spontaneous ventilation in managing the difficult pediatric airway [83]. In typical clinical practice, however, the difficult pediatric airway is managed after anesthetic induction and with maintenance of spontaneous ventilation.

### Devices to Aid in Difficult Airway Management

The difficult airway can be successfully managed with the aid of a number of available devices. These devices include the flexible fiberoptic bronchoscope, indirect laryngoscopes, and SGAs.

The flexible fiberoptic bronchoscope is the "gold standard" in navigating a difficult tracheal intubation [7] and is available in an ultra-thin 2.2 mm external diameter size that is suitable for the newborn airway [87]. Video and optical lanyngoscopes are a more recently available option to guide tracheal intubation when direct laryngoscopy is not feasible. A wide variety of designs are available, and all combine a blade with a video camera or fiberoptic bundle to facilitate laryngeal visualization for oral and/or nasotracheal intubation. Also, if mouth opening permits, an SGA may be used as a primary [64–65] or temporary means to secure the airway. These devices do not require optimal anatomic positioning to achieve adequate

**Table 14.2** Craniofacial syndromes grouped by functional abnormality

| Functional abnormality | Craniofacial syndrome | Physical features contributing to difficult airway | Possible airway management strategies |
|---|---|---|---|
| Subglottic abnormality | Crouzon, Apert, Pfeiffer Syndromes [65–67] | Facial/maxillary hypoplasia; prematurely fused cranial sutures | Oro- or nasopharyngeal airway; SGA; CPAP; consider indirect laryngoscopy in patients who have undergone previous corrective surgery or who have a rigid external distraction device |
| | Pierre Robin sequence [68] | Mandibular hypoplasia; relative macroglossia/glossoptosis; ± cleft palate | Prone positioning; video laryngoscopy; lightwand, paraglossal approach with gum-elastic bougie; SGA to overcome upper airway obstruction; SGA-assisted flexible fiberoptic intubation |
| | Treacher Collins syndrome [69,70] | Mandibular, maxillary, and zygomatic hypoplasia; small mouth; temporomandibular joint abnormalities | Video laryngoscopy; SGA to overcome upper airway obstruction; SGA-assisted fiberoptic intubation |
| | Hemifacial/bilateral facial microsomia/ Goldenhar's syndrome [70–73] | Mandibular, maxillary, and malar hypoplasia; facial asymmetry; cleft-like extension on affected sides(s) of the face  Goldenhar's syndrome: cervical spine defects | SGA to overcome upper airway obstruction; SGA-assisted fiberoptic intubation, videolaryngoscopy; lightwand |
| Abnormality of the entire airway, including the glottis | Mucopolysacchariodoses [68,74–77] | Mucopolysaccharide deposits causing macroglossia, thickened oropharyngeal, laryngeal, and nasal mucosae. Restricted temporomandibular joint mobility, narrow trachea | Avoidance of neuromuscular blocking agents until airway is secured; SGA; SGA-assisted flexible fiberoptic intubation; elective tracheostomy; surgical airway backup |
| Subglottic abnormality | Down syndrome [68, 78–80] | Subglottic stenosis, macroglossia, hypotonia, atlantoaxial instability | Straight blade; video laryngoscopy; use of smaller diameter TTs than calculated; neutral neck position |
| | Larsen syndrome [81,82] | Subglottic stenosis; laryngotracheomalacia; short neck; cephalad larynx; cervical spine instability | Use of smaller diameter TTs than calculated; neutral neck position |
| | Fraser syndrome | Subglottic stenosis, webbing, or atresia (may make intubation impossible) | Use of smaller diameter TTs than calculated; SGA as primary means of ventilation |

SGA, Supraglottic airway; CPAP, continuous positive airway pressure; TT, tracheal tube.
Source: [63,64].

ventilation [88]. However, when used as a means to achieve tracheal intubation, the assistance of visualization techniques as opposed to blind intubation may prove more successful [89].

Table 14.3 highlights the strengths and limitations of using these devices to manage the difficult airway.

## The Unanticipated Difficult Airway

The unanticipated difficult airway often becomes known after anesthetic induction. A preplanned structured approach facilitates successful navigation of the situation, though management should ultimately be guided by the patient's condition and available resources.

129

**Table 14.3** Devices to aid in difficult airway management of the infant and neonate

| Device | Strengths | Limitations |
|---|---|---|
| Flexible fiberoptic bronchoscope [7,68,83,87, 90–94] | • Allows for tracheal intubation via oral or nasal route or through an SGA<br>• Useful in patients with limited mouth opening<br>• Permits lower airway examination<br>• Assists in positioning bronchial blockers<br>• Most sizes have a suction port to remove secretions in the airway<br>• Working channel allows for delivery of local anesthesia | • Difficult to manipulate, particularly the ultra-thin bronchoscope (<3.0 mm OD)<br>• Ultra-thin bronchoscope lacks a suction port<br>• Image may be obscured by blood and secretions in the airway<br>• Steep learning curve, regular practice needed to maintain proficiency<br>• Higher cost, delicate, and costly to repair<br>• Time intensive to setup and clean up |
| Indirect laryngoscope [68,95–104]<br>GlideScope™<br>Stortz DCI™<br>Truview PCD™<br>Airtraq™<br>Pentax Airway Scope (AWS)™<br>Optical stylets: Bonfils Intubation Stylet and Shikani Optical Stylet | • Less head and neck movement required vs. direct laryngoscopy<br>• Improved glottic views compared with direct laryngoscopy<br>• Laryngeal inlet may be visualized without alignment of the oral, pharyngeal, and laryngeal axis<br>• LEDs of the GlideScope and Pentax AWS prevent fogging by providing heat<br>• Most devices have a quick learning curve | • Airway visualization may be obscured due to blood and secretions<br>• Difficult to manipulate TT through the glottis<br>• Risk of failure with altered neck anatomy associated with a mass, radiation changes, or a surgical scar<br>• Evidence for the efficacy of some devices in managing the difficult infant airway is lacking |
| Supraglottic airway devices [7,64, 68,89, 105, 106, 107–112]<br>Air-Q™<br>Classic LMA™<br>Supreme LMA™<br>Proseal LMA™<br>i-gel™ | • Useful alternative when mask ventilation is difficult<br>• Functions as a conduit for tracheal intubation<br>• Adequate and efficient ventilation: does not rely on optimal device positioning even in the difficult airway<br>• Devices with gastric drain tubes are available to help protect against regurgitation of gastric contents<br>• air-Q can accommodate cuffed TTs | • Two-step process when used as a conduit for intubation<br>• Classic LMA may produce delayed airway obstruction in neonates<br>• Narrow lumen of LMA Supreme restricts TT insertion and fiberoptic intubation<br>• Narrower lumen of LMA ProSeal restricts TT insertion |

LMA, laryngeal mask airway; TT, tracheal tube: LED, light-emitting diode.

Achieving adequate mask ventilation alone may be difficult. In this scenario, consider recruiting help and attempting a two-handed bag-mask technique. Alternatively, the SGA is a useful rescue device when mask ventilation or intubation are unsuccessful [113].

Difficult intubation may also be an issue. If direct laryngoscopy proves impractical, methods of indirect visualization are useful in increasing the frequency of successful intubation and successful first attempt intubation [113]. Additionally, an SGA may be used as a conduit for tracheal intubation [113]. However, care should be taken to avoid an excessive number of intubation attempts as even gentle instruments may cause iatrogenic injury to the fragile infant airway [83]. When these methods fail to adequately ventilate

and oxygenate the patient, a surgical airway may be a necessary. Figure 14.1 is a proposed algorithm for management of the unanticipated difficult airway in the child.

## Cannot Intubate, Cannot Ventilate

The "cannot intubate, cannot ventilate" situation can be a very stressful scenario to encounter, particularly because there are limited rescue options for infants. Both surgical tracheostomy and percutaneous cricothyroid puncture are invasive and high-risk [83]. Ideally, the assistance of an otolaryngologist should be solicited for creating a surgical airway [83]. However, if help is not close at hand, the more efficient, but risky, method for invasive tracheal access is needle

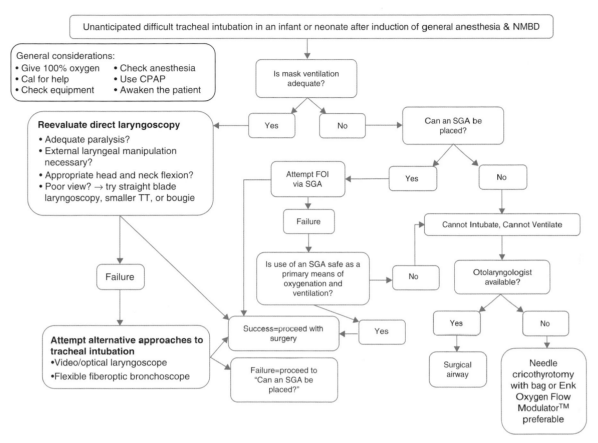

**Figure 14.1** A proposed algorithm for management of the unanticipated difficult airway in the child. Source: adapted from Difficult Airway Society. Paediatric Difficult Airway Guidelines for: Difficult Mask Ventilation; Unanticipated Difficult Intubation; and Cannot Intubate and Cannot Ventilate. CPAP, continuous positive airway pressure; FOI, fiberoptic intubation; NMBD, neuromuscular blocking drug; SGA, supraglottic airway device; TT, tracheal tube.

cricothyrotomy [83,114]. This procedure has limited efficacy in infants [83,115]. This is due in part to their proportionately smaller cricothyroid membrane, which restricts the size of the transtracheal catheter that may be used for oxygenation [83,116]. There is also a high incidence of complications associated with this procedure, such as posterior tracheal wall puncture, and esophageal puncture [114,117].

If needle cricothyrotomy is necessary, procedure-specific equipment such as the Ventilation-Catheter (VBM, Medizintechnik GmBH, Sula and Neckar, Germany) may be used with either bag or jet ventilation [114]. In the resource-limited setting, a makeshift device composed of a large-bore intravenous catheter, a syringe, and 3.0 mm internal diameter tracheal tube will suffice with bag ventilation [114]. The Enk Oxygen Flow Modulator™ (Cook Medical, Bloomington, IN, USA) is a lower-pressure jet ventilation system that can provide adequate oxygenation utilizing standard wall oxygen, with a lower risk of barotrauma [114]. However, current knowledge suggests that jet ventilation through transtracheal catheters is associated with serious complications and barotrauma [19,118], and further evidence is needed to elucidate whether or not these devices minimize pressure-related complications [119].

## Management for Tongue–Lip Adhesion and Mandibular Distraction Osteogenesis

Mandibular distraction osteogenesis (MDO) and tongue–lip adhesion are common surgical interventions to relieve upper airway obstruction in infants and neonates with craniofacial deformities. A difficult airway should be anticipated in these patients.

Nasal intubation is preferred for both MDO and tongue–lip adhesion as it minimizes disturbance to the surgical field. While awake fiberoptic intubation is the most conservative approach to achieve ventilation in these patients, lack of patient cooperation may make it unfeasible. A more practical option involves mask induction followed by asleep fiberoptic intubation. Use of a nasopharyngeal airway during nasal fiberoptic intubation in small children with difficult airways may help overcome obstruction and allow the clinician to provide CPAP, analogous to using an SGA for fiberoptic intubation [120]. If an ultra-thin flexible fiberoptic bronchoscope is available, a TT may be advanced over the scope for successful intubation of the infant or neonate [121]. However, if this approach is unsuccessful, or only a larger diameter scope is available, a guidewire may be used to facilitate intubation [122]. The guidewire is threaded through the working channel of a larger diameter bronchoscope, the bronchoscope is withdrawn and an airway exchange catheter can be placed over the guidewire to allow for railroading of the TT over it.

Retrograde nasotracheal intubation is also an alternative to achieve adequate ventilation in neonates and infants [123,124]. The airway is first secured orally, typically via SGA-assisted tracheal intubation. After the SGA is removed, a smaller TT is placed into the nose and the end is exited out of the mouth. It is then telescoped into the larger TT and secured with a suture. Both TTs are pulled retrograde out of the nose and separated, leaving the larger TT trans-nasal.

It should be noted that glossoptosis may make intubation difficult in patients with Pierre Robin sequence. In this case, the tongue can be held with Magill forceps during intubation [122], or nasotracheal intubation may be performed in the prone position. Jaw thrust is another helpful maneuver to increase airway patency.

# References

1. Bruce IA, Rothera MP. Upper airway obstruction in children. *Pediatr Anesth*. 2009;19:88–99.

2. Stocks J. Respiratory physiology during early life. *Monaldi Arch Chest Dis*. 1999;54:358–64.

3. Hammer J, Eber E. The peculiarities of infant respiratory physiology. In Hammer J, Eber E, editors, *Paediatric Pulmonary Function Testing*. Basel: Karger Books; 2005.

4. Mortensen A, Lenz K, Abildstrom H, Lauritsen TL. Anesthetizing the obese child. *Paediatr Anaesth*. 2011;21:623–9.

5. Harless JRR, Bhananker SM. Pediatric airway management. *Int J Crit Illn Inj Sci*. 2014;4:65–70.

6. Adewale L. Anatomy and assessment of the pediatric airway. *Paediatr Anaesth*. 2009;19(Suppl 1):1–8.

7. Sims C, von Ungern-Sternberg BS. The normal and the challenging pediatric airway. *Paediatr Anaesth*. 2012;22:521–6.

8. Carr RJ, Beebe DS, Belani KG. The difficult pediatric airway. In *Seminars in Anesthesia, Perioperative Medicine and Pain*. New York: Elsevier; 2001; 219–27.

9. Abramson Z, Susarla S, Troulis M, Kaban L. Age-related changes of the upper airway assessed by 3-dimensional computed tomography. *J Craniofac Surg*. 2009;20(Suppl 1):657–63.

10. Dalal PG, Murray D, Messner AH, et al. Pediatric laryngeal dimensions: an age-based analysis. *Anesth Analg*. 2009;108:1475–9.

11. Dalal PGMD, Feng A, Molter D, McAllister J. Upper airway dimensions in children using rigid videobronchoscopy and a computer software: description of a measurement technique. *Pediatr Anesth*. 2008;18:645–53.

12. Hudgins PA, Siegel J, Jacobs I, Abramowsky CR. The normal pediatric larynx on CT and MR. *AJNR Am J Neuroradiol*. 1997;18:239–45.

13. Litman RS, McDonough JM, Marcus CL, Schwartz AR, Ward DS. Upper airway collapsibility in anesthetized children. *Anesth Analg*. 2006;102:750–4.

14. Litman RS, Weissend EE, Shibata D, Westesson PL. Developmental changes of laryngeal dimensions in unparalyzed, sedated children. *Anesthesiology*. 2003;98:41–5.

15. Brambrink AM, Braun U. Airway management in infants and children. *Best Pract Res Clin Anaesthesiol*. 2005;19:675–97.

16. Neuhaus D, Schmitz A, Gerber A, Weiss M. Controlled rapid sequence induction and intubation: an analysis of 1001 children. *Paediatr Anaesth*. 2013;23:734–40.

17. Gencorelli FJ, Fields RG, Litman RS. Complications during rapid sequence induction of general anesthesia in children: a benchmark study. *Paediatr Anaesth*. 2010;20:421–4.

18. Chua C, Schmölzer GM, Davis PG. Airway manoeuvres to achieve upper airway patency during mask ventilation in newborn infants: an historical perspective. *Resuscitation*. 2012;83:411–16.

19. Hagberg C, Georgi R, Krier C. Complications of managing the airway. *Best Pract Res Clin Anaesthesiol*. 2005;19:641–59.

20. Ris HB, Krueger T. Video-assisted thoracoscopic surgery and open decortication for pleural

empyema. *Multimed Man Cardiothorac Surg*. 2006. doi: mmcts.2004.000273

21. Campos JH. Progress in lung separation. *Thorac Surg Clin*. 2005;15:71–83.

22. Dimitriou G, Greenough A, Pink L, et al. Effect of posture on oxygenation and respiratory muscle strength in convalescent infants. *Arch Dis Child Fetal Neonatal Ed*. 2002;86:F147–50.

23. Hammer GB. Single-lung ventilation in infants and children. *Paediatr Anaesth*. 2004;14:98–102.

24. Heaf DP, Helms P, Gordon I, Turner HM. Postural effects on gas exchange in infants. *N Engl J Med*. 1983;308:1505–8.

25. Rowe R, Andropoulos D, Heard M, et al. Anesthetic management of pediatric patients undergoing thoracoscopy. *J Cardiothorac Vasc Anesth*. 1994;8:563–6.

26. Hammer GB, Fitzmaurice BG, Brodsky JB. Methods for single-lung ventilation in pediatric patients. *Anesth Analg*. 1999;89:1426–9.

27. Tan GM, Tan-Kendrick AP. Bronchial diameters in children: use of the Fogarty catheter for lung isolation in children. *Anaesth Intensive Care*. 2002;30:615–18.

28. Mansell A, Bryan C, Levison H. Airway closure in children. *J Appl Physiol*. 1972;33:711–14.

29. Brodsky JB. Lung separation and the difficult airway. *Br J Anaesth*. 2009;103(Suppl 1): i66–75.

30. Baraka A, Dajani A, Maktabi M. Selective contralateral bronchial intubation in children with pneumothorax or bronchopleural fistula. *Br J Anaesth*. 1983;55:901–4.

31. Bastien JL, O'Brien JG, Frantz FW. Extraluminal use of the Arndt pediatric endobronchial blocker in an infant: a case report. *Can J Anaesth*. 2006;53:159–61.

32. Hammer GB, Manos SJ, Smith BM, Skarsgard ED, Brodsky JB. Single-lung ventilation in pediatric patients. *Anesthesiology*. 1996;84:1503–6.

33. Borchardt RA, LaQuaglia MP, McDowall RH, Wilson RS. Bronchial injury during lung isolation in a pediatric patient. *Anesth Analg*. 1998;87:324–5.

34. Sutton CJ, Naguib A, Puri S, Sprenker CJ, Camporesi EM. One-lung ventilation in infants and small children: blood gas values. *J Anesth*. 2012;26:670–4.

35. Kamaya H, Krishna PR. New endotracheal tube (Univent tube) for selective blockade of one lung. *Anesthesiology*. 1985;63:342–3.

36. Marciniak B, Fayoux P, Hebrard A, et al. Fluoroscopic guidance of Arndt endobronchial blocker placement for single-lung ventilation in small children. *Acta Anaesthesiol Scand*. 2008;52:1003–5.

37. Yoneda KY, Louie S, Shelton DK. Mediastinal tumors. *Curr Opin Pulm Med*. 2001;7:226–33.

38. Lee EY. Evaluation of non-vascular mediastinal masses in infants and children: an evidence-based practical approach. *Pediatr Radiol*. 2009;39(Suppl 2):S184–90.

39. Merten DF. Diagnostic imaging of mediastinal masses in children. *AJR Am J Roentgenol*. 1992;158:825–32.

40. King RM, Telander RL, Smithson WA, Banks PM, Han MT. Primary mediastinal tumors in children. *J Pediatr Surg*. 1982;17:512–20.

41. Ravitch M. Mediastinal cysts and tumors. In *Pediatric Surgery*. Chicago, IL: Year Book Medical Publishers;1986; 602–18.

42. Azarow KS, Pearl RH, Zurcher R, Edwards FH, Cohen AJ. Primary mediastinal masses: a comparison of adult and pediatric populations. *J Thorac Cardiovasc Surg*. 1993;106:67–72.

43. Sannoh S, Quezada E, Merer DM, Moscatello A, Golombek SG. Cystic hygroma and potential airway obstruction in a newborn: a case report and review of the literature. *Cases J*. 2009;2:48.

44. Seibert JJ, Marvin Jr. WJ, Rose EF, Schieken RM. Mediastinal teratoma: a rare cause of severe respiratory distress in the newborn. *J Pediatr Surg*. 1976;11:253–5.

45. Song TB, Kim CH, Kim SM, et al. Fetal axillary cystic hygroma detected by prenatal ultrasonography: a case report. *J Korean Med Sci*. 2002;17:400–2.

46. Hammer GB. Anaesthetic management for the child with a mediastinal mass. *Paediatr Anaesth*. 2004;14:95–7.

47. Pullerits J, Holzman R. Anaesthesia for patients with mediastinal masses. *Can J Anaesth*. 1989;36:681–8.

48. Slinger P, Karsli C. Management of the patient with a large anterior mediastinal mass: recurring myths. *Curr Opin Anaesthesiol*. 2007;20:1–3.

49. Neuman GG, Weingarten AE, Abramowitz RM, et al. The anesthetic management of the patient with an anterior mediastinal mass. *Anesthesiology*. 1984;60:144–7.

50. Anghelescu DL, Burgoyne LL, Liu T, et al. Clinical and diagnostic imaging findings predict anesthetic complications in children presenting with malignant mediastinal masses. *Paediatr Anaesth*. 2007;17:1090–8.

51. Gautam PL, Kaur M, Singh RJ, Gupta S. Large mediastinal tumor in a neonate: an anesthetic challenge. *J Anesth*. 2012;26:124–7.

52. Robie DK, Gursoy MH, Pokorny WJ. Mediastinal tumors: airway obstruction and management. *Semin Pediatr Surg*. 1994;3:259–66.

53. Yamashita M, Chin I, Horigome H, Umesato Y, Tsuchida M. Sudden fatal cardiac arrest in a child with an unrecognized anterior mediastinal mass. *Resuscitation*. 1990;19:175–7.

54. Viswanathan S, Campbell CE, Cork RC. Asymptomatic undetected mediastinal mass: a death during ambulatory anesthesia. *J Clin Anesth*. 1995;7:151–5.

55. Toda N, Murakami N, Ando T, et al. [Anesthetic management in two infants undergoing hemilaminectomy for giant mediastinal neuroblastoma]. *Masui*. 2007;56:158–62.

56. Ferrari LR, Bedford RF. Anterior mediastinal mass in a pregnant patient: anesthetic management and considerations. *J Clin Anesth*. 1989;1:460–3.

57. Sibert KS, Biondi JW, Hirsch NP. Spontaneous respiration during thoracotomy in a patient with a mediastinal mass. *Anesth Analg*. 1987;66:904–7.

58. Piro AJ, Weiss DR, Hellman S. Mediastinal Hodgkin's disease: a possible danger for intubation anesthesia. Intubation danger in Hodgkin's disease. *Int J Radiat Oncol Biol Phys*. 1976;1:415–19.

59. Polaner DM. The use of heliox and the laryngeal mask airway in a child with an anterior mediastinal mass. *Anesth Analg*. 1996;82:208–10.

60. Barnett TB. Effects of helium and oxygen mixtures on pulmonary mechanics during airway constriction. *J Appl Physiol*. 1967;22:707–13.

61. Ferrari LR, Bedford RF. General anesthesia prior to treatment of anterior mediastinal masses in pediatric cancer patients. *Anesthesiology*. 1990;72:991–5.

62. Heinrich S, Birkholz T, Ihmsen H, et al. Incidence and predictors of difficult laryngoscopy in 11,219 pediatric anesthesia procedures. *Pediatr Anesth*. 2012;22:729–36.

63. de Beer D, Bingham R. The child with facial abnormalities. *Curr Opin Anaesthesiol*. 2011; 24:282–8.

64. Jagannathan N, Sequera-Ramos L, Sohn L, et al. Elective use of supraglottic airway devices for primary airway management in children with difficult airways. *Br J Anaesth*. 2014;112:742–8.

65. Morris GP, Cooper MG. Difficult tracheal intubation following midface distraction surgery. *Paediatr Anaesth*. 2000;10:99–102.

66. Barnett S, Moloney C, Bingham R. Perioperative complications in children with Apert syndrome: a review of 509 anesthetics. *Paediatr Anaesth*. 2011;21:72–7.

67. Roce J, Frawley G, Heggie A. Difficult tracheal intubation induced by maxillary distraction devices in craniosynostosis syndromes. *Paediatr Anaesth*. 2002;12:227–34.

68. Duggan L, Jagannathan N. *Unique airway issues in the pediatric population*. In Hung O, Murphy M., editors. *Management of the Difficult and Failed Airway*, 2nd edn. New York: McGraw-Hill; 2012.

69. Pean D, Desdoits A, Asehnoune K, Lejus C. Airtraq laryngoscope for intubation in Treacher Collins syndrome. *Paediatr Anaesth*. 2009;19:698–9.

70. Milne AD, Dower AM, Hackmann T. Airway management using the pediatric GlideScope in a child with Goldenhar syndrome and atypical plasma cholinesterase. *Paediatr Anaesth*. 2007;17:484–7.

71. Xue FS, Yang QY, Liao X, He N, Liu HP. Lightwand guided intubation in paediatric patients with a known difficult airway: a report of four cases. *Anaesthesia*. 2008;63:520–5.

72. Shukry M, Hanson RD, Koveleskie JR, Ramadhyani U. Management of the difficult pediatric airway with Shikani Optical Stylet. *Paediatr Anaesth*. 2005;15:342–5.

73. Johnson CM, Sims C. Awake fibreoptic intubation via a laryngeal mask in an infant with Goldenhar's syndrome. *Anaesth Intensive Care*. 1994;22:194–7.

74. Khan FA, Khan FH. Use of the laryngeal mask airway in mucopolysaccharidoses. *Paediatr Anaesth*. 2002;12:468.

75. Walker RW, Allen DL, Rothera MR. A fibreoptic intubation technique for children with mucopolysaccharidoses using the laryngeal mask airway. *Paediatr Anaesth*. 1997;7:421–6.

76. Diaz JH, Belani KG. Perioperative management of children with mucopolysaccharidoses. *Anesth Analg*. 1993;77:1261–70.

77. Osthaus WA, Harendza T, Witt LH, et al. Paediatric airway management in mucopolysaccharidosis 1: a retrospective case review. *Eur J Anaesthesiol*. 2012;29:204–7.

78. Chin CJ, Khami MM, Husein M. A general review of the otolaryngologic manifestations of Down syndrome. *Int J Pediatr Otorhinolaryngol*. 2014;78:899–904.

79. Shott SR. Down syndrome: analysis of airway size and a guide for appropriate intubation. *Laryngoscope*. 2000;110:585–92.

80. Infosino A. Pediatric upper airway and congenital anomalies. *Anesthesiol Clin North Am*. 2002;20:747–66.

81. Malik P, Choudhry DK. Larsen syndrome and its anaesthetic considerations. *Paediatr Anaesth*. 2002;12:632–6.

82. Stevenson GW, Hall SC, Palmieri J. Anesthetic considerations for patients with Larsen's syndrome. *Anesthesiology*. 1991;75:142–4.

83. Sunder RA, Haile DT, Farrell PT, Sharma A. Pediatric airway management: current practices and future directions. *Paediatr Anaesth*. 2012;22:1008–15.

84. Weiss M, Engelhardt T. Cannot ventilate – paralyze! *Pediatr Anesth*. 2012;22:1147–9.

85. Jagannathan N, Sohn LE, Suresh S. Glossopharyngeal nerve blocks for awake laryngeal mask airway insertion in an infant with Pierre-Robin syndrome: can a glidescope come to the rescue? *Paediatr Anaesth.* 2009;19:189–90.

86. Asai T, Nagata A, Shingu K. Awake tracheal intubation through the laryngeal mask in neonates with upper airway obstruction. *Paediatr Anaesth.* 2008;18:77–80.

87. de Blic J, Delacourt C, Scheinmann P. Ultrathin flexible bronchoscopy in neonatal intensive care units. *Arch Dis Child.* 1991;66:1383–5.

88. Foucher-Lezla A, Lehousse T, Monrigal JP, Granry JC, Beydon L. Fibreoptic assessment of laryngeal positioning of the paediatric supraglottic airway device I-Gel. *Eur J Anaesthesiol.* 2013;30:441–2.

89. Jagannathan N, Kozlowski RJ, Sohn LE, et al. A clinical evaluation of the intubating laryngeal airway as a conduit for tracheal intubation in children. *Anesth Analg.* 2011;112:176–82.

90. Bandla HP, Smith DE, Kiernan MP. Laryngeal mask airway facilitated fibreoptic bronchoscopy in infants. *Can J Anaesth.* 1997;44:1242–7.

91. Lesmes C, Siplovich L, Katz Y. Fiberoptic bronchoscopy in children using the laryngeal mask airway. *Pediatr Surg Int.* 2000;16:179–81.

92. Vijayasekaran D, Gowrishankar NC, Kalpana S, et al. Lower airway anomalies in infants with laryngomalacia. *Indian J Pediatr.* 2010;77:403–6.

93. Neustein SM. The use of bronchial blockers for providing one-lung ventilation. *J Cardiothorac Vasc Anesth.* 2009;23:860–8.

94. Ramesh S. Fiberoptic airway management in adults and children. *Indian J Anaesth.* 2005;49:293–9.

95. Bhardwaj N, Jain K, Rao M, Mandal AK. Assessment of cervical spine movement during laryngoscopy with Macintosh and Truview laryngoscopes. *J Anaesthesiol Clin Pharmacol.* 2013;29:308–12.

96. Griesdale DE, Chau A, Isac G, et al. Video-laryngoscopy versus direct laryngoscopy in critically ill patients: a pilot randomized trial. *Can J Anaesth.* 2012;59:1032–9.

97. Aziz MF, Healy D, Kheterpal S, et al. Routine clinical practice effectiveness of the Glidescope in difficult airway management: an analysis of 2,004 Glidescope intubations, complications, and failures from two institutions. *Anesthesiology.* 2011;114:34–41.

98. Paolini JB, Donati F, Drolet P. Review article: video-laryngoscopy: another tool for difficult intubation or a new paradigm in airway management? *Can J Anaesth.* 2013;60:184–91.

99. Cheyne DR, Doyle P. Advances in laryngoscopy: rigid indirect laryngoscopy. *F1000 Med Rep.* 2010;2:61.

100. Pott LM, Murray WB. Review of video laryngoscopy and rigid fiberoptic laryngoscopy. *Curr Opin Anaesthesiol.* 2008;21:750–8.

101. Serocki G, Bein B, Scholz J, Dorges V. Management of the predicted difficult airway: a comparison of conventional blade laryngoscopy with video-assisted blade laryngoscopy and the GlideScope. *Eur J Anaesthesiol.* 2010;27:24–30.

102. Ciccozzi A, Angeletti C, Guetti C, et al. GlideScope and Frova Introducer for difficult airway management. *Case Rep Anesthesiol.* 2013;2013:717928.

103. Holm-Knudsen R. The difficult pediatric airway: a review of new devices for indirect laryngoscopy in children younger than two years of age. *Paediatr Anaesth.* 2011;21:98–103.

104. Savoldelli GL, Schiffer E, Abegg C, et al. Learning curves of the Glidescope, the McGrath and the Airtraq laryngoscopes: a manikin study. *Eur J Anaesthesiol.* 2009;26:554–8.

105. Scheller B, Schalk R, Byhahn C, et al. Laryngeal tube suction II for difficult airway management in neonates and small infants. *Resuscitation.* 2009;80:805–10.

106. Whyte SD, Cooke E, Malherbe S. Usability and performance characteristics of the pediatric air-Q(R) intubating laryngeal airway. *Can J Anaesth.* 2013;60:557–63.

107. Wong DT, Yang JJ, Mak HY, Jagannathan N. Use of intubation introducers through a supraglottic airway to facilitate tracheal intubation: a brief review. *Can J Anaesth.* 2012;59:704–15.

108. Jagannathan N, Roth AG, Sohn LE, et al. The new air-Q intubating laryngeal airway for tracheal intubation in children with anticipated difficult airway: a case series. *Paediatr Anaesth.* 2009;19:618–22.

109. Jagannathan N, Sommers K, Sohn LE, et al. A randomized equivalence trial comparing the i-gel and laryngeal mask airway Supreme in children. *Paediatr Anaesth.* 2013;23:127–33.

110. Jagannathan N, Fiadjoe JE. Supraglottic airways for pediatric patients: an overview. *Anesthesiology News.* 2013

111. Cook TM, Gatward JJ, Handel J, et al. Evaluation of the LMA Supreme in 100 non-paralysed patients. *Anaesthesia.* 2009;64:555–62.

112. Patel B, Bingham R. Laryngeal mask airway and other supraglottic airway devices in paediatric practice. *Continuing Education in Anaesthesia, Critical Care & Pain.* 2009;9:6–9.

113. Apfelbaum JL, Hagberg CA, Caplan RA, et al. Practice guidelines for management of the difficult

airway: an updated report by the American Society of Anesthesiologists Task Force on Management of the Difficult Airway. *Anesthesiology*. 2013;118:251–70.

114. Cote CJ, Hartnick CJ. Pediatric transtracheal and cricothyrotomy airway devices for emergency use: which are appropriate for infants and children? *Paediatr Anaesth*. 2009;19(Suppl 1):66–76.

115. Cook T, Woodall N, Harper J, Benger J. Major complications of airway management in the UK: results of the Fourth National Audit Project of the Royal College of Anaesthetists and the Difficult Airway Society. Part 2: intensive care and emergency departments. *Br J Anaes*. 2011;106:632–42.

116. Navsa N, Tossel G, Boon J. Dimensions of the neonatal cricothyroid membrane: how feasible is a surgical cricothyroidotomy? *Pediatr Anesth*. 2005;15:402–6.

117. Stacey J, Heard A, Chapman G, et al. The "Can't Intubate Can't Oxygenate" scenario in pediatric anesthesia: a comparison of different devices for needle cricothyroidotomy. *Pediatr Anesth*. 2012;22:1155–8.

118. Cook TM, Bigwood B, Cranshaw J. A complication of transtracheal jet ventilation and use of the Aintree intubation catheter during airway resuscitation. *Anaesthesia*. 2006;61:692–7.

119. Ahmad Y, Turner M. Transtracheal jet ventilation in patients with severe airway compromise and stridor. *Br J Anaesth*. 2011;106:602.

120. Holm-Knudsen R, Eriksen K, Rasmussen LS. Using a nasopharyngeal airway during fiberoptic intubation in small children with a difficult airway. *Pediatr Anesth*. 2005;15:839–45.

121. Kleeman P-P, Jantzen J-PH, Bonfils P. The ultra-thin bronchoscope in management of the difficult paediatric airway. *Can J Anaesth*. 1987;34:606–8.

122. Howardy-Hansen P, Berthelsen P. Fibreoptic bronchoscopic nasotracheal intubation of a neonate with Pierre Robin syndrome. *Anaesthesia*. 1988;43:121–2.

123. Smallman B, Ball R, Tatum S. A novel technique of retrograde nasal intubation for the Pierre Robin sequence infant with a known difficult airway. *Paediatr Anaesth*. 2009;19:919–21.

124. Portnoy JE, Tatum S. Retrograde nasal intubation via the cleft in Pierre-Robin sequence neonates: a case series. *Int J Pediatr Otorhinolaryngol*. 2009;73:1828–32.

Chapter

# 15

# Fluid and Transfusion Management

Justin Long, Tiffany Frazee, and Hubert Benzon

Management of fluids, blood products, and electrolytes in infants and children requires special attention to detail and constant vigilance. While the kidneys and neuroendocrine systems are responsible for fluid and electrolyte homeostasis, they are not fully developed at birth. Fluid compartment volumes throughout the body vary with age as well. As such, management of fluid resuscitation changes throughout infancy and childhood. In term infants, 17 percent will urinate in the delivery room and 90 percent will urinate in the first 24 hours.

## Body Fluid Compartments

The body water compartment models that are most commonly utilized today are products of deuterium oxide dilution studies done over 60 years ago, which remain the best information available today. Total body water (TBW) rapidly changes throughout the first nine months of life. Term neonates have a TBW that is about 80 percent of total body weight while a very low birth weight (VLBW) preterm infant may have a TBW that is 90 percent of the total body weight [1].

At birth, extracellular volume (ECV) and intracellular volume (ICV) do not have the same proportional relationship that is observed after about three months of age into adulthood. In the peripartum period, ECV is best estimated as two-thirds of TBW, while ICV is one-third (an inverted relationship compared to what occurs after three months of age). In order for this relative fluid balance to change, there must be loss of fluid from the extracellular compartment, since the absolute ICV remains relatively steady. This loss of fluid is most pronounced during the first week of life: 5–10 percent of the birth weight of a healthy, term infant is lost. The fluid is lost in the form of transcutaneous losses and diuresis through natriuresis. Thus, fluid management must be more customized for the neonatal period while broader generalizations can be made later in infancy.

One important determinant of TBW, especially in the neonate, is the body fat percentage, since fat is largely anhydrous. While a VLBW preterm infant at 28 weeks gestation will have about 1 percent body fat, a term infant has approximately 10 percent body fat [2]. The result is that percentage body water is higher in premature infants, especially those that are VLBW. While this has widespread implications for pharmacology, electrolyte balance, and nutritional requirements, those topics are covered elsewhere. For the purposes of fluid management, it implies that fluid requirements may be greater than anticipated due to increased insensible losses, faster metabolic rate, immature kidney concentrating ability, and growth.

Formulas for accurate calculation of TBW are presented in Table 15.1; use age, height, gender, and weight for calculation of TBW.

## Intravascular Blood Volume

Plasma accounts for about one-fifth of ECV. Red blood cell volume is part of ICV. Rather than calculating intravascular volume each time from the TBW, there are accepted estimations of intravascular volume on an ml kg$^{-1}$ basis that change based on age. Full-term neonates are estimated to have an intravascular blood volume of 90 ml kg$^{-1}$ [4]. Preterm, VLBW, or critically ill infants have a higher percentage total body water and a higher intravascular blood volume, estimated to be about 100 ml kg$^{-1}$ [5]. The estimated total intravascular volume continues to decrease on an ml kg$^{-1}$ basis until adulthood, when 70 ml kg$^{-1}$ is the generally accepted estimation of intravascular volume. Estimates of intravascular blood volume by age are presented in Table 15.2.

## Electrolyte Balance

Sodium, as the primary determinant of serum osmolality, largely determines the distribution of water throughout the extracellular compartment, including

**Table 15.1** Total body water calculation based on gender, height, and weight

0 to 3 months of age: $TBW = 0.887 \times (Wt)^{0.83}$

3 months to 13 years: $TBW = 0.0846 \times 0.95^{[if\ female]} \times (Ht \times Wt)^{0.65}$

Children > 13 years: $TBW = 0.0758 \times 0.84^{[if\ female]} \times (Ht \times Wt)^{0.69}$

Source: [3].

**Table 15.2** Intravascular volume estimates based on weight

| Age group | Intravascular volume |
| --- | --- |
| Preterm infants | 100 ml kg$^{-1}$ |
| Full-term neonates | 90 ml kg$^{-1}$ |
| Infants and toddlers | 80 ml kg$^{-1}$ |
| School-age children | 75 ml kg$^{-1}$ |
| Adolescents and adults | 70 ml kg$^{-1}$ |

Source: [6].

intravascular volume. Homeostatic mechanisms to increase intravascular volume largely affect retention of sodium and water. Therefore, decreases in intravascular volume are brought about through loss of sodium and water.

In utero, the fetus has a high urine output, despite low blood flow to the kidneys and low glomerular filtration rate (GFR), due to almost no retention capability for sodium and water. By term, however, the kidneys are capable of conserving a great deal of the sodium and glomurulotubular balance is reached. All nephrons are developed fully by 36 weeks' gestation, but renal blood flow (RBF) is still not high enough to produce a GFR that is consistent with adult GFR.

In preterm infants, however, the nephrons have not yet fully matured and glomerulotubular balance is not yet intact. Renal blood flow does increase postpartum and GFR increases, but the nephrons are not capable of balanced resorption of sodium. Therefore, sodium is not reabsorbed in proportion with GFR. There is also a poor response of the distal tubule to mineralocorticoids in preterm infants [7]. The result is natriuresis and diuresis, increasing their susceptibility to hyponatremia and hypovolemia. Other mechanisms of kidney immaturity result in the neonate being incapable of adult levels of urine concentration until approximately two years of age [8].

The neonatal kidney's diluting capacity matures more rapidly. During the first 24 hours of life a neonate may be unable to increase water excretion appropriately [9]. Diluting capacity is fully mature about one month postpartum.

# Fluid Requirements for Maintenance and Resuscitation

In order to calculate the fluid needed for any given patient, the anesthesiologist must keep in mind several issues. Fluid deficit, metabolic requirements, insensible loss, blood loss, and other outputs must all be considered in order to make an estimation of the fluid requirements of a particular patient. No formulas can precisely predict the fluid required in any given patient undergoing any particular procedure. Rather, fluid management often becomes part of the art of anesthesia.

The long used formula for estimating the maintenance fluid requirements for a child is derived from a study by Holliday and Segar in 1957 [10]. This formula provides the starting point for the calculation of fluid deficit and basic fluid requirements in healthy children. It was never intended to be the sole guidance for fluid administration to every hospitalized child, but many have expanded the conclusions in this paper beyond their original intent. This resulted in another paper by the same authors in 2004 that suggested that resuscitation fluid be isotonic and given in boluses as initial resuscitation while maintenance fluid should be given that is hypotonic to prevent excess salt wasting [11].

When maintenance fluid estimates were initially calculated, they were based on metabolic rate calculations and obligatory urine output estimates. However, the critically ill patient can have severe perturbations in both metabolic rate and urine output. The maintenance fluid estimates used today are still derived from Holliday and Segar. The 4–2–1 rule of maintenance fluid calculation is that there should be 4 ml kg$^{-1}$ h$^{-1}$ for the first 10 kg of body weight, an additional 2 ml kg$^{-1}$ for the next 10 kg of body weight, and an additional 1 ml kg$^{-1}$ for the remainder of weight over 20 kg. The suggested fluid would be a hypotonic, glucose-containing solution after initial resuscitation has been undertaken, since daily requirements for sodium, chloride, and potassium were also calculated based on metabolic rate and obligatory urine loss.

It is generally accepted in the operating room that metabolic rate falls under anesthesia, especially if hypothermia is observed or induced. Therefore, it is a common practice to decrease the rate of glucose administration in the operative environment, compared with glucose administration to a hospitalized child in another setting. Furthermore, the stress response to surgery further increases serum glucose levels. This topic is covered in greater detail in Chapter 6, Glucose Control.

While the 4–2–1 rule is generally used to calculate the fluid deficit of a child, isotonic fluid solutions should be used for resuscitative efforts. The most common fluid deficit encountered in the operating room is the fasting time for those children presenting to surgery from home. It is calculated by multiplying the maintenance fluid rate and total fasting time for liquids [12]. This deficit should be replaced over the first portion of a long case, but can be replaced faster in patients in whom there are no reasons to suspect heart disease. More specifically, it has been suggested that the first half of the deficit be replaced over the first hour of surgery and the other half over the following two hours. A simplification of this is to assume an average fasting time of 6–8 hours and administer to children under four years of age 25 ml kg$^{-1}$ and children four years or older 15 ml kg$^{-1}$ of isotonic solution [13]. However, current common practice is to give maintenance IV fluids to inpatients awaiting surgery and to encourage outpatients presenting for surgery to drink clear liquids until two hours before surgery, based on the ASA guidelines for preoperative fasting [14]. Therefore, those bolus estimations are probably an overestimation of fluid deficit.

Since the 4–2–1 rule was calculated based on estimations of metabolism and did not account for the body's compensatory mechanisms for fasting, it may be that this is also an overestimation of the actual fluid deficit. In healthy adults, there is evidence that their intravascular volume is maintained even with prolonged fasting times, but this is probably not the case with neonates [15].

In some conditions, increased fluid loss is obvious, such as in cases of diarrhea or vomiting. But, some fluid deficits are more insidious, such as encountered with burns or with significant capillary leak that can occur with strangulated hernia, gastroschisis, or sepsis. Since the fluid that needs to be replaced in these scenarios is most similar to the extracellular environment, the resuscitation is best accomplished with crystalloid solutions most similar in osmolality and solute makeup to ECV, such as lactated Ringer's. Some have recommended initial resuscitation volumes of approximately 40 ml kg$^{-1}$ for cases of severe dehydration [16]. In cases where renal impairment is suspected, potassium-free fluids may be indicated.

The low birth weight (LBW) and VLBW infants will have three well-described phases of urine output. First, the first day of life is a low intake and low urine output state – therefore body weight is stable. Days two and three of life are characterized by diuresis, independent of any fluid intake. Then days four and five are when urine output begins to vary more directly with fluid intake. Premature infants who are treated with excess fluids have a higher incidence of respiratory distress, necrotizing enterocolitis, left ventricular failure, and patent ductus arteriosus [17]. Because renal function, insensible water losses, and metabolism change rapidly in the newborn, it can be difficult to apply a generic formula to all neonates for daily fluid requirements. Based on practical experience, neonatologists have developed recommendations for fluid management in the first seven days of life (Table 15.3).

Even though diuresis and natriuresis are concerns during the neonatal period, it is relatively easy to encounter fluid overload in the operative setting. From a practical standpoint, use of large-bore IV tubing may result in flush volumes that are larger than the hourly maintenance fluid requirements for a neonate. Use of heated humidifiers in the ventilator circuit may deliver a large, insensible volume of fluid that is readily absorbed through the lungs. Intravenous solutions hung to gravity, even with a volumetric burette, are easily administered in full before their rates of infusion are realized by the provider.

From a practical standpoint, neonates undergoing surgical procedures are likely to be inpatients. They have IV access and are likely to be receiving a hypotonic, glucose-containing solution for maintenance. Others will arrive to the operating room on total parenteral nutrition (TPN) with or without lipid infusions. Lipid infusions can almost always be safely discontinued for surgery and should be discontinued in most cases (burns may represent an important exception to this rule). A general approach to the glucose management and to the maintenance fluid management is to maintain the infusion either at maintenance rates or half maintenance rates by the 4–2–1 rule. All other fluid given for insensible losses, volume resuscitation, and blood loss should be isotonic or hypertonic crystalloid solutions or colloid solutions like albumin, in order to avoid hyperglycemia [18]. Maintenance of this hypotonic solution also ensures that there is at least some free water available for elimination of other solute load from

**Table 15.3** Daily fluid requirements during first week of life (ml kg$^{-1}$ day$^{-1}$)

| Birth weight | Day 1 | Day 2 | Day 3 | Day 4 | Day 5 | Day 6 | Day 7 |
|---|---|---|---|---|---|---|---|
| <1000 g | 80 | 100 | 120 | 130 | 140 | 150 | 160 |
| 1000–1500 g | 80 | 95 | 110 | 120 | 130 | 140 | 150 |
| >1500 g | 60 | 75 | 90 | 105 | 120 | 135 | 150 |
| Source: [8]. | | | | | | | |

resuscitation, since neonates and infants are unable to concentrate urine at adult levels.

Frequent intraoperative glucose monitoring is indicated. Glucose management may also be complicated by the large amounts of dextrose in stored blood products. TPN and maintenance fluids may also contain potassium, which may become a concern if rapid transfusion of blood products is anticipated.

Fluid resuscitation may be needed due to intraoperative losses. There is great ongoing loss when the exposed surface area, as a percentage of the child's total surface area, is high. The classic example is dressing changes for burns. While the burn is covered in wet gauze, there is little ongoing loss to the environment. When the burn is exposed to the operating environment, the losses can be extraordinary. While this direct evaporative loss may not be as important in older children, this can represent an enormous loss of fluid from an infant.

There can be great variations in capillary leak induced by surgical injury, and this amount of fluid can also be very difficult to quantify. This fluid is generally described as third space losses, which is a shift of fluid into a nonfunctional extracellular space that is not in equilibrium with the intravascular compartment [19]. It was suggested that the greater the trauma related to the surgery, the greater this third space shift would become. Furthermore, redistribution of blood flow, induced by anesthetics, patient positioning, venous stasis, and temperature regulation may lead to greater relative intravascular volume depletion even in the most minimally invasive cases.

Ongoing blood loss is the most direct cause of intravascular volume depletion. As a general rule, 3 ml of isotonic crystalloid solution should be provided for each 1 ml of blood loss. However, between dilution of existing intravascular blood and even moderate amounts of blood loss, neonates have a limited capacity for replacement of blood volume with crystalloid alone. Colloid may also be used, 1 ml for each 1 ml of blood loss [20]. However, the most direct replacement

of blood loss is with blood products, to be discussed later in this chapter.

There have been some studies to suggest fluid management for a variety of cases. One such case is gastroschisis, in which fluid requirements are quite high in the first day of life. Where the neonate usually requires minimal fluid during the first 24 hours of life, neonates with gastroschisis require 150 ml + 35 ml kg$^{-1}$ over the first 24 hours, 75 percent of which was crystalloid and 25 percent of which was colloid in this particular study [21]. Depending on the level of trauma expected in a particular surgical procedure, 1 ml kg$^{-1}$ h$^{-1}$ to 15 ml kg$^{-1}$ h$^{-1}$ has been suggested for replacement of continued intraoperative losses. For premature neonates undergoing laparotomy for necrotizing enterocolitis, up to 50 ml kg$^{-1}$ h$^{-1}$ has been utilized in the literature [22]. In a more general sense, small surgical procedures with mild tissue trauma may have third space and evaporative losses of about 3–4 ml kg$^{-1}$ h$^{-1}$, while large abdominal procedures may lead to more significant losses of 10 ml kg$^{-1}$ h$^{-1}$ or more [23].

## Colloid and Hypertonic Solutions

Colloids are a valuable adjunct for intravascular volume replacement. As they generally remain intravascular for longer, the amount of colloid needed for the same intravascular volume replacement versus isotonic crystalloid is less. Colloids that are generally available are albumin, as 5 percent or 25 percent solution, and hydroxyethyl starches (HESs). While dextrans are commercially available, they are not often used because of their negative coagulation effects and increased risk of anaphylaxis [24]. Gelatins are commercially available as well, but their use was discontinued in the United States in 1978 because of hypersensitivity reactions [25].

Albumin 5 percent solution is osmotically equivalent to an equal volume of plasma. Thus, the 25 percent solution is five times more osmotically active.

Otherwise stated, 100 ml of 5 percent albumin increases plasma volume by 100 ml, while 25 percent albumin may increase plasma volume by 300–500 ml [26]. The volume-limiting benefit of albumin may not be as certain in the setting of significant tissue trauma, as capillary leak may allow albumin to translocate extravascularly and osmotically draw fluid into the interstitium.

Albumin use in the pediatric population is perhaps most well-studied in infants. Albumin has long been considered the standard colloid against which all others are measured and, as of 2001, was still the most commonly used colloid in children [27,28]. Its long history in clinical use is likely due to its benign side-effect profile. It has been shown in adults to have minimal effects on the coagulation cascade as long as total dose is below 25 percent of blood volume [29] and carries no risk of disease transmission [30]. It has almost no contraindications aside from increased mortality rates when used in adults for initial resuscitation after traumatic brain injury.

The use of albumin intraoperatively versus crystalloid has really only been studied in children undergoing cardiopulmonary bypass [31,32]. Hence, there is not much guidance for its use other than generic dosing, which is 10–20 ml kg$^{-1}$ for 5 percent albumin [33] and 2.5–5 ml kg$^{-1}$ for 25 percent albumin [34]. In hypoalbuminemic patients who are also hypotensive, replacement of albumin may be calculated by the following equation [35]:

$$\text{Albumin dose (g)} = (2.5 \text{ g dl}^{-1} - \text{patient's albumin concentration}) \times (\text{patient weight [kg]}) \times 0.8$$

HESs are synthetic colloids that may be used for volume expansion. They are osmotically active and too large for diffusion through most capillary beds into the intravascular space. They are degraded in the bloodstream by amylase and ultimately eliminated renally. Depending on the HES solution, they have a half-life of 2–6 hours [36]. The side-effects include impairment of the coagulation cascade, renal toxicity, and pruritus [37].

There are three HES solutions currently available in the United States: Hespan, Hextend, and Voluven. Each are 6 percent HES solutions, but they have different molecular structures that change the half-life of their effect on volume as well as their tendency to affect coagulation parameters. Hextend and Hespan have a longer half-life of 5–6 hours, and Hextend has

fewer effects on the coagulation cascade than Hespan [38]. Voluven has minimal effects on the coagulation cascade, but boasts a half-life of only 2–3 hours [39]. Voluven has no renal side-effects [40].

There are several studies of HES solutions in pediatric patients, demonstrating their safety and capacity for volume expansion. Importantly, a study in 26 neonates undergoing central line placement revealed there was no increase in creatinine or bleeding with the use of HES versus albumin [41]. Another study of 316 children with normal baseline coagulation and renal function were infused 5–15 ml kg$^{-1}$ of Voluven and no serious adverse reactions such as anaphylaxis, renal failure, or clotting disorder were observed [42]. These, among other studies, lend credit toward HES use for volume expansion in even the smallest of patients. The product inserts for Hextend and Hespan suggest that the approximate maximum dose that should be used is 20 ml kg$^{-1}$ for adults, but that pediatric trials are unavailable [43]. The product insert for Voluven indicates a maximum dose of 50 ml kg$^{-1}$ regardless of age group [44]. Large-scale adult studies have questioned renal toxicity and mortality rates in patients treated with HES. As a result of these studies, the US Food and Drug Administration (FDA) and several international organizations have recommended limiting the use of HES [45].

Hypertonic saline is increasing in use in the perioperative setting across many practices. It is a valuable tool in resuscitation because of its hypertonicity and, therefore, its ability to increase plasma volume. Hypertonic saline has more traditionally been used for the treatment of acute or severe hyponatremia and cerebral edema in neurotrauma. There have been two studies in children that revealed increased cerebral perfusion pressure in the three days after traumatic brain injury when using hypertonic saline versus lactated Ringer's solution [46,47]. The use of hypertonic saline in children was not associated with renal failure in a previous study of its effects on intracranial pressure [48]. Many institutions have a limit on what rate of infusion may be used for various concentrations of hypertonic saline, but this is poorly studied and generally sodium levels should be followed during therapy and should not exceed 155 mEq/L.

There are no reports in the literature of normonatremic patients suffering from central pontine myelinolysis as a result of hypertonic saline use. If 3 percent NaCl is used, the chloride load can be quite high and this leads to a non-anion gap metabolic acidosis.

However, many institutions make buffered solutions in which acetate is used to buffer some of the sodium in solution rather than all chloride. Acetate is then metabolized to bicarbonate, which helps offset the metabolic acidosis often seen in children receiving large chloride loads. In adult trauma literature, there is evidence that hypertonic saline modulates the immune system dysfunction that is related to trauma [49].

Hypertonic saline may induce vascular damage when it is injected into small peripheral veins. Up to 3 percent hypertonic saline has been used regularly without a central line. When mixed with red blood cells for transfusion, hypertonic saline can induce hemolysis. Similarly, the hypertonicity of fluid may cause tissue damage if a significant infiltration occurs. There are only a few case reports of successful use of hypertonic saline in neonates, and it should only be considered in cases of extreme hyponatremia.

## Postoperative Fluid Management

Postoperative administration of hypotonic fluid is common [50]. The traditional teaching that led to this practice is based on the aforementioned work by Holliday and Segar. Neonates may not be capable of eliminating any excess solute provided due to immature urine concentrating ability. Thus, the traditional practice has been to administer hypotonic fluid to children postoperatively.

Syndrome of inappropriate antidiuretic hormone secretion (SIADH) is a common response to the stress state induced by surgery. Taken with the fact that "routine" postoperative labs are not typically obtained and hypotonic fluids are routinely administered, hyponatremia may be a real risk to patients postoperatively. In fact, there are reports of significant harm coming to children in that situation [51]. Hyponatremia is difficult to identify clinically due to the general symptoms encountered: nausea, vomiting, headache, and lethargy. However, a meta-analysis comparing hypotonic fluids versus isotonic fluids in all hospitalized children showed the odds of developing hyponatremia after administration of hypotonic IV fluid were 17 times greater than isotonic fluid, and resulted in greater patient morbidity [52]. Another recent meta-analysis confirmed that postoperative children receiving hypotonic fluids were much more likely to develop hyponatremia than those receiving isotonic fluid [53].

In a clinical trial looking at the type of maintenance IV fluid to administer postoperatively to pediatric patients, excluding children under six months of age, it was concluded that the administration of isotonic fluid, rather than traditional hypotonic fluids, decreases the risk of postoperative hyponatremia. There was no difference in postoperative ADH levels or in risk of adverse events between the groups that received isotonic or hypotonic fluids postoperatively. Isotonic fluids did not increase the risk of hypernatremia [54]. While there is not currently enough evidence to completely change postoperative fluid administration practices, there may be additional evidence in the future that hypotonic fluids are not desirable postoperatively. Because of the unpredictable response of neonatal patients to hypotonic and isotonic solutions, it is recommended that serum electrolytes be measured in post-surgical neonates receiving intravenous hydration.

## Physiologic Anemia and Anemia of Prematurity

At birth, the normal neonate has a hemoglobin concentration of approximately 17 g dl$^{-1}$, a hematocrit of 55 percent, and large red blood cells. Within one week, the hemoglobin and hematocrit begin to fall from approximately 17 g dl$^{-1}$ at birth to 9–11 g dl$^{-1}$ at 8–12 weeks. This expected decrease in hemoglobin and hematocrit is termed *physiologic anemia of infancy*. Although the drop seems dramatic, this anemia is asymptomatic in the healthy neonate.

Decreased erythropoiesis early in the neonatal period is largely responsible for this physiologic anemia. Erythropoietin is made in the fetal liver and later in the kidneys. It is synthesized in response to low oxygen tension. When oxygen tension rises at birth, erythropoietin synthesis decreases. In the first 4–6 months, hemoglobin F is also replaced with hemoglobin A and levels of 2,3-diphosphoglycerate (2,3-DPG) climb. The change in conformation of the predominant hemoglobin along with more 2,3-DPG increases the P50 from 19 mmHg to 27 mmHg and shifts the oxyhemoglobin dissociation curve to the right [55]. As this shift occurs, the increased oxygen delivery to tissues continues to contribute to decreased erythropoiesis. As red blood cells lose the enzymatic function needed to maintain their deformable membrane, they become fragile and destructible. In the setting of decreased erythropoiesis, destroyed red blood cells are not replaced, and anemia further ensues.

At 8–12 weeks, oxygen needs begin to exceed oxygen delivery. In response to lower oxygen tension, erythropoietin gene expression increases, erythropoiesis resumes, and hemoglobin and hematocrit levels rise to near adult levels over the next six months.

In preterm infants, hemoglobin decreases weeks earlier, falls further, and takes longer to recover without treatment. During anemia of prematurity, hemoglobin reaches a nadir of 7–8 g dl$^{-1}$ by 3–6 weeks of age. Unlike the physiologic anemia of infancy, this is often symptomatic, causing arrhythmias, respiratory distress and apnea, and inadequate weight gain. Erythropoietin synthesis has not yet converted from the liver, where EPO gene expression is less responsive to hypoxia, to the kidney, where it is more responsive. As a result, in spite of symptomatic low oxygen tension, erythropoiesis remains decreased and anemia continues.

While healthy term infants require no treatment for physiologic anemia, preterm neonates often receive transfusions for anemia of prematurity. Studies of liberal and restrictive transfusion parameters in preterm neonates have been conflicting. While some have shown no increased morbidity or mortality with restrictive transfusion therapy [56], at least one has shown more frequent adverse neurologic outcomes with a restrictive strategy [57]. In the absence of an established optimal hemoglobin target, premature neonates should be transfused based on their clinical condition while taking into consideration baseline hemoglobin, increased oxygen affinity of residual Hgb F, and expected blood volume for age.

## Transfusion Guidelines

Very young children have smaller total blood volume, decreased production of erythropoietin in response to anemia, and immature humoral systems that render them less capable of forming antibodies to antigenic red blood cells [58,59]. Because of these physiologic differences, very young children are transfused under different guidelines than those greater than four months. Historically, in fact, premature neonates were transfused simply to replace blood loss from frequent phlebotomy. While this is no longer recommended, patients in this age group are still among the most frequently transfused in the hospital [60,61].

The following are current guidelines for transfusion of red blood cells in patients less than four months of age [62]:

Hct <20 percent with low reticulocyte count and symptoms of anemia.

Hct <30 percent with an infant on <35 percent hood $O_2$, $O_2$ per nasal cannula, CPAP, or IMV with mechanical ventilation with mean airway pressure <6 cmH$_2$0.

Hct <30 percent with an infant with significant apnea, bradycardia, tachycardia, tachypnea, or poor weight gain.

Hct <45 percent with an infant on ECMO or with congenital heart disease.

Hct <35 percent with an infant on >35 percent $O_2$ or on CPAP/IMV with mandatory ventilation with mean airway pressure ≥ 6 cmH$_2$O.

The indications for transfusion of red blood cells to older infants and children are similar to those in adults [62]:

Emergency surgery in patients with significant preoperative anemia.

Preoperative anemia when other corrective therapy is not available.

Intraoperative blood loss ≥15 percent total blood volume.

Hct <24 percent in perioperative period with signs and symptoms of anemia while on chemo/radiation or with chronic congenital or acquired symptomatic anemia.

Acute blood loss with hypovolemia not responsive to other therapy.

Hct <40 percent with severe pulmonary disease or ECMO.

Sickle cell disease with cerebrovascular accident, acute chest syndrome, splenic sequestration, recurrent priapism, or preoperatively to reach Hb 10 g dl$^{-1}$.

In the intraoperative period, a calculation of maximum allowable blood loss is often useful in determining when to transfuse. This method uses estimated blood volume, initial hematocrit, and lowest allowable hematocrit to determine how much blood a patient can lose before transfusion is necessary [63]:

$$MABL = EBV \times (Hi - Hf) / Hav$$

The decision to transfuse cannot be based on the predetermined lowest allowable hemoglobin alone, however. In the setting of rapid blood loss, expected ongoing blood loss, and in the face of clinical signs of decreased oxygen-carrying capacity, it may be necessary to transfuse at higher hemoglobin values.

Many studies have investigated transfusion triggers in critically ill adults, but far fewer have been performed in pediatric patients. In 1999, a landmark trial by Herbert et al. found a higher in-hospital mortality rate and higher estimates of severity of multiple organ dysfunction and nosocomial infections in adult patients transfused for a hemoglobin less than 10 g dl$^{-1}$ as compared to those transfused for a hemoglobin less than 7 g dl$^{-1}$ [64]. There was no difference in 30-day mortality between the groups.

A study performed in 2007 of critically ill pediatric patients found similar results. Those transfused according to a liberal (transfusion for hemoglobin less than 9.5 g dl$^{-1}$) strategy received 44 percent more transfusions than those transfused according to a restrictive strategy (transfusion for hemoglobin less than 7 g dl$^{-1}$); but there was no significant difference in percentage of patients with new or worsening multiple organ dysfunction syndrome or death between the two groups [65]. This suggests that a transfusion threshold hemoglobin of 7 g dl$^{-1}$ may be appropriate in critically ill children who are not actively bleeding.

In any case, the indication for red blood cell transfusion is to increase oxygen-carrying capacity in order to ensure adequate oxygen delivery to tissues. We see this in the aforementioned transfusion criteria, which highlight clinical scenarios in which tissue oxygen delivery is compromised or at risk. Therefore, the assessment of a child's clinical picture is as important as any laboratory value in making the decision to transfuse.

## Unique Populations

### Congenital Heart Disease

Pediatric patients with uncorrected cyanotic congenital heart disease require more hemoglobin – higher oxygen-carrying capacity – to ensure adequate oxygen delivery to tissues. Intracardiac shunts result in the delivery of desaturated blood to tissues and polycythemia develops due to increased erythropoietin in response to low tissue oxygen tension. Although it is common practice to maintain hemoglobin levels between 13 and 18 g dl$^{-1}$ in these patients, there are few data to support this [66]. As in all cases, an assessment of the child's clinical picture must be used to determine when to transfuse.

## Sickle Cell Disease

Sickle cell disease is a hereditary hemoglobinopathy that results from a single point mutation on the hemoglobin β-A gene, the gene that codes for beta globulin chains of hemoglobin A. This mutation results in production of hemoglobin S, which deforms or sickles the erythrocyte when deoxygenated [67]. Clinically, this sickling results in chronic hemolytic anemia, intermittent vaso-occlusion causing tissue anoxia and severe pain, and progressive organ damage. When the infant is around 4–5 months of age, the baby or fetal hemoglobin is replaced by sickle hemoglobin and the cells begin to sickle. Often the first manifestations of sickle cell disease in the infant is painful swelling of the hands and feet.

In 1955, the first major review of the anesthetic implications of sickle cell disease found a high rate of serious and even potentially fatal exacerbations of the disease after surgery [68].

Patients with sickle cell disease continue to have a 10 percent perioperative mortality rate and a 50 percent rate of serious disease-related postoperative complications – acute chest syndrome, painful crisis, and neurologic events [65]. Diluting hemoglobin S concentrations to less than 30 percent has been advised by some as a way to decrease the perioperative morbidity and mortality [69]. However, a study comparing a restrictive transfusion strategy (transfusion for hemoglobin less than 10 g dl$^{-1}$) with a liberal strategy (transfusion to dilute hemoglobin S to less than 30 percent) found no difference in the incidence of aforementioned major perioperative complications between the two groups in spite of the fact that the restrictive transfusion group had hemoglobin S concentrations of 59 percent compared with the liberal group's 31 percent [65]. These results suggest that diluting the hemoglobin S concentration may not reduce the rate of complications perioperatively.

The next question concerns the lowest acceptable preoperative hemoglobin in the sickle cell patient. A recent randomized trial compared preoperative transfusion with no preoperative transfusion in children and adults with hemoglobin SS or S-β-thalassemia sickle cell disease undergoing low and medium risk surgery [65]. The trial was terminated when the investigators found a marked increase in severe adverse events – primarily acute chest syndrome – in the group who was not transfused preoperatively. They concluded that patients with a preoperative hemoglobin less than 9 g dl$^{-1}$ should be transfused to decrease the risk of acute chest syndrome in the perioperative period.

Certain types of operations and patient characteristics seem to be associated with an increased incidence of perioperative complications in patients with sickle cell disease. A review of 1079 procedures found no complications with tonsillectomy and adenoidectomies, but complication rates of 16.9 percent for hysterectomies and Cesarean sections and 18.6 percent for dilation and curettage [65]. Increased age, recent complications, pregnancy, infection, and inpatient status also seem to be associated with increased sickle cell-related morbidity in the perioperative period [70]. However, in children undergoing cholecystectomies, a younger age increased the risk of developing acute chest syndrome. [71]

Therefore, type of surgery and patient characteristics must be taken into account along with preoperative hemoglobin in the decision to transfuse the sickle cell patient. Finally, the benefits of red blood cell therapy in sickle cell disease patients much be weighed with the costs of repeated transfusion, including iron overload and the risk of alloimmunization.

## Thalassemia

The beta thalassemias are a group of inherited disorders characterized by decreased production of alpha globulin chains of hemoglobin [72]. Severe anemia occurs due to hemolysis and ineffective erythropoiesis, and patients with severe disease are transfusion-dependent [73]. Maintenance of hemoglobin levels of 9–10 g dl$^{-1}$ allows for normal growth and development and reduces bone deformities and hepatosplenomegaly from extramedullary hematopoiesis [65,74]. Unfortunately, repeated transfusions lead to iron overload. In fact, cardiac death from iron overload is the primary cause of death in this hemoglobinopathy; patients must be treated with chelation therapy beginning in childhood [75].

## Preparation of Products

## Cytomegalovirus-Seronegative Blood Components

Cytomegalovirus rarely causes serious illness in the immunocompetent host [76], but immunosuppression can allow for uncontrolled viral replication and

serious disease [77]. Infants born to seronegative mothers have historically been transfused with CMV-seronegative blood. These recommendations were based on a study of preterm neonates that showed that transfusing CMV-seronegative blood products to multi-transfused low weight (<1200 g) neonates of seronegative mothers reduced the risk for CMV infection [78].

Low birth weight neonates, HIV-infected patients, recipients of seronegative allogeneic organ or hematopoietic stem cell transplants, pregnant women, and those receiving intrauterine transfusions should receive CMV-negative products. Patients with Hodgkin and non-Hodgkin lymphoma, recipients of immunosuppressive therapy, candidates for autologous hematopoietic stem cell transplantation, and those with hereditary or acquired cellular immunodeficiency can be considered for CMV-negative red blood cells.

## Leukocyte Reduction

Leukocyte reduction is the filtration of leukocytes from donor blood products prior to transfusion. Over 80 percent of the blood products transfused to pediatric patients in the United States have been leuko-reduced in spite of few studies demonstrating benefit [79]. The process reduces the transmission of CMV [65], HLA alloimmunization, and febrile hemolytic transfusion reactions. Patients with congenital hemolytic anemias (sickle cell disease and thalassemia) and hypoproliferative anemias who are likely to need multiple transfusions should be transfused with leuokocyte-reduced red blood cells in order to prevent alloimmunization [65]. Because of their immature immune systems, however, neonates less than four months of age rarely become alloimmunized. They also infrequently suffer from febrile transfusion reactions. As such, leukocyte reduction of blood products for neonates remains controversial. A study of LBW (<1250 g) premature infants before and after implementation of universal leukocyte reduction found no difference in mortality or rate of bacteremia. There was, however, a decrease in retinopathy of prematurity, bronchopulmonary dysplasia, and length of hospital stay after leuko-reduction [65]. This evidence supports continued leukocyte reduction for the youngest, smallest patients.

## Irradiation

While leukocyte reduction may also decrease the risk of transfusion-associated graft-versus-host disease

(TA-GvHD), blood products must be irradiated in order to inactivate T-cells in the donated blood product and prevent the development of TA-GvHD. TA-GvHD occurs when transfused T-lymphocytes attack host HLA-incompatible lymphoid tissue and host T-lymphocytes fail to mount an appropriate response [80]. This can occur not only in immunocompromised patients but also in immunocompetent recipients who share HLA antigens with the donor [65]. The disease carries a high rate of fatality from infection as the host's bone marrow become hypoplastic [81].

Although it is not an absolute indication, neonates less than four months of age who may have undiagnosed cellular immune deficiency often receive irradiated fresh blood products. Low birth weight neonates (<1200 g), neonates receiving exchange transfusion, and those on extracorporeal membrane oxygenation should receive irradiated products. Patients with congenital cell-mediated immunodeficiencies, Hodgkin disease, acute lymphocytic leukemia, those receiving purine analogue therapy, and patients receiving direct donations from relatives or HLA-matched donors *must* have irradiated products, as should patients receiving hematopoietic stem cell transplants, intrauterine or postintrauterine transfusions, and immunocompromised organ transplant recipients [65].

## Washing

Washing blood products removes or reduces plasma, anticoagulant-preservative solutions, and high levels of potassium. While it is not used routinely, children and infants who may be predisposed to hyperkalemia may preferentially receive washed products. In addition, the process of irradiation increases the potassium in the blood product, which should then be washed before transfusion to infants to avoid hyperkalemia.

## Age of Blood

While some institutions transfuse red blood cell products less than seven days old to neonates, others use a dedicated unit until the expiration date to reduce donor exposure. A study comparing the use of fresh versus standard-issue red blood cell transfusion in premature infants found no difference in outcome [65].

## Platelets

Platelets are necessary to maintain an intact endothelial barrier to prevent spontaneous bleeding and, in higher levels, for hemostasis after vascular injury to control surgical bleeding. Patients of all ages are at risk for spontaneous hemorrhage at platelet counts <10 000/μl [65]. If active bleeding is occurring or an invasive procedure is imminent, platelet counts of 50 000/μl are usually required [82]. For those patients with platelets counts between 50 000/μl and 100 000/μl, platelets do not need to be given prophylactically but should be immediately available in case of microvascular bleeding during invasive procedures [66]. In some clinical settings, in which even small amounts of bleeding could be catastrophic, the platelet transfusion trigger is higher [83]. In neurosurgery, for example, patients may be transfused for platelet count <100 000/μl, even without active bleeding [63].

Critically ill preterm infants are a population that deserves particular attention here. These patients have an immature subependymal matrix prone to rupture, putting them at risk of intracranial hemorrhage [61,84]. Specific transfusion guidelines for these infants are locally defined, but recommendations suggest transfusing them when platelet counts fall below 60 000/μl [85]. However, a randomized controlled trial comparing transfusion to platelet count >150 000/μl versus >50 000/μl found no significant difference in the incidence of intracranial hemorrhage between the groups [65]. Therefore, as with all transfusions, the risks and potential benefits must be weighed on a case-by-case basis after careful clinical assessment.

Platelets can be collected in one of two ways. They can be derived from whole-blood donations and then pooled with 5–7 other donors. Alternatively, they can be collected from a single donor through apheresis. The later method produces approximately the same number of platelets but reduces exposure to multiple donors [86]. Plasma-incompatible, whole-blood-derived platelets contain very small volumes of plasma compared to the total plasma volume of an adult patient. As such, these transfusions do not lead to clinically significant hemolysis. However, apheresed platelets and whole-blood platelets given to small patients should be ABO compatible to avoid a hemolytic reaction. Rh antigens are not expressed on platelets, so Rh(D) matching is not necessary for apheresis platelets. Whole-blood-derived platelets contain enough red blood cells to cause Rh alloimmunization, so platelets from Rh(D) negative donors are preferentially given to Rh(D) negative recipients of childbearing age.

There are several important logistical considerations in the transfusion of platelets. Pediatric patients are typically administered 10–15 ml kg$^{-1}$ to increase their platelet count by 30 000 to 90 000/μl. However, this dose is currently being studied and discussed. In light of recent evidence suggesting lower doses may achieve adequate hemostasis, the dose may be reduced in the future [87,88]. When given in anticipation of an invasive procedure, platelets should be transfused just prior to the procedure. They should only be filtered by large-pore filters (>150 μm) and should be stored at room temperature. Recent evidence suggests, though, they may be safely infused through a warmer during transfusion [89].

## Fresh Frozen Plasma and Cryoprecipitate

Fresh frozen plasma (FFP) is the fluid portion of whole-blood containing all of the coagulation factors in normal concentrations. Fresh frozen plasma is indicated to replace factors during massive blood transfusion, to correct a severely prolonged prothrombin time prior to an invasive procedure or during active bleeding, to emergently reverse warfarin, or as replacement therapy when specific factor concentrates are not available. Preterm infants and neonates most often receive FFP to treat factor deficiencies from vitamin K deficiency and in cases of hemorrhagic disease of the newborn in which coagulation factors are depleted. Unfortunately, it is also often transfused without evidence-based justification in cases where no coagulopathy exists and a colloid would be more appropriate for resuscitation [90].

Cryoprecipitate is prepared from FFP by thawing the product and separating the precipitated protein.

This contains 20–50 percent of the Factor VIII from the original FFP, von Willebrand factor, approximately 250 mg of fibrinogen, and Factor XIII. It is indicated in cases of hypofibrinogenemia, dysfibrinogenemia, or Factor XIII deficiency, but is no longer used to treat hemophilia A or von Willebrand disease [91,92]. Infants usually only require 1 unit and children 1–2 units per 10 kg to raise fibrinogen 60–100 mg dl$^{-1}$.

## Coagulation Disorders and Their Specific Treatment

About 1 in 5000 males is born with hemophilia every year [93]. The severity of bleeding with these coagulopathies is proportional to the degree of factor deficiency [94]. Those with milder disease may only bleed with trauma or surgery, but children with more severe disease may bleed spontaneously [95]. Children with these inherited factor deficiencies were historically treated with pooled plasma, putting them at high risk for contracting viral hepatitis and HIV. Transmission rates have now been greatly reduced, however, due to more effective virus removal and inactivation and the use of recombinant factors. Patients with hemophilia A are treated with Factor VIII. Similarly, children with the much less common hemophilias B, or Factor IX deficiency, are transfused with recombinant Factor IX or purified Factor IX products.

Table 15.4 lists specific guidelines for factor repletion in hemophilia A and B.

Von Willebrand disease (vWD) results from an abnormal amount, structure, or function of von Willebrand Factor (vWF), a glycoprotein that acts to facilitate platelet adhesion and transport Factor VIII,

**Table 15.4** Specific guidelines for factor repletion in hemophilia A and B

| Site of hemorrhage | Target Factor VIII or IX level (percent) | Treatment duration (days) |
| --- | --- | --- |
| Muscle | 30–50 | 1–2 |
| Joint | 50–80 | 1–2 |
| Gastrointestinal tract | 40–60 | 10–14 |
| Oral mucosa | 30–50 | 2–3 |
| Epistaxis | 30–50 | 2–3 |
| Hematuria | 30–100 | 1–2 |
| Retroperitoneal | 80–100 | 7–10 |
| Central nervous system | 80–100 | 14 |
| Trauma or surgery | 80–100 | 14 |
| Source: [94]. | | |

preventing its degradation. It was once thought to be more common than hemophilia, but may be as rare as 1 case per 10 000 people. Children with vWF often suffer from bruising, epistaxis, and menorrhagia due to impaired platelet adhesion. Unlike in hemophilia, however, they do not develop hemarthrosis. They may have prolonged bleeding time and activated partial thromboplastin time (aPPT) depending on the Factor VIII level, but the most sensitive and specific diagnostic lab test is the platelet function assay [65].

Milder forms of hemophilia A and vWD often do not require factor replacement as they can be treated with desmopressin in older children and adults. Desmopressin (DDAVP) is a synthetic analogue of vasopressin [96]. A dose of 0.3 µg kg$^{-1}$ IV increases Factor VIII:vWF two-fold to three-fold in 30–60 minutes [97]. When DDAVP is ineffective, as in vWD type 2 in which it may increase abnormal vWF or worsen thrombocytopenia, Factor VIII:vWF concentrates such as Humate-P are used [92]. DDAVP is also not given to young children and infants because of the risk of free water retention, hyponatremia, and seizures. Finally, in the perioperative period, consultation with a child's hematologist is important in establishing the appropriate dose of DDAVP or Humate-P.

# Complications Associated With Transfusion

## Infection

When seeking consent from patients and their families for product transfusion, providers learn that there is perhaps no more feared complication than the risk of infection – particularly the risk of infection with HIV. In spite of the patient concern, however, the risk of acquiring a major viral infection from a transfusion is extremely low. Donor-screening, eliminating the use of products from self-identified high-risk donors, and viral testing of products has ensured that the incidence of viral transmission is now so low as to be almost nonexistent (Table 15.5).

As viral infectious risk has fallen, the risk of bacterial infections has gained attention. Of the 694 transfusion-related deaths between 1985 and 1999, 11.1 percent were due to bacterial contamination [65]. *Yersinia enterocolitica* is the most prevalent contaminant of stored red blood cells [98] and the risk of contamination is directly related to length of storage [65,99].

**Table 15.5** Viral infection risk

| Disease | Incidence with transfusion |
| --- | --- |
| Hepatitis B virus | 1 in 137 000 |
| Hepatitis C virus | <1 in 1 000 000 |
| Human immunodeficiency virus | <1 in 1 900 000 |
| Human T lymphotropic virus types I and II | 1 in 250 000 to 1 in 2 000 000 |
| Source: [65]. | |

Because platelets are stored at room temperature, the risk of bacterial growth in these products is higher and their shelf life is only five days. There is also evidence of greater infectious risk when pooled donors are used than when an apheresed unit from a single donor is given. *Staphylococcus aureus*, *Klebsiella pneumoniae*, *Serratia marcescens*, and *Staphylococcus epidermidis* are among the most common causes of death from bacterial infection following platelet transfusion. The mortality rate from platelet-related bacterial infection is 26 percent [100].

## Hyperkalemia and Hypocalcemia

During storage and with aging, red blood cells leak potassium into the extracellular fluid. Although there does not seem to be clinically significant hyperkalemia when packed red blood cells are given slowly through peripheral IV access [65], the Perioperative Cardiac Arrest Registry reported eight hyperkalemic cardiac arrests related to blood transfusion [101]. With the rapid administration of large volumes of whole-blood or packed red blood cells, especially through a central venous catheter, hyperkalemia can develop [102]. This may be more likely to occur in infants and small children in whom it is easy to transfuse products at a rate >1.5–2 ml kg$^{-1}$ min$^{-1}$. Therefore, it is especially important to be vigilant to ongoing intraoperative blood loss, avoiding situations in which massive, rapid transfusion of products is necessary.

When products do need to be given, they should be warmed and infused through peripheral intravenous access. When massive transfusion is necessary, newer products – those that have spent less time in storage leaking potassium – should be used whenever possible. Further, if fresh products are not available, to the extent that time permits, washing the RBCs can be done to reduce the extracellular potassium. Hyperkalemia is also worse in units that have been irradiated. As such, these units can be stored for less time and need to be washed prior to administration to very young patients. Finally, when the infusion rate is greater than 1.5–2 ml kg$^{-1}$ min$^{-1}$, the ECG should be monitored for peaked T waves and treatment for hyperkalemia – calcium, sodium bicarbonate, albuterol, insulin, and glucose – should be readily available.

Stored blood components are anticoagulated with citrate, which chelates ionized calcium. Upon transfusion, the citrate is taken up by all cells but cleared primarily in the liver. In cases of massive transfusion, especially with whole-blood or FFP, citrate is transfused faster than the body can clear it, causing a decrease in the concentration of ionized calcium [103,104]. The ionized calcium falls enough to decrease cardiac contractility when the citrated product is transfused faster than 1.5–2 ml kg$^{-1}$ min$^{-1}$ [65]. When citrated products do need to be delivered at a rapid rate, exogenous calcium should be administered. Neonates and small infants may not eliminate citrate as rapidly, putting them at particular risk for hypocalcemia. Also, owing to its clearance in the liver, citrate toxicity may develop more readily in patients with hepatic dysfunction and during the anhepatic phase of liver transplantation [105].

## Transfusion-Related Acute Lung Injury

The leading cause of transfusion-related death in the United States is transfusion-related acute lung injury (TRALI) [106]. The estimated risk of TRALI is 1 in 5000 transfusions, and it is most commonly associated with FFP [65]. TRALI is thought to be caused by an interaction between antibodies from the donor interacting with leukocyte antigens in the recipient, resulting in neutrophil activation in the pulmonary vascular bed. Clinically, its symptoms resemble acute respiratory distress syndrome – dyspnea, hypoxia, noncardiogenic pulmonary edema – and typically begin 4–6 hours after transfusion. Supportive therapy is indicated and 90 percent of patients recover [64].

## Monitoring Intravascular Volume Status

Because ongoing losses, including blood loss, may be especially significant in the neonate or infant, estimation of intravascular volume status is difficult. Blood loss estimation is made quite difficult because small amounts are difficult to quantify and these small amounts may be significant, given low body weights of the patients. There has even been some interest in the use of cameras to detect and estimate blood loss. However, invasive monitoring of volume status, estimates of fluid losses, and clinician vigilance are the tools most readily available in the operating arena at this time and those monitors most frequently used in infants and neonates will be discussed here.

Central venous pressure (CVP) has been a long-accepted standard for the monitoring of intravascular volume status. The physiologic basis for this monitor is that superior vena cava (SVC) pressures approximate right atrial pressures (RAP), which reflect right ventricular preload [107]. However, placement of a central venous catheter (CVC) carries risks including arterial puncture, pneumothorax, and infection [108]. Patient factors become very important when deciding the site of CVC placement. It may be very difficult to place a subclavian line in a very small patient using anatomical landmarks. Ultrasound can be used to facilitate CVC placement and may reduce complications associated with insertion [109].

Peripherally inserted central catheters (PICCs) can also be easily inserted for monitoring and access purposes. Their advantage over traditional central lines is a low or similar infection rate, decreased complications of placement, and decreased need for general anesthesia to facilitate placement [110]. While the course it takes during placement is less predictable, this can be overcome with use of fluoroscopy. PICC lines can also provide another reliable route to monitoring of CVP.

Traditionally, the SVC was the most trusted site for CVP monitoring, but some alternatives have been studied. Measuring CVP in the inferior vena cava (IVC) has been shown to correlate well with RAP as measured in infants and children in the cardiac catheterization laboratory [111]. Peripheral venous pressure (PVP) has been studied and correlates well with CVP in infants, children, and adults [112]. PVP has also been shown to correlate well with CVP in infants and children with congenital heart disease and in children undergoing major surgical procedures [113,114]. However, neither bedside ultrasonographic measurement of the IVC to abdominal aorta (AA) ratio nor the IVC collapsibility index correlated well with CVP in acutely ill children [115].

Use of CVP as a monitor for intravascular volume status has been called into question by several studies.

Specific concerns with CVP include its susceptibility to problems with venous return, right ventricular compliance, left ventricular failure, peripheral venous tone, patient position, valvular heart disease, increased abdominal pressure, and pulmonary vascular disease. Trends are likely to be more useful for interpretation than discrete measurements of CVP [116].

Transpulmonary indicator dilution (TID) has been advocated in neonates and infants, though there have not been large trials regarding outcomes. Transpulmonary indicator dilution has been validated in infants and children as an accurate measurement of cardiac output and systemic vascular resistance (SVR) [117]. Transpulmonary indicator dilution has been shown to more accurately indicate changes in intravascular volume status than CVP [118]. Many of the commercially available TID devices also utilize arterial pulse contour analysis to provide continuous cardiac output monitoring. Measurement of cardiac output and mixed venous oxygen saturation by pulmonary artery (PA) catheterization is rare in neonates and infants due to the high associated complication rate [119].

Arterial pulse pressure variation (PPV) and systolic pressure variation (SPV) are other common methods to estimate changes in intravascular volume status. More specifically, PPV and SPV are useful measures of fluid responsiveness. The principle behind these methods is that greater arterial pulse pressure changes with positive pressure ventilation will occur because of a greater drop in right ventricular preload, a greater increase in right ventricular afterload, and a decrease in left ventricular afterload [120]. In cases where wide swings in intravascular volume status are anticipated, an arterial line is often placed. Since these methods require only an arterial pressure waveform for analysis, it is a valuable tool that adds little to the required monitors or equipment for the procedure. Its reliability is decreased in the setting of spontaneous respiration, arrhythmias, pulmonary hypertension, right heart failure, low tidal volume, and open chest [121]. Systolic pressure variation greater than 10 mmHg is indicative of a fluid responsive state [122].

Urine output is a frequently utilized monitor for intravascular volume status. Despite renal system immaturity, the neonate and infant will restrict urine output in response to decreases in intravascular volume. Oliguria, less than 1 ml kg$^{-1}$ h$^{-1}$ in infants and 0.5 ml kg$^{-1}$ h$^{-1}$ in children, is often, but not always, indicative of hypovolemia [123]. Confounding factors include other hypotensive states that decrease GFR, SIADH, intrinsic renal failure, and mechanical problems with urinary catheters. However, in the presence of other physical signs, oliguria can be a useful monitor of intravascular volume status.

Echocardiography is a reasonable monitor in the intraoperative setting. With a variety of probe sizes available, even very small neonates can be monitored safely with transesophageal echocardiography. If the chest is unobscured by the surgery, transthoracic echocardiography may also be used, but not continuously. Inferior vena cava measurement, SVC collapsability, ventricular filling, systolic left ventricular cavity obliteration, and left ventricular end-diastolic area have all been described as methods for diagnosing hypovolemia [124].

# Vascular Access Strategies

Vascular access can be challenging in neonates and infants. The process of obtaining access is challenging and the management of that access remains difficult. To further complicate matters, many neonates and infants who present for surgery have had multiple prior access sites.

Traditional peripheral intravenous (PIV) access is the most common technique encountered. When vasculature cannot be easily located visually or by palpation, there are several technologies to aid in vein localization. Anatomy-based techniques are popular, where PIV access is attempted without visualization, palpation, or the aid of a medical device. Common sites to attempt this method of PIV cannulation are the great saphenous vein, the cephalic vein ("intern's" vein), veins on the dorsum of the hand, and antecubital venous access because of their more consistent anatomy.

The external jugular vein is frequently utilized in a difficult access situation. However, the vein is quite mobile and carries the additional risk of pneumothorax or carotid cannulation. The mobility of the site also results frequently in catheter dislodgement. Scalp veins are also utilized in this age group, whereas they are frequently not utilized in older children or adults. Scalp veins are also prone to dislodgement, infiltrations are not inconsequential, and temporal artery cannulation is possible. Surgical cut-down for peripheral venous access is another possibility, but it is difficult, time-consuming, and associated with increased patient morbidity.

Several technologies have been made available for PIV cannulation in neonates and infants. Ultrasound is a frequently used technology and has been studied versus the anatomical-based approach to difficult PIV access. It was found that both techniques are effective in venous cannulation, but ultrasound was faster and more likely to be successful on the first attempt than the "blind" technique [125]. Transillumination is another technique useful in neonates and infants for PIV placement [126]. Local warming of proposed cannulation sites and epidermal nitroglycerin have been used to increase success of percutaneous PIV insertion [127,128]. Near-infrared (NIR) vein scanners are available in several different commercial variants. They emit NIR light and reveal a vein map because the light is scattered by forward flow of blood. The light scatter is detected by the device and a vein map is projected on the patient to facilitate PIV insertion [129].

Central venous access is frequently utilized in neonates and infants without incidence. One of the most common methods of central venous access in neonates are umbilical venous catheters (UVCs). Traditionally, the biggest risks have been malposition and infection, but one study has advocated that long-term use of UVCs does not necessarily increase risk of infection over replacing the UVC with a PICC [130]. The umbilical vein is 2–3 centimeters long and then joins the left branch of the portal vein. At this juncture, the ductus venosus arises, which bypasses the liver and joins the IVC just distal to its entry into the atrium. The ideal position for the UVC is in the IVC, but in emergency situations the catheter can be placed shallowly in the umbilical vein, though care must be taken to avoid hyperosmolar solutions which can cause liver necrosis. Umbilical arterial catheters (UACs) can also be placed. The umbilical arteries are a direct continuation of the internal iliac arteries and thus a UAC will pass through the umbilical artery to the internal iliac artery, then go behind the bladder to reach the aorta. The UAC should be placed high enough within the aorta (above the diaphragm) to avoid inadvertently occluding the celiac axis, renal arteries, or superior mesenteric arteries. PICC lines can be placed in even the smallest of neonates, frequently using the femoral site for cannulation. Midline catheters are similarly inserted in the deep veins of the upper arm, but terminate outside the thorax, as opposed to centrally.

Traditional sites for CVC placement are the same as in older children and adults: femoral, subclavian, and internal jugular. While the external jugular is sometimes used to place a CVC, difficulty is often encountered in navigating the catheter into the central circulation [131]. Adult studies have generally shown the subclavian site to have the lowest risk of infection, but in children it has been identified that the more important risk factors for infection are younger age and duration of CVC use [132]. Complications related to insertion are highest with the subclavian site and complications related to maintaining the central line were more common in younger children and in the femoral site of access [133] [134]. A systematic review of central line literature suggested that implanted ports may be more often recommended in children than in adults for longer periods of use, and that central line placement be routinely confirmed with radiograph given the high risk of malposition in children [135].

Intraosseous (IO) lines are frequently used in critically ill neonates and infants, and are safe to place [136,137]. They should be considered when other routes of intravenous access have been unsuccessfully attempted. In neonatal emergencies, they are faster to place than a UVC [138]. There are reports of IO lines being successfully placed and used in the perioperative period [139]. However, IO lines are not without complications, which include fat embolism, infection, fractures, and malposition or dislodgement. Malposition or dislodgement can result in a compartment syndrome [140]. Intraoperative dislodgement would be especially concerning, given the ongoing difficulty in vascular access at this point, with very little access to the patient under surgical drapes. While the decision to employ an IO line should be approached with caution, this important route to vascular access should be considered.

# References

1. Friis-Hansen, B. Body water compartments in children: changes during growth and related changes in body composition. *Pediatrics*. 1961;28:169–81.

2. Hawkes CP, Hourihane JO, Kenny LC, et al. Gender- and gestational age-specific body fat percentage at birth. *Pediatrics*. 2011;128(3):e645–51.

3. Morgenstern BZ, Mahoney DW, Warady BA. Estimating total body water in children on the basis of height and weight: a reevaluation of the formulas of Mellits and Cheek. *J Am Soc Nephrol*. 2002. 13(7):1884–8.

4. Linderkamp O, Versmold HT, Riegel KP, Betke K. Estimation and prediction of blood volume in infants and children. *Eur J Pediatr*. 1977;125(4):227–34.

5. Cassady G. Plasma volume studies in low birth weight infants. *Pediatrics*. 1966;38(6):1020–7.

6. Feldschuh J, Enson Y. Prediction of the normal blood volume: relation of blood volume to body habitus. *Circulation.* 1977;56(4 Pt 1):605–12.

7. Schlondorff D, Weber H, Trizna W, Fine LG. Vasopressin responsiveness of renal adenylate cyclase in newborn rats and rabbits. *Am J Physiol.* 1978;234(1):F16–21.

8. Chawla D, Agarwal R, Deorari AK, Paul VK. Fluid and electrolyte management in term and preterm neonates. *Indian J Pediatr.* 2008;75(3):255–9.

9. Aperia A, Zetterstrom R. Renal control of fluid homeostasis in the newborn infant. *Clin Perinatol.* 1982;9(3):523–33.

10. Holliday MA, Segar WE. The maintenance need for water in parenteral fluid therapy. *Pediatrics.* 1957;19(5):823–32.

11. Holliday MA, Friedman AL, Segar WE, Chesney R, Finberg L. Acute hospital-induced hyponatremia in children: a physiologic approach. *J Pediatr.* 2004;145(5):584–7.

12. Furman EB, Roman DG, Lemmer LA, et al. Specific therapy in water, electrolyte and blood-volume replacement during pediatric surgery. *Anesthesiology.* 1975;42(2):187–93.

13. Berry F. *Practical aspects of fluid and electrolyte therapy.* In Berry F, editor. *Anesthetic Management of Difficult and Routine Pediatric Patients.* New York: Churchill Livingstone; 1986; 107–35.

14. American Society of Anesthesiologists. Practice guidelines for preoperative fasting and the use of pharmacologic agents to reduce the risk of pulmonary aspiration: application to healthy patients undergoing elective procedures: an updated report by the American Society of Anesthesiologists Committee on Standards and Practice Parameters. *Anesthesiology.* 2011;114(3):495–511.

15. Jacob M, Chappell D, Conzen P, Finsterer U, Rehm M. Blood volume is normal after pre-operative overnight fasting. *Acta Anaesthesiol Scand.* 2008;52(4):522–9.

16. Friedman AL. Pediatric hydration therapy: historical review and a new approach. *Kidney Int.* 2005;67(1):380–8.

17. Bell EF, Warburton D, Stonestreet BS, Oh W. Effect of fluid administration on the development of symptomatic patent ductus arteriosus and congestive heart failure in premature infants. *N Engl J Med.* 1980;302(11):598–604.

18. Srinivasan G, Jain R, Pildes RS, Kannan CR. Glucose homeostasis during anesthesia and surgery in infants. *J Pediatr Surg.* 1986;21(8):718–21.

19. Shires T, Williams J, Brown F. Acute change in extracellular fluids associated with major surgical procedures. *Ann Surg.* 1961;154:803–10.

20. Liumbruno GM, Bennardello F, Lattanzio A, et al. Recommendations for the transfusion management of patients in the peri-operative period: II. The intra-operative period. *Blood Transfus.* 2011;9(2):189–217.

21. Mollitt DL, Ballantine TV, Grosfeld JL, Quinter P. A critical assessment of fluid requirements in gastroschisis. *J Pediatr Surg.* 1978;13(3):217–19.

22. Murat I Dubois MC. Perioperative fluid therapy in pediatrics. *Paediatr Anaesth.* 2008;18(5):363–70.

23. Campbell IT, Baxter J, Tweedie I, et al. IV fluids during surgery. *Br J Anaesth.* 1990;65(5):726–9.

24. de Jonge E Levi M. Effects of different plasma substitutes on blood coagulation: a comparative review. *Crit Care Med.* 2001. 29(6):1261–7.

25. Nearman HS Herman ML. Toxic effects of colloids in the intensive care unit. *Crit Care Clin.* 1991;7(3):713–23.

26. De Gaudio AR. Therapeutic use of albumin. *Int J Artif Organs.* 1995;18(4):216–24.

27. Schwarz U. Intraoperative fluid therapy in infants and young children. *Anaesthesist.* 1999;48(1):41–50.

28. Soderlind M, Salvignol G, Izard P, Lönnqvist PA. Use of albumin, blood transfusion and intraoperative glucose by APA and ADARPEF members: a postal survey. *Paediatr Anaesth.* 2001;11(6):685–9.

29. Tobias MD, Wambold D, Pilla MA, Greer F. Differential effects of serial hemodilution with hydroxyethyl starch, albumin, and 0.9% saline on whole blood coagulation. *J Clin Anesth.* 1998;10(5):366–71.

30. McClelland DB. Safety of human albumin as a constituent of biologic therapeutic products. *Transfusion.* 1998;38(7):690–9.

31. Boldt J, Knothe C, Schindler E, et al. Volume replacement with hydroxyethyl starch solution in children. *Br J Anaesth.* 1993;70(6):661–5.

32. Riegger LQ, Voepel-Lewis T, Kulik TJ, et al. Albumin versus crystalloid prime solution for cardiopulmonary bypass in young children. *Crit Care Med.* 2002;30(12):2649–54.

33. B.H. Corporation. BUMINATE 5% [albumin (human)]: prescribing information, 2009.

34. B.H. Corporation. BUMINATE 25% [albumin (human)]: prescribing information, 2009.

35. Liumbruno GM, Bennardello F, Lattanzio A, et al. Recommendations for the use of albumin and immunoglobulins. *Blood Transfus.* 2009;7(3):216–34.

36. Bailey AG, McNaull PP, Jooste E, Tuchman JB. Perioperative crystalloid and colloid fluid management in children: where are we and how did we get here? *Anesth Analg.* 2010;110(2):375–90.

37. Wilkes MM, Navickis RJ, Sibbald WJ. Albumin versus hydroxyethyl starch in cardiopulmonary bypass surgery: a meta-analysis of postoperative bleeding. *Ann Thorac Surg.* 2001. 72(2):527–33.; discussion 534.

38. Martin G, Bennett-Guerrero E, Wakeling H, et al. A prospective, randomized comparison of thromboelastographic coagulation profile in patients receiving lactated Ringer's solution, 6% hetastarch in a balanced-saline vehicle, or 6% hetastarch in saline during major surgery. *J Cardiothorac Vasc Anesth.* 2002;16(4):441–6.

39. Kozek-Langenecker SA. Effects of hydroxyethyl starch solutions on hemostasis. *Anesthesiology.* 2005. 103(3):654–60.

40. Fenger-Eriksen C, Hartig Rasmussen C, Kappel Jensen T, et al. Renal effects of hypotensive anaesthesia in combination with acute normovolaemic haemodilution with hydroxyethyl starch 130/0.4 or isotonic saline. *Acta Anaesthesiol Scand.* 2005;49(7):969–74.

41. Liet JM, Bellouin AS, Boscher C, Lejus C, Rozé JC. Plasma volume expansion by medium molecular weight hydroxyethyl starch in neonates: a pilot study. *Pediatr Crit Care Med.* 2003;4(3):305–7.

42. Sumpelmann R, Kretz FJ, Luntzer R, et al. Hydroxyethyl starch 130/0.42/6:1 for perioperative plasma volume replacement in 1130 children: results of a European prospective multicenter observational postauthorization safety study (PASS). *Paediatr Anaesth.* 2012;22(4):371–8.

43. Hospira. Hextend and 6% Hetastarch in 0.9% sodium chloride injection, 2006.

44. Hospira. Voluven (6% hydroxyethyl starch 130/0.4 in 0.9% sodium chloride injection), for administration by intravenous infusion: Highlights Of Prescribing Information, FDA, 2007.

45. F.S. Communication. Hydroxyethyl starch solutions: FDA safety communication – boxed warning on increased mortality and severe renal injury and risk of bleeding, 2013.

46. Fisher B, Thomas D, Peterson B. Hypertonic saline lowers raised intracranial pressure in children after head trauma. *J Neurosurg Anesthesiol.* 1992;4(1):4–10.

47. Simma B, Burger R, Falk M, Sacher P, Fanconi S. A prospective, randomized, and controlled study of fluid management in children with severe head injury: lactated Ringer's solution versus hypertonic saline. *Crit Care Med.* 1998;26(7):1265–70.

48. Peterson B, Khanna S, Fisher B, Marshall L. Prolonged hypernatremia controls elevated intracranial pressure in head-injured pediatric patients. *Crit Care Med.* 2000;28(4):1136–43.

49. Junger WG, Coimbra R, Liu FC, et al. Hypertonic saline resuscitation: a tool to modulate immune function in trauma patients? *Shock.* 1997;8(4):235–41.

50. Snaith R, Peutrell J, Ellis D. An audit of intravenous fluid prescribing and plasma electrolyte monitoring: a comparison with guidelines from the National Patient Safety Agency. *Paediatr Anaesth.* 2008;18(10):940–6.

51. Arieff AI, Ayus JC, Fraser CL. Hyponatraemia and death or permanent brain damage in healthy children. *BMJ.* 1992;304(6836):1218–22.

52. Choong K, Kho M, Menon K, Bohn D. Hypotonic versus isotonic saline in hospitalised children: a systematic review. *Arch Dis Child.* 2006;91(10):828–35.

53. Foster BA, Tom D, Hill V. Hypotonic versus isotonic fluids in hospitalized children: a systematic review and meta-analysis. *J Pediatr.* 2014;165:163–9.

54. Choong K, Arora S, Cheng J, et al. Hypotonic versus isotonic maintenance fluids after surgery for children: a randomized controlled trial. *Pediatrics.* 2011;128(5):857–66.

55. Oski FA. The unique fetal red cell and its function. E. Mead Johnson Award address. *Pediatrics.* 1973;51(3):494–500.

56. Kirpalani H, Whyte RK, Andersen C, et al. The Premature Infants in Need of Transfusion (PINT) study: a randomized, controlled trial of a restrictive (low) versus liberal (high) transfusion threshold for extremely low birth weight infants. *J Pediatr.* 2006;149(3):301–7.

57. Bell EF, Strauss RG, Widness JA, et al. Randomized trial of liberal versus restrictive guidelines for red blood cell transfusion in preterm infants. *Pediatrics.* 2005;115(6):1685–91.

58. DePalma L, Luban NL. Blood component therapy in the perinatal period: guidelines and recommendations. *Semin Perinatol.* 1990;14(5):403–15.

59. Stockman JA, 3rd, Graeber JE, Clark DA, et al. Anemia of prematurity: determinants of the erythropoietin response. *J Pediatr.* 1984;105(5):786–92.

60. Ramasethu J, Luban N. Red blood cell transfusion in the newborn. *Semin Neonatol.* 1999;4:5–16.

61. Strauss RG. Transfusion therapy in neonates. *Am J Dis Child.* 1991;145(8):904–11.

62. Roseff SD, Luban NL, Manno CS. Guidelines for assessing appropriateness of pediatric transfusion. *Transfusion.* 2002. 42(11):1398–413.

63. Desmet L, Lacroix J. Transfusion in pediatrics. *Crit Care Clin.* 2004;20(2):299–311.

64. Hebert PC, Wells G, Blajchman M, et al. A multicenter, randomized, controlled clinical trial of transfusion requirements in critical care: transfusion requirements

in critical care investigators, Canadian Critical Care Trials Group. *N Engl J Med*. 1999;340(6):409–17.

65. Lacroix J, Hebert PC, Hutchison JS. Transfusion strategies for patients in pediatric intensive care units. *N Engl J Med* 2007;356(16):1609–19.

66. Mauermann W, Haile D, Flick R. Blood conservation. In Davis P,Cladis F, Motoyama E, editors. *Smith's Anesthesia for Infants and Children*. Philadelphia, PA: Elsevier; 2011; 395–417.

67. Hahn E, Gillespie E. Sickle cell anemia. *Arch Intern Med*. 1927; 39:233–4.

68. Shapiro ND Poe MF. Sickle-cell disease: an anesthesiological problem. *Anesthesiology*. 1955;16(5):771–80.

69. Bhattacharyya N, Wayne AS, Kevy SV, Shamberger RC. Perioperative management for cholecystectomy in sickle cell disease. *J Pediatr Surg*. 1993;28(1):72–5.

70. Firth PG, Head CA. Sickle cell disease and anesthesia. *Anesthesiology*. 2004. 101(3):766–85.

71. Kokoska ER, West KW, Carney DE, et al. Risk factors for acute chest syndrome in children with sickle cell disease undergoing abdominal surgery. *J Pediatr Surg*. 2004;39(6):848–50.

72. Muncie HL Jr., Campbell J. Alpha and beta thalassemia. *Am Fam Physician*. 2009;80(4):339–44.

73. Rund D Rachmilewitz E. Beta-thalassemia. *N Engl J Med*. 2005;353(11):1135–46.

74. Old J, Olivieri N, Thein S. Diagnosis and management of thalassaemia. In Weatherall D, Clegg B, editors. *The Thalassaemia Syndromes*. Oxford: Blackwell Science; 2001; 630–85.

75. Modell B, Khan M, Darlison M. Survival in beta-thalassaemia major in the UK: data from the UK Thalassaemia Register. *Lancet*. 2000;355(9220):2051–2.

76. Sissons JG, Carmichael AJ. Clinical aspects and management of cytomegalovirus infection. *J Infect*. 2002. 44(2):78–83.

77. Zaia JA, Sissons JG, Riddell S, et al. Status of cytomegalovirus prevention and treatment in 2000. *Hematology Am Soc Hematol Educ Program*. 2000;2000:339–55.

78. Yeager AS, Grumet FC, Hafleigh EB, et al. Prevention of transfusion-acquired cytomegalovirus infections in newborn infants. *J Pediatr*. 1981;98(2):281–7.

79. Fergusson D, Hébert PC, Barrington KJ, Shapiro SH. Effectiveness of WBC reduction in neonates: what is the evidence of benefit? *Transfusion*. 2002;42(2):159–65.

80. Billingham RE. The biology of graft-versus-host reactions. *Harvey Lect*. 1966;62:21–78.

81. Schroeder ML. Transfusion-associated graft-versus-host disease. *Br J Haematol*. 2002;117(2):275–87.

82. McVay PA, Toy PT. Lack of increased bleeding after paracentesis and thoracentesis in patients with mild coagulation abnormalities. *Transfusion*. 1991;31(2):164–71.

83. Chan KH, Mann KS, Chan TK. The significance of thrombocytopenia in the development of postoperative intracranial hematoma. *J Neurosurg*. 1989;71(1):38–41.

84. Sacher RA, Luban NL, Strauss RG. Current practice and guidelines for the transfusion of cellular blood components in the newborn. *Transfus Med Rev*. 1989;3(1):39–54.

85. Andrew M Brooker L, *Hemorrhagic complications in the newborn*. In Petz L, et al., editors. *Clinical Practice of Transfusion Medicine*. New York: Churchill Livingstone; 1996; 647–84.

86. Fasano R Luban NL. Blood component therapy. *Pediatr Clin North Am*. 2008;55(2):421–45.

87. Heddle NM, Wu C, Vassallo R, et al. Adjudicating bleeding events in a platelet dose study: impact on outcome results and challenges. *Transfusion*. 2011;51(11):2304–10.

88. Estcourt LJ, Stanworth SJ, Murphy MF. Prophylactic platelet transfusions. *Curr Opin Hematol*. 2010;17(5):411–17.

89. Konig G, Yazer MH, Waters JH. Stored platelet functionality is not decreased after warming with a fluid warmer. *Anesth Analg*. 2013; 117(3):575–8.

90. Stanworth SJ, Brunskill SJ, Hyde CJ, Murphy MF, McClelland DB. Appraisal of the evidence for the clinical use of FFP and plasma fractions. *Best Pract Res Clin Haematol*. 2006;19(1):67–82.

91. Manco-Johnson MJ, Riske B, Kasper CK. Advances in care of children with hemophilia. *Semin Thromb Hemost*. 2003;29(6):585–94.

92. Federici AB. Management of von Willebrand disease with factor VIII/von Willebrand factor concentrates: results from current studies and surveys. *Blood Coagul Fibrinolysis*. 2005;16(Suppl. 1):S17–21.

93. Soucie JM, Evatt B, Jackson D. Occurrence of hemophilia in the United States: The Hemophilia Surveillance System Project Investigators. *Am J Hematol*. 1998;59(4):288–94.

94. Brown DL. Congenital bleeding disorders. *Curr Probl Pediatr Adolesc Health Care*. 2005;35(2):38–62.

95. Martlew VJ. Peri-operative management of patients with coagulation disorders. *Br J Anaesth*. 2000;85(3):446–55.

96. Sutor AH. Desmopressin (DDAVP) in bleeding disorders of childhood. *Semin Thromb Hemost.* 1998;24(6):555–66.

97. Richardson DW Robinson AG. Desmopressin. *Ann Intern Med.* 1985;103(2):228–39.

98. Centers for Disease Control and Prevention. Red blood cell transfusions contaminated with *Yersinia enterocolitica* – United States, 1991–1996, and initiation of a national study to detect bacteria-associated transfusion reactions. *MMWR Morb Mortal Wkly Rep.* 1997;46(24):553–5.

99. Goodnough LT, Brecher ME, Kanter MH, AuBuchon JP. Transfusion medicine. Second of two parts – blood conservation. *N Engl J Med.* 1999;340(7):525–33.

100. Goldman M Blajchman MA. Blood product-associated bacterial sepsis. *Transfus Med Rev.* 1991;5(1):73–83.

101. Bhananker SM, Ramamoorthy C, Geiduschek JM, et al. Anesthesia-related cardiac arrest in children: update from the Pediatric Perioperative Cardiac Arrest Registry. *Anesth Analg.* 2007;105(2):344–50.

102. The Pediatric Anesthesia Quality Improvement Initiative. Hyperkalemia Statement, 2011. Available at: http://wakeupsafe.org/Hyperkalemia_statement .pdf.

103. Bunker JP. Metabolic effects of blood transfusion. *Anesthesiology.* 1966;27(4):446–55.

104. Dzik WH Kirkley SA. Citrate toxicity during massive blood transfusion. *Transfus Med Rev.* 1988;2(2):76–94.

105. Davis PJ, Cook DR. Anesthetic problems in pediatric liver transplantation. *Transplant Proc.* 1989;21(3):3493–6.

106. Kleinman S, Caulfield T, Chan P, et al. Toward an understanding of transfusion-related acute lung injury: statement of a consensus panel. *Transfusion.* 2004;44(12):1774–89.

107. Mark JB. Central venous pressure monitoring: clinical insights beyond the numbers. *J Cardiothorac Vasc Anesth.* 1991;5(2):163–73.

108. Greenberg S, Murphy G, Vender J. *Standard monitoring techniques.* In Barash P, et al., editors. *Clinical Anesthesia.* Philadelphia, PA: Elsevier Saunders; 2009; 697–714.

109. Maecken T, Grau T. Ultrasound imaging in vascular access. *Crit Care Med.* 2007;35(5 Suppl):S178–85.

110. Westergaard B, Classen V, Walther-Larsen S. Peripherally inserted central catheters in infants and children: indications, techniques, complications and clinical recommendations. *Acta Anaesthesiol Scand.* 2013;57(3):278–87.

111. Lloyd TR, Donnerstein RL, Berg RA. Accuracy of central venous pressure measurement from the abdominal inferior vena cava. *Pediatrics.* 1992. 89(3):506–8.

112. Amar D, Melendez JA, Zhang H, et al. Correlation of peripheral venous pressure and central venous pressure in surgical patients. *J Cardiothorac Vasc Anesth.* 2001;15(1):40–3.

113. Amoozgar H, Ajami G, Borzuoee M, et al. Peripheral venous pressure as a predictor of central venous pressure in continuous monitoring in children. *Iran Red Crescent Med J.* 2011;13(5):342–5.

114. Anter AM, Bondok RS. Peripheral venous pressure is an alternative to central venous pressure in paediatric surgery patients. *Acta Anaesthesiol Scand.* 2004;48(9):1101–4.

115. Ng L, Khine H, Taragin BH, et al. Does bedside sonographic measurement of the inferior vena cava diameter correlate with central venous pressure in the assessment of intravascular volume in children? *Pediatr Emerg Care.* 2013;29(3):337–41.

116. Al-Khafaji A, Webb A. Fluid resuscitation. *BJA, Contin Educ Anaesth Crit Care Pain.* 2004;4:127–31.

117. Tibby SM, Hatherill M, Marsh MJ, et al. Clinical validation of cardiac output measurements using femoral artery thermodilution with direct Fick in ventilated children and infants. *Intensive Care Med.* 1997;23(9):987–91.

118. Schiffmann H, Erdlenbruch B, Singer D, et al. Assessment of cardiac output, intravascular volume status, and extravascular lung water by transpulmonary indicator dilution in critically ill neonates and infants. *J Cardiothorac Vasc Anesth.* 2002;16(5):592–7.

119. Introna RP, Martin DC, Pruett JK, Philpot TE, Johnston JF. Percutaneous pulmonary artery catheterization in pediatric cardiovascular anesthesia: insertion techniques and use. *Anesth Analg.* 1990;70(5):562–6.

120. Michard F. Changes in arterial pressure during mechanical ventilation. *Anesthesiology.* 2005;103(2):419–28.; quiz 449–5.

121. Durand P, Chevret L, Essouri S, Haas V, Devictor D. Respiratory variations in aortic blood flow predict fluid responsiveness in ventilated children. *Intensive Care Med.* 2008;34(5):888–94.

122. Rick JJ, Burke SS. Respirator paradox. *South Med J.* 1978;71(11):1376–8.

123. Arant BS, Jr. Postnatal development of renal function during the first year of life. *Pediatr Nephrol.* 1987;1(3):308–13.

124. Singh S, Kuschner WG, Lighthall G. Perioperative intravascular fluid assessment and monitoring: a

narrative review of established and emerging techniques. *Anesthesiol Res Pract*. 2011;2011:231493.

125. Benkhadra M, Collignon M, Fournel I, et al. Ultrasound guidance allows faster peripheral IV cannulation in children under 3 years of age with difficult venous access: a prospective randomized study. *Paediatr Anaesth*. 2012;22(5):449–54.

126. Bellotti GA, Bedford RF, Arnold WP. Fiberoptic transillumination for intravenous cannulation under general anesthesia. *Anesth Analg*. 1981;60(5):348–51.

127. Lenhardt R, Seybold T, Kimberger O, Stoiser B, Sessler DI. Local warming and insertion of peripheral venous cannulas: single blinded prospective randomised controlled trial and single blinded randomised crossover trial. *BMJ*. 2002;325(7361):409–10.

128. Teillol-Foo WL, Kassab JY. Topical glyceryl trinitrate and eutectic mixture of local anaesthetics in children: a randomised controlled trial on choice of site and ease of venous cannulation. *Anaesthesia*. 1991;46(10):881–4.

129. Chiao FB, Resta-Flarer F, Lesser J, et al. Vein visualization: patient characteristic factors and efficacy of a new infrared vein finder technology. *Br J Anaesth*. 2013;110(6):966–71.

130. Butler-O'Hara M, Buzzard CJ, Reubens L, et al. A randomized trial comparing long-term and short-term use of umbilical venous catheters in premature infants with birth weights of less than 1251 grams. *Pediatrics*. 2006;118(1):e25–35.

131. Nicolson SC, Sweeney MF, Moore RA, Jobes DR. Comparison of internal and external jugular cannulation of the central circulation in the pediatric patient. *Crit Care Med*. 1985;13(9):747–9.

132. Garcia-Teresa MA, Casado-Flores J, Delgado Domínguez MA, et al. Infectious complications of percutaneous central venous catheterization in pediatric patients: a Spanish multicenter study. *Intensive Care Med*. 2007;33(3):466–76.

133. Karapinar B, Cura A. Complications of central venous catheterization in critically ill children. *Pediatr Int*. 2007;49(5):593–9.

134. Casado-Flores J, Barja J, Martino R, Serrano A, Valdivielso A. Complications of central venous catheterization in critically ill children. *Pediatr Crit Care Med*. 2001;2(1):57–62.

135. de Jonge RC, Polderman KH, Gemke RJ. Central venous catheter use in the pediatric patient: mechanical and infectious complications. *Pediatr Crit Care Med*. 2005;6(3):329–39.

136. Ellemunter H, Simma B, Trawoger R, Maurer H. Intraosseous lines in preterm and full term neonates. *Arch Dis Child Fetal Neonatal Ed*. 1999;80(1):F74–5.

137. Jaimovich DG, Kecskes S. Intraosseous infusion: a re-discovered procedure as an alternative for pediatric vascular access. *Indian J Pediatr*. 1991;58(3):329–34.

138. Rajani AK, Chitkara R, Oehlert J, et al. Comparison of umbilical venous and intraosseous access during simulated neonatal resuscitation. *Pediatrics*. 2011;128(4):e954–8.

139. Stewart FC, Kain ZN. Intraosseous infusion: elective use in pediatric anesthesia. *Anesth Analg*. 1992. 75(4):626–9.

140. Galpin RD, Kronick JB, Willis RB, Frewen TC. Bilateral lower extremity compartment syndromes secondary to intraosseous fluid resuscitation. *J Pediatr Orthop*. 1991;11(6):773–6.

Chapter

# 16

# Neonatal Ventilation Strategies

Gerhard K. Wolf

## Introduction

Neonatal lung injury differs from acute lung injury (ALI) in older children and adults in a number of ways. Neonatal respiratory failure is the endpoint of several disease pathways. For instance, respiratory failure in the preterm infant is associated primarily with surfactant deficiency and is lacking the inflammatory and infectious properties of ALI in older patients. Persistent pulmonary hypertension (PPHN) of the newborn is caused by pulmonary artery hypertension, and in PPHN physiology, fetal circulation (systemic pulmonary artery pressures and a persistent ductus arteriosus with shunting) usually persists in the setting of acidosis, hypoxemia, infection, and thermal stress of the neonate. Meconium aspiration syndrome is associated with surfactant inactivation and lung inflammation.

In contrast to adult respiratory failure, nonconventional modes of ventilation such as high-frequency ventilation (HFV), the use of inhaled nitric oxide (iNO), and extracorporeal membrane oxygenation (ECMO) have a long tradition in neonatal ventilation, are used more liberally in neonates compared to the adult clinical arena, and are associated with improved outcomes in selected neonatal patient populations.

## Monitoring and Goals of Gas Exchange

Pulse oximetry is commonly used to monitor oxygenation in neonates. However, $SpO_2$ is an unreliable tool with regards to detecting hyperoxia. If $SpO_2$ is above 95–96 percent, the corresponding $PaO_2$ may be above 90–100 mmHg, raising concerns for increased oxygen toxicity in neonates. The ideal transcutaneous saturation in neonates during mechanical ventilation should probably be around 90–95 percent. In the SUPPORT trial, a transcutaneous saturation of 85–89 percent was associated with increased mortality compared to a saturation of 91–95 percent, with no difference in the rate of severe retinopathy [1]. In neonates

with pulmonary hypertension and large right-to-left shunts, such as patients with PPHN or congenital diaphragmatic hernia, a difference in pre- and postductal saturations is observed. The preductal saturation is usually measured with an arterial line or probe on the right arm. The postductal saturation is usually measured by a left-arm arterial line, a lower extremity arterial line, or an umbilical artery catheter, as the tip of the umbilical artery catheter is usually in the aorta, reflecting a postductal saturation. In cases with significant shunting, treatment is usually adapted to target a preductal saturation of 85–95 percent and a postductal saturation above 70 percent.

Ventilation is noninvasively monitored by end-tidal carbon dioxide or transcutaneous carbon dioxide sensors. The presence of end-tidal $CO_2$ is a function of pulmonary blood flow. Increased amounts of pulmonary dead space usually accounts for a large gap between arterial and end-tidal carbon dioxide measurements. If pulmonary dead space increases, the end-tidal $CO_2$ is considerably lower than the arterial $CO_2$. Low cardiac output, low pulmonary blood flow (such as in pulmonary hypertension), and airway obstruction can also lead to low or even absent end-tidal $CO_2$ levels, despite correct tracheal position of the endotracheal tube. Regarding goals for $CO_2$ levels, some degree of permissive hypercapnia is an accepted strategy, indicated by a pH above 7.25 and a $CO_2$ level less than 60 mmHg. Hyperventilation, on the other hand, may lead to an alkalosis, resulting in cerebral vasoconstriction, low cerebral blood flow, and the potential for intracerebral hemorrhage.

## Setting Up Ventilation Parameters for Neonates

### Conventional Ventilation

Limiting delivered tidal volumes and optimizing alveolar recruitment, thus minimizing atelectrauma

[2] and volutrauma [3], is one of the main strategies of lung protective ventilation in neonates with acute lung injury. Most centers attempt to limit peak inspiratory pressures to 25 cmH$_2$O, and start with a peak inspiratory pressure of 15–20 cmH$_2$O and a PEEP level of 3–5 cmH$_2$O. Respiratory rate is usually adjusted to achieve PaCO$_2$ levels of 45–60 mmHg. During conventional ventilation, tidal volumes are usually targeted to be 6 ml kg$^{-1}$ body weight, with a level of positive end-expiratory pressure that allows the FiO$_2$ to be weaned under 0.6 [3]. Lower tidal volumes have shown to be lung protective compared to larger tidal volumes in neonatal and adult patients. The inspiratory time is usually set at 0.3–0.4 seconds. During pressure-controlled ventilation with a decelerating inspiratory flow, the decelerating flow at the end of inspiration can be used to determine the ideal inspiratory time: the flow at the end of inspiration should reach the baseline. A noncompliant lung usually requires a shorter inspiratory time (0.2–0.3 seconds), a compliant lung a longer inspiratory time (0.4 seconds). In premature neonates, this effect can be observed before and after application of exogenous surfactant: prior to surfactant, the lung has a lower compliance, requiring a shorter inspiratory time; after surfactant, lung compliance increases, resulting in a longer inspiratory time during pressure-controlled ventilation with decelerating inspiratory flow.

Persistent hypercapnia and respiratory acidosis in neonates in the absence of obstructive physiology is often associated with obstructed endotracheal tubes. The inner diameter of neonatal endotracheal tubes may be as small as 2.0–2.5 mm. Often, suctioning the endotracheal tube does not improve the hypercapnia and the suction catheter may pass easily through the endotracheal tube. However, in this circumstance, changing out the endotracheal tube may be warranted. Figure 16.1 shows a 2.5 mm endotracheal tube after removal with large amounts of mucous narrowing the internal orifice. This infant had suffered from persistent respiratory acidosis, and was weaned to extubation shortly after endotracheal tube change.

## High-Frequency Ventilation

High-frequency ventilation allows sustained recruitment of atelectatic lung units while delivering small tidal volumes. High-frequency ventilation can be delivered through slightly different options. High-frequency oscillatory ventilation (HFOV),

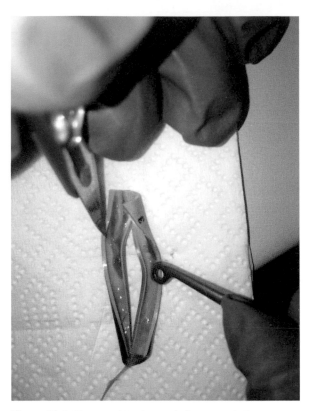

**Figure 16.1** Obstructed ETT (2.5 mm) after removal. This premature baby had persistent respiratory acidosis and hypercapnia. Expiratory flow curves and end-tidal CO$_2$ tracing showed no characteristic signs of obstruction. Suctioning of the endotracheal tube was possible without problems. Regardless, the ETT showed severe obstruction by mucous and debris. The infant was extubated within 24 h after changing the ETT. Photograph by Gerhard Wolf.

high-frequency jet ventilation, and high-frequency flow interruption all have in common that small (1–3 ml kg$^{-1}$) tidal volumes approximating the anatomical dead space are delivered at rates exceeding the normal respiratory rate (3–20 Hz, 180–1200 breaths per minute). Data from a neonatal trial indicated a small benefit of HFOV in terms of pulmonary outcome for very low birth weight infants. Although no improvement in mortality or ventilator-free days during HFOV has been shown, there is a large body of evidence that HFOV is a safe strategy of ventilation allowing rapid and effective recruitment of lung volume [4].

## Mechanisms of Gas Exchange During HFOV

While HFOV is frequently used in the neonatal intensive care unit, it appears physiologically

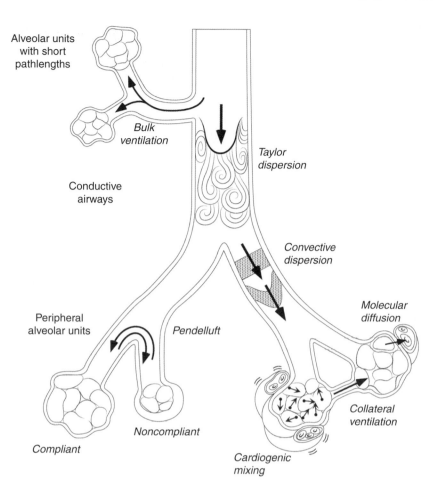

**Figure 16.2** Mechanisms of gas exchange during high-frequency ventilation. Source: [6].

Alveolar units with short pathlengths

Bulk ventilation

Taylor dispersion

Conductive airways

Convective dispersion

Peripheral alveolar units

Pendelluft

Molecular diffusion

Collateral ventilation

Compliant

Noncompliant

Cardiogenic mixing

counterintuitive that this modality of ventilation produces both adequate oxygenation and removal of $CO_2$. The physiology of HFV is sometimes explained with the spontaneous respiratory physiology of panting dogs, who are capable of respiratory rates of 5–6 Hz (240–300 breaths per minute) while they are panting. Adequate gas exchange in dogs is maintained despite small tidal volumes during rapid breathing [5]. However, this model of comparison is lacking the important fact that during spontaneous respiration, a negative inspiratory pressure is generated, whereas during HFV, positive pressure is applied. In reality, during HFOV, gas exchange is achieved by a number of different mechanisms, which all interact with each other in the neonatal lung. The various modes of gas exchange are different in the larger airways, the proximal alveoli, and on the alveolar level (Figure 16.2).

In the proximal lung units with short path lengths, direct ventilation of alveoli by bulk flow is predominant. Even small tidal volumes reach the most

proximal alveolar units directly, resulting in direct ventilation of this fraction of lung units. This mode of gas exchange closely resembles conventional ventilation, and, to use the earlier example, is probably the predominant mode of ventilation in panting dogs.

In large airways such as the trachea and the left and right main stem bronchus, Taylor-type dispersion and convective dispersion occur. Taylor, in 1953, described the dispersion of particles in the presence of laminar flow [7]. When the velocity of gas flow increases, the initial planar surface of a gas column transforms into a parabolic surface, allowing a greater amount of longitudinal mixing and dispersion. The center of the parabolic gas column is believed to travel faster than the outer areas, allowing further diffusion and mixing downstream. Turbulence occurring when this gas column reaches a bifurcation partly replaces laminar mixing, resulting in dispersion of gas molecules, further contributing to gas exchange. Convective dispersion occurs when a uniform column of air is transformed into a parabolic shape. Air molecules undergo mixing as molecules in the center of the gas column move to the tip of the parabolic shape and the molecules near the wall stay behind.

In the peripheral airways and the alveoli, Pendelluft, molecular diffusion, and cardiogenic mixing play the main role. Pendelluft (from German: pendel = pendulum and luft = air) means that gas moves between compliant and noncompliant lung units, resulting in regional mixing. Pendelluft is believed to occur during both inspiration and expiration. At end-expiration, air moves from the compliant to the noncompliant lung unit, as the compliant unit has a higher time constant and is still emptying when the noncompliant area is already empty. At end inspiration, air moves from the noncompliant area, which secondary to a lower time constant is filled earlier, to the compliant area, which is still filling [8]. Passive diffusion of gas molecules through the alveolo-capillary membrane (molecular diffusion) and cardiac-induced pressure changes in the vascular bed (cardiogenic mixing) both add to gas mixing on the alveolar level. Both mechanisms of gas exchange occur during any form of ventilation and are not unique to HFOV [4].

## Setting Up and Maintaining HFOV in Neonates

### Indication and General Considerations

High-frequency ventilation is considered in the setting of failing conventional ventilation in patients with acute lung injury. In addition, HFV is considered when potentially lung-injurious ventilator settings are applied. This is usually indicated by arterial hypoxemia despite peak inspiratory pressures of >25 cmH$_2$O or oxygenation indices (FiO$_2$ × mean airway pressure × 100/ PaO$_2$) of >13 on two or more arterial blood gas analyses within a six-hour time period. Unlike older children or adults, neonates can breathe spontaneously during HFV, as the bias flow of the system is sufficiently high to support spontaneous ventilation in neonatal, but not pediatric or adult patients.

### Considerations for Exclusion

Diseases with increased airway resistance, as seen in bronchiolitis and reactive airway disease, are generally associated with decreased ventilation, hypercarbia, and air trapping. The application of an aggressive recruitment strategy may increase the incidence of air trapping, hypercarbia, and the risk of extrapulmonary leak such as pneumothorax, pneumomediastinum, and air dissection into the abdomen. Hypotension is a relative contraindication, and neonates with hypotension should be adequately volume-resuscitated and stabilized on vasopressors before the initiation of HFOV, as the transition to higher mean airway pressures may compromise right arterial preload [4].

### Initial Settings

To improve alveolar recruitment upon the transition to HFOV, the initial mean airway pressure on HFOV is usually set 5 cmH$_2$O higher than the last mean airway pressure during conventional ventilation. Lung hyperinflation should be avoided by cautious increase of mean airway pressure. The mean airway pressure is increased by increments of 1 cmH$_2$O until arterial oxygenation improves. A chest radiograph is taken after transitioning to HFOV to confirm adequate lung expansion. Hyperinflation is manifested by lung expansion of more than nine ribs and flattened diaphragms. The FiO$_2$ is usually set at 0.6–1.0 upon the transition to HFOV, and gradually weaned over time.

## Management of Gas Exchange During HFV

### Alveolar Recruitment, Oxygenation, and Ventilation

Optimal lung volume during HFOV is achieved during the lowest mean airway pressure that produces oxygenating efficiency, maintains lung volume, and avoids overdistention [9]. Alveolar recruitment is usually associated with improving gas exchange as mean airway pressure is increased [10,11], whereas subsequent overdistention may be signified by again decreasing oxygenation as the mean airway pressure is further increased. Alveolar ventilation is a function of the rate of oscillations and the squared tidal volume ($V_{CO_2} = f \times Vt^2$) [12,13]. Tidal volume contributes more to CO$_2$ elimination than frequency, as tidal volume is squared in the formula. Increasing the amplitude leads to increasing tidal volumes and improves CO$_2$ elimination. Conversely, decreasing the amplitude decreases CO$_2$ elimination by directly decreasing delivered tidal volume. Decreasing the rate during HFV makes the oscillations more effective and tidal volumes may increase; that is why decreasing the rate increases $CO_2$ elimination during HFV. This is in sharp contrast to the physiology during conventional ventilation, where decreasing the rate decreases minute ventilation and therefore decreases $CO_2$ elimination.

# Extracorporeal Membrane Oxygenation

Extracorporeal membrane oxygenation provides mechanical support for neonates in cardiac or respiratory failure not responding to conventional therapy.

It has been offered to more than 26,000 neonates worldwide to date. The use of ECMO for neonatal respiratory failure has been declining since the early 1990s, associated with the development of advanced ventilator management, including iNO, surfactant, lung protective conventional ventilation, and HFV. The classic ECMO indications in the 1990s, such as meconium aspiration syndrome and PPHN, are now usually successfully managed without ECMO. The use of cardiac ECMO has increased.

The indications for neonatal ECMO are reversible respiratory failure, vasopressor-resistant shock physiology, low cardiac output syndrome not responding to conventional therapy, and air leak not manageable with optimized ventilator support and chest drainage. In neonates with congenital heart defects or congenital diaphragmatic hernia, ECMO is often provided as a bridge until definite treatment has been provided and the physiology of the neonate has been stabilized. Veno-venous ECMO is usually provided for respiratory failure, whereas veno-arterial ECMO is provided for combined respiratory and circulatory failure. Of note, total anomalous venous pulmonary venous (TAPVR) return should be excluded prior to ECMO. First, TAPVR often mimics respiratory failure with hypoxia and bilateral opacities on chest X-ray, but treatment is obviously cardiac surgery rather than respiratory support alone. Second, once on veno-arterial ECMO, the pulmonary veins have minimal flow into the left atrium and establishing the diagnosis of TAPVR by ECHO may be impossible.

Access is usually gained through the right carotid artery and the right internal jugular vein for veno-atrial ECMO, or via a double lumen venous cannula in the right internal jugular vein for veno-venous ECMO. In cardiac ECMO, access is usually gained via sternotomy. Arterial perfusion to the brain as well as venous drainage are impaired by the ECMO cannulas. Arterial perfusion is maintained in neonates via collateral circulation through the circle of Willis. The carotid artery is often ligated after separation from ECMO, although reconstruction of the carotid artery can be successfully performed. During ECMO, ventilator settings are usually weaned to minimal settings to allow the lung to rest and recover. However, during veno-venous ECMO, oxygenation via the circuit alone may be insufficient, and ventilator settings need to be increased as the neonate's own lungs may need to contribute to gas exchange [14].

# References

1. SUPPORT Study Group of the Eunice Kennedy Shriver NICHD, et al. Target ranges of oxygen saturation in extremely preterm infants. *N Engl J Med.* 2010;362(21):1959–69.

2. Chu EK, Whitehead T, Slutsky AS. Effects of cyclic opening and closing at low- and high-volume ventilation on bronchoalveolar lavage cytokines. *Crit Care Med.* 2004;32(1):168–74.

3. Hernandez LA, Peevy KJ, Moise AA, Parker JC. Chest wall restriction limits high airway pressure-induced lung injury in young rabbits. *J Appl Physiol.* 1989;66(5):2364–8.

4. Wolf GK, Arnold JH. High-frequency oscillation in paediatric respiratory failure. *Pediatr Child Health.* 2007;17(3):77–81.

5. Meyer M, Hahn G, Buess C, Mesch U, Piiper J. Pulmonary gas exchange in panting dogs. *J Appl Physiol.* 1989;66(3):1258–63.

6. Courtney SE, Durand DJ, Asselin JM, et al. High-frequency oscillatory ventilation versus conventional mechanical ventilation for very-low-birth-weight infants. *N Engl J Med.* 2002;347(9):643–52.

7. Taylor GI. The dispersion of soluble matter in solvent flowing slowly through a tube. *Proc R Soc London.* 1953;223:446–68.

8. Chang HK. Mechanisms of gas transport during ventilation by high-frequency oscillation. *J Appl Physiol.* 1984;56(3):553–63.

9. Brazelton TB, 3rd, Watson KF, Murphy M, et al. Identification of optimal lung volume during high-frequency oscillatory ventilation using respiratory inductive plethysmography. *Crit Care Med.* 2001;29(12):2349–59.

10. Maggiore SM, Jonson B, Richard JC, et al. Alveolar derecruitment at decremental positive end-expiratory pressure levels in acute lung injury: comparison with the lower inflection point, oxygenation, and compliance. *Am J Respir Crit Care Med.* 2001, 164(5):795–801.

11. Ranieri VM, Eissa NT, Corbeil C, et al. Effects of positive end-expiratory pressure on alveolar recruitment and gas exchange in patients with the adult respiratory distress syndrome. *Am Rev Respir Dis.* 1991;144(3 Pt 1):544–51.

12. Kamitsuka MD, Boynton BR, Villanueva D, Vreeland PN, Frantz ID 3rd. Frequency, tidal volume, and mean airway pressure combinations that provide adequate gas exchange and low alveolar pressure during high frequency oscillatory ventilation in rabbits. *Pediatr Res.* 1990;27(1):64–9.

13. Boynton BR, Hammond MD, Fredberg JJ, et al. Gas exchange in healthy rabbits during high-frequency oscillatory ventilation. *J Appl Physiol.* 1989;66(3):1343–51.

14. Wolf GK, Arnold JH. Extracorporeal membrane oxygenation. In: Cloherty JP, Stark AR, editors. *Manual of Neonatal Care*, 6th edn. Philadelphi, PA: Wolters Kluwer; 2007; 346–52.

Chapter

**17**

# Anesthetic-Induced Neurotoxicity

Dusica Bajic and Sulpicio G. Soriano

## Historical Background on Anesthetic Management of Infants

The perioperative anesthetic management of infants has greatly evolved over the past 25 years. Prior to the mid-1980s, it was assumed that infants did not perceive pain due to the relative immaturity of the developing central nervous system. Furthermore, use of volatile anesthetics was limited because of their cardiac depressant effects and the inability to precisely monitor the hemodynamic and respiratory parameters in very young infants. Thus, neonatal surgery was managed with a minimal "anesthetic" approach: nitrous oxide and muscle relaxant (Liverpool Technique). However, it was demonstrated that in premature and full-term newborns, neuroanatomic nociceptive pathways were present from the periphery to the cortex. Studies indicated that even preterm babies mount a substantial stress response to surgery under anesthesia with nitrous oxide and muscle relaxant, and that prevention of this response by fentanyl or inhalational agents suggested an improved postoperative outcome [1–4]. Furthermore, it was also demonstrated that increased neonatal metabolic (epinephrine and norepinephrine) and hormonal (insulin and glucagon) responses to cardiac surgery in neonates were extreme and associated with a high mortality rate [5]. We now know that as early as 24 weeks' gestation, painful stimuli are associated with physiologic, hormonal, and metabolic markers of the stress response [6]. Our better understanding of the neurobiology of pain pathways development coupled with the evidence that pain in infants during surgery is associated with increased stress responses and increased mortality led to a significant change in perioperative anesthetic management of the youngest surgical patients. It involved not only administration of volatile anesthetics, but analgesics as well, with a goal to prevent pain sensation as well as the stress responses to surgery. Several studies

demonstrated that painful stimulation in unanesthetized newborns, especially in preterm infants, leads to long-term effects. These long-term effects of early painful stimulation may involve permanent changes in pain processing and impaired brain development [7–9], including altered pain sensitivity and maladaptive behavior later in life [10,11]. Today, providing anesthesia and preventing pain and stress responses in the youngest of patients is considered a standard of anesthesia practice. Withholding anesthetics during painful procedures in infants is considered unethical.

## What is Known About Anesthetic Effects on the Developing Brain?

Nationwide inpatient data in the United States indicate that 1.5 million infants, defined as those under 12 months of age, undergo surgery every year. Since millions of children and infants undergo anesthesia and/or sedation for surgery and painful procedures [12], significant concerns have been raised regarding the potential neurotoxic effects of sedative, analgesic, and anesthetic agents on the developing brain [13–16]. Specifically, these concerns are based on recent research findings in the field of neurobiology of anesthetic and sedative drug effects on the developing brain using different animal models. Hence as the preeminent controversy in pediatric anesthesiology: Developmental neurotoxicity after anesthetic exposure in the immature/developing brain [17].

During normal brain development, neurons are produced in excess; the elimination of as much as 50–70 percent of neurons and progenitor cells is critical for achieving normal brain morphology, brain size, and viability of the organism [18]. It is well known that neurons undergo programmed cell death (apoptosis) during the brain maturation period, which can be triggered by both physiological and pathological stimuli [19–24]. Disruption of physiological apoptotic cell death during development leads to brain malformations and premature death in rodent models [25]. Another essential process in the developing central nervous system is the formation of synaptic connections between neurons. Therefore, the critical period of neurodevelopment is also marked by a period of synaptogenesis. The pruning of neurons and synapses is activity-dependent. Gaba-aminobutyric acid (GABA), N-methyl-d-asparate (NMDA), and opioid receptors all have a direct role in neuronal migration, differentiation, and central nervous system maturation. Although the exact mechanism of general anesthesia is not entirely understood, alterations of synaptic transmission involving GABA type A receptors and/or NMDA receptors seem to play an important role.

It is plausible that drugs that either alter neuronal activity or affect the neuronal number will have some impact on final brain morphology and function. In many animal studies, apoptosis was used as a surrogate marker implicating neurotoxicity of anesthetics and sedating agents.

The landmark research report revealed potential neurotoxic effects of anesthetics on the developing rat brain [26]. Blockade of NMDA receptors with the antagonist MK801 (an agent similar to ketamine) resulted in widespread neuronal apoptosis in the brains of week-old rats (corresponding to the peak synaptogenesis period and the most vulnerable period in this species). Subsequently, a combination of midazolam, nitrous oxide, and isoflurane for six hours in the same animal model of seven-day-old rat pups caused widespread apoptosis, changes in hippocampal synaptic function, and was associated with long-term persistent memory and learning impairments [27]. These reports fueled laboratory investigations of other anesthetic and sedative drugs used in clinical practice. In fact, all commonly used anesthetics, such as benzodiazepines, ketamine, propofol, nitrous oxide, and isoflurane, have all been shown to exacerbate neuronal cell death. For a list of studies, please refer to Loepke and Soriano's recent review report [28]. Of those, a number of recent studies were conducted in nonhuman primates. These reports demonstrated enhanced apoptosis by isoflurane [29], but also confirmed differences in effects depending on the age of exposure [30] and duration of exposure to injectable anesthetic/analgesic (e.g., ketamine) [31].

Common themes are: (1) prolonged and repeated exposure to anesthetics/sedating agents, and (2) the use of combinations of different types of anesthetics (drugs with different mechanism of action), may contribute to an increased apoptotic effect in different animal models. Despite the abundance of valid research reports, the pattern of detrimental neurobehavioral effects is inconsistent and has not been shown in all experiments. This variability of the long-term effects was attributed to sensitivity of different brain regions to different anesthetic/sedating agents [27,32–34].

## Difficulties in Extrapolating Data from Animal Models to Human

The empirical evidence supporting the neurotoxicity of anesthetic and sedative drugs in experimental animal models serves as the basis for our concern with potential harm imposed by anesthetic and sedative drugs on humans. Based on shared neurobiology, potential developmental neurotoxicity of anesthetics and analgesics depend on several factors: (1) dose of the drug; (2) developmental age of the patient; (3) duration of exposure; and (4) presence or absence of pain [17]. However, there are several factors to be taken into account that limit simple translation of data obtained in animal models to neurobiology of human development and to current clinical practice.

### Drug Dose

Species differences are well documented with respect to appropriate dose of certain drugs. Specifically, anesthetic requirement for injectable anesthetics are much higher in rodents than in humans, by a factor of 10 for ketamine and a factor of 100 for both propofol and morphine. The dose of inhalational agents, such as isoflurane, is about 2–3 times higher in rats than humans. Furthermore, even with respect to the animal studies, results are conflicting depending on the dose of drug administered (e.g., ketamine). Neurocognitive dysfunctions were reported after injections of high or repeated doses [26,35–38], but not in those cases with a smaller dose resulting in lower plasma concentrations [30,35,36].

### Critical Period and Duration of Drug Exposure

The window of vulnerability to drugs coincides with the developmental period of synaptogenesis, also known as the brain growth spurt period. The association of rat and human developmental stages depends upon several endpoints such as the number of brain cells, degree of myelination, brain growth rate, synaptogenesis, as well as measures related to more contemporary neuroinformatics [39–41]. In rodents, this critical period of neuronal differentiation and synaptic development is limited to a time window up to the fourth postnatal week [42–44]. The most vulnerable period for anesthesia-induced neurodegeneration appears to be very brief in animals, occurring during the first postnatal week in small rodents. In humans, the brain growth spurt, characterized by synaptogenesis and accompanied by dendritic and axonal growth, as well as myelination of the subcortical white matter, extends from the last trimester of pregnancy up to the first few years of postnatal life [45]. In fact, the newborn rat model at one week of life has been extensively used in relation to early (premature, neonatal, and infant) development in humans [46–48]. Thus, it is difficult to simply extrapolate comparative developmental trajectory of rats (days to weeks) to humans (years) [49,50]. A five-hour anesthesia exposure in a rat covers a significant proportion of the animal's period of development and may not have the same effect as five-hour exposure in a human. As of now, the critical period of human brain development is still undetermined, although some experts argue it lasts until 2–5 years of life.

## Translating the Neurobehavioral Effects

Neurobehavioral tests in rodents and even in monkeys tend to be very crude (e.g., fear conditioning, spatial reference memory, water/maze-based memory consolidation tests, short-term memory, early long-term memory, etc.). It is possible that anesthesia exposure may have subtle effects in humans that cannot be detected in animal models.

## Presence or Absence of Pain

As described earlier, untreated pain and stress can have detrimental effects on the developing brain. Untreated pain in animal models was also shown to be associated with enhanced apoptosis [51]. Unfortunately, the majority of animal studies were conducted without surgery or painful stimulation. Only one limited study reported no effects of painful stimulus (e.g., tail clamping) on degree of apoptosis [52]. In contrast, other studies found a decrease in apoptosis after ketamine administration in a rodent model of chronic inflammatory pain [51,53]. In animal models,

nociceptive stimulation causes less apoptosis than general anesthesia.

In summary, translation of data from animal studies to the neurotoxic effects of anesthetics used in pediatric practice has yet to be established and can only be made if the mechanisms of both anesthesia and neurotoxicity are the same (for a review, see [54]).

## Clinical Studies

As described in recent review articles addressing the topic of anesthesia and neurotoxicity of the developing brain [28,55], no studies report structural brain abnormalities in children after anesthesia. It is impossible to histologically examine the brains of infants who were exposed to anesthetic drugs (the way animal brains were analyzed). Furthermore, there are no imaging techniques that are sensitive enough to detect neuroapoptosis. Certainly, even if the imaging technology were available, data interpretation would be complicated by the fact that the infants would have to undergo sedation/anesthesia to obtain the images [55]. Neurodevelopmental outcome studies are possible in children, but must be carefully designed to minimize bias and confounding factors. Specifically, neurodevelopmental outcome could be defined as the presence of neurodevelopmental disorders, such as autism, mental retardation, language delay, learning disability, or attention deficit hyperactivity disorder [56–58]. Several studies report association between surgery and an increased risk of poor neurobehavioral outcome [59–61]. According to one recent report, even infants with a relatively minor procedure, such as pyloric stenosis repair, have an increased risk of poor developmental outcome [62]. However, due to many confounding factors (e.g., age, severity of disease, surgery), the precise role of anesthesia, analgesia, and/or sedation is very difficult to determine [55]. There is only a paucity of studies that evaluated the neurocognitive outcomes of infants who have received prolonged or repetitive exposure to general anesthesia or sedation. In the NOPAIN trial, Anand et al. [63] noted that there was a poorer neurologic outcome as well as increased mortality in premature infants sedated for prolonged periods of time with midazolam compared to placebo or morphine.

Since 2007, several studies have attempted to examine the association between surgery and anesthesia in the clinical setting. Each of these studies relies on retrospective examinations of existing databases. The first of these studies published by Wilder and colleagues from the Mayo Clinic examined an existing cohort of children born between 1976 and 1982 whose complete medical and school records were retrospectively reviewed for evidence of any type of learning disability [64]. These studies were conducted to determine whether those who were exposed to anesthesia before four years of age were more likely to have any type of learning disability than those not exposed. The authors found that those with a single exposure were not at increased risk, although those with two or more exposures were at significantly increased risk, and that risk increased with duration of exposure. Subsequently, the same group re-examined the cohort with a goal to reduce the potential for confounding factors (comorbid conditions), providing reassurance that the findings were not related to an excess of disease in the exposed group [65]. The findings of this study were very similar to those of the previous study; the children exposed two or more times before their third birthday were at nearly twice the risk for a learning disability as those not exposed. A third study using this same cohort examined the risk of attention deficit hyperactivity disorder, and found similar results while controlling for comorbidity [66]. Another study in older children also showed long-term differences in language and cognitive function after exposure to anesthesia [67]. Another group by Di Maggio et al. examined a birth cohort from 1999 through 2002 enrolled in the New York Medicaid Program [68,69]. After correcting for age, sex, and complicating birth-related conditions, children who had hernia repair were more than twice as likely to be diagnosed with developmental or behavioral disorder. A study from Denmark examined the risk of poor neurodevelopmental outcome and hernia repair [70]. After correcting for sex, birth weight, parental and maternal age, and education, no difference was reported in academic performance between those who underwent a hernia repair and those who did not. Another study by Iowa researchers reported that the duration of anesthesia and surgery correlated negatively with school performance scores between children undergoing surgery in infancy [71]. The impact of anesthesia and surgery on educational assessments have been examined in large databases from national registries in Canada and Sweden. In contrast to the previous reports on smaller populations, these "large data" assessments reveal that children less than three years old were equivalent to the non-exposed cohort, while older children had statistically significant decrements in their educational assessments [72,73].

Interpretation of these cohort studies has several limitations [55]. Although retrospective chart reviews may give some information about gross neurological and learning deficits, in most cases the information is incomplete and, thus, it is difficult to draw accurate conclusions. The biggest concern is the presence of confounding factors. Adjustment for these factors can only partly remove this effect. This is because adjustment for the many, likely unknown, confounding factors is impossible. An important next step is to conduct well-designed prospective clinical studies. Prospective measurement of outcome following a research protocol ensures that data collection will be consistent for all children.

Two high-profile multicenter clinical trials, the GAS (General Anesthesia compared to Spinal anesthesia) and PANDA (Pediatric Anesthesia and NeuroDevelopment Assessment) trials have recently published their findings. The GAS trial is a randomized controlled trial that provided strong evidence that an hour of exposure in infancy does not result in neurologic deficit as measurable at two years of age [74]. However, an assessment at two years of age does not rule out an effect on higher executive function, cognition, and memory. The five-year follow-up evaluation is underway and will provide more data on cognitive outcomes. The PANDA study prospectively examined the impact of inguinal hernia surgery in infants under 36 months of age on an extensive battery of neurocognitive tests [75]. When compared to a sibling cohort naïve to surgery and general anesthesia, no significant differences in these neurocognitive domains were detected. Both of these negative studies only examined the impact of short exposures to general anesthesia and surgery. This does not rule out an effect with longer exposures. These findings are consistent with the lack of toxicity and neurobehavioral deficits after short exposures to anesthetics in laboratory animals.

## Clinical Practice in the Light of Basic Science and Epidemiological Studies

Caution should be applied in simply translating and extrapolating available preclinical data to current anesthesia perioperative management. Despite the evidence for widespread neuronal cell death in newborn animals, a clinical marker of anesthesia-induced neurotoxicity has yet to be identified in children. Being that we still lack the overt clinical evidence for impairment in neurodevelopment of children following anesthetic and sedating drug administration, there is no reason to easily dismiss the animal data and reports from limited clinical studies. On the other side, pediatric anesthesiologists do not have any alternative to current anesthesia practice for care of premature and term neonates and infants.

This brings us to a difficult question: Should we change our clinical practice [76]?

These concerns were addressed at the March 29, 2007 public hearing of the Anesthesia and Life Support Drugs Advisory Committee of the US Food and Drug Administration (transcript is available at [77]). After reviewing the preclinical data on anesthetic-induced neurotoxicity, the US Food and Drug Administration Advisory Committee issued the following statement: "[although] there are no adequate data to extrapolate the animal finding to humans" the well-understood risks of anesthesia (respiratory and hemodynamic morbidity) continue to be the overwhelming consideration in designing an anesthetic, and the understood risks of delaying surgery are the primary reasons to determine the timing. Despite these parallel risks associated with general anesthesia, the FDA published a cautionary communication on the use of anesthetic and sedative drugs in patients aged three years and under [78]. Certainly, young children usually do not undergo surgery unless the procedure is vital to their health. In some instances, however, postponing a necessary procedure may itself lead to significant health problems and may not be an option for the majority of children [79,80]. Therefore, pediatric anesthesiologists should use the currently available knowledge to guide their practice.

## How to Address Concerned Family Members

All families vary in regard to what information is desired when it comes to anesthetic care of their children. Parental desire for anesthetic information has been studied and virtually all studies report that the vast majority of parents want to know about the risks of anesthesia, including severe and rare risks such as death [81]. Furthermore, it was reported that both parents [82] and children [83] most often want

detailed information on well-defined, readily apparent, and largely short-term concerns such as: pain, nausea, anesthetic induction, and emergence. Since these studies addressed risks that are accepted and short-term, rather than those that are hypothetical and long-term, it is difficult to extend these data to the issue of anesthetic neurotoxicity.

It should be clinicians' practice to take an individualized approach by discussing anesthetic risks in general terms and inviting parents and older children to ask for additional, more specific information. No mention of anesthetic-related neurologic injury is typically made unless parents or children specifically ask [84]. When asked, emphasis should be placed on the following: (1) unknown risk of neurologic injury in the context of all risk associated with anesthesia and surgery; (2) the low rate of harm associated with anesthesia; and (3) the lack of compelling data clearly implicating anesthetic drugs in subsequent cognitive deficits of children.

## Summary and Conclusions

It is important to understand that physiologic pruning of redundant neurons is an integral part of normal brain development. A plethora of research reports published over the last two decades demonstrating enhanced apoptotic cell death and long-term developmental dysfunctions in animal models implicate potential detrimental effect of anesthetics on brain development. However, the clinical phenotype of anesthesia-induced neurocognitive impairment still remains elusive. Considering that infants and children mostly undergo life-saving procedures, postponing the surgery is not usually a reasonable option. Certainly, in all such instances, providing anesthesia and preventing pain and stress responses in the youngest of patients is considered a standard of anesthesia practice.

## References

1. Anand KJ, Sippell WG, Aynsley-Green A. Pain, anaesthesia, and babies. *Lancet*. 1987;2(8569):1210.

2. Anand KJ, Sippell WG, Aynsley-Green A. Randomised trial of fentanyl anaesthesia in preterm babies undergoing surgery: effects on the stress response. *Lancet*. 1987;1(8524):62–6.

3. Anand KJ, Sippell WG, Schofield NM, Aynsley-Green A. Does halothane anaesthesia decrease the

metabolic and endocrine stress responses of newborn infants undergoing operation? *Br Med J (Clin Res Ed)*. 1988;296(6623):668–72.

4. Hickey PR, Hansen DD. High-dose fentanyl reduces intraoperative ventricular fibrillation in neonates with hypoplastic left heart syndrome. *J Clin Anesth*. 1991;3(4):295–300.

5. Anand KJ, Hansen DD, Hickey PR. Hormonal-metabolic stress responses in neonates undergoing cardiac surgery. *Anesthesiology*. 1990;73(4):661–70.

6. Lee SJ, Ralston HJ, Drey EA, Partridge JC, Rosen MA. Fetal pain: a systematic multidisciplinary review of the evidence. *JAMA*. 2005;294(8):947–54.

7. Vinall J, Miller SP, Chau V, et al. Neonatal pain in relation to postnatal growth in infants born very preterm. *Pain*. 2012;153(7):1374–81.

8. Brummelte S, Grunau RE, Chau V, et al. Procedural pain and brain development in premature newborns. *Ann Neurol*. 2012;71(3):385–96.

9. Johnston CC, Stevens BJ. Experience in a neonatal intensive care unit affects pain response. *Pediatrics*. 1996;98(5):925–30.

10. Anand KJ, Scalzo FM. Can adverse neonatal experiences alter brain development and subsequent behavior? *Biol Neonate*. 2000;77(2):69–82.

11. Taddio A, Katz J. The effects of early pain experience in neonates on pain responses in infancy and childhood. *Paediatr Drugs*. 2005;7(4):245–57.

12. DeFrances CJ, Cullen KA, Kozak LJ. National Hospital Discharge Survey: 2005 annual summary with detailed diagnosis and procedure data. *Vital Health Stat*. 13. 2007(165):1–209.

13. Olney JW, Young C, Wozniak DF, Jevtovic-Todorovic V, Ikonomidou C. Do pediatric drugs cause developing neurons to commit suicide? *Trends Pharmacol Sci*. 2004;25(3):135–9.

14. Soriano SG, Anand KJ, Rovnaghi CR, Hickey PR. Of mice and men: should we extrapolate rodent experimental data to the care of human neonates? *Anesthesiology*. 2005;102(4):866–8; author reply 8–9.

15. Todd MM. Anesthetic neurotoxicity: the collision between laboratory neuroscience and clinical medicine. *Anesthesiology*. 2004;101(2):272–3.

16. Olney JW, Young C, Wozniak DF, Ikonomidou C, Jevtovic-Todorovic V. Anesthesia-induced developmental neuroapoptosis: does it happen in humans? *Anesthesiology*. 2004;101(2):273–5.

17. Soriano SG. Thinking about the neurotoxic effects of sedatives on the developing brain. *Pediatr Crit Care Med*. 2010;11(2):306–7.

18. Buss RR, Oppenheim RW. Role of programmed cell death in normal neuronal development and function. *Anat Sci Int*. 2004;79(4):191–7.

19. Blaschke AJ, Staley K, Chun J. Widespread programmed cell death in proliferative and postmitotic regions of the fetal cerebral cortex. *Development*. 1996;122(4):1165–74.

20. Oppenheim RW. Cell death during development of the nervous system. *Annu Rev Neurosci*. 1991;14:453–501.

21. Rabinowicz T, de Courten-Myers GM, Petetot JM, Xi G, de los Reyes E. Human cortex development: estimates of neuronal numbers indicate major loss late during gestation. *J Neuropathol Exp Neurol*. 1996;55(3):320–8.

22. Raff MC, Barres BA, Burne JF, et al. Programmed cell death and the control of cell survival: lessons from the nervous system. *Science*. 1993;262(5134):695–700.

23. Rakic S, Zecevic N. Programmed cell death in the developing human telencephalon. *Eur J Neurosci*. 2000;12(8):2721–34.

24. Nijhawan D, Honarpour N, Wang X. Apoptosis in neural development and disease. *Annu Rev Neurosci*. 2000;23:73–87.

25. Kuida K, Zheng TS, Na S, et al. Decreased apoptosis in the brain and premature lethality in CPP32-deficient mice. *Nature*. 1996;384(6607):368–72.

26. Ikonomidou C, Bosch F, Miksa M, et al. Blockade of NMDA receptors and apoptotic neurodegeneration in the developing brain. *Science*. 1999;283(5398):70–4.

27. Jevtovic-Todorovic V, Hartman RE, Izumi Y, et al. Early exposure to common anesthetic agents causes widespread neurodegeneration in the developing rat brain and persistent learning deficits. *J Neurosci*. 2003;23(3):876–82.

28. Loepke AW, Soriano SG. An assessment of the effects of general anesthetics on developing brain structure and neurocognitive function. *Anesth Analg*. 2008;106(6):1681–707.

29. Brambrink AM, Evers AS, Avidan MS, et al. Isoflurane-induced neuroapoptosis in the neonatal rhesus macaque brain. *Anesthesiology*. 2010;112(4):834–41.

30. Slikker W, Jr., Zou X, Hotchkiss CE, et al. Ketamine-induced neuronal cell death in the perinatal rhesus monkey. *Toxicol Sci*. 2007;98(1):145–58.

31. Brambrink AM, Evers AS, Avidan MS, et al. Ketamine-induced neuroapoptosis in the fetal and neonatal rhesus macaque brain. *Anesthesiology*. 2012;116(2):372–84.

32. Fredriksson A, Ponten E, Gordh T, Eriksson P. Neonatal exposure to a combination of N-methyl-D-aspartate and gamma-aminobutyric acid type A receptor anesthetic agents potentiates apoptotic

neurodegeneration and persistent behavioral deficits. *Anesthesiology*. 2007;107(3):427–36.

33. Stratmann G. Review article: neurotoxicity of anesthetic drugs in the developing brain. *Anesth Analg*. 2011;113(5):1170–9.

34. Stratmann G, Sall JW, May LD, et al. Isoflurane differentially affects neurogenesis and long-term neurocognitive function in 60-day-old and 7-day-old rats. *Anesthesiology*. 2009;110(4):834–48.

35. Hayashi H, Dikkes P, Soriano SG. Repeated administration of ketamine may lead to neuronal degeneration in the developing rat brain. *Paediatr Anaesth*. 2002;12(9):770–4.

36. Scallet AC, Schmued LC, Slikker W, Jr., et al. Developmental neurotoxicity of ketamine: morphometric confirmation, exposure parameters, and multiple fluorescent labeling of apoptotic neurons. *Toxicol Sci*. 2004;81(2):364–70.

37. Wang C, Sadovova N, Hotchkiss C, et al. Blockade of N-methyl-D-aspartate receptors by ketamine produces loss of postnatal day 3 monkey frontal cortical neurons in culture. *Toxicol Sci*. 2006;91(1):192–201.

38. Fredriksson A, Archer T, Alm H, Gordh T, Eriksson P. Neurofunctional deficits and potentiated apoptosis by neonatal NMDA antagonist administration. *Behav Brain Res*. 2004;153(2):367–76.

39. Clancy B, Darlington RB, Finlay BL. Translating developmental time across mammalian species. *Neuroscience*. 2001;105(1):7–17.

40. Clancy B, Finlay BL, Darlington RB, Anand KJ. Extrapolating brain development from experimental species to humans. *Neurotoxicology*. 2007;28(5):931–7.

41. Quinn R. Comparing rat's to human's age: how old is my rat in people years? *Nutrition*. 2005;21(6):775–7.

42. De Felipe J, Marco P, Fairen A, Jones EG. Inhibitory synaptogenesis in mouse somatosensory cortex. *Cereb Cortex*. 1997;7(7):619–34.

43. Micheva KD, Beaulieu C. Quantitative aspects of synaptogenesis in the rat barrel field cortex with special reference to GABA circuitry. *J Comp Neurol*. 1996;373(3):340–54.

44. Micheva KD, Beaulieu C. Development and plasticity of the inhibitory neocortical circuitry with an emphasis on the rodent barrel field cortex: a review. *Can J Physiol Pharmacol*. 1997;75(5):470–8.

45. Huttenlocher PR, Dabholkar AS. Regional differences in synaptogenesis in human cerebral cortex. *J Comp Neurol*. 1997;387(2):167–78.

46. Dekaban AS. Changes in brain weights during the span of human life: relation of brain weights to body heights and body weights. *Ann Neurol*. 1978;4(4):345–56.

47. Dobbing J. Undernutrition and the developing brain: the relevance of animal models to the human problem. *Am J Dis Child*. 1970;120(5):411–15.

48. Dobbing J, Sands J. Quantitative growth and development of human brain. *Arch Dis Child*. 1973;48(10):757–67.

49. Andersen SL. Trajectories of brain development: point of vulnerability or window of opportunity? *Neurosci Biobehav Rev*. 2003;27(1–2):3–18.

50. Andersen SL, Navalta CP. Altering the course of neurodevelopment: a framework for understanding the enduring effects of psychotropic drugs. *Int J Dev Neurosci*. 2004;22(5–6):423–40.

51. Anand KJ, Garg S, Rovnaghi CR, et al. Ketamine reduces the cell death following inflammatory pain in newborn rat brain. *Pediatr Res*. 2007;62(3):283–90.

52. Shih J, May LD, Gonzalez HE, et al. Delayed environmental enrichment reverses sevoflurane-induced memory impairment in rats. *Anesthesiology*. 2012;116(3):586–602.

53. Liu JR, Liu Q, Li J, et al. Noxious stimulation attenuates ketamine-induced neuroapoptosis in the developing rat brain. *Anesthesiology*. 2012;117(1):64–71.

54. Davidson A, Flick RP. Neurodevelopmental implications of the use of sedation and analgesia in neonates. *Clin Perinatol*. 2013;40(3):559–73.

55. McCann ME, Bellinger DC, Davidson AJ, Soriano SG. Clinical research approaches to studying pediatric anesthetic neurotoxicity. *Neurotoxicology*. 2009;30(5):766–71.

56. Jacobson JL, Jacobson SW. Methodological issues in research on developmental exposure to neurotoxic agents. *Neurotoxicol Teratol*. 2005;27(3):395–406.

57. Susser E, Bresnahan M. Epidemiologic approaches to neurodevelopmental disorders. *Mol Psychiatry*. 2002;7(Suppl 2):S2–3.

58. Winneke G. Appraisal of neurobehavioral methods in environmental health research: the developing brain as a target for neurotoxic chemicals. *Int J Hyg Environ Health*. 2007;210(5):601–9.

59. Laing S, Walker K, Ungerer J, Badawi N, Spence K. Early development of children with major birth defects requiring newborn surgery. *J Paediatr Child Health*. 2011;47(3):140–7.

60. Gischler SJ, Mazer P, Duivenvoorden HJ, et al. Interdisciplinary structural follow-up of surgical newborns: a prospective evaluation. *J Pediatr Surg*. 2009;44(7):1382–9.

61. Ludman L, Spitz L, Lansdown R. Intellectual development at 3 years of age of children who underwent major neonatal surgery. *J Pediatr Surg*. 1993;28(2):130–4.

62. Walker K, Halliday R, Holland AJ, Karskens C, Badawi N. Early developmental outcome of infants with infantile hypertrophic pyloric stenosis. *J Pediatr Surg*. 2010;45(12):2369–72.

63. Anand KJ, Barton BA, McIntosh N, et al. Analgesia and sedation in preterm neonates who require ventilatory support: results from the NOPAIN trial. Neonatal Outcome and Prolonged Analgesia in Neonates. *Arch Pediatr Adolesc Med*. 1999;153(4):331–8.

64. Wilder RT, Flick RP, Sprung J, et al. Early exposure to anesthesia and learning disabilities in a population-based birth cohort. *Anesthesiology*. 2009;110(4):796–804.

65. Flick RP, Katusic SK, Colligan RC, et al. Cognitive and behavioral outcomes after early exposure to anesthesia and surgery. *Pediatrics*. 2011;128(5):e1053–61.

66. Sprung J, Flick RP, Katusic SK, et al. Attention-deficit/hyperactivity disorder after early exposure to procedures requiring general anesthesia. *Mayo Clin Proc*. 2012;87(2):120–9.

67. Ing C, DiMaggio C, Whitehouse A, et al. Long-term differences in language and cognitive function after childhood exposure to anesthesia. *Pediatrics*. 2012;130(3):e476–85.

68. DiMaggio C, Sun LS, Kakavouli A, Byrne MW, Li G. A retrospective cohort study of the association of anesthesia and hernia repair surgery with behavioral and developmental disorders in young children. *J Neurosurg Anesthesiol*. 2009;21(4):286–91.

69. DiMaggio C, Sun LS, Li G. Early childhood exposure to anesthesia and risk of developmental and behavioral disorders in a sibling birth cohort. *Anesth Analg*. 2011;113(5):1143–51.

70. Hansen TG, Pedersen JK, Henneberg SW, et al. Academic performance in adolescence after inguinal hernia repair in infancy: a nationwide cohort study. *Anesthesiology*. 2011;114(5):1076–85.

71. Block RI, Thomas JJ, Bayman EO, et al. Are anesthesia and surgery during infancy associated with altered academic performance during childhood? *Anesthesiology*. 2012;117(3):494–503.

72. O'Leary JD, Janus M, Duku E, et al. A population-based study evaluating the association between surgery in early life and child development at primary school entry. *Anesthesiology*. 2016;125(2):272–9.

73. Glazt P, Sandin RH, Pedersen NL, et al. Association of anesthesia and surgery during childhood with long-term academic performance. *JAMA Pediatr*. 2016;171(1):e163470.

74. Davidson AJ, Disma N, de Graaff JC, et al. Neurodevelopmental outcome at 2 years of age after general anaesthesia and awake-regional anaesthesia in infancy (GAS): an international multicentre, randomised controlled trial. *Lancet*. 2015;387:239–50.

75. Sun LS, Li G, Miller TL, et al. Association between a single general anesthesia exposure before age 36 months and neurocognitive outcomes in later childhood. *JAMA*. 2016;315(21):2312–20.

76. Anand KJ. Anesthetic neurotoxicity in newborns: should we change clinical practice? *Anesthesiology*. 2007;107(1):2–4.

77. Food and Drug Administration. Anesthetic and life support drugs: advisory committee meeting, 2007. Available at: www.fda.gov/ohrms/dockets/ac/07/transcripts/2007-4285t1.pdf.

78. Food and Drug Administration. FDA review results in new warnings about using general anesthetics and sedation drugs in young children and pregnant women. Drug Safety Communication, 2016.

79. Food and Drug Administration. Anesthesia: is it safe for young brains?, 2016. Available at: www.fda.gov/forconsumers/consumerupdates/ucm364078.htm.

80. Dr. Roizen's Advice Smart Tots: www.smarttots.org/aboutus/drRoizensAdvice.html.

81. Litman RS, Perkins FM, Dawson SC. Parental knowledge and attitudes toward discussing the risk of death from anesthesia. *Anesth Analg*. 1993;77(2):256–60.

82. Wisselo TL, Stuart C, Muris P. Providing parents with information before anaesthesia: what do they really want to know? *Paediatr Anaesth*. 2004;14(4):299–307.

83. Fortier MA, Chorney JM, Rony RY, et al. Children's desire for perioperative information. *Anesth Analg*. 2009;109(4):1085–90.

84. Nemergut ME, Aganga D, Flick RP. Anesthetic neurotoxicity: what to tell the parents? *Paediatr Anaesth*. 2014;24(1):120–6.

# New Anesthetic Agents on the Horizon

Thomas Weismueller and Kai Matthes

## Introduction

Every year six million children, including 1.5 million infants, receive general anesthesia for a surgical procedure within the United States [1]. In particular, premature infants are often in need of multiple surgical procedures, thereby requiring multiple general anesthetics.

Despite this being an essential practice, most anesthetics routinely administered to neonates and infants have not been adequately tested for safety or efficacy. A growing body of evidence indicates that exposure to anesthetic drugs may be harmful to the developing brain of very young children [2–4]. Controversy exists regarding to what extent long-term neurodevelopmental outcome is impacted by the repeated exposure to general anesthesia. Yet it seems to be clear that the effects of anesthesia are most detrimental in the age group of neonates and infants, as well as very old patients.

Against this background it appears prudent to push for the development of new anesthetic drugs with a better neuroprotective pharmacologic profile.

## Xenon

The noble gas xenon has been around in anesthesia practice for more than 60 years. The name xenon derives from the Greek term for *stranger*, reflecting its rarity. As a colorless, heavy, odorless gas, xenon constitutes 0.0018 percent of the earth's atmosphere.

Xenon was discovered in 1898 by Sir William Ramsay and Morris Travers, who purified the inert gas by fractional distillation from air. Yet, it was not until 1951 when it was used for the first time as an anesthetic agent by Cullen and Cross [5]. Since then, xenon has been considered as the closest candidate for an ideal anesthetic gas. High costs in the purification process that involves liquefaction of air and subsequent fractional distillation make xenon an expensive anesthetic.

Since 1990 xenon has regained attention as more studies were published examining clinical aspects of xenon anesthesia. Xenon has favorable kinetic characteristics: it is inflammable, not explosive, and does not undergo metabolism. Furthermore, it does not contribute to atmospheric pollution. Xenon does not affect hepatic and renal function and is not teratogenic or fetotoxic [6–8].

## Mechanism of Action

The N-methyl-D aspartate (NMDA) receptor antagonist xenon blocks the NMDA receptor competitively at its glycine co-agonist binding site. This inhibition is considered to be the main mechanism for xenon's anesthetic and neuroprotective properties [9]. The NMDA receptor is an ionotropic receptor that is activated by the binding of glutamate. Glutamate is the main excitatory neurotransmitter, yet constant activation of the NMDA receptor has been found to contribute to neuronal death in the setting of ischemia or stroke [5].

In addition, other ionotropic transmembrane receptors such as the α-amino-3-hydroxy-5-methyl-4-isoxazolepropionic acid receptor (AMPA) might contribute to xenon's anesthetic and analgesic action as well, yet their precise role is not fully understood [10].

## Pharmacokinetics

The blood partition coefficient of xenon is 0.115 and therefore significantly lower than any of the other to-date known inhalational anesthetics [11]. The minimum alveolar concentration (MAC) of xenon has been estimated as 63–71 percent [12].

Very short induction and emergence times have been demonstrated in various studies [13,14]. This might be advantageous in an outpatient setting as well as any other clinical scenario where fast-tracking is desirable.

One of the many reasons why xenon regained attention is its cardio protective profile: Systolic blood pressure is maintained at baseline values during xenon anesthesia [15]. Ventricular function as assessed by transesophageal echocardiography is unchanged [16]. In a guinea pig ventricular muscle model, no effect on cardiac contractility could be observed under xenon exposure. In contrast, isoflurane led to a 30 percent decrease in myocardial contractility in the same study [17].

Great hemodynamic stability was also observed in adults with markedly reduced ejection fraction who underwent cardioverter/defibrillator implantation [18]. Pilot studies examining the safety feasibility of xenon anesthesia in children undergoing cardiac catheterization are currently on the way [19].

## Neuroprotection, Therapeutic Hypothermia

To date, several studies demonstrate xenon's role acting as a neuroprotective agent by inhibiting apoptotic neuronal signaling pathways. An activation of NMDA receptors may lead to initiation and progression of apoptosis in the context of cerebral hypoxia and ischemia.

Xenon reduces NMDA receptor signaling through its antagonistic property and also limits ischemia-induced neurotransmitter release [5].

Subanesthetic doses of xenon were shown to be beneficial in a neonatal hypoxia-ischemia model in rats, where three hours of xenon exposure following hypoxia-ischemia provided short-term neuroprotection [20]. Other studies investigated xenon as a preconditioning agent: preexposure to xenon for two hours revealed a decrease in infarction size and improved neurological function in neonatal hypoxic-ischemic rats [21].

Recently a clinical feasibility study was conducted in England in which 14 infants were subjected to hypothermia and ventilated with 50 percent xenon for a time period of up to 18 hours for the treatment of neonatal encephalopathy. The neurodevelopmental outcome of these infants was assessed after 18 months and showed no adverse effects in comparison to the subgroup of infants that was treated with hypothermia alone. The authors concluded that it is feasible and safe to do a randomized type II outcome study to examine a potential therapeutic benefit of xenon in

newborns suffering from moderate to severe neonatal encephalopathy [22].

## Mechanisms of Analgesia

Analgesic properties of xenon were first described by Lachman et al. in 1990. This study demonstrated lower fentanyl supplementation in patients who underwent xenon anesthesia for routine surgery in comparison to a control group that received nitrous oxide, which was found to have significantly higher narcotic requirements [23].

Xenon appears to be at least three times more potent in blocking the responses to surgical incision than nitrous oxide at the same concentration.

NMDA receptors are the main target of xenon and, as such, play an important role in postoperative and inflammatory pain. Inhibition of AMPA receptors via xenon might contribute to the antinociceptive effects of this gas as seen in a rat model in which inhibition of AMPA receptors in cortical neurons led to inhibition of pain sensitization [24].

## Toxicity

All volatile anesthetics are harmful to the ozone layer. Nitrous oxide is a very potent greenhouse gas, being 230 times more potent than carbon dioxide. The naturally occurring noble gas xenon lacks all these harmful environmental effects.

Besides its cardio- and neuroprotective properties, xenon has no impact on coagulation and platelet function [25]. Renal and hepatic function are not affected. Xenon is not fetotoxic or teratogenic. Taken together, xenon has the features of an idle gas, yet high costs and its scarcity are currently limiting clinical use. It has been estimated that xenon's expenses for two hours of anesthesia are around $300, whereas conventional volatile anesthetics cost around $10 for the same time use [5]. More studies are necessary to better understand how xenon anesthesia relates to clinical outcome and potential reduction in hospital stay duration and decreased need for postoperative intensive care. The development of more refined low-flow and closed-circuit systems will help to limit the costs of xenon anesthesia.

Xenon's advantages as a neuro- and cardioprotective agent, as well as its other clinically favorable features and non-toxic chemical properties, should ultimately lead to innovations in the medical gas field that will aim to establish xenon as a readily available gas in daily anesthesia practice.

## Remimazolam

Remimazolam is a new ultra-short-acting benzodiazepine that is highly selective for the $GABA_A$ receptor. It is metabolized by tissue esterases and as such promises a more predictable offset of action. Rapid onset of dose-dependent sedation and rapid recovery were demonstrated in Phase I clinical trials. Similar to remifentanyl, the short, context-sensitive half-time of remimazolam seems to be insensitive to the infusion duration. Phase II studies are currently on the way.

## Etomidate Analogs

Etomidate is a well-known short-acting induction agent that provides rapid onset of anesthesia with minimal cardiovascular depression. It is metabolized in the liver by ester hydrolysis. Side-effects of etomidate are pain on injection, postoperative nausea and vomiting, myoclonus, and, most concerning of all, adrenocortical suppression via $11\beta$-hydroxylase inhibition. Increased mortality after a single dose of etomidate has been found in critically ill patients with sepsis [26]. New analogs of etomidate were designed to address the problem of adrenocortical suppression. Three analogs are briefly introduced here.

Methoxycarbonyl (MOC) etomidate is an etomidate analog with a half-life of a few minutes. Rapid metabolism leads to accumulation of MOC etomidate carboxylic acid (MOC-ECA), which is 350 times less potent as a hypnotic metabolite and as an inhibitor of adrenocortical steroid synthesis. Follow-up studies have showed that high infusion rates are required for this drug to maintain hypnosis, which results in an accumulation of MOC-ECA with prolonged recovery times.

A more promising etomidate analog appears to be cyclopropyl MOC etomidate (CPMM). This is a spacer-linked etomidate ester which is eight times more potent than MOC etomidate. Animal studies indicate that it doesn't suppress adrenocortical function. Clinical usefulness has yet to be investigated in humans.

MOC-carboetomidate shows potent hypnotic activity together with reduced adrenal suppression and good hemodynamic stability. However, onset time is slow due to water insolubility.

In order to improve rapid metabolism together with no adrenal suppression, as of now etomidate analogs need further optimization: Improved rapid metabolism, meaning rapid recovery from hypnosis, minimal cardiovascular suppression, and no adrenal suppression are the main goals for novel etomidate analog drug design.

## Sugammadex

Sugammadex is a modified $\gamma$-cyclodextrin that was discovered in 2007. It inhibits steroidal neuromuscular blockers (NMBAs) by encapsulating them. The ability to encapsulate NMBAs is strongest for rocuronium. Sugammadex exhibits no cholinergic effects such as seen with neostigmine. The co-administration of an antimuscarinic agent such as atropine is not necessary. Multiple clinical trials reported a rapid and safe reversal of varying degrees of neuromuscular blockade. Sugammadex was approved for use in the European Union in summer 2008. Concerns about its potential side-effects on bone and tooth modeling as well as safety in pediatric and parturient populations resulted in non-approval of this drug by the FDA.

## Neosaxitoxin

Neosaxitoxin (neoSTX) belongs to the group of paralytic shellfish toxins that reversibly block voltage-gated sodium channels at the neuronal level. Less cardiotoxicity in comparison to amide local anesthetic agents has been observed. This is likely due to neosaxitoxin's lower affinity for cardiac sodium channel receptors.

Furthermore, prolonged duration of local anesthesia has been demonstrated with neoSTX: whereas commonly available local anesthetics rarely last longer than a few hours after wound infiltration, this new compound was shown to last beyond 24 hours, with a single dose injection following laparoscopic cholecystectomy [27]. No serious adverse reactions including systemic neoSTX effects were observed in a first randomized double-blind trial that was conducted in Chile. Recently, the FDA approved neoSTX for a phase I clinical study on healthy volunteers within the United States. This current trial aims to provide more refined dose escalation and safety data in line with FDA standards.

# References

1.  Lee JH, Zhang J, Wei L, Yu SP. Neurodevelopmental implications of the general anesthesia in neonate and infants. *Exp Neurol*. 2015;272:50–60.

2.  Flick RP, Nemergut ME, Christensen K, Hansen TG. Anesthetic-related neurotoxicity in the young and outcome measures: the devil is in the details. *Anesthesiology*. 2014;120(6):1303–5.

3.  Flick RP, Katusic SK, Colligan RC, et al. Cognitive and behavioral outcomes after early exposure to anesthesia and surgery. *Pediatrics*. 2011;128(5):e1053–61.

4.  Ing CH, DiMaggio CJ, Malacova E, et al. Comparative analysis of outcome measures used in examining neurodevelopmental effects of early childhood anesthesia exposure. *Anesthesiology*. 2014;120(6):1319–32.

5.  Esencan E, Yuksel S, Tosun YB, et al. XENON in medical area: emphasis on neuroprotection in hypoxia and anesthesia. *Med Gas Res*. 2013;3(1):4.

6.  Reinelt H, Marx T, Kotzerke J, et al. Hepatic function during xenon anesthesia in pigs. *Acta Anaesthesiol Scand*. 2002;46(6):713–16.

7.  Bedi A, Murray JM, Dingley J, Stevenson MA, Fee JP. Use of xenon as a sedative for patients receiving critical care. *Crit Care Med*. 2003;31(10):2470–7.

8.  Lane GA, Nahrwold ML, Tait AR, et al. Anesthetics as teratogens: nitrous oxide is fetotoxic, xenon is not. *Science*. 1980;210(4472):899–901.

9.  Franks NP, Dickinson R, de Sousa SL, Hall AC, Lieb WR. How does xenon produce anaesthesia? *Nature*. 1998;396(6709):324.

10. Giacalone M, Abramo A, Giunta F, Forfori F. Xenon-related analgesia: a new target for pain treatment. *Clin J Pain*. 2013;29(7):639–43.

11. Goto T, Suwa K, Uezono S, et al. The blood-gas partition coefficient of xenon may be lower than generally accepted. *Br J Anaesth*. 1998;80(2):255–6.

12. Sanders RD, Franks NP, Maze M. Xenon: no stranger to anaesthesia. *Br J Anaesth*. 2003;91(5):709–17.

13. Goto T, Saito H, Shinkai M, et al. Xenon provides faster emergence from anesthesia than does nitrous oxide–sevoflurane or nitrous oxide–isoflurane. *Anesthesiology*. 1997;86(6):1273–8.

14. Nakata Y, Goto T, Morita S. Comparison of inhalation inductions with xenon and sevoflurane. *Acta Anaesthesiol Scand*. 1997;41(9):1157–61.

15. Coburn M, Kunitz O, Baumert JH, et al. Randomized controlled trial of the haemodynamic and recovery effects of xenon or propofol anaesthesia. *Br J Anaesth*. 2005;94(2):198–202.

16. Luttropp HH, Romner B, Perhag L, et al. Left ventricular performance and cerebral haemodynamics during xenon anaesthesia: a transoesophageal echocardiography and transcranial Doppler sonography study. *Anaesthesia*. 1993;48(12):1045–9.

17. Stowe DF, Rehmert GC, Kwok WM, et al. Xenon does not alter cardiac function or major cation currents in isolated guinea pig hearts or myocytes. *Anesthesiology*. 2000;92(2):516–22.

18. Baumert JH, Falter F, Eletr D, et al. Xenon anaesthesia may preserve cardiovascular function in patients with heart failure. *Acta Anaesthesiol Scand*. 2005;49(6):743–9.

19. Devroe S, Lemiere J, Van de Velde M, et al. Safety and feasibility of xenon as an adjuvant to sevoflurane anaesthesia in children undergoing interventional or diagnostic cardiac catheterization: study protocol for a randomised controlled trial. *Trials*. 2015;16(1):74.

20. Dingley J, Tooley J, Porter H, Thoresen M. Xenon provides short-term neuroprotection in neonatal rats when administered after hypoxia-ischemia. *Stroke*. 2006;37(2):501–6.

21. Ma D, Hossain M, Pettet GK, et al. Xenon preconditioning reduces brain damage from neonatal asphyxia in rats. *J Cereb Blood Flow Metab*. 2006;26(2):199–208.

22. Dingley J, Tooley J, Liu X, et al. Xenon ventilation during therapeutic hypothermia in neonatal encephalopathy: a feasibility study. *Pediatrics*. 2014;133(5):809–18.

23. Lachmann B, Armbruster S, Schairer W, et al. Safety and efficacy of xenon in routine use as an inhalational anaesthetic. *Lancet*. 1990;335(8703):1413–15.

24. Haseneder R, Kratzer S, Kochs E, et al. The xenon-mediated antagonism against the NMDA receptor is non-selective for receptors containing either NR2A or NR2B subunits in the mouse amygdala. *Eur J Pharmacol*. 2009;619(1–3):33–7.

25. de Rossi LW, Horn NA, Baumert JH, et al. Xenon does not affect human platelet function in vitro. *Anesth Analg*. 2001;93(3):635–40.

26. Chan CM, Mitchell AL, Shorr AF. Etomidate is associated with mortality and adrenal insufficiency in sepsis: a meta-analysis. *Crit Care Med*. 2012;40:2945–53.

27. Rodríguez-Navarro AJ, Berde CB, Wiedmaier G, et al. Comparison of neosaxitoxin versus bupivacaine via port infiltration for postoperative analgesia following laparoscopic cholecystectomy: a randomized, double-blind trial. *Regional Anesthes Pain Med* 2011;36:103–9.

## Chapter 19

# Monitoring of the Newborn and Young Infant Under Anesthesia

Michael R. King, Samuel Rodriguez, and Kathleen Chen

One of the key duties of the anesthetist, monitoring requires an advanced level of understanding of both how monitors work as well as how to interpret their data. An additional level of complexity is added when monitoring infants and children, as their physiology changes rapidly with age and may involve various abnormalities due to congenital disease.

Although monitors play a key role in the modern operating room, it cannot be overemphasized that keeping one's eyes on the patient remains the most important method of detecting the evolution of critical events and evaluating the adequacy of the airway, breathing, and circulation. The goal of this chapter is to review commonly used and newly introduced monitors, the unique considerations of these monitors in pediatric patients, and how the information they provide can help detect critical events and guide management during anesthesia.

## Central Nervous System Monitoring

A variety of monitors exist for the measurement of neurologic physiology and function. While these are most often used in cardiac and neurologic surgery, several are also becoming more common for use in general procedures as technology has improved in the area of noninvasive monitoring.

## Intracranial Pressure Monitoring

Intracranial pressure (ICP) monitors, or ventricular catheters, are invasive monitors that sit inside the ventricle, where they can be used for continuous ICP monitoring, as well as drainage of cerebrospinal fluid (CSF) for therapeutic reduction of ICP. Infants often will not require them as open fontanelles allow for expansion of the intracranial contents without an increase in ICP, but they may be indicated in older children at risk for a pathologic increase in ICP. In general ICP is considered normal if less than 15 mmHg. It is typically 2–6 mmHg in term neonates and even

lower in premature infants. Measuring both the mean arterial pressure (MAP) and ICP allows for calculation of cerebral perfusion pressure (CPP), which is defined as the difference between MAP and ICP. A high ICP decreases the CPP and can put the brain at risk for ischemia, thus monitoring of CPP is of utmost importance in patients with neurologic trauma or intracranial pathology. It has been suggested that children with traumatic brain injury should have their CPP maintained between 40 and 65 mmHg [1], a goal that can be guided by continuous pressure monitoring. As they are invasive monitors, ventricular catheters may cause hemorrhage or infection, and thus will typically be placed only in critically ill patients who may require intervention.

## Electroencephalography

The electroencephalogram (EEG) utilizes a variable number of scalp electrodes to report electrical changes due to brain activity. Unprocessed EEG contains a wealth of information about neurologic function and can be used for monitoring in a variety of procedures, such as surgery on the carotid artery or epileptic foci, but requires specialized personnel for interpretation and is beyond the scope of most anesthesiologists. However, anesthesia produces characteristic changes in EEG function that give clues about the depth of anesthesia. Patterns such as burst suppression and electrical silence are easy to recognize as signs of an overanesthetized patient, while increased muscle activity in the non-relaxed patient suggests light anesthesia and impending movement.

Processed EEG, which includes proprietary monitoring systems such as the bispectral index (BIS®) or SEDline®, attempts to simplify unprocessed EEG into a more interpretable form. BIS monitors process EEG data using a propriety algorithm into a number from 0 (electrical silence) to 100 (full wakefulness) to report a level of consciousness [2]. BIS may be used for sedation monitoring and has been shown to correlate with clinical depth of sedation in children [3]. It also appears to correlate with depth of sevoflurane anesthesia in a manner similar to adults [4]. BIS can, however, be affected by developmental status – compared with neurodevelopmentally normal children, in children with cerebral palsy the same pattern of change is seen in response to anesthesia but overall BIS values are lower [5]. In infants BIS values are significantly lower for a given level of clinical sedation than in older children [6]. The use of BIS to prevent awareness during anesthesia has received considerable attention and remains controversial [7–9]. Although rates of awareness in children are similarly low to those in adults [10], no study has evaluated it for this purpose in pediatric patients.

## Near-Infrared Spectroscopy

Using principles similar to those used for pulse oximetry, near-infrared spectroscopy (NIRS) utilizes near-infrared light to measure oxyhemoglobin and deoxyhemoglobin saturations in the cerebral vessels. The NIRS probe is placed on the scalp, where a light source emits two wavelengths of near-infrared light that traverse through the soft tissue of the scalp and the brain (Figure 19.1). The scattering and absorption of light is received by detectors where changes in hemoglobin saturation are analyzed and a saturation value known as the regional cerebral oxygen

saturation index ($rSO_2i$) is produced for both the right and left hemispheres. Although baseline readings are of limited value, an acute decrease in $rSO_2i$ suggests an imbalance between cerebral metabolism and blood flow. In general, a decrease in $rSO_2i$ of greater than 20 percent or an $rSO_2i$ reading of less than 50 percent is considered a threshold for intervention, with the goal of intervention being an increase in cerebral blood flow or a decrease in cerebral metabolic requirements depending on the most likely source of the disruption.

Clinically, NIRS has been used in pediatric cardiac surgery, neurosurgery, and intensive care. A study of 20 pediatric cardiac surgical patients showed that $rSO_2i$ correlated well with mixed-venous oxygen saturation [11], suggesting it could be used as a marker for overall tissue oxygenation. In contrast to pulse oximetry, NIRS analyzes not just pulsatile blood flow but also nonpulsatile (i.e., venous) flow. Because of this, it can be used during states of nonpulsatile flow, such as cardiopulmonary bypass, and is of particular use in monitoring cerebral oxygenation during bypass and deep hypothermic circulatory arrest. Changes in NIRS signals were used in one case to diagnose aortic cannula malpositioning during cardiac surgery, which likely avoided a neurologic disaster [12]. A study looking at deep hypothermic circulatory arrest observed a smaller increase in cerebral oxygen saturation at the initiation of hypothermic cardiopulmonary

**Figure 19.1** NIRS probe applied to the scalp. Near-infrared light of multiple wavelengths is emitted from a light source. The scalp and brain detector receive scattered and absorbed light from these tissues and output regional cerebral saturations.

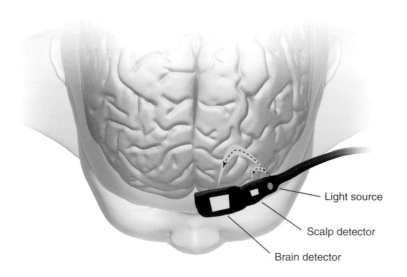

Light source

Scalp detector

Brain detector

bypass in patients who had postoperative neurologic changes [13].

Although NIRS is standard practice for pediatric cardiac surgery in many institutions, at this point the literature lacks a large study clearly demonstrating improved clinical outcomes with NIRS monitoring. This may be due to the fact that although NIRS can accurately identify a decrease in cerebral oxygenation, the provider must still diagnose and successfully treat the cause. NIRS sensors must be placed on the skin of the forehead and therefore hair, hematomas, or skull abnormalities may decrease the quality of signals. The requirement for forehead placement also makes NIRS unable to reliably detect changes in the posterior circulation.

## Transcranial Doppler Sonography

Transcranial Doppler (TCD) signals monitor blood velocities to the brain via ultrasound signals through the skull. Typically probes are placed over the middle cerebral arteries where they can relay information regarding cerebral blood flow or embolic events, making TCD particularly popular for monitoring during cardiopulmonary bypass. The utility of TCD lies in its ability to detect changes in flow velocities [14], which can alert the user to acute changes in flow due to events such as hypotension or bypass cannula misplacement. However, the velocities themselves are poorly predictive of actual flow [15]. Like the precordial Doppler, TCD can detect embolic events and has been used during cardiac surgery in children [16].

TCD is limited by the need for operator skill to recognize changes in flow, and a lack of regular use reduces accuracy [17]. Signals can also be difficult to obtain in patients with thicker skull bones, although as infants and neonates have less-developed skulls they are among the easiest patients in which to obtain signals.

## Evoked Potential Monitoring

Evoked potential (EP) monitoring is similar to EEG in that it uses electrical activity in the nervous system to monitor function. In contrast to EEG, which monitors spontaneous electrical activity in the brain, EPs result from artificial stimuli initiated at electrodes placed at specific peripheral monitoring sites throughout the body. An individual trained in EP monitoring typically places the leads and monitors nerve function periodically throughout the surgery to detect changes

in neurologic function that may result from surgical manipulation. Important parameters of EPs include latency, defined as the length of time from stimulus to peak amplitude of the evoked response, and amplitude, which is the difference in voltages of the most positive and most negative peaks of deflection from the baseline reference potential.

The most commonly used forms of EPs in monitoring are brainstem auditory-evoked potentials (BAEPs), somatosensory-evoked potentials (SSEPs), and motor-evoked potentials (MEPs). BAEPs monitor the response to sounds and therefore can be affected by changes in much of the auditory pathway, including the cochlear, afferents of the vestibulocochlear nerve, and the brainstem. Brainstem auditory-evoked potentials are thus useful in neurosurgery and otorhinolaryngology, particularly in procedures around the skull base or involving the ear canal.

Somatosensory-evoked potentials are a monitor of peripheral afferent function. Recording takes place over the brain, and common stimulation sites include the ulnar, median, tibial, and common peroneal nerves. The technique is useful for monitoring for injury during complex spine procedures, such as scoliosis surgery, where its use has been demonstrated to decrease postoperative neurologic deficits [18]. Because their peripheral nerves are shorter, pediatric patients often have better signals than adults, and a decrease in amplitude of 50 percent or an increase in latency of 10 percent from baseline is defined as a change significant enough to warrant intervention.

Whereas SSEPs monitor afferent peripheral nerves, MEPs monitor efferent peripherals and can be combined with SSEPs for spine surgery to increase the sensitivity and predictive value versus SSEP alone [19]. MEP signals originate at electrodes over the scalp and motor potentials are elicited and recorded in the muscles of the hands and legs. A 50 percent decrease in amplitude is considered a significant change.

The use of EP monitoring requires several anesthetic considerations. Deepening an anesthetic can reduce the quality of EP signals, with MEPs affected the most and BAEPs the least. Volatile anesthetics have the largest effect on EP signals, thus these cases are performed using a total intravenous anesthetic when possible. MEPs also preclude the use of muscle relaxants and may be unreliable in patients with a preexisting neuromuscular deficit.

## Neuromuscular Junction Monitoring

Because of their increased oxygen consumption and decreased respiratory reserve relative to adults, neuromuscular monitoring should be considered in all patients receiving nondepolarizing neuromuscular blockers (NDNMBs) when preparing for reversal or extubation. The major consideration in neonates and infants is that acetylcholine receptors are immature even at term, and continue to mature with age, which results in altered responses of infants and children to NDNMBs [20].

Neuromuscular blockade can be monitored by a variety of techniques. Qualitative clinical signs of strength, such as deep respirations, coughing, and thrashing, are good indicators of function. In infants, brow furrowing and hip flexion also are promising signs of activity, but clinical tests requiring language comprehension, such as a five-second head lift or hand squeeze, are impossible in infants and usually difficult in young children. As a result, it is prudent to use a twitch monitor before extubation of a patient who has recently received a NDNMB. Twitch monitors consist of two electrodes placed along a motor nerve connected to a source of current. The current is then applied between the electrodes along the nerve to stimulate acetylcholine release. Under ordinary circumstances this causes the innervated muscle to twitch, but if NDNMBs are present in the neuromuscular junction the twitch will be diminished or absent. The most popular locations to monitor include the ulnar nerve, facial nerve, posterior tibial nerve, and peroneal nerve, all of which are located close to the skin and innervate muscles that cause easily identifiable twitches. Larger children may have a large amount of subcutaneous fat which acts as an insulator and limits signal transmission to the nerve, sometimes to the point where a twitch cannot be elicited.

Twitches can be produced in a variety of patterns, most commonly the train-of-four (TOF). Current is applied a total of four times over two seconds (a frequency of 2 Hz) to produce four muscle twitches, and the ratio of the strength of the fourth twitch is compared to the first. A patient who has received a NDNMB will have a progressive decrease in the strength of each twitch until strength has returned. Zero twitches are ideal for intubation, while a ratio of 0.95 or greater is ideal for extubation. Premature babies and neonates have immature neuromuscular junctions and will often have decreased ratios at baseline in the first months of life, thus extubation criteria may need to be altered in this age group [21,22].

Other twitch patterns include the single twitch, tetany, and post-tetanic stimulation. The single twitch is less sensitive than the TOF at detecting residual blockade as it does not include further twitches to detect fade. Tetany applied at 50, 100, or 200 Hz will produce fade if blockade is present, but is very stimulating and not recommended if the patient is lightly anesthetized. A post-tetanic twitch is performed with a 5 s period of tetany followed by single twitches at 1 Hz. A patient who lacks a single twitch may have one after a period of tetany due to an increase in acetylcholine synthesis triggered by the tetany [23], making the post-tetanic twitch the earliest sign of the return of neuromuscular function. Like the TOF, post-tetanic stimulation is also less effective in infants with immature neuromuscular junctions.

## Cardiovascular Monitoring

Anesthetists utilize similar cardiovascular monitors in neonates and infants as they use in adults. However, cardiac physiology and the vital signs change rapidly in the first year of life (Table 19.1), and an understanding of neonatal physiology is required for proper interpretation of commonly monitored parameters. In addition, the small size of infants makes placement of some invasive monitors difficult and their potential for congenital cardiac pathology requires flexibility in interpretation.

## Precordial Stethoscope

Although less commonly used in the twenty-first century, the precordial stethoscope is an enormously useful monitor in pediatrics for detecting both cardiovascular and respiratory events. Typically the stethoscope is taped over the apex of the patient's heart to free the hands of the anesthetist, and a fitted earpiece is placed in the anesthetist's ear. Airway events such as apnea, bronchospasm, or obstruction, which are prevalent during mask induction, are detected more quickly than with the pulse oximeter or electrocardiogram (ECG). Changes in heart rate, blood pressure, or myocardial contractility can be detected as a change in the volume of heart sounds [25]. The precordial stethoscope does, however, require experience for proper interpretation and relies on sometimes subtle qualitative changes in volume that can be difficult to detect in the modern, noisy operating room.

**Table 19.1** Normal ranges for heart rate and blood pressure in healthy, nonanesthetized infants

| Age | Heart rate (beats min−1) | Blood pressure (mmHg) |
|---|---|---|
| Premature | 120–170 | 55–75/35–45 |
| 0–3 months | 100–150 | 65–85/45–55 |
| 3–6 months | 90–120 | 70–90/50–65 |
| 6–12 months | 80–120 | 80–100/55–65 |
| 1–3 years | 70–110 | 90–105/55–70 |
| Source: [24]. | | |

## Esophageal Stethoscope

The esophageal stethoscope is similar to the precordial stethoscope in practice, but sits in the esophagus instead of over the heart. It is obviously less useful for induction as placement requires an anesthetized, intubated patient. However, it is more convenient for intraoperative use. It detects the same events that a precordial stethoscope can, and recent work has shown it is also effective for detecting residual flow in patent ductus arteriosus closure [26]. As with any oropharyngeal invasive device, there is potential for trauma to the esophagus, airways, or displacement of the endotracheal tube.

## Electrocardiography

The basis of ECG monitoring is the detection of electric potentials originating from the heart across various vectors on the chest. It is used continuously during anesthesia to detect a variety of changes in cardiac function that may result from anesthetic or surgical factors. In pediatrics the most common ECG changes are arrhythmias, thus patients are typically monitored with three leads that best display P-waves and QRS complexes. Ventricular leads, which are used to detect ischemia in adults, are often omitted due to the rarity of coronary artery pathology in pediatric patients. However, there are some conditions, such as Williams syndrome, that may involve coronary pathology and thus warrant the use of ventricular leads.

The arrhythmias most common in children are supraventricular tachycardia (SVT), atrial tachyarrhythmias, and sinus bradycardia [27]. Supraventricular tachycardia may be encountered during periods of high stimulation, such as intubation with light anesthesia. Atrial arrhythmias are seen in congenital heart disease with structural abnormalities.

Sinus bradycardia is often the result of hypoxia and severe sinus bradycardia, also commonly seen on mask induction in children with Down syndrome. Halothane classically can cause various arrhythmias, but is no longer commonly used.

## Indirect Arterial Pressure Measurement

Blood pressure (BP) can be monitored noninvasively via auscultation or oscillometry. Automatic oscillometric monitors are typically used during surgery and checked every 3–5 minutes. Oscillometric monitors measure BP by finding the pressure below which pulsatile flow returns in the artery, the systolic blood pressure (SBP), and the pressure at which the pulsatility in the artery has its highest amplitude, the MAP. Oscillometric monitors do not measure diastolic blood pressure (DBP) – it is instead calculated from the SBP and MAP and is frequently underestimated in children.

Noninvasive measurements are painless and easy in asleep and awake children, but can cause ischemic damage including nerve palsies and skin breakdown if repeated too frequently over the course of a long surgery. Cuff placement can affect the accuracy of noninvasive monitors. Placement on the distal arm or leg tends to overestimate SBP while underestimating DBP, although the MAP should be similar throughout the body in the absence of vascular disease. It has also long been known that a small cuff can overestimate the BP [28]. To avoid this, a cuff that is two-thirds to three-quarters in width of the upper arm length or, alternatively, a cuff that is wide enough to cover 40 percent of the upper arm circumference, should be chosen. Some cuffs come in sizes labeled "Infant," "Neonate," etc., but selecting a cuff merely based on age often yields an inappropriately sized cuff and therefore less accurate readings [29].

## Direct Arterial Blood Pressure Measurement

For some procedures, or in the presence of some comorbidities where hemodynamics can change quickly, intermittent noninvasive blood pressure measurement may not be sufficient for safety. Other cases may require frequent blood sampling that would require multiple peripheral draws, which can be notoriously difficult in infants. In these cases placement of an indwelling arterial catheter is indicated.

Insertion of arterial catheters is described below and typically is performed with a 22- or 24-gauge intravenous catheter, although in older children and adults a 20-gauge is often used. The benefit of a larger catheter is a lower rate of clotting or kinking. After insertion, an arterial catheter is attached to pressurized, saline-filled tubing to ensure that retrograde flow, which can lead to exsanguination, does not occur. The tubing contains a transducer that is normalized to atmospheric pressure at the level of the aortic root or external auditory meatus, depending on whether the clinician wishes to monitor the pressures at the heart or brain, respectively. A monitor displays the arterial pressures transmitted through the tubing to the transducer. A typical arterial tracing in a normotensive patient has a brisk upstroke with a dicrotic notch, which diminishes the more peripheral the location of the arterial catheter. As a general rule, the further from the heart a catheter is placed, the higher the SBP will be and the lower the DBP will be, but the MAP should stay constant. A dampened tracing suggests catheter kinking, excessively long pressure tubing, or the presence of a clot on the tip of the tubing, but it is essential to assume any tracing or pressure reading is real until proven otherwise in order to expedite treatment in case a significant physiologic change has actually occurred.

## Placement Techniques

Insertion of arterial catheters can be difficult in neonates. The artery is typically identified by one of three methods: palpation, ultrasound, or directly via surgical cut-down. Palpation is the most common method and is easiest in older children as their blood pressures increase and arteries enlarge, making the pulse easier to feel. One hand is used to locate the pulse while the other drives the catheter until a flash of blood is seen. The catheter can then be threaded in or can be placed with the Seldinger technique. For the Seldinger technique, the needle is often advanced through the back of the artery. The needle is then removed and the catheter pulled back until blood return is seen, confirming its placement in the lumen of the artery. At this point a wire is guided through the catheter into the lumen of the artery and the catheter is advanced over it into place. This method is especially useful in infants and neonates because they often do not have a palpable pulse. In the absence of a pulse, the needle is often advanced blindly and pulled back, repeated

in different locations until blood return is finally obtained.

Insertion with ultrasound is a newer technique that is becoming more popular in infants due to their poor peripheral pulses. The ultrasound is first used to identify the targeted artery, either in a transverse or "out-of-plane" approach (Figure 19.2), or a longitudinal or "in-plane" approach. The needle is then advanced under ultrasound visualization as it enters the artery and is placed either with a wire or direct threading. Current literature on the efficacy of ultrasound-guided arterial line placement is mixed, with some studies on radial artery catheterization suggesting no improvement in the speed of placement [30] while others suggest that it improves speed, decreases the number of attempts required for placement, and decreases the rate of hematomas [31,32]. As practitioners become more facile with ultrasound technology it is likely that ultrasound placement will become more common, especially in neonates and infants.

Surgical cut-down, the process of dissecting tissue down until the artery can be directly visualized and cannulated, is effective as both a first-line placement as well as when other methods have failed (Figure 19.2). Although it is the standard method for placement in small infants at many institutions, it has been associated with increased rates of complications, which will be discussed in a later section.

## Cannulation Locations

Arterial lines can be placed in a variety of peripheral arteries, the most popular of which is the radial. The technique is performed at the radial aspect of the wrist, where the radial artery is straight, superficial, and palpably pulsatile. Radial artery cannulation is considered safe because of collateral flow to the hand from the ulnar artery – limb ischemia is extremely rare, but it is nonetheless advisable to check for collateral flow by observing perfusion with compression of the radial artery (Allen's test) prior to attempting placement. Radial arteries and all other upper extremity arterial lines may have different readings on the right and left sides in infants with pathology involving the aortic arch, such as coarctation of the aorta. In such conditions the right radial artery is preferred as the brachiocephalic trunk leaves the aortic arch the earliest and has the highest likelihood of branching before the lesion. Surgically altered anatomy, such as a Blalock–Taussig shunt, may also affect pressures depending on

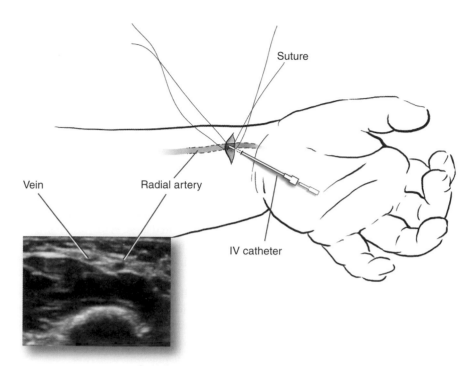

**Figure 19.2** Surgical cut-down and ultrasound approaches to radial artery catheterization. The cut-down utilizes direct visualization after dissection to the level of the radial artery. Ultrasound imaging can be used to locate the artery and the IV catheter observed to enter the vessel in a two-dimensional slice.

the site and should be considered accordingly. Some congenital syndromes, such as Down syndrome, are also associated with abnormalities in the radial arteries. One study of Down syndrome patients found one or more abnormalities in 16 percent of patients' forearm arterial trees [33].

An alternative to the radial artery in the upper extremity is the brachial artery, which is larger and often has a better pulse than the radial [34]. Although considered safe, it is important to remember that the brachial is an end-artery and occlusion will stop blood flow to the entire extremity in the absence of collateral circulation. The artery is found at the medial aspect of the antecubital fossa and is easiest to cannulate there.

Other commonly chosen arteries are the temporal, femoral, posterior tibial, and dorsalis pedis. The temporal artery can be found at the temple and is occasionally used in neonates, but is difficult to place well and is easily displaced by a moving child. The femoral artery is found just distal to the inguinal ligament between the pubic tubercle and anterior superior iliac spine. As it is the largest peripheral artery it is the easiest to cannulate, making it a popular choice in small neonates and infants or in emergent situations. The posterior tibial is found posterior to the medial malleolus and the dorsalis pedis is found on the dorsum

of the foot. As they are the farthest point in the body from the heart, both arteries will have grossly overestimated SBPs and underestimated DBPs. Placement should never be attempted in both a dorsalis pedis and posterior tibial artery on the same limb as the arteries form a collateral network and blocking both would cut all circulation to the foot.

A unique option for catheterization in the neonate is the umbilical artery, which compared to other artery choices offers both major benefits and potentially devastating complications. As it is used in neonates that are usually in an intensive care setting who may need months of inpatient treatment, the umbilical artery is often used first as it spares other sites that may be needed for catheterization in the future. It is the only artery that also can be a route for medication administration. Umbilical catheters are placed by identifying and puncturing one of the two umbilical arteries on the umbilical cord and advancing a catheter into the descending aorta. As the neonate is very small, even a slight movement of the catheter can result in occlusion of major vessels and ischemia. A short list of things that can be occluded by umbilical catheters includes the iliac, femoral, and brachial arteries, chambers of the heart itself, and, if it were to traverse a patent ductus arteriosus, the pulmonary artery. Catheters can also cause infection, embolic events, vascular puncture and hemorrhage, and arrhythmias [35].

## Risk/Safety Profile of Arterial Lines

In general, arterial lines are very safe and have a low rate of infection – lowest if inserted with sterile technique [36,37]. As it is highly invasive, the cut-down technique is associated with a higher rate of infection [38].

A concern in children who will undergo multiple arterial cannulations, such as those with congenital heart disease, is occlusion and eventual scarring of the artery. Pediatric patients have higher rates of arterial occlusion after catheter placement; however, this typically resolves several days after removal. Placement by the cut-down technique or prolonged catheterization makes occlusion less likely to resolve [39]. Hematoma formation is another threat to arterial flow that may be reduced with fewer arterial punctures and, potentially, the use of ultrasound for placement [31]. Blood loss must also not be forgotten during placement and subsequent blood draws, especially in neonates and small infants with low blood volumes. Losses during sampling draws can be decreased by using shorter lengths of tubing between the artery and the stopcock. Blood loss can also be a result of low pressure in the tubing due to a disconnection from the pressure bag or a lack of pressure in the bag, with either scenario having the potential to cause life-threatening hemorrhage.

## Central Venous Access and Central Venous Pressure

Obtaining central venous access is indicated when there is a lack of adequate peripheral access, the need for vasopressors or other medications that are hazardous when administered peripherally, measurement of central venous pressure (CVP), and, during high-risk cases, aspiration of air emboli from the heart. Central lines are placed most often in the internal jugular, femoral, or subclavian veins, but can also be inserted into the external jugular or basilar veins in some cases. In neonates the umbilical vein can be accessed in a similar method as the umbilical artery. Umbilical vein catheters have many of the same hazards as their arterial counterparts, most notably potential migration and subsequent venous obstruction in the liver.

## Placement of Central Venous Catheters

The techniques for locating large veins in infants are similar to those used in adults. The basilar, external jugular, and umbilical veins can be directly visualized for puncture. The palpation and landmark techniques used for subclavian, femoral, and internal jugular lines in adults can be used in the same manner in pediatric patients, although it should be noted that the internal jugular vein is often located more cephalad in infants than in older children and adults. Ultrasound-guided line placement was widely used in infants before becoming routine in adults, can be used to locate any of the commonly cannulated large veins, and has been demonstrated to improve success rates, reduce carotid artery punctures, and increase the speed of placement [40,41].

Regardless of how the vein is located, the Seldinger technique is typically used to place the line. A needle attached to a syringe with negative pressure applied by the inserter is advanced until blood is aspirated into the syringe, confirming placement in the vein. The syringe is then removed and a wire advanced into the vein so the needle can be removed; during this stage it is essential that the ECG be monitored as the wire can cause arrhythmias if it is advanced too far and comes into contact with the walls of the heart. After widening the opening in the skin with a skin blade, a dilator is inserted over the wire and then removed to clear a path for the catheter. The catheter is then advanced into place and the wire removed. Catheters placed in the basilar, external jugular, internal jugular, and subclavian veins may have distal tips capable of reaching the heart. Care must be taken to make sure the tip of the catheter does not sit within the heart – to accomplish this, central venous catheters that are going to be used long-term are often placed in the operating room under fluoroscopy. If the clinician wishes to monitor CVP, the catheter should terminate at the junction between the superior vena cava and the right atrium.

The complications of central lines are the same as those in adults. Infection is a common complication and unless placed in an emergency all central venous lines should be inserted using sterile preparation, draping, and technique. Catheter migration into the heart may cause arrhythmia and all catheters should have placement confirmed radiographically. Pneumothorax is a concern for internal jugular and subclavian lines. Bleeding can also be significant if

CVP is high or placement is prolonged. Inferior vena cava thrombosis was detected in six of 56 children with femoral lines in one study [42]. All of these children had their catheters for more than six days, and it is thus recommended that catheters be monitored for thrombosis or changed after six days.

## Measurement of CVP

A properly placed central line can be used to obtain CVP, the pressure recorded at the junction of the right atrium and superior vena cava. Continuous monitoring of pressure in the central vein creates a tracing with three ascents: the a-wave, which is caused by atrial contraction; the c-wave, which is caused by ventricular contraction and upward tricuspid displacement; and the v-wave, which is the result of rapid venous filling against a closed tricuspid valve. The number reported as the CVP is the value obtained at end-expiration and has long been used as a surrogate marker for volume status. Recent work in adults [43] has called into question whether CVP correlates with volume status, although many still use it in conjunction with other data to assess volume status.

## Pulmonary Artery Catheters

Although infrequently placed in pediatric patients, pulmonary artery catheters can provide useful measurement of cardiac output, mixed venous oxygen saturation, and pressures in the right atrium, right ventricle, and pulmonary artery. This information can be useful, especially in the setting of abnormal cardiac physiology, particularly in cardiac surgical patients with severe pulmonary hypertension or anatomical defects [44]. However, interpretation in these children requires a flexible interpretation of normal values as significant shunting or anatomical abnormalities can result in major changes in readings at baseline.

Pulmonary artery catheters are placed through central venous catheters, typically an internal jugular, subclavian, or femoral line. The size of infants makes placement extremely difficult and is fraught with complications including infection, arrhythmia, pulmonary artery rupture, and bleeding. A recent review [45] showed that although there was no increase in mortality from pulmonary artery catheter placement, there was also little evidence in favor of placement in pediatric patients.

## Transesophageal Echocardiography

Transesophageal echocardiography (TEE) is an increasingly utilized method for monitoring cardiac function during both cardiac and noncardiac surgery. Its efficacy has been demonstrated in cardiac surgery for diagnosing intraoperative problems and guiding medical and surgical therapy [46]. Transesophageal echocardiography must be used cautiously in infants and neonates because the heavy probe can cause compression of vascular and respiratory structures, as well as esophageal perforation and vagal responses. As a result, its use is limited to situations where TEE information may change the course of a procedure or provide vital diagnostic or physiologic information.

## Respiratory Monitoring

Neonates and infants have multiple anatomic and physiologic features that make them prone to perioperative respiratory events. At birth a neonate has a rate of oxygen consumption twice that of an adult, a smaller functional residual capacity while anesthetized, and a variety of airway features that leave little room for error during anesthesia. After anesthesia, many remain at a high risk for respiratory events including apnea of prematurity [47]. A strong understanding and awareness of respiratory monitors is therefore essential for pediatric anesthesiologists.

## Pulse Oximetry

The pulse oximeter determines oxygen saturation via a probe placed on a peripheral location, often a finger or toe, sometimes the earlobe or forehead. The probe emits light at two specific wavelengths, which are absorbed differently by oxygenated and deoxygenated blood, allowing the oximeter to determine the percentage of hemoglobin that is oxygenated via an algorithm. The pulse oximeter also uses plethysmography to determine pulsatile flow and report saturation information during systolic beats. In this way, the pulse oximeter is also a sensitive monitor of peripheral perfusion.

The pulse oximeter has been used in children since early in its clinical life. One of the first studies on the effectiveness of the pulse oximeter was performed on children and showed that practitioners blinded to pulse oximetry data had more hypoxic events and were slower to identify hypoxic events than those who had the data available, although there was no difference in overall morbidity [48]. A follow-up study that added capnography [49] identified the pulse oximeter as the best monitor for identifying desaturation events and a serviceable one for detecting events typically identified by capnography, such as esophageal intubation or endotracheal tube kinking, although capnography and pulse oximetry together showed the best overall results.

Several considerations are relevant for accurate pulse oximetry use in pediatrics. The pulse oximeter is disrupted by any kind of motion [50], making it somewhat impractical in awake children such as those being induced via mask. Skin color and thickness minimally affect accuracy. Environmental factors can affect pulse oximeter signals. Electrocautery and some types of lighting can interfere with readings [50]. Nail polish, especially blue and green in color, can artificially decrease oximeter readings [51]. Stereotactic guidance systems, often used for neurosurgical procedures, use infrared light and disrupt pulse oximeter signals [52], although this can be averted by placing an opaque wrapping over a probed finger. If there is concern for inaccurate readings during a procedure, two pulse oximeters are often used in different locations.

Pigments within the bloodstream also affect oximeter signals based on their light absorption spectra. Intravenous dyes, such as methylene blue, indigo carmine, and indocyanine green can all falsely decrease readings [50]. Abnormal hemoglobins and related pigments may also alter readings. Fetal hemoglobin, carboxyhemoglobin, and bilirubin do not affect signals, but the presence of methemoglobin will decrease readings, classically to 85 percent, regardless of the actual saturation [50]. If methemoglobin or carboxyhemoglobin levels are suspected to be high they can be detected by multiwave pulse oximeters (CO-oximeters) that use extra wavelengths of light to identify different forms of hemoglobin [53,54].

Placement of pulse oximeters requires special attention in infants with congenital heart disease. Pulse oximeters are designed to be most accurate at higher saturations and tend to lose accuracy at lower ones, especially saturations lower than 80 percent [55], which may limit their use in children with cyanotic lesions or lung disease. Patients with patent ductus arteriosus may have a variety of readings depending on where the probe is placed. A preductal probe on the hand or ear will report preductal saturations and is useful for monitoring cerebral oxygenation. A postductal probe placed on the foot will report postductal

saturations, which is especially important in conditions with significant right-to-left shunting, such as persistent pulmonary hypertension of the newborn. In practice, however, a difference in saturations is not always seen, as the ductus arteriosus often attaches distal to where the left subclavian artery leaves the aorta. A study of newborns revealed no significant decrease in left-hand pulse oximeter saturations during the first four hours of life [56].

# Capnography

By continuously sampling the $CO_2$ levels near the endotracheal tube and graphing the levels in real time, the $CO_2$ analyzer creates an accurate graphical representation of the patient's ventilation, known as the capnograph. Carbon dioxide analyzers use infrared light to measure the $CO_2$ content in the expired gas. The sample can be taken from either a sidestream analyzer, which removes gas from the circuit and analyzes in a separate unit, or via a mainstream analyzer that detects gas in the circuit via a cuvette that is inserted into the tubing. Mainstream analyzers are less prone to obstruction but require cuvette sterilization and replacement. Although they rely on small tubing that can be obstructed with condensation or secretions, sidestream analyzers are the most common in practice today.

Capnography is used in anesthesia to monitor gas exchange during anesthesia with or without an endotracheal tube. When used to guide mechanical ventilation settings, continuous capnography has been shown to decrease intraoperative hyper- and hypoventilation in children [49]. The monitor is also accurate for monitoring respiration during sedation via long tubing with nasal cannula or facemask when the patient may not be immediately accessible, such as during MRI procedures [57]. Capnography is also used to diagnose events manifested by altered end-tidal $CO_2$ readings, such as esophageal intubation, hypoventilation, circulatory arrest, pulmonary embolism, or bronchospasm [58,59]. Hypercarbia is among the most sensitive signs for malignant hyperthermia and the capnograph can be used to both diagnose and guide treatment [60]. Endotracheal tube kinking or disconnection is also easily detected [61].

Capnography can be difficult in children due to their size and respiratory physiology, both of which contribute to widening of the alveolar $CO_2$ ($PACO_2$) to end-tidal $CO_2$ ($ETCO_2$) gradient. Sidestream analyzers typically aspirate 50 ml min$^{-1}$, and fresh gas can be entrained if tidal volumes are low and the aspiration rate nears the expiratory flow rate – thus smaller children tend to have higher $PACO_2$ to $ETCO_2$ gradients [62]. Small tidal volumes also mean that to ensure minimal mixing with fresh gas, the sampling should be done as close to the patient as possible. The shape of the capnograph is often rounded at the peaks and troughs in pediatric patients, which is an artifact that can be caused by high respiratory rate or leak around an uncuffed tube. Cardiopulmonary pathology can also result in underreported $CO_2$ levels, such as in the presence of a left-to-right shunt or severely decreased cardiac output.

## Inhaled and End-Tidal Gas Monitoring

In most modern anesthesia machines, the sidestream aspirator used to deliver $CO_2$ for capnography is also used to deliver gases for analysis of inhaled anesthetics, nitrous oxide, and oxygen by infrared spectroscopy. Monitoring of oxygen allows for avoidance of delivery of a hypoxic gas mixture while monitoring of inhaled agents helps prevent over- or underanesthetizing the patient. Although the monitor may reliably report the concentration of inhaled anesthetic, this information should not be mistaken for a measurement of the depth of anesthesia, which requires an assimilation of information from physical examination and various monitors by the anesthesiologist. Pediatric patients come for surgery at many stages of development and the level of anesthetic needed for each will vary.

Older anesthesia machines may use mass spectroscopy to measure end-tidal gases, which allows for the measurement of end-tidal nitrogen ($ETN_2$). End-tidal nitrogen can be used to determine when nitrogen washout has been satisfactorily completed during preoxygenation, and was shown to detect air emboli more quickly than $ETCO_2$ in a canine model [63]. As modern anesthesia machines almost exclusively use infrared spectroscopy for gas analysis, $ETN_2$ is rarely used in today's practice.

## Temperature Monitoring

Neonates and infants are at a high risk for intraoperative hypothermia; a full discussion of temperature regulation is found in Chapter 8. The induction of general anesthesia relaxes the body's tight control of core temperature, making patients vulnerable to various forms of heat loss in the operating room: radiant heat loss to the cold operating room; conductive loss from cold intravenous fluids or blood products; evaporative heat loss from exposed skin or viscera or from the airways during mechanical ventilation; and convective heat loss to the air or breathing circuit [64]. Conversely, hyperthermia can also be a threat due to aggressive warming techniques or malignant hyperthermia. Because pediatric patients have a high surface area to volume ratio and often have less fat tissue for insulation, temperature monitoring and modulation with appropriate warming or cooling mechanisms is standard for most procedures and essential for those involving tight temperature control, such as procedures requiring cardiopulmonary bypass.

The most common thermometers used in operating rooms are disposable thermistors or thermocouples. A thermistor contains a semiconductor that changes resistance with a change in temperature. A thermocouple is a circuit made of two different metals as electrodes. One of the electrodes is kept at a fixed temperature while the other is placed distally on the probe and used to measure the patient's temperature. The difference in temperatures creates a gradient in the circuit that results in the flow of current, with the degree of flow used to determine the temperature on the probe. Thermistors and thermocouples can be used for monitoring in essentially any location. Skin temperature can also be monitored by liquid crystal thermometry. These thermometers are typically strips placed on the forehead that change color when a specific temperature is reached, but they are typically less accurate and should be reserved for simple procedures where tight temperature control is not essential [65].

The location to monitor temperature is based on accuracy, safety, ease of placement, and operative considerations. For most procedures the goal of temperature monitoring is to reflect the core temperature, which is the temperature of central tissues that receive the majority of the blood flow. Peripheral tissues are often cooler than the core compartment and in general the more peripheral the site, the greater the discrepancy with core temperature due to environmental factors [66].

Nasopharyngeal monitoring is considered safe in the absence of anatomic defects in the region (e.g., basilar skull fracture) and accurately reflects core temperature when placed in contact with the soft palate. It is ideal for monitoring of brain temperature during cardiopulmonary bypass. Nasopharyngeal monitors can lose accuracy if they are not placed in contact with the soft palate, are placed too high in the oropharynx, or come into contact with cold respiratory gases, such as when an uncuffed tube with a significant leak is placed.

Esophageal probes also accurately reflect core temperature and are easy to place. They can be combined with an esophageal stethoscope as a single piece of equipment to insert. Ideally they should be placed in the distal esophagus where the heart sounds are loudest. In small children, esophageal probes can come into close contact with the airways, which can skew the measurement based on inspired air temperature [67]. It may also be less accurate during cardiac or thoracic procedures with an open chest.

The axilla is a convenient, noninvasive location for temperature monitoring that can accurately reflect core temperature if placed correctly [67]. It is essential that the probe is in tight contact with the skin for an accurate reading. Axillary probes come into contact with several mechanisms that can reduce their accuracy, such as intravenous fluids being infused through the ipsilateral arm or external warming blankets.

The skin is an easy, noninvasive monitoring location that is considered less accurate than the others mentioned, especially as the sensor is placed in more peripheral locations [67]. A recent study suggested that measuring skin temperature over the carotid artery accurately reflected core temperature provided that a correction factor of 0.52 °C was added to the reading [68].

Rectal temperature is considered accurate for procedures that do not involve heating or cooling of the abdomen or pelvis. Accuracy can also be lowered by large amounts of stool in the rectum which reduce contact with the mucosa. Rectal probes cannot be placed in patients with an imperforate anus and should be avoided in patients at risk for serious damage should trauma occur to the rectum, such as those with friable tissues (e.g., inflammatory bowel disease) or coagulopathy. Rectal temperatures also lag esophageal and nasopharyngeal measurements in active cooling and warming during cardiopulmonary bypass procedures [69].

Bladder temperature can be measured via a probe inserted as part of a Foley catheter. It is accurate in most conditions but, similar to rectal monitoring, it lags other locations during rapid changes in cardiopulmonary bypass procedures [69].

Pulmonary artery catheters provide very accurate measurements of core temperature, but as pulmonary artery catheters are infrequently placed and involve considerable risks of perforation or arrhythmia, they are uncommonly used. During cardiopulmonary bypass the catheter is isolated from circulation and unusable.

The tympanic membrane is traditionally used as the gold standard for temperature monitoring as it approximates the temperature of the hypothalamus [70], although it has not been shown that hypothalamic temperature reflects core temperature. The probe is inserted into the external auditory canal but should not contact the tympanic membrane itself, as it can cause damage to the delicate structures within the ear. This location is used infrequently for continuous monitoring as studies have demonstrated that other sites can accurately reflect core temperature with easier placement and less risk [66,67].

# References

1. Kochanek PM, Carney N, Adelson PD, et al. Guidelines for the acute medical management of severe traumatic brain injury in infants, children, and adolescents: second edition. *Pediatr Crit Care Med.* 2012;13(S1):S1–82.

2. Sigl JC, Chamoun NG. An introduction to bispectral analysis for the electroencephalogram. *J Clin Monit.* 1994;10(6):392–404.

3. Sadhasivam S, Ganesh A, Robison A, Kaye R, Watcha MF. Validation of the bispectral index monitor for measuring depth of sedation in children. *Anesth Analg.* 2006;102(2):383–8.

4. Denman WT, Swanson EL, Rosow D, et al. Pediatric evaluation of the bispectral index (BIS) monitor and correlation of BIS with end-tidal sevoflurane concentration in infants and children. *Anesth Analg.* 2000;90(4):872–7.

5. Choudhry DK, Brenn BR. Bispectral index monitoring: a comparison between normal children and children with quadriplegic cerebral palsy. *Anesth Analg.* 2002;95(6):1582–5.

6. Malviya S, Voepel-Lewis T, Tait AR, et al. Effect of age and sedative agent on the accuracy of bispectral index in detecting depth of sedation in children. *Pediatrics.* 2007;120(3):461–70.

7. Myles PS, Leslie K, McNeil J, Forbes A, Chan MT. Bispectral index monitoring to prevent awareness during anaesthesia: the B-Aware randomised controlled trial. *Lancet.* 2004;363(9423):1757–63.

8. Avidan MS, Zhang L, Burnside BA, et al. Anesthesia awareness and the bispectral index. *NEJM*. 2008;358:1097–108.

9. Avidan MS, Jacobsohn E, Glick D, et al. Prevention of intraoperative awareness in a high-risk surgical population. *NEJM*. 2011;365:591–600.

10. Davidson AJ, Huang GH, Czarnecki C, et al. Awareness during anesthesia in children: a prospective cohort study. *Anesth Analg*. 2005;100(3):653–61.

11. Tortoriello TA, Stayer SA, Mott AR, et al. A noninvasive estimation of mixed venous oxygen saturation using near-infrared spectroscopy by cerebral oximetry in pediatric cardiac surgery patients. *Paediatr Anaesth*. 2005;15:495–503.

12. Gottlieb EA, Fraser CD Jr., Andropoulos DB, Diaz LK. Bilateral monitoring of cerebral oxygen saturation results in recognition of aortic cannula malposition during pediatric congenital heart surgery. *Paediatr Anaesth*. 2006;16(7):787–9.

13. Kurth CD, Steven JM, Nicolson SC. Cerebral oxygenation during pediatric cardiac surgery using deep hypothermic circulatory arrest. *Anesthesiology*. 1995;82(1):74–82.

14. Burrows FA, Bissonnette B. Monitoring the adequacy of cerebral perfusion during cardiopulmonary bypass in children using transcranial Doppler technology. *J Neurosurg Anesthesiol*. 1993;5(3):209–12.

15. Kontos HA. Validity of cerebral arterial blood flow calculations from velocity measurements. *Stroke*. 1989;20(1):1–3.

16. O'Brien JJ, Butterworth J, Hammon JW, et al. Cerebral emboli during cardiac surgery in children. *Anesthesiology*. 1997;87(5):1063–9.

17. Shen Q, Stuart J, Venkatesh B, et al. Inter observer variability of the transcranial Doppler ultrasound technique: impact of lack of practice on the accuracy of measurement. *J Clin Monit Comput*. 1999;15(3–4):179–84.

18. Nuwer MR, Dawson EG, Carlson LG, Kanim LE, Sherman JE. Somatosensory evoked potential spinal cord monitoring reduces neurologic deficits after scoliosis surgery: results of a large multicenter survey. *Electroencephalogr Clin Neurophysiol*. 1995;96(1):6–11.

19. Hyun SJ, Rhim SC, Kang JK, Hong SH, Park BR. Combined motor- and somatosensory-evoked potential monitoring for spine and spinal cord surgery: correlation of clinical and neurophysiological data in 85 consecutive procedures. *Spinal Cord*. 2009;47(8):616–22.

20. Meakin GH. Neuromuscular blocking drugs in infants and children. *Contin Educ Anaesth Crit Care Pain*. 2007;7:143–7.

21. Goudzousian NG. Maturation of neuromuscular transmission in the infant. *Br J Anaesth*. 1980;52:205–14.

22. Goudzousian NG, Crone RK, Todres ID. Recovery from pancuronium blockade in the neonatal intensive care unit. *Br J Anaesth*. 1981;53:1303–9.

23. Gwinnutt CL, Meakin G. Use of the post-tetanic count to monitor recovery from intense neuromuscular blockade in children. *Br J Anaesth*. 1988;61:547–50.

24. Kliegman RM, Stanton B, St. Geme J, Schor N, Behrman R. *Nelson Textbook of Pediatrics*, 19th edn. Philadelphia, PA: Elsevier Saunders; 2011.

25. Manecke GR Jr., Nemirov MA, Bicker AA, Adsumelli RN, Poppers PJ. The effect of halothane on the amplitude and frequency characteristics of heart sounds in children. *Anesth Analg*. 1999;88(2):263–7.

26. Nezfati MH, Soltani G, Kahrom M. Esophageal stethoscope: an old tool with a new role, detection of residual flow during video-assisted thoracoscopic patent ductus arteriosus closure. *J Pediatr Surg*. 2010;45(11):2141–5.

27. Doniger SJ, Sharieff GQ. Pediatric dysrhythmias. *Pediatr Clin North Am*. 2006;53(1):85–105.

28. Karvonen MJ, Telivuo LJ, Jaervinen EJ. Sphygmomanometer cuff size and the accuracy of indirect measurement of blood pressure. *Am J Cardiol*. 1964;13:688–93.

29. Arafat M, Mattoo TK. Measurement of blood pressure in children: recommendations and perceptions on cuff selection. *Pediatrics*. 1999;104:e30.

30. Ganesh A, Kaye R, Cahill AM, et al. Evaluation of ultrasound-guided radial artery cannulation in children. *Pediatr Crit Care Med*. 2009;10(1):45–8.

31. Ishii S, Shime N, Shibasaki M, Sawa T. Ultrasound-guided radial artery catheterization in infants and small children. *Pediatr Crit Care Med*. 2013;14(5):471–3.

32. Schwemmer U, Arzet HA, Trautner H, et al. Ultrasound-guided arterial cannulation in infants improves success rate. *Eur J Anaesth*. 2006;23(6):476–80.

33. Lo RN, Leung MP, Lau KC, Yeung CY. Abnormal radial artery in Down's syndrome. *Arch Dis Child*. 1986;61(9):885–90.

34. Schindler E, Kowald B, Suess H, et al. Catheterization of the radial or brachial artery in neonates and infants. *Paediatr Anaesth*. 2005;15(8):677–82.

35. Green C, Yohannan MD. Umbilical arterial and venous catheters: placement, use, and complications. *Neonatal Netw*. 1998;17(6):23–8.

36. Furfaro S, Gauthier M, Lacroix J, et al. Arterial catheter-related infections in children: a 1-year cohort analysis. *Am J Dis Child.* 1991;145(9):1037–43.

37. Ducharme FM, Gauthier M, Lacroix J, Lafleur L. Incidence of infection related to arterial catheterization in children: a prospective study. *Crit Care Med.* 1988;16(3):272–6.

38. Band JD, Maki DG. Infections caused by arterial catheters used for hemodynamic monitoring. *Am J Med.* 1979;67(5):735–41.

39. Miyasaka K, Edmonds JF, Conn AW. Complications of radial artery lines in the paediatric patient. *Can Anaesth Soc J.* 1976;23(1):9–14.

40. Verghese ST, McGill WA, Patel RI, et al. Ultrasound-guided internal jugular venous cannulation in infants: a prospective comparison with the traditional palpation method. *Anesthesiology.* 1999;91(1):71–7.

41. Chuan WX, Wei W, Yu L. A randomized-controlled study of ultrasound prelocation vs anatomical landmark-guided cannulation of the internal jugular vein in infants and children. *Paediatr Anaesth.* 2005;15(9):733–8.

42. Shefler A, Gillis J, Lam A, et al. Inferior vena cava thrombosis as a complication of femoral vein catheterization. *Arch Dis Child.* 1995;72(4):343–5.

43. Marik PE, Baram M, Vahid B. Does central venous pressure predict fluid responsiveness? A systematic review of the literature and the tale of seven mares. *Chest.* 2008;134(1):172–8.

44. Damen J, Wever JE. The use of balloon-tipped pulmonary artery catheters in children undergoing cardiac surgery. *Intensive Care Med.* 1987;13(4):266–72.

45. Perkin RM, Anas N. Pulmonary artery catheters. *Pediatr Crit Care Med.* 2011;12(Suppl. 4):S12–20.

46. Bettex DA, Schmidlin D, Bernath MA, et al. Intraoperative transesophageal echocardiography in pediatric congenital cardiac surgery: a two-center observational study. *Anesth Analg.* 2003;97(5):1275–82.

47. Cote CJ, Zaslavsky A, Downes JJ, et al. Postoperative apnea in former preterm infants after inguinal herniorrhaphy: a combined analysis. *Anesthesiology.* 1995;82(4):809–22.

48. Cote CJ, Goldstein EA, Cote MA, Hoaglin DC, Ryan JF. A single-blind study of pulse oximetry in children. *Anesthesiology.* 1988;68(2):184–8.

49. Cote CJ, Rolf N, Liu LM, et al. A single-blind study of combined pulse oximetry and capnography in children. *Anesthesiology.* 1991;74(6):980–7.

50. Ralston AC, Webb RK, Runciman WB. Potential errors in pulse oximetry: III. Effects of interferences, dyes, dyshaemoglobins and other pigments. *Anaesthesia.* 1991;46(4):291–5.

51. Cote CJ, Goldstein EA, Fuchsman WH, Hoaglin DC. The effect of nail polish on pulse oximetry. *Anesth Analg.* 1988;67(7):683–6.

52. van Oostrom JH, Mahla ME, Gravenstein D. The Stealth Station Image Guidance System may interfere with pulse oximetry. *Can J Anaesth.* 2005;52(4):379–82.

53. Annabi EH, Barker SJ. Severe methemoglobinemia detected by pulse oximetry. *Anesth Analg.* 2009;108(3):898–9.

54. Suner S, Partridge R, Sucov A, et al. Non-invasive pulse CO-oximetry screening in the emergency department identifies occult carbon monoxide toxicity. *J Emerg Med.* 2008;34(4):441–50.

55. Webb RK, Ralston AC, Runciman WB. Potential errors in pulse oximetry: II. Effects of changes in saturation and signal quality. *Anaesthesia.* 1991;46(3):207–12.

56. Rüegger C, Bucher HU, Mieth RA. Pulse oximetry in the newborn: is the left hand pre- or post-ductal? *BMC Pediatr.* 2010;10:35.

57. Mason KP, Burrows PE, Dorsey MM, Zurakowski D, Krauss B. Accuracy of capnography with a 30 foot nasal cannula for monitoring respiratory rate and end-tidal CO2 in children. *J Clin Monit.* 2000;16:259–62.

58. Williamson JA, Webb RK, Cockings J, Morgan C. The Australian Incident Monitoring Study: the capnograph – applications and limitations. An analysis of 2000 incident reports. *Anaesth Intensive Care.* 1993;21(5):551–7.

59. Westhorpe RN, Ludbrook GL, Helps SC. Crisis management during anaesthesia: bronchospasm. *Qual Saf Health Care.* 2005;14:e7.

60. Baudendistel L, Goudsouzian N, Cote C, Strafford M. End-tidal CO2 monitoring: its use in the diagnosis and management of malignant hyperthermia. *Anaesthesia.* 1984;39(10):1000–3.

61. Cote CJ, Liu LM, Szyfelbein SK, et al. Intraoperative events diagnosed by expired carbon dioxide monitoring in children. *Can Anaesth Soc J.* 1986;33(3 Pt 1):315–20.

62. Badgwell JM, McLeod ME, Lerman J, Creighton RE. End-tidal PCO2 measurements sampled at the distal and proximal ends of the endotracheal tube in infants and children. *Anesth Analg.* 1987;66(10):959–64.

63. Matjasko J, Petrozza P, Mackenzie CF. Sensitivity of end-tidal nitrogen in venous air embolism detection in dogs. *Anesthesiology.* 1985;63(4):418–23.

64. Nilsson K. Maintenance and monitoring of body temperature in infants and children. *Paediatr Anaesth.* 1991;1:13–20.

65. Burgess GE 3rd, Cooper JR, Marino RJ, Peuler MJ. Continuous monitoring of skin temperature using a liquid-crystal thermometer during anesthesia. *South Med J.* 1978;71:516–18.

66. Cork RC, Vaughan RW, Humphrey LS. Precision and accuracy of intraoperative temperature monitoring. *Anesth Analg.* 1983;62:211–14.

67. Bissonnette B, Sessler DI, LaFlamme P. Intraoperative temperature monitoring sites in infants and children and the effect of inspired gas warming on esophageal temperature. *Anesth Analg.* 1989;69:192–6.

68. Jay O, Molgat-Seon Y, Chou S, Murto K. Skin temperature over the carotid artery provides an accurate noninvasive estimation of core temperature in infants and young children during general anesthesia. *Pediatr Anesth.* 2013;23(12):1109–16.

69. Moorthy SS, Winn BA, Jallard MS, et al. Monitoring urinary bladder temperature. *Heart Lung.* 1985:14:90–3.

70. Benzinger TH. Heat regulation: homeostasis of central temperature in man. *Physiol Rev.* 1969;49:671–759.

Chapter

# 20

# Anesthesia for Neurosurgical Procedures

Roby Sebastian and Craig D. McClain

## Introduction

The central nervous system (CNS) is a complicated network of neurons that integrates a myriad of sensory input from both inside and outside the body and effects motor responses. The CNS consists of neurons, oligodendrites, and support cells such as microglia. Abnormal CNS development can result in devastating injury to young children, making the administration of general anesthesia very challenging. In order to successfully care for children undergoing neurosurgical procedures, it is essential to understand the interaction between the disordered CNS and the anesthetic milieu. In this chapter we review the general principles of anesthetic management of infants and neonates undergoing neurosurgical procedures. The purpose of this chapter is not to give recipes for treating infants and neonates for various neurosurgical procedures. Rather, we hope to give the reader an understanding of the variety of anesthetic considerations when caring for babies that are neurosurgical patients.

## Development of the Central Nervous System

Many of the neurosurgical conditions seen in infants occur because of abnormal fetal development. Thus a basic understanding of the embryologic development of the nervous system is helpful to comprehend the variety of neurologic conditions that affect young infants and neonates.

## Beginning of the Nervous System

During the third week of fetal development, the ectoderm differentiates into the neuroplate. This neuroplate folds upon itself to form the neural groove. There are two neural folds which form along each side of the neural groove. Neurulation begins at the fourth week of development, when the neural folds fuse dorsally to create the neural tube. The spinal ganglia, cranial nerves, and components of the peripheral and autonomic nervous system are derived from neural crest cells which are located adjacent to the neural folds. The neural tube fuses in a central to caudal and central to cranial direction, creating the neural canal. The small holes remaining at each end of the neural tube fuse at days 25 and 27 days concomitantly with the development of the vascular supply to the neural tube. The ventricular system and central canal of the CNS develops from the neural canal, with the walls of the neural tube forming the brain and spinal cord.

## Development of the Spinal Cord

The spinal cord develops from the caudal end of the neural tube, with the neural canal becoming the central canal at about ten weeks' gestation. The cells of the neural tube differentiate into two different layers; the ependymal layer which becomes neurons, astrocytes, and oligodendrocytes, and the marginal layer which becomes the white matter as axons grow into this area from spinal cord neurons. The sulcus limitans is a longitudinal groove which forms on each side of the fetal spinal cord. This groove forms a separation between the dorsal or afferent portion of the spinal cord from the ventral or efferent portion of the spinal cord. The mesenchymal cells surrounding the protospinal cord differentiate into the dura mater, pia mater, and arachnoid mater. These meninges become fluid filled as cerebrospinal fluid (CSF) is produced during the fifth week of development, which forms the subarachnoid space.

As the spinal cord is developing, the cranial portion of the neural tube undergoes rapid growth and turning, with the neural canal forming the cranial ventricular canal. It is believed by many authors that normal development of the ventricular canal system is dependent of the caudal closure of the neural tube, which causes an increase in intraluminal pressure which stimulates brain growth and ventricular enlargement. This is one possible explanation for the finding that infants with open neural tube defects of the spinal cord, such as meningomyeloceles, very often have associated abnormalities of their brain and ventricular system.

## Physiology

### Intracranial Contents

After infancy the cranial vault should be considered a closed space that is normally occupied by three components: the brain and interstitial fluid comprising 80 percent of the volume; the CSF comprising 10 percent of the volume; and the blood comprising 10 percent of the total volume. The Monro-Kellie hypothesis, which states that the sum of all intracranial components are constant, necessitates that an increase in the volume of one component demands a decrease in volume of one or two of the remaining components in children in whom the sutures and fontanelles are closed. Infants with their unfused sutures and open fontanelles can tolerate slow increases in intracranial volumes [1]. Thus a child with an increase in head circumference should be evaluated for a space-occupying brain lesion or hydrocephalus even if there are no signs of increased intracranial pressure. Rapid increases in the volume of CSF or growth of a space-occupying lesion such as a brain tumor even in a young infant will overwhelm the infant's ability to increase the size of his cranial volume, leading to brain herniation as a result of acute elevations of intracranial pressure (ICP).

### Intracranial Pressure

The normal ICP in children is <15 mmHg and < 6mmHg in infants. The normal ICP for premature infants is not known. In infants with open fontanelles, the ICP may remain normal even in the setting of significant intracranial pathology. Careful physical examination should always include an examination of the fontanelles. Full or bulging fontanelles can be a sign of intracranial disease. Often the first sign of intracranial disease in an infant is a normal steady state ICP with occasional ICP pressure waves. These pressure waves should never be considered normal.

Other infants will manifest an elevation of ICP despite open fontanelles. These elevations of ICP can cause either cerebral ischemia and/or brain herniation leading to secondary brain injury. Elevations of the ICP without concomitant elevations of mean arterial pressure (MAP) will result in a decrease in cerebral perfusion pressure (CPP), which can result in cerebral ischemia.

With a decrease in CPP, cerebral blood flow (CBF) decreases. This results in decreased delivery of metabolic substrates and oxygen. Cell damage then occurs, which leads to cell death and an increase in inflammatory mediators, a cascade causing further increases in extracellular water and exacerbating the elevation in ICP. As CPP falls, neuronal dysfunction and ultimately cell death occur [1].

In addition to decreasing cerebral perfusion pressure, elevations of ICP can lead to brain herniation. This occurs when intracranial contents herniate from one compartment into another, leading to further brain ischemia and injury. Transtentorial herniation occurs when the temporal lobe displaces into the infratentorial space. Infants will show signs of hemiparesis, pupillary dilation, and eventual loss of consciousness. This is a medical emergency that will lead to death if the condition is not expeditiously relieved. The clinical signs of elevated ICP are less reliable in infants and children. Infants may exhibit signs of papilledema, hypertension, and bradycardia, but have normal ICP. Or infants with elevated ICP may show no clinical signs at all [2,3]. Classically, young children with chronically elevated ICP will have headaches, irritability, decreased oral intake, and morning emesis without papilledema [4]. Late signs include alterations in the level of consciousness, with children exhibiting abnormal responses to painful stimuli [2]. Depending on the level of obtundation, general anesthesia or sedation may be needed to evaluate these patients. Imaging studies are most commonly done, such as cranial X-rays, computed tomography (CT), and magnetic resonance imaging (MRI). These studies often reveal a decrease or obliteration of the lateral ventricles, hydrocephalus, midline shift, and/or obliteration of the third and fourth ventricles.

### Cerebrospinal Fluid

Cerebrospinal fluid is produced by the choroid plexus at the rate of 0.35 ml per minute in both infants and adults [5,6], resulting in approximately 500 ml produced per day in adults [5]. However, the total volume of CSF in the subarachnoid space in adults is only 100–150 ml, meaning that the CSF is replaced several times during the day. The overall volume of

CSF in infants and children is much less than in adults because the subarachnoid space is much smaller. Cerebrospinal fluid production is only marginally affected by elevated ICP.

Arachnoid villi within the subarachnoid space absorb the CSF, which enters the venous system via one-way valves between the subarachnoid space and the sagittal sinus. There is also a limited amount of reabsorption that occurs through the ependymal lining of the ventricles. The rate of reabsorption increases with elevation of ICP. Obstruction of the arachnoid villi or obstruction within the ventricular system can lead to decreased absorption. Pathologic processes such as inflammation, infection, intracranial hemorrhage, congenital malformations, and CSF absorption and ICP elevations [2].

## Intracranial Compliance

It is important to estimate the amount of intracranial compliance that an infant or child has before administering a general anesthetic. Intracranial compliance is defined as the ratio of change of ICP over change of intracranial volume. In infants who have greater abilities to compensate for increases in cranial volumes because of their open fontanelles, it is difficult to assess the degree of additional compensation available if needed for general anesthesia. Once the ICP is elevated, it is reasonable to assume that compensatory mechanisms have been overridden. But infants with normal ICP may be at high risk for brain injury with even the small increases in cranial volumes/CBF that may occur with certain anesthetic techniques. Assessment of the fontanelles to determine whether the fontanelle is full in infants suspected of having intracranial pathology is essential before administering a general anesthetic. Although infants have higher compliance than adults because of their sutures and open fontanelles, children have lower compliance than adults. This is thought to be due to a higher ratio of brain water content, less CSF volume, and a higher ratio of brain content to intracranial capacity [1]. Infants with fused cranial sutures are at higher risk than normal infants for developing ICP elevations.

## Cerebral Blood Volume and Cerebral Blood Flow

The cranial compartment most easily manipulated by anesthesiologists is the cerebral blood volume (CBV),

though this compartment only represents 10 percent of the total volume of the cranial contents. Most of the CBF by volume is contained in the low-pressure, high-capacitance venous system. Initially increases in intracranial volume are met with decreases in CBV. Often, venous blood shifts from intracranial to extracranial, as seen in infants with hydrocephalus who develop distended scalp veins [7].

In a normal adult, the CBF is approximately 55 ml per 100 g of brain tissue per minute, which represents approximately 15 percent of the adult cardiac output [8–10]. The CBF is almost double in children, at approximately 100 ml per 100 g of brain tissue per minute, which represents about 25 percent of cardiac output [11,12]. Infants and young children in general have a larger portion of their cardiac output devoted to cerebral perfusion than do adults. Neonates and premature infants appear to have a lower CBF at about 40 ml per 100 g per minute than any other age group. The reasons for this are unclear. There is also greater variability of CBF in neonates and premature infants depending on the physical state of the infant. Cerebral blood flow is decreased during sleep and feeding states [12,13].

Cerebral blood flow in the nonanesthetized state is usually very closely coupled with cerebral metabolic rate for oxygen ($CMRO_2$), which is known as cerebral autoregulation. In adults, $CMRO_2$ is approximately 3.5–4.5 ml $O_2$ per 100 g per minute; in children it is higher, but in premature infants it is lower [11]. Most general anesthetics will depress the $CMRO_2$ by as much as 50 percent, but in very young premature infants these same general anesthetics can be excitotoxic, leading to an increase in $CMRO_2$ [14]. Inadequate CBF will lead to conditions that result in acidosis, such as hypoxemia, hypercarbia, and ischemia. These conditions increase the hydrogen ion concentration within the cerebral blood vessels, which will cause cerebral dilation and thereby increase CBF and CBV. When there is a loss of coupling between $CMRO_2$ and CBF, cerebral autoregulation is impaired. CBF then becomes pressure passive, meaning it varies with the system MAP.

## Cerebrovascular Autoregulation

### Effects of Blood Pressure

Cerebrovascular autoregulation refers to the ability of the brain to have a relatively constant CBF within a MAP range. This range is believed to be between 50 and 150 mmHg in older children and adults. In infants the lower limit of autoregulation is unknown, but studies have shown that there is a decrease in CBF when the MAP in infants less than six months of age is less than 40 mmHg. Cerebral autoregulation can be diminished or abolished by a variety of physiologic disturbances, including extreme prematurity, acidosis, sepsis, cerebral edema, tumors, various medications, and vascular anomalies.

Although the absolute lower limits of autoregulation are undefined in premature and term infants, and are likely to vary within that population, most neonatal intensive care units try to maintain the MAPs in mmHg of their patients as equal to or higher than the gestational age in weeks of the infant. It should be assumed that in critically ill infants there is a loss of cerebral autoregulation and systemic blood pressures should be maintained to ensure adequate cerebral perfusion [15].

Neonates are particularly susceptible to hypoxic events when MAP is too low. Further, these patients are particularly sensitive to drugs that depress myocardial function. The end result is that without meticulous management of blood pressure and ventilation to normocapnia, neonates and infants can suffer significant neurologic injury [16]. We have been conditioned to worry about the neurocognitive effects of anesthetic agents by the relatively recent myriad of literature. Anesthesiologists must first ensure that adequate physiologic parameters are maintained in order to achieve the best possible outcomes in neonates and small children.

### Effects of Oxygen

Oxygen tension also affects CBF at the extremes, with CBF remaining constant over a wide range of oxygen tensions. In adults, when the partial pressure is less than 50 mmHg, CBF begins to increase to the point that at a $PaO_2$ of 15 mmHg the CBF is four times normal in an effort to maintain $O_2$ delivery [17]. This extreme increase in CBF will result in an increase in CBV, which in turn will result in an increase in ICP if the intracranial compliance is low. Hyperoxia conversely will lead to a decrease in CBF. Adults breathing 100 percent $O_2$ will have a 10 percent decrease in CBF while neonates breathing 100 percent $O_2$ will have up to a 33 percent decrease in CBF [9,10,18]. Hyperoxia has many adverse effects on neonates, especially premature neonates, so it is essential to balance adequate oxygen delivery with potential oxygen toxicity.

### Effects of Carbon Dioxide

Carbon dioxide tension and CBF are related in a linear fashion. In adults, a 1 mmHg increase in $PaCO_2$ increases CBF by approximately 2 ml per 100 g per minute [19]. Medically induced hyperventilation will lead to a decrease in CBF and CBV and thus ultimately decrease ICP for a short period of time, and is the basis of treating elevated ICP patients with hyperventilation. Elevations in $PaCO_2$ will increase CBF. There is growing evidence that medically induced hyperventilation is on balance detrimental to most patients, including infants with brain injury, and is generally reserved to acutely treat high spikes of ICP. Cerebral ischemia can be exacerbated in brain-injured children who are treated with moderate hyperventilation for elevations of ICP [20].

## Perioperative Management

## Preoperative Evaluation

It is important to realize that the perioperative period is extremely stressful to both child and family. Parents have concerns about both the immediate risks of general anesthesia as well as the long-term consequences of their infant undergoing a prolonged general anesthetic for a neurosurgical procedure. These issues should be addressed during the preoperative interview in a reassuring manner. A very careful history and review of systems with an emphasis on the neurologic system is essential to obtain from the parents. In addition, it is very important to obtain a history of any coexisting diseases such as pulmonary and cardiac anomalies, prematurity, or evidence of difficult airway issues. Physical examination should focus on the airway, cardiac, pulmonary, and neurologic systems. A thorough history and review of symptoms with particular emphasis on neurological symptoms should be obtained from the parent. A focused physical examination with particular emphasis to the neurological system should be done.

Emergent neurosurgical procedures in infants pose special challenges. In most cases, the infants should be considered as a "full stomach" and airway precautions should be taken to prevent pulmonary aspiration. There may not be resources available to do a complete preoperative evaluation in neonates suspected of having congenital cardiac disease. A transthoracic echocardiogram along with pre- and postductal oxygen saturation on both room air and 100 percent oxygen can discriminate between cardiac and pulmonary disease.

For elective procedures, infants and neonates are fasted before general anesthesia in order to decrease the risk of pulmonary aspiration. It is important to minimize fasting time to decrease the risk of developing dehydration and hypoglycemia. For routine procedures, fasting times for clear liquids should be no more than two hours and for young infants intraoperative glucose monitoring should occur if the infants are not receiving intravenous glucose solutions intraoperatively.

As part of the preoperative evaluation, the anesthesiologist providing care for the infant should evaluate all neuroimaging studies that have been done on the infant in order to assess the type of lesion, location, the presence of intracranial hypertension, the vascular supply, and the risk of perioperative herniation. Most major neurosurgical procedures in infants are associated with intraoperative blood loss. Accordingly, it is necessary to type and crossmatch blood for intraoperative use. It is also important for the anesthesiologist to confer with the surgeon about special neurophysiologic monitoring that may be done intraoperatively in order to plan the optimal general anesthetic.

## Vascular Access and Monitoring

Obtaining adequate intravenous access before incision is essential to conducting a safe general neurosurgical anesthetic. Once the procedure has commenced it is very difficult to place intravenous lines. Two relatively large-bore intravenous lines (larger than 22 gauge) are usually adequate for most procedures. Central venous access can be obtained if peripheral access is difficult. In general, femoral venous access is preferable to internal or external jugular venous access because they are technically easier to place and there is no concern about obstructing cerebral venous drainage. A single lumen central line is preferable to a multilumen central line if rapid transfusion of fluid and blood products is anticipated.

Placement of an intra-arterial catheter for blood sampling and monitoring is also very helpful for procedures in which significant blood loss is anticipated.

The most commonly accessed vessel is the radial artery, but dorsalis pedis and posterior tibialis can also be easily accessed. It is important to zero the transducer at the level of the infant's head in order to get an estimate of the cerebral perfusion pressure (CPP).

Infants undergoing craniotomies, especially in the head-up position, are at increased risk of venous air embolism so precordial Doppler is recommended in addition to standard ASA monitors. During some procedures, electroencephalographic (EEG) and neurophysiologic monitoring are used. Consultation with both the surgeon and neurophysiologist is necessary to coordinate the general anesthetic care.

Keeping the infant warm during neurosurgical procedures can be difficult. Because the head of a neonate is large in comparison with the rest of the body and a larger percentage of cardiac output is directed to the head and upper body, the neonate is at particular risk for significant heat loss during surgery. It is important to use warming lights and forced-air warming blankets, and to keep the operating room temperature high to prevent heat loss. Monitoring core temperature either esophageally or rectally is necessary. Intraoperative hyperthermia should also be scrupulously avoided.

## Induction of Anesthesia and Airway Management

The most commonly used inhalational agent for children who are neurologically stable and lack intravenous access is sevoflurane. It lends itself to a rapid and smooth induction without significant myocardial depression and cardiovascular instability. Because inhalational inductions can be accompanied by respiratory depression leading to hypercarbia that could worsen elevated ICP, the anesthesiologist should be prepared to assist in ventilation relatively early during induction. Infants that are cardiovascularly unstable or who have already been accessed intravenously should have an intravenous induction with a rapid-acting hypnotic agent such as etomidate for unstable infants and propofol for stable infants. Although ketamine is a useful medication for infants with cardiovascular instability who are not neurologically compromised, it is not ideal for neurosurgical procedures. It will cause an increase in cerebral metabolism, CBF, and ICP, so it should be used cautiously in this patient population.

For emergency procedures in which the infant is felt to be at risk for pulmonary aspiration, a rapid sequence technique using succinylcholine or a large dose of a nondepolarizing medication such as rocuronium can be used. Care must be taken to ensure there are no contraindications to the use of succinylcholine, such as malignant hyperthermia, myopathies, or denervation diseases.

Elevations of ICP can occur with laryngeal intubation, so it is important to make sure that the anesthetic depth is appropriate before airway manipulation. In infants, a nasal intubation is often more easily secured and less likely to be inadvertently displaced during the surgery, especially when the infant is placed in the prone position.

## Maintenance of Anesthesia

### Positioning

Positioning with head pins such as the Mayfield clamp is not possible in infants because of the thinness of the infant skull. Padded headholders such as the horseshoe are most commonly used, but are not as stable as head pins. Even in a neutral position, infants are at risk for venous air embolus (VAE) because of the size of their cranium. A precordial Doppler device placed on the right sternal border of the heart will monitor for VAE. A distinctive windmill murmur will be appreciated when there is a VAE, which should prompt the surgeon to flood the field with irrigation fluid, and seal any obvious sites for air entry. The anesthesiologist should also administer a fluid bolus even if there is no evidence of cardiovascular instability. Meticulous care should be taken in positioning young infants to prevent peripheral nerve injuries and skin breakdown during prolonged procedures.

## Effect of Anesthesia on the Developing Brain

Most general anesthetics have been implicated in animal models in causing long term neurocognitive deficits. In particular, prolonged exposure to agents that are gamma amino butyric acid (GABA) receptor antagonists and those that are NMDA receptor agonists has caused neuroapoptosis and long-term deficits in monkeys, rats, and mice. Although this particular issue is one of the most important in contemporary pediatric anesthesia, a thorough discussion is

beyond the scope of this chapter and will be addressed elsewhere in this text.

## Blood and Fluid Management

Neurosurgical cases are difficult to manage in young children, in part because fluid management is critical. Over-hydration is very possible in young children with excellent intravenous access, which can lead to excessive cerebral edema. Procedures on the cranium tend to be accompanied by intraoperative hemorrhage that is very difficult to estimate in young children by examination of the suction canisters and drapes. Frequent measured arterial blood gases and hematocrits are an important method to estimate intravascular fluid volume and red blood cell mass. Antifibrinolytics such as tranexamic acid can be administered to ameliorate blood loss in certain patient populations such as children undergoing major orthopedic and craniofacial procedures [21,22].

It should be assumed that the blood–brain barrier is disrupted during neurosurgical procedures. So the choice of intravenous fluids may affect cerebral perfusion, cerebral edema, water and sodium homeostasis, and serum glucose concentration. It is not known whether osmotic or oncotic pressure gradients are more important in preventing cerebral edema, but most investigators lean toward using crystalloid solutions rather than colloid solutions during neurosurgery. Since the goal is to provide a solution that is hypertonic (or at least not hypotonic) to plasma, lactated Ringer's solution, which has an osmolality of 273 mOsm $L^{-1}$ (normal serum osmolality being 285–290 mOsm $L^{-1}$) is not ideal for neurosurgery. Normal saline, which is slightly hypertonic with an osmolality of 308 mOsm $L^{-1}$, is a better choice for neurosurgical procedures, even though it can lead to a hyperchloremic acidosis if large volumes are infused [23]. Osmotic and loop diuretics can be used to transiently induce dehydration when surgical exposure is difficult or there is a dangerous elevation of ICP. Care must be taken to avoid systemic hypotension due to peripheral vasodilation caused by diuretics, which can diminish cerebral perfusion pressure. Very young patients can benefit from slow glucose administration during neurosurgical procedures. In patients with altered glucose metabolism, such as those treated with hyperalimentation, who are diabetics, or poorly nourished, the addition of glucose intravenously may also be necessary. However, hyperglycemia during procedures has been associated with increasing cerebral infarct size during cerebral ischemia, so avoiding both hyper- and hypoglycemia is important [24].

## Specific Lesions and Situations

### Hydrocephalus

Hydrocephalus, affecting about 2 in 1000 live births, is a condition in which there is excessive accumulation of CSF around or within the brain. It can be caused by too much CSF production, too little CSF resorption, or a blockage within the cerebral ventricular system that causes a build-up of fluid. Communicating hydrocephalus occurs when the blockage of CSF flow is downstream of the ventricles. Noncommunicating hydrocephalus or obstructive hydrocephalus occurs when the flow of CSF is blocked along one of the passages connecting the ventricles. During infancy, the most common symptoms of hydrocephalus are a rapid increase in head circumference, irritability, sleepiness, vomiting, and downward deviation of the eyes (sunsetting). It is treated by shunting from the ventricles or spinal cord to the abdominal cavity or atria. There is a one-way valve within the shunt that prevents CSF from flowing back into the ventricles. Some infants with hydrocephalus can be treated neuroendoscopically with the creation of a ventriculostomy on the floor of the third ventricle. Complications of ventricular shunts include failures, infections, and disconnections.

### Epilepsy

Surgical treatment for epilepsy is being done more commonly in infants. Lesions associated with epilepsy include focal malformations of cortical development, tumors, Sturge–Weber syndrome, epidermal nevus syndrome, and vascular malformations and infarctions. Surgical treatment of focal lesions has a success rate of infants being seizure-free of approximately 60 percent. Infants operated on at a young age and for infantile spasms had the most improvement of developmental quotients [25].

### Myelomeningocele

Myelomeningocele occurs when the neural tube fails to fold normally in the third to fourth week of gestation. It occurs in about 1 in 1000 live births in the United States. The infant is at increased risk for infection, so generally closure of the meningomyelocele occurs on the first day of life. It can be associated with other congenital anomalies so a thorough preoperative evaluation is warranted. About 20 percent of cases at birth are associated with hydrocephalus, but eventually 80 percent of patients with meningomyelocele will require ventricular shunting for hydrocephalus. The lesion must be protected prior to closure with sterile warm, wet dressings. Intubation can be accomplished in the lateral position or with the infant supine on foam cushions that shield the meningomyelocele from any pressure. Postoperatively, infants must be in the prone position.

## Brain and Spinal Cord Tumors

See Chapter 30 on neonatal and infant tumors.

## References

1. Arieff AI, Ayus JC, Fraser CL. Hyponatraemia and death or permanent brain damage in healthy children. *BMJ*. 1992;304:1218–22.

2. Bruce DA, Berman WA, Schut L. Cerebrospinal fluid pressure monitoring in children: physiology, pathology and clinical usefulness. *Adv Pediatr*. 1977;24:233–90.

3. Marshall LF, Smith RW, Shapiro HM. The influence of diurnal rhythms in patients with intracranial hypertension: implications for management. *Neurosurgery*. 1978;2:100–2.

4. Chaves-Carballo E, Gomez MR, Sharbrough FW. Encephalopathy and fatty infiltration of the viscera (Reye-Johnson syndrome): a 17-year experience. *Mayo Clin Proc*. 1975;50:209–15.

5. Minns RA, Brown JK, Engleman HM. CSF production rate: "real time" estimation. *Z Kinderchir*. 1987;42(Suppl 1):36–40.

6. Blomquist HK, Sundin S, Ekstedt J. Cerebrospinal fluid hydrodynamic studies in children. *J Neurol Neurosurg Psychiatry*. 1986;49:536–48.

7. Di Rocco C, McLone DG, Shimoji T, Raimondi AJ. Continuous intraventricular cerebrospinal fluid pressure recording in hydrocephalic children during wakefulness and sleep. *J Neurosurg*. 1975;42:683–9.

8. Lassen NA, Christensen MS. Physiology of cerebral blood flow. *Br J Anaesth*. 1976;48:719–34.

9. Lassen NA, Hoedt-Rasmussen K. Human cerebral blood flow measured by two inert gas techniques: comparison of the Kety–Schmidt method and the intra-arterial injection method. *Circ Res*. 1966;19:681–94.

10. Kety SS, Schmidt CF. The nitrous oxide method for the quantitative determination of cerebral blood flow in man: theory, procedure and normal values. *J Clin Invest*. 1948;27:476–83.

11. Kennedy C, Sokoloff L. An adaptation of the nitrous oxide method to the study of the cerebral circulation in children: normal values for cerebral blood flow and cerebral metabolic rate in childhood. *J Clin Invest*. 1957;36:1130–7.

12. Mehta S, Kalsi HK, Nain CK, Menkes JH. Energy metabolism of brain in human protein-calorie malnutrition. *Pediatr Res*. 1977;11:290–3.

13. Milligan DW. Cerebral blood flow and sleep state in the normal newborn infant. *Early Hum Dev*. 1979;3:321–8.

14. Settergren G, Lindblad BS, Persson B. Cerebral blood flow and exchange of oxygen, glucose, ketone bodies, lactate, pyruvate and amino acids in infants. *Acta Paediatr Scand*. 1976;65:343–53.

15. Lou HC, Lassen NA, Friis-Hansen B. Impaired autoregulation of cerebral blood flow in the distressed newborn infant. *J Pediatr*. 1979;94:118–21.

16. Rahilly PM. Effects of 2% carbon dioxide, 0.5% carbon dioxide, and 100% oxygen on cranial blood flow of the human neonate. *Pediatrics*. 1980;66:685–9.

17. Rogers MC, Nugent SK, Traystman RJ. Control of cerebral circulation in the neonate and infant. *Crit Care Med*. 1980;8:570–4.

18. Kety SS, Schmidt CF. The effects of altered arterial tensions of carbon dioxide and oxygen on cerebral blood flow and cerebral oxygen consumption of normal young men. *J Clin Invest*. 1948;27:484–92.

19. Coles JP, Fryer TD, Coleman MR, et al. Hyperventilation following head injury: effect on ischemic burden and cerebral oxidative metabolism. *Crit Care Med*. 2007;35:568–78.

20. Lassen NA. Control of cerebral circulation in health and disease. *Circ Res*. 1974;34:749–60.

21. Goobie SM, Zurakowski D, Proctor MR, et al. Predictors of clinically significant postoperative events after open craniosynostosis surgery. *Anesthesiology*. 2015;122:1021–32.

22. Goobie SM, Meier PM, Pereira LM, et al. Efficacy of tranexamic acid in pediatric craniosynostosis surgery: a double-blind, placebo-controlled trial. *Anesthesiology*. 2011;114:862–71.

23. Scheingraber S, Rehm M, Sehmisch C, Finsterer U. Rapid saline infusion produces hyperchloremic acidosis in patients undergoing gynecologic surgery. *Anesthesiology*. 1999;90:1265–70.

24. Mekitarian Filho E, Carvalho WB, Cavalheiro S, et al. Hyperglycemia and postoperative outcomes in pediatric neurosurgery. *Clinics*. 2011;66(9):1637–40.

25. Loddenkemper T, Holland KD, Stanford LD, et al. Developmental outcome after epilepsy surgery in infancy. *Pediatrics*. 2007;119:930–5.

**Chapter**

# 21

# Anesthesia for Otolaryngologic Procedures in Infants and Neonates

T. Anthony Anderson, Richard Anderson, and Charles Nargozian

## Choanal Atresia and Stenosis

Choanal atresia and stenosis are congenital defects resulting in abnormal narrowing or blockage of the nasal passages(s), typically by excess bone (90 percent) or membranous tissue (10 percent) which does not recanalize during fetal development. Unilateral stenosis/atresia may be asymptomatic, remaining undiagnosed until later in life, or masquerade as chronic sinusitis. However, bilateral stenosis is a serious problem for the obligate nasal breathing neonate that results in respiratory distress marked by severe chest wall retractions during inspiration at rest and relief of the obstruction when the infant cries [1]. In addition, the infant is also unable to breathe and nurse simultaneously. Insertion of an oral airway or endotracheal intubation may be needed to treat severe obstruction until a surgical consult can be done [2,3]. The diagnosis is suspected after failure to pass a feeding nasogastric tube through either nare. Radiographic confirmation is accomplished by a computerized tomography (CT) scan. The incidence of this defect is 1:7000 births. The ratio of male:female as well as bilateral:unilateral is 1:2. Patients with CHARGE syndrome account for 50 percent of the bilateral cases.

Numerous methods of surgical correction have been described using trans-palatal, trans-septal, trans-antral, sublabial trans-nasal, and trans-nasal approaches [4–6]. Traditional surgical correction involves puncturing the occluding tissue followed by dilating the opening and stenting it to prevent closure. The stent is removed after 5–12 weeks, with longer duration resulting in better results [7]. An alternative method to avoid using a stent is to administer oral steroids for five days followed by a month of intranasal steroids [6]. Newer methods of correction utilize a trans-nasal endoscopic approach to remove the membranous or bony tissue with or without the use of a helium:YAG laser. Anesthetic considerations start with evaluation of associated defects, including the possibility of congenital cardiac disease. General orotracheal anesthesia is performed with required safety considerations if a laser is used. Hemodynamic parameters should be closely monitored as the use of cocaine or other vasoconstrictive agents to decrease bleeding and aid visualization may cause hypertension and/or arrhythmias. Operative complications include cerebrospinal fluid (CSF) leak if excess bone is removed, respiratory distress should the stent become occluded, and re-stenosis.

## Laryngeal and Tracheal Issues

### Tracheal Stenosis

Tracheal stenosis may be congenital, iatrogenic, or the result of a disease process [1]. It may be classified as being general hypoplasia, funnel-shaped, or segmental [2]. Complete tracheal atresia is a very rare entity that is incompatible with life and is mentioned for completeness. Other congenital problems include complete tracheal rings involving one to all rings and a complete cartilaginous sleeve. The abnormal tracheal structure causes problems with airflow and interferes with clearance of secretions, causing stridor, retractions, and wheezing which may be associated with repeat episodes of pneumonia. Treatment of short segments is by surgical excision and re-anastomosis. Longer segments require more extensive procedures or possibly tracheal autograft. Innovative solutions using 3D printing and biologic materials, e.g., stem cells, to replace the defective trachea are starting to be reported.

Iatrogenic causes of tracheal stenosis are almost exclusively caused by prolonged intubation. Mucosal injury may be caused by high transmural pressure of the inflated cuff of an endotracheal tube, which interferes with perfusion of the mucosa. Mucosal damage is compounded by up-and-down movement of the endotracheal tube, leading to scarring and circumferential contraction. The damaged segment can be small or extensive. Small segments can be treated by dilation, while large segments require excision or posterior cartilage graft to keep the segment from re-stricturing.

## Tracheomalacia/Bronchomalacia

Tracheomalacia describes the collapse of the airway when tracheal structures are unable to keep the airway patent in response to transmural airway pressures during respiration. Primary tracheomalacia is caused by an abnormal ratio of the cartilaginous to the membranous section of a tracheal ring. During expiration the posterior membranous section collapses into the lumen of trachea causing a variable degree of obstruction. Primary malacia is often seen in premature and newborn infants and usually resolves by two years of age. Severe cases, however, may require prolonged CPAP, intubation, or tracheostomy for treatment.

Secondary tracheal malacia may result from congenital abnormal vasculature, which may compress the trachea at various locations. Other etiologies include compression by an enlarged heart secondary to cardiac defects, bronchopulmonary dysplasia, or a tracheoesophageal fistula. Abnormal development of the major vessels may present as a double aortic arch, pulmonary vascular sling, aberrant right subclavian artery, and right-sided aortic arch [8]. The unifying feature of these conditions is that the trachea is compressed between two vascular structures that cause an increased ratio of the cartilaginous to membranous section of the compressed tracheal rings. Congenital cardiac lesions usually involve the left main stem bronchus, which is normally located between the left pulmonary artery and the left atrium, along with the left pulmonary veins. Cardiac lesions that lead to increased pulmonary pressure and/or left atrial enlargement can encroach on the left main stem bronchus causing malacia. Eighty-six percent of tracheal esophageal fistulas are type C, which consists of proximal esophageal atresia with a distal esophageal fistula to the trachea. The triad of widened cartilages, ballooning of the posterior wall, and collapse of the distal tracheal lumen in one or both bronchi is seen on endoscopy.

The severity of respiratory symptoms associated with tracheomalacia varies. Patients will present with stridor, dysphagia, wheezing, chronic cough, inability to handle secretions, recurrent pneumonias, atelectasis, and cyanotic apneic spells. An inability to wean from mechanical ventilation or the failure of tracheal extubation or tracheostomy decannulation may indicate underlying tracheomalacia. Diagnostic studies include chest radiograph, esophagram, chest CT with dynamic studies, bronchoscopy, and possibly angiography. Treatment may require long-term ventilation and/or surgical correction. Surgical procedures include splinting, stenting, aortopexy, resection, and correction of the underlying problem.

## Bronchogenic Cysts

Bronchogenic cysts are the result of abnormal budding of the bronchial tree, which develops independently of normal alveolar formation and growth. They contain ciliated epithelium and pseudostratified columnar epithelium [8]. They may be connected to the bronchial airways, and for that reason spontaneous respiration during anesthesia is preferred. Anticholinergic premedication to decrease secretions and topical local anesthesia are useful adjuncts for sedation. Most often they present in infants as wheezing, cough, or respiratory distress. Airway obstruction may occur if they enlarge. Diagnosis is by radiograph or CT of the chest. Surgical excision is indicated.

## Pulmonary Sequestration

Pulmonary sequestration is a collection of abnormal pulmonary tissue that is abnormally connected to the tracheobronchial tree. It may be extralobar or intralobar. The arterial blood supply originates from the systemic circulation from below the diaphragm, but venous drainage may differ. The extralobar type may have its own pleural cavity and systemic venous drainage whereas the intralobar type has no pleural membrane and venous blood drains into the pulmonary circulation. Like other pulmonary problems, it may present with infection, mass effect, and other symptoms. Plain radiographs, CT, MRI, and angiography are used for diagnosis. Treatment is surgical excision.

## Congenital Cystic Adenomatoid Malformation

Congenital cystic adenomatoid malformations (CCAMs) are benign cystic lesions that appear during fetal development. They are classified as microcytic, macrocytic, or solid, but differ from bronchopulmonary sequestration by the fact that they do not have a systemic arterial supply. They are found during fetal ultrasonography. The lesions may shrink and disappear or continue to enlarge as the fetus grows. Large lesions may cause fetal distress by causing contralateral lung hypoplasia, cardiovascular collapse, maternal polyhydramnios, and fetal hydrops. For large lesions, fetal surgery, which includes thoracocentesis, thoracoamniotic shunting, or resection utilizing an ex utero intrapartum therapy (EXIT) procedure, may be life-saving. Smaller lesions may wait until after birth to be excised as these lesions may undergo malignant degeneration.

### Anesthetic Considerations for Tracheal and Pulmonary Issues

The primary anesthetic consideration is to maintain adequate inspiratory and expiratory air flow through the tracheal branchial tree. Stenotic lesions limit air passage and increase the work of breathing by causing nonlaminar flow. Inhalational induction is prolonged and is best accomplished by using a slow respiratory rate with high concentration of anesthetic gas. Malacia of the tracheobronchial tree leads to collapse of the lumen as transmural pressures change during inspiration and expiration, depending on whether the segment is intrathoracic or extrathoracic. Intrathoracic segments are stented open during inspiration and collapse during expiration. Use of end-expiratory pressure, PEEP or CPAP, keeps the airway patent throughout the respiratory cycle. Thorough intraoperative monitoring and maintenance of deep anesthesia to prevent coughing, laryngospasm, or bronchospasm should be the anesthetic goals for all cases. Mass lesions cause compression of the adjacent lung parenchyma and tracheobronchial structures. Patient positioning may have a dramatic effect on the ability to ventilate the lungs and dictate surgical positioning. Likewise, hypoventilation increases collapse of the distal alveolar segments. Maintaining adequate inflation pressures is necessary to prevent the resultant hypoxia. Finally, for lesions that connect to the tracheobronchial tree, positive pressure ventilation may cause expansion of the lesion. This in turn may increase any mass effect. Spontaneous ventilation should be used in this situation until the connection is severed.

## Cystic Lesions

Dermoid cysts are structures lined by epithelium which contain various elements derived from epithelium along embryonic fusion plates [9]. They range from 1 to 4 cm in size, are commonly found on the forehead, lateral eye, or neck, and can be fixed or mobile. Most are subcutaneous although there can be

extension intracranially or intraorbitally. Treatment is surgical excision so preoperative CT or MR scan to rule out extension is recommended. A tunneled endoscopic approach starting behind the hairline to avoid facial scarring can be utilized.

Thyroglossal duct cysts occur along the tract by which the thyroid descends during embryonic development from the base of the tongue to the normal thyroid position. They are typically noticed as a midline neck mass following an upper respiratory infection, or become primarily infected [10]. These cysts often move when swallowing and can track though the hyoid bone [3]. Preoperative ultrasound is recommended. Treatment is excision to prevent further infection. Recurrence is more likely if the child is under two years of age or has had two or more infections [11].

Branchial cleft cysts are derived from sequestration of first and second branchial cleft elements, resulting in cysts, sinuses, and tags. The incidence is sporadic, although there are reports of autosomal inheritance with equal male to female frequency, and 10 percent are bilateral [9]. These lesions usually present as soft tissue masses along the border of the sternocleidomastoid muscle. First branchial arch cysts are usually high in the neck. The more common second arch cysts are lower in the neck and often communicate with the tonsillar fossa. The less common third arch cysts are low in the neck and can communicate with the pyriform sinus. Branchial cleft cysts usually present after an upper respiratory infection as a tender mass. After treatment of the cysts with antibiotics they are excised in order to prevent reinfection and the possibility of carcinoma [10].

## Vascular Malformations

### Hemangioma

Hemangiomas are the most common benign tumors in infants [12]. This abnormal collection of blood vessels is characterized by having increased activity of endothelium and mast cells during the growth phase. They can be superficial, "capillary or strawberry" or deep, "cavernous" and can occur in any organ. They may not be present at birth, but appear within a few weeks and rapidly expand for 6–12 months. It is during this growth phase that they are invasive, causing ulceration, expansion, and may involve a vital organ [12]. After the growth phase finishes, they will slowly involute over a period of years. Hemangiomas may be multicentric; so affected patients should be thoroughly evaluated for other lesions. Large segmental hemangiomas about the face may be part of PHACE syndrome (posterior fossa malformation, hemangiomas, arterial abnormalites, cardiac defects, and eye anomalies). Kasabach–Merritt syndrome is the occurrence of hemangioma, thrombocytopenia, and coagulopathy. Treatment with propranolol may slow the rate of growth. Prednisone is very effective in causing rapid involution. Superficial lesions may be treated by laser excision while surgical excision may be needed for others.

### Other Vascular Malformations

Unlike hemangiomas, vascular malformations are characterized as having normal growth of the endothelium and mast cells. They grow proportionately with the rest of the body and do not involute [2]. These vascular malformations can be associated with various syndromes such as Klippel–Trenaunay–Weber, Struge–Weber, Maffucci, and Parkes–Weber. All vascular malformations should be thoroughly evaluated using MR/CT scan, Doppler ultrasonography, and contrast radiography to delineate the type and extent of the lesion.

## Venous Malformations

Venous malformations are the most common vascular malformations. They present as soft, compressible, blue-colored structures. They are found predominantly about the head and neck. A high percentage of larger lesions have associated deep cerebral malformations that should be investigated. Treatment with sclerotherapy is highly successful, especially when surgical excision would be disfiguring or impossible.

## Arteriovenous Malformations

Arteriovenous malformations (AVMs) are the most serious vascular lesions. They can cause high-output heart failure or may spontaneously rupture. Dental extraction in the presence of a mandibular AVM has been known to lead to massive bleeding. Treatment of an AVM is sclerotherapy, quickly followed by surgical excision to prevent new arterial channels from opening.

## Lymphatic Malformations

Lymphatic malformations are the result of primary lymph sacs that do not coalesce with the rest of the lymphatic system. The resultant cystic structures may be small, microcystic, or large, macrocystic, also termed cystic hygroma. Microcystic lymphangioma are invasive and ill-defined, extending through various tissues and organs. Macrocystic tend to be well circumscribed, although both elements can coexist. Lymphatic malformations present early in life and expand as lymph accumulates within the cysts. Cystic hygromas occur in about 1:12 000 live births, and are located in the posterior triangle of the neck, cephalad to the clavicle [3]. The cyst may extend from the skin internally to the mucosa of the trachea. Lesions can be life-threatening if the trachea becomes compressed [11]. If detected in utero by ultrasonography, the airway may be secured intrapartum while the umbilical vessels are still attached, via an EXIT procedure. Surgical excision is necessary for treatment in most cases. A chest radiograph, ultrasonography, and MR/CT scan are needed to delineate the extent of the lesion. Sclerotherapy may be effective, although for macrocystic lesions a new sclerosing agent, OK432, has been very effective.

### Anesthetic Considerations for Vascular Malformations

Airway management and blood loss are the two major considerations. As a large percentage of all vascular malformations occur in the head and neck region, problems arise resulting in distortion of facial structures and causing difficulty with mask ventilation, tracheal intubation, and ventilation/respiratory mechanics. Venous and lymphatic malformations can become disfiguring and grow to large size. They may interfere with the fit of the facemask, making inhalational induction of anesthesia difficult or impossible. Alternatively, when located within the neck or thorax, compression and deviation of the airway is common. Fortunately, typically these malformations are compressible, allowing for instrumentation and the passage of an endotracheal tube. However, they can swell and become non-compressible in response to surgical manipulation, sclerotherapy, or infection. Tracheal extubation should be delayed until airway swelling has subsided, which may require several days after surgery. Hemangiomas and arteriovenous malformations may also present in, or around, the airway. Hemangiomas are friable and thus bleed easily. Endotracheal lesions may ooze if traumatized by an endotracheal tube. Arteriovenous malformations may also bleed if manipulated. The bleeding, however, will be brisk, heavy, and potentially life-threatening.

Airway management should be directed to avoid manipulating or touching the malformation.

Blood loss during excision of large hemangiomas can be misleading in the small infant or child. Bleeding occurs at a steady slow rate and is controlled by direct pressure. For the small infant near the physiologic hematocrit nadir, the transfusion threshold may be reached quickly. Mucosal paleness or tachycardia may be signs that a repeat hematocrit is needed for determination if red cell transfusion is warranted. Large venous or mixed lesions may result in large blood volume loss, especially since tourniquets cannot be used in head and neck procedures. Large-bore venous access and possibly an arterial line are needed. Arteriovenous malformations always present the possibility of massive blood loss. Preoperative embolization decreases the risk of bleeding, but an arterial line is mandatory for anything but the smallest lesions.

## Craniofacial Problems

Structural abnormalities of the head and neck comprise a diverse set of congenital problems that may be grouped in numerous ways. Syndromes resulting from abnormal ossification of bony structures include Crouzon's (craniofacial dysotosis), Apert (acrocephalosyndactyly), and Treacher Collins (mandibulofacial dysotosis) syndromes. A defining feature of Crouzon's and Apert syndromes is the premature closure of cranial sutures and that of the skull base, resulting in midface hypoplasia. The small nares and choanal stenosis cause these patients to be nearly obligate mouth breathers with a high incidence of sleep apnea. Those with Treacher Collins syndrome have midface abnormalities caused by nonfusion and hyoplasic development of the maxilla, mandible, and auditory structures. These patients have a high incidence of glossoptosis with associated Robin sequence.

Other abnormalities are the result of lack of development of bone or soft tissue. These include oculoauriculovertebral syndrome (hemifacial microsomia, Goldenhar's syndrome), hemifacial atrophy (Romberg syndrome), and congenital facial diplegia (Moebius syndrome). In Goldenhar's syndrome, the first and second brachial arch structures of the ear and mandible are affected to various degrees. Loss of tissue results in distortion of the face and airway, which worsens with unbalanced growth. Romberg syndrome patients are normal at birth, with progressive atrophy and distortion of the facial features with growth. The congenital palsies of the cranial nerves of Moebius syndrome result in difficulties with feeding, speech, and expression. The mouth opening is usually small.

## Anesthetic Considerations

Airway management is the major anesthetic concern of these patients as they typically are difficult to bag-mask ventilate, difficult to intubate, or both. Patients with midface hypoplasia have high resistance to nasal breathing and are essentially mouth breathers. Standard airway maneuvers, which close the mouth to get a better mask fit, increase the degree of obstruction. Care should be taken to keep the mouth open to allow for air passage. Early insertion of an oral airway is helpful. Topical anesthesia applied to the oral cavity prior to induction anesthesia will minimize the risk of laryngospasm from the early insertion of the oral airway.

Other patients who have mandibular hypoplasia or associated Robin sequence are at high risk of airway obstruction and difficult tracheal intubation. Alternative methods other than direct laryngoscopy to secure the airway include insertion of a laryngeal mask airway (LMA), fiberoptic instrumentation, and surgical instrumentation. Also see 'Robin sequence' below.

## Cleft Lip and Palate

Cleft lip and palate are the most common congenital anomalies, occurring in 1 in 500 live births [13]. They may occur singly, together, as part of a syndrome, or the result of Robin sequence. The exact causative genetic factors are unknown but there is a strong familial inheritance. The problems associated with cleft lip/palate include difficulties with breathing, feeding, speaking, hearing, and general psychological well-being. The repair of the cleft lip may be staged or done as a primary repair. A dentomaxillary appliance may be inserted prior to repair to align the discontinuous alveolar ridges of the palate. Correction of the cleft palate should be performed before the child starts speaking. Some surgeons will use the Rose positon, resting the patient's head in their lap, for the palate repair. Similarly, some will use a balsam of Peru-soaked pack sewn on the palate repair to promote wound healing. This dressing effectively obstructs the oral airway and thus patients must breathe nasally postoperatively.

## Robin sequence

Robin sequence is defined by the three findings of micrognathia, glossoptosis, and airway obstruction. It was Pierre Robin who first identified the airway obstruction as being the result of glossoptosis as the posteriorly displaced tongue contacts the pharyngeal wall. Cleft palate occurs in 90 percent of Robin sequence patients as the displaced tongue mechanically interferes with closure of the palatal plates. Both the airway obstruction and the cleft palate are the result of micrognathia. Robin sequence may occur by itself or be associated with any syndrome that includes micrognathia.

These patients may have failure to thrive as the result of chronic hypoxia, increased work of breathing, and poor feeding. Treatment is directed at relieving the airway obstruction. Nonsurgical modalities include using the prone position with or without a nasopharygeal airway. Surgical therapies include tongue–lip adhesion, mandibular distraction, and tracheostomy. Additional alimentation may be provided via a feeding tube or a gastrostomy tube. If the Robin sequence is not associated with a syndrome, the mandible eventually will grow to near normal size, alleviating the airway obstruction. However, if associated with a syndrome, the mandible may remain hypoplastic.

### Anesthetic Considerations

Patients with cleft lip or palate usually do not have airway management problems unless they are associated with other facial abnormalities. Airway obstruction may occur during inhalational induction if the tongue falls posteriorly into the cleft palate. Obstruction is relieved by insertion of an oral airway. Tracheal intubation is likewise without problem unless a bilateral cleft exists. The midline prolabial segment is angulated forward and upward, interfering with insertion of the laryngoscope and alignment of the axis of larynx visualization. Oral RAE endotracheal tubes are preferred as they don't distort the facial symmetry around the upper lip. When properly inserted, the distance from the bend in the tube to the tip is a fixed distance. Flexion of the neck may move the tip into a mainstem bronchus. Secondarily, RAE tubes are not easily suctioned and are easily clogged.

The safe induction of anesthesia and tracheal intubation for Robin sequence patients is always a problem. General anesthesia relaxes the oropharyngeal musculature, augmenting the airway obstruction. Techniques that bypass the obstruction allow safe inhalational anesthesia. These include awake insertion of an LMA or insufflation of anesthesia gas after insertion of a nasal pharyngeal airway/endotracheal tube within the nasopharynx. The second step is to safely secure the airway with an endotracheal tube. Options include intubating through the LMA, use of a glidescope once the patient is anesthetized, or using a fiberoptic bronchoscope for nasal/oral intubation with the patient breathing spontaneously.

## Myringotomy and Tympanostomy Tubes

Otitis media, commonly called an "ear infection," is a very common diagnosis and is the most common indication for pediatric outpatient antimicrobial therapy in the United States [14]. Recurrent otitis media may result in fibrosis and scarring of the middle ear, formation of a cholesteatoma, and conductive hearing loss. The treatment of recurrent otitis media is drainage via a myringotomy, a small incision in the tympanic membrane, followed by the insertion of a small tube to facilitate drainage. The tubes are naturally extruded in 6–12 months, although retained tubes may be surgically removed. The procedure is generally less than ten minutes in duration. General anesthesia is commonly administered using an inhalation agent by mask for induction and maintenance. Intravenous (IV) access is generally not required. The postoperative pain is mild and can be addressed with acetaminophen, ketorolac, or intranasal fentanyl. As always, a careful preoperative history and physical is important to discover comorbid conditions, the most common being cleft palate.

## Middle Ear Surgery

### Cholesteatoma

A cholesteatoma is squamous epithelium and its accumulated debris within the middle ear and pneumatized temporal bone. It may be characterized as congenital or acquired, with or without an infection. Acquired cholesteatoma is the most common etiology as the result of middle ear disease and is seen in older children. Congenital cholesteatoma is usually diagnosed by a pediatrician and is differentiated from the acquired form by being diagnosed in infancy or early childhood, in patients with no history of prior ruptured eardrums. Treatment is surgical excision either by a tympanoplasty or can be more extensive with a mastoidectomy. A general anesthetic with a secure airway and IV access are required for the surgery.

The patient is positioned supine with the head rotated laterally for exposure of the affected side. Care should be used for patients with limited neck range of motion or those at risk for cervical instability (e.g., patients with trisomy 21). For these patients, consideration for lateral decubitus positioning may be warranted. The facial nerve is usually monitored, necessitating avoidance of long-acting neuromuscular blocking agents. Sevoflurane and/or isoflurane are generally used, but nitrous oxide should be avoided. Tympanometry has shown increased fluctuations in middle ear pressure when nitrous is added to other inhaled anesthetics [15]. Diffusion of nitrous oxide into the middle ear will increase the pressure, causing outward movement of the tympanic membrane. Once the nitrous oxide is turned off, the rapid absorption of gas will create negative pressure, resulting in backward displacement of the tympanic membrane and disrupting the surgical repair. The movement may also be significant enough to cause disarticulation of the ossicles, leading to conductive hearing loss than can persist for several weeks postoperatively. The incidence of postoperative nausea and vomiting (PONV) after tympanoplasty is greater than 50 percent in some studies, although rarely occurs in infants, and the use of nitrous oxide may be contributory. Both dexamethasone and ondansetron have been shown to be efficacious as prophylactic agents for the treatment of PONV [16] in older children. If possible, a deep extubation is desirable to facilitate a smooth wake-up without excessive coughing or head movement.

## Cochlear Implants

Cochlear implants are a popular and effective treatment for children with severe to profound sensorineural hearing loss. Unlike hearing aids which simply amplify sounds, the cochlear implants transform acoustic energy into electrical energy and stimulate the remaining inner ear neurons, partially restoring the child's hearing. The surgical procedure involves attaching an internal processor to the mastoid process and connecting the electrodes to the cochlear neurons. There has been a trend toward earlier placement, with the procedure being performed on children as young as six months of age. The procedure is best completed in tertiary care centers where experienced pediatric surgeons, anesthesiologists, and perioperative care teams can take care of these young children [17].

The procedure requires a general anesthetic with a secure airway for children, though sedation with regional techniques has been used in adults. Use of muscle relaxation for optimal surgical conditions should be discussed with the surgeon as intraoperative facial nerve monitoring may be used. After insertion into the cochlear nerve, the implant is calibrated by two electrically evoked potentials, the evoked stapedius reflex threshold (ESRT) and the evoked compound action potential (ECAP). The ESRT is the loudest stimulus than can be tolerated without pain, while the ECAP is the smallest stimulus that can be perceived as sound. Volatile anesthetics suppress the ESRT in a dose-dependent fashion, resulting in inaccurate calibration, and a stimulus which may be painful when awake. Propofol does not cause this decrement and can be safely used, making it prudent to switch to a total intravenous anesthesia (TIVA) for the calibration portion of the procedure [18]. If volatile anesthetics are used early in the procedure it is important to communicate with the surgeon about the concentration and timing of the inhaled agent in relation to the actual implantation. Alternatively, the device can be calibrated when awake postoperatively, though this is very difficult in an infant. As with tympanoplasty, the PONV rate can be quite high and prophylactic antiemetic agents should be utilized in children older than one year.

## Chronic Sinusitis/Rhinosinusitis

### Sinus Development in Children

At birth, neonates have pea-sized ethmoid and maxillary sinuses. During the second year of life, the sphenoid sinuses begin to develop, and after age eight the frontal sinuses develop. All reach adult size by adolescence. The paranasal sinuses are very commonly infected in young children, with about 10 percent of upper respiratory infections being complicated by paranasal sinusitis. Diagnosis is usually made in children with a cold lasting longer than 10–14 days, often with a low fever. Sinusitis symptoms are uncommon in infants and should lead to suspicion of immunologic deficiencies, congenital abnormalities, and

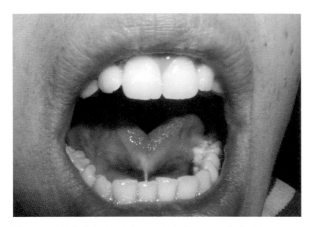

**Figure 21.1** Ankyloglossia in an adult. Photography by Klaus D. Peter.

the possibility of foreign bodies in the nasal cavity. Endoscopic sinus surgery is rarely done in infants. Occasionally adenoidectomies are done in infants to alleviate chronic sinus congestion.

## Tongue Tie Ankyloglossia

The term ankyloglossia (AG), commonly called a tongue tie, is Greek for "curved tongue." It has an incidence as high as 10 percent in some studies. The condition is somewhat controversial as not all clinicians agree on the definition or its clinical significance. Ankyloglossia is essentially a short, tight, thickened, lingual frenulum which may reduce tongue mobility, making speech articulation and breastfeeding difficult. (Figure 21.1) In infants with difficulty breastfeeding, release of ankyloglossia has been shown to improve the ability to latch onto the breast and feed effectively. It may also reduce maternal discomfort with breast feeding. Some clinicians have suggested that ankyloglossia is linked to the development of malocclusion and gingival recession, but the data are inconclusive [19].

The frenulum naturally recedes between six months and six years of age so observation for some years may be indicated. The timing of the procedure is therefore quite variable and is aimed to relieve symptoms. For speech issues, there are very few data to support prophylactic intervention and limited data to support intervention in those with breastfeeding issues. A simple frenotomy can be carried out very quickly with local anesthetic as the frenulum is often poorly vascularized and innervated. Laser procedures have been described as well. A tighter and

more vascular frenulum may require a more extensive frenectomy or frenuloplasty, including possible division of the genioglossus muscle with a Z-plasty of the remaining tissue [20]. In an older child, this may be possible with local anesthesia, but younger children require general anesthesia

There are no literature recommendations to guide specific anesthetic management. Anesthetic technique should be discussed with the surgeon and based on the length of the procedure, the need for mouth opening, and the need to secure the airway. Short procedures may be done with inhalational mask anesthesia, just removing the mask to allow the surgeon brief access. Longer procedures may need to have the airway secured with an oral endotracheal tube or LMA. As always, a detailed history and physical should be completed, with special attention to comorbid conditions as there have been reported associations with an X-linked cleft palate condition.

## Iatrogenic Problems

### Tracheal Stenosis

Tracheal stenosis may be congenital in etiology, but is more commonly an unfortunate consequence of prolonged intubation in a neonate, even if the endotracheal tube is appropriately sized. The stenosis may be glottic or subglottic, with the latter being much more serious and difficult to intervene upon surgically. Flexible or rigid bronchoscopy is often performed to visualize the site of the lesion and the surrounding anatomy. In combination with CT imaging and bronchoscopy, intubation with the largest endotracheal tube (ETT) that allows an audible leak provides information regarding the diameter of the stenosed portion.

If the stenosis is mild, a simple dilation or laser tracheoplasty may be the only needed intervention. With more severe lesions, invasive reconstructive procedures are indicated. One approach is the anterior cricoid split procedure. This is essentially a cricoid incision that uses an endotracheal tube as a stent. The incision begins just inferior to the thyroid cartilage and traverses the cricoid, continuing into the second tracheal ring. Sutures are then placed through the incision, allowing it to heal over the ETT tube with a slightly larger diameter. The ETT may be left in place for 1–2 weeks while the incision heals.

A more invasive larynogotracheoplasty involves a longer midline incision of the trachea from the inferior portion of the thyroid cartilage to the third or fourth tracheal ring. Following the incision, cartilage grafts are sewn in place to increase the diameter of the lumen. A stent is sometimes needed for mechanical support as the healing takes place. Revisions, excisions of scar tissue, and further procedures are often needed after tracheal surgery.

## Vocal Cord Paralysis

Vocal cord paralysis is a common diagnosis in both adults and pediatric patients. While birth trauma, postoperative nerve dysfunction, and cardiac malformations are some potential etiologies, most patients carry a diagnosis of idiopathic vocal cord paralysis. Inspiratory stridor with hoarseness or a weak abnormal cry is frequently the presenting symptom in unilateral paralysis. Bilateral paralysis results in significant airway obstruction, stridor with a normal cry, aspiration, and difficulty with phonation. Bilateral paralysis is frequently comorbid with posterior fossa lesions and Arnold–Chiari malformation as stretching of the vagus nerve over the jugular foramen leaves it open to injury and paralysis. A tracheostomy may be required for severe obstructive symptoms and aspiration until an underlying cause can be diagnosed and surgical correction performed.

When inducing anesthesia, continuous positive pressure should be gently applied, abolishing the stridor, and stenting the airway open for easy ventilation. A direct laryngoscopy often provides very little information other than seeing if the vocal cord is paramedian and immobile. A fiberoptic intubation in the appropriate candidate provides better visualization, and allows a view of the glottis as well. The paralyzed vocal cord will *not* narrow the airway so a normal-sized ETT can be used.

Postoperative swelling and edema can make a well-compensated infant with a vocal cord lesion more stridulous and increase the work of breathing. Care should be taken to complete an atraumatic intubation with an appropriately sized ETT. The cuff pressure should not be above 20–25 mmHg. If there is concern about airway swelling, consider leaving the infant intubated or administer steroids.

## Adenoids and Tonsils

The tonsillectomy, often performed with an adenoidectomy, is one of the most common pediatric procedures in the United States, but is rarely done in children less than one year. However, there is a recent trend to consider adenotonsillectomy in infants as a primary treatment for obstructive sleep apnea [21]. The efficacy of this treatment is unclear, with several studies showing good benefit from adenotonsillectomy in infants but others showing a greater persistence of OSA after adenotonsillectomy and a higher incidence of postoperative complications despite an improved apnea hypopnea index (AHI) [22,23]. Because of the possibility of worsening OSA in the immediate postoperative period, most institutions will admit infants to the intensive care unit postoperatively.

### Intraoperative Considerations

The procedure is generally quite fast, typically less than 30 minutes. A variety of surgical techniques are used, including the guillotine and snare, ultrasonic coblation, cold dissection, hot dissection, and the use of electrocautery. In small children, anesthesia is usually induced by mask, using a breathdown technique, after which IV access is established. The airway is secured with an ETT, which may be an oral RAE tube or an armored ETT. The use of an LMA has also been shown to be effective. Tracheal extubation can be accomplished when the patient is awake, either in the supine or lateral head-down position. Alternatively, deep extubation can be utilized, with care given to maintain the patient's airway and prevent aspiration. Postoperative airway complications include laryngospasm and bleeding, which make mask ventilation and reintubation more difficult. Postoperative airway manipulation can disturb the friable tissues, contributing to postoperative hemorrhage.

The use of electrocautery increases the risk of an airway fire. Fire prevention includes keeping the $FiO_2$ below 0.3, using only short bursts of cautery, and covering the eyes with wet gauze. The use of a special ETT (discussed below) will help reduce the risk of a fire.

### Analgesia and PONV

There is a paucity of information about the optimal analgesic plans for infants after tonsillectomy. Analgesia is important to ensure a smooth wake-up without excessive crying and agitation, but narcotics should be used cautiously in infants postoperatively, especially those that have a history of obstructive sleep apnea. Small doses should be used until the infant is awake and able to breathe and maintain a patent airway. A variety of nonopioid techniques can be used in all children. A recent study of 161 children (non-infants) found that a single dose of IV ibuprofen (10 mg kg$^{-1}$) given preoperatively significantly reduced postoperative fentanyl requirements with no increase in the incidence of postoperative hemorrhage [24]. A 2013 Cochrane review on the effect of nonsteroidal anti-inflammatory drugs (NSAIDs) on postoperative bleeding after pediatric tonsillectomy found a non-significant increase in the risk of bleeding requiring surgical intervention, no significant increase in the risk of bleeding requiring nonsurgical intervention, and less PONV [25]. Regional techniques have been found to be effective and opioid-sparing. A block of the auricular branch of the vagus nerve with 0.2 ml of 0.25 percent bupivacaine was as effective as 2 µg ml$^{-1}$ of intranasal fentanyl, with no differences in postoperative pain score, rescue analgesics, PONV, or time to discharge [26].

A recent Cochrane review, updated in 2011, found that a single dose of dexamethasone (dose range 0.15–1.0 mg kg$^{-1}$) not only reduced the PONV rate by approximately one-half, but increased the likelihood of progressing to a solid diet on post-op day one and reduced VAS pain scores without any significant adverse effects [27]. Ondansetron is frequently used in conjunction with dexamethasone for PONV prophylaxis in older children.

### Postoperative Complications

The major postoperative concerns after adenoidectomy and tonsillectomy include respiratory issues and hemorrhage. Minor issues include PONV, pain, and poor oral intake. Uvular edema or amputation can occur, but are rare.

Younger children, under three years of age, are more prone to respiratory complications including apnea, breath holding, and supraglottic obstruction. Due to the increased likelihood of needing airway interventions, patients under two years of age are usually not considered candidates for ambulatory tonsillectomies.

The incidence of postoperative hemorrhage is 3–5 percent and is the most common indication for a return to the operating room. The time frame is bimodal, occurring in the first 24 hours or at 7–10 days postoperatively. Disruption of the eschar, either spontaneously or from mechanical trauma (i.e., eating, coughing, etc.) can result in significant bleeding. Volume status should be evaluated preoperatively and fluid resuscitation started. An intraosseous line can be used if there is failure of venous access. The urine

output, heart rate, blood pressure, and hydration of mucous membranes can be used to judge the volume status, in addition to lab values. After fluid resuscitation, induction of anesthesia requires a rapid sequence induction (RSI) as swallowed blood constitutes a full stomach. Visualization of the airway may be difficult if bleeding is brisk, and at least two working suction catheters should be available to the anesthesiologist during induction and intubation. Sometimes the only indication of the location of the larynx is the presence of air bubbles to guide ETT placement. Blood transfusion can be given if necessary.

## Laser Procedures and Suspension Laryngoscopy

The most common application for lasers in pediatrics involves airway surgery for recurrent papillomatosis. These benign tumors are the result of a human papilloma virus and may occur anywhere on the laryngeal tissues, including the true vocal cords. To facilitate visualization and access to the glottic region, the infant is often placed in suspension laryngoscopy after the induction of general anesthesia. Depending on the size, location, and characteristics of the lesions, they may cause varying degrees of obstruction. Thus, inhalational induction with spontaneous ventilation is the preferred anesthetic technique. As the anesthesiologist slowly takes over the child's breathing, an IV is placed and airway management addressed.

Visualization of the larynx is accomplished using suspension laryngoscopy. Prior to suspension, propofol (2–3 mg kg$^{-1}$) should be given as this is quite stimulating. Glycopyrolate and/or atropine should be available to treat bradycardia caused by pressure on the larynx. Once in suspension laryngoscopy, the airway can be managed via several techniques including: (1) conventional ETT intubation, (2) intermittent apnea, (3) jet ventilation, and (4) tubeless spontaneous ventilation. The plan for the airway should be discussed with the surgeon prior to induction of anesthesia. The decision to secure the airway is based on the size and location of the tumor, as well as the surgeon's need for space while applying the laser to the lesions. Anterior laryngeal lesions are generally not obstructed by the ETT, while posterior lesions will be blocked by the ETT lying directly over the posterior vocal cords and laryngeal structures.

Intermittent apnea is a technique that involves repeated intubations and extubations, which are facilitated by suspension laryngoscopy. During intubation periods, the patient can be hyperventilated and well-oxygenated. The tube can be removed, giving unrestricted access to the glottis. Periods of up to two minutes are generally tolerated quite well. This technique works well for shorter cases where anterior lesions require the absence of an ETT. Due to the apnea, a TIVA is preferable for maintenance of anesthesia.

Jet ventilation is a technique that allows ventilation while maintaining an unrestricted view of the glottis and a quiescent operating field. It requires a special jet ventilator to insufflate the lungs by altering the driving pressure, $FiO_2$, and frequency. A $CO_2$ monitor can be attached to a side port of the suspension laryngoscopy device to monitor the presence of exhaled $CO_2$. Chest rise and $SpO_2$ are used to judge the adequacy of the ventilation. Obese children and those with stiffened chest walls may not show much of a rise in the chest. When in doubt, an arterial blood gas (ABG) can be sent to assess the adequacy of ventilation and other ventilation strategies may need to be considered. In addition to inadequate ventilation, other risks of jet ventilation include gastric insufflation with potential aspiration, pneumothorax, and pneumomediastinum.

Lasers are the second most common cause of operating room fires. The gas mixture and route of delivery are important considerations for laser procedures. Aside from the standard PVC tubes, which are flammable, there are a variety of ETTs available to help reduce the risk of airway fires. These include red rubber tubes that can be wrapped in metallic tape, non-latex tubes, and several ETTs manufactured specifically for laser procedures (see table 3 from [28]). Though routinely used uneventfully in adults, these special ETTs have a large outer diameter and may not be appropriate for infants or children with a partially obstructed airway. It is important to note that the metallic tape-wrapped ETTs are safer than unwrapped tubes, but the cuff remains vulnerable to the laser. Any time lasers are being used, the $FiO_2$ should be less than 0.3, the eyes and face should be covered with wet sponges, and constant communication should be maintained between the surgeon and anesthesiologist. If possible, jet ventilation or tubeless techniques should be used to reduce the risk of fires [28]. Dexamethasone is typically given, 0.5 mg kg$^{-1}$, to reduce airway swelling as all airway procedures produce varying degrees of controlled injury and inflammation.

# References

1. Chesnutt MSPT, Tavan ET. Pulmonary disorders. In: Papadakis MAMS, Rabow MW, editors. *Current Medical Diagnosis & Treatment*. New York: McGraw-Hill; 2014.

2. Albanese CTSK Pediatric surgery. In: GM D, editor. *Current Diagnosis & Treatment: Surgery*, 13th edn. New York: McGraw-Hill; 2010.

3. Yoon PJKP, Friedman NR Ear, nose, & throat. In: Hay WWJ, Levin MJ, Deterding RR, Abzug MJ, Sondheimer JM, editors. *Current Diagnosis & Treatment: Pediatrics*, 21st edn. New York: McGraw-Hill; 2012.

4. Abdullah B, Hassan S, Salim R. Transnasal endoscopic repair for bilateral choanal atresia. *Malays J Med Sci.* 2006;13(2):61–3.

5. Asma A, Roslenda AR, Suraya A, Saraiza AB, Aini AA. Management of congenital choanal atresia (CCA) after multiple failures: a case report. *Med J Malaysia.* 2013;68(1):76–8.

6. Schoem SR. Transnasal endoscopic repair of choanal atresia: why stent? *Otolaryngol Head Neck Surg.* 2004;131(4):362–6.

7. Friedman NR, Mitchell RB, Bailey CM, Albert DM, Leighton SE. Management and outcome of choanal atresia correction. *Int J Pediatr Otorhinolaryngol.* 2000;52(1):45–51.

8. Austin J, Ali T. Tracheomalacia and bronchomalacia in children: pathophysiology, assessment, treatment and anaesthesia management. *Paediatr Anaesth.* 2003;13(1):3–11.

9. Thomas VDSN, Lee KK, Swanson NA Benign epithelial tumors, hamartomas, and hyperplasias. In: Goldsmith LAKS, Gilchrest BA, Paller AS, Leffell DJ, Wolff K, editors. *Fitzpatrick's Dermatology in General Medicine*, 8th edn. New York: McGraw-Hill; 2012.

10. Shah RNCT, Shores CG Infections and disorders of the neck and upper airway. In: Tintinalli JESJ, Ma O, Cline DM, Cydulka RK, Meckler GD, editors. *Tintinalli's Emergency Medicine: A Comprehensive Study Guide*, 7th edn. New York: McGraw-Hill; 2011.

11. Hackam DJGT, Wang KS, Newman KD, Ford HR Pediatric surgery. In: Brunicardi FAD, Billiar TR, Dunn DL, et al., editors. *Schwartz's Principles of Surgery*, 9th edn. New York: McGraw-Hill; 2012.

12. Usatine RPSM, Chumley HS, Mayeaux EJ Jr. Childhood hemangiomas and vascular malformations. In: *The Color Atlas of Family Medicine*, 2nd edn. New York: McGraw-Hill; 2013.

13. Losee JEGM, Rubin J, Wallace CG, Wei F Plastic and reconstructive surgery. In: Brunicardi FAD, Billiar TR, Dunn DL, et al., editors. *Schwartz's Principles of Surgery*, 9th edn. New York: McGraw-Hill; 2010.

14. McDonald S, Langton Hewer CD, Nunez DA Grommets (ventilation tubes) for recurrent acute otitis media in children. *Cochrane Database Syst Rev*. 2008;4: CD004741.

15. Chinn K, Brown OE, Manning SC, Crandell CC. Middle ear pressure variation: effect of nitrous oxide. *Laryngoscope*. 1997;107(3):357–63.

16. Eidi M, Kolahdouzan K, Hosseinzadeh H, Tabaqi R. A comparison of preoperative ondansetron and dexamethasone in the prevention of post-tympanoplasty nausea and vomiting. *Iran J Med Sci*. 2012;37(3):166–72.

17. Jöhr M, Ho A, Wagner CS, Linder T. Ear surgery in infants under one year of age: its risks and implications for cochlear implant surgery. *Otology & Neurotology*. 2008. 29(3):310–13.

18. Baidya KD, Dehran M. Anaesthesia for cochlear implant surgery. *Trends Anaesth Crit Care*. 2011;1:90–4.

19. Suter VG, Bornstein MM. Ankyloglossia: facts and myths in diagnosis and treatment. *J Periodontol*. 2009;80(8):1204–19.

20. Kupietzky A, Botzer E. Ankyloglossia in the infant and young child: clinical suggestions for diagnosis and management. *Pediatr Dent*. 2005;27(1):40–6.

21. Hamada, M, Iida M, Nota J, et al. Safety and efficacy of adenotonsillectomy for obstructive sleep apnea in infants, toddlers and preschool children. *Auris Nasus Larynx*. 2015;42(3):208–12.

22. Brigance, JS, Miyamoto RC, Schilt P. Surgical management of obstructive sleep apnea in infants and young toddlers. *Otolaryngol Head Neck Surg*. 2009;140(6):912–16.

23. Mitchell, RB, Kelly J. Outcome of adenotonsillectomy for obstructive sleep apnea in children under 3 years. *Otolaryngol Head Neck Surg*. 2005;132(5):681–4.

24. Moss JR, Watcha MF, Bendel LP, et al. A multicenter, randomized, double-blind placebo-controlled, single dose trial of the safety and efficacy of intravenous ibuprofen for treatment of pain in pediatric patients undergoing tonsillectomy. *Pediatr Anesth*. 2014;24:483–9.

25. Lewis SR, Nicholson A, Cardwell ME, Siviter G, Smith AF Nonsteroidal anti-inflammatory drugs and perioperative bleeding in paediatric tonsillectomy. *Cochrane Database Syst Rev*. 2013;7:CD00359.

26. Voronov P, Tobin MJ, Billings K, et al. Postoperative pain relief in infants undergoing myringotomy and tube placement: comparison of a novel regional anesthetic block to intranasal fentanyl – a pilot analysis. *Pediatr Anesth*. 2008;18(12):1196–201.

27. Steward D, Grisel J, Meinzen-Derr J Steroids for improving recovery following tonsillectomy in children. *Cochrane Database Syst Rev*. 2011;8:CD003997.

28. Dhar P, Malik A. Review: anesthesia for laser surgery in ENT and the various ventilatory techniques. *Trends Anaesth Crit Care*. 2011;1(2):60–6.

## Chapter 22

# Anesthesia for Plastic Surgery

Petra M. Meier

## Introduction

Congenital structural anomalies in the head and neck usually require surgical correction and pose special problems for the anesthesiologist. Management of these infants is best accomplished by an interdisciplinary team of pediatric specialists in plastic surgery, neurosurgery, otolaryngology, ophthalmology, maxillofacial surgery, and pediatric intensive care. Many infants are syndromic and will necessitate multiple procedures. Often there are airway problems and congenital heart anomalies that require careful assessment and anesthetic management.

## Cleft Lip and Palate (CL/P)

Cleft lip, with or without cleft palate, is among the most common congenital malformation and presents in a wide spectrum of severity. The incidence is 3.6/1000 in Native Americans, 2/1000 in Asians, 1/1000 in Caucasians, and 0.3/1000 in African Americans. Ninety percent of cleft lips are unilateral and two-thirds are on the left side. Isolated cleft palate (CP) is considered genetically different: It occurs in 0.5/1000 births, more commonly in girls, whereas CL/P occurs more often in boys. Associated anomalies are more frequent in CP (~50 percent) versus CL/P (~10 percent). These infants present with anemia, malnutrition secondary to feeding difficulties, repeated respiratory infections, and impairment in speech.

## Classification

*Cleft lip* is categorized as *unilateral* or *bilateral* and designated as *incomplete* when the skin of the upper lip is not fully separated or *complete* when the defect involves the nasal floor and alveolus (Figure 22.1).

*Cleft of the palate* occurs in two major forms: soft palate only, which may extend into the posterior hard palate; and complete defect of the soft/hard palate,

which is either unilateral or bilateral. The type and extent of palatal clefting is categorized by the Veau classification (Figure 22.2). Submucous CP is a minor form characterized by bifid uvula, thin soft palate due to incomplete muscular formation and a notch in the posterior edge of the hard palate. There is also an occult submucous CP that appears to be intact but can cause hypernasal speech.

## Surgical Procedures and Timing

Many cleft lip and palate centers use some form of preoperative dentofacial orthopedic manipulation of the maxillary segments for the infant with unilateral and bilateral complete CL/P. A surgical alternative is a preliminary lip adhesion (labial closure) if the cleft is especially wide or if dentofacial orthopedics is not available.

Surgical closure of a *cleft lip* is usually performed at 4–5 months of age, when the infant is gaining satisfactory weight, and is free of any oral, respiratory, or systemic infection. The most commonly used technique for a unilateral CL is the rotation-advancement method of Millard. Repair of a bilateral CL is often accomplished synchronously with nasal and alveolar closure. Some surgeons stage the correction of the bilateral deformity. Most surgeons repair a CL while standing.

*Cleft palate* should be repaired at 8–10 months of age, because the incidence of velopharyngeal insufficiency increases after this age. Normal speech becomes increasingly unlikely if palatal repair is delayed beyond one year of age. Closure involves elevating mucoperiosteal flaps from the underlying palatal shelves and approximating these flaps in the midline, including dissection and retro-positioning of the levator muscles. Some centers employ a z-plasty palatal closure (Furlow technique). Most surgeons sit while undertaking repair of the CP.

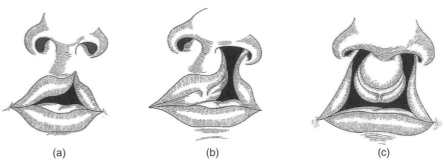

(a)                    (b)                    (c)

**Figure 22.1** Types of cleft lip: (a) unilateral incomplete; (b) unilateral complete; (c) bilateral complete. Adapted and reprinted with permission from Dr. John B. Mulliken [1]. Used with permission from the People's Medical Publishing House, USA.

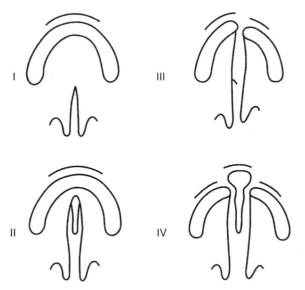

**Figure 22.2** Veau classification: soft palate only (Veau I); soft/hard palate (Veau II); unilateral complete cleft lip/palate (Veau III); bilateral complete cleft lip/palate (Veau IV). Adapted and reprinted with permission from Dr. John B. Mulliken [1]. Used with permission from the People's Medical Publishing House, USA.

Usually the infants are discharged on the second postoperative day after CL repair and after CP on postoperative day 2–4.

## Associated Conditions

Every infant with CL/P or CP should be assessed for other associated anomalies. There is a long list of syndromes associated with CL/P and CP. Cleft lip/palate centers report that up to 30 percent of affected infants have other anomalies [2]. These congenital anomalies tend to be under-diagnosed at birth and early infancy, especially in those infants with a less severe expression of a genetic disorder. Associated anomalies include malformations of the upper and lower limbs or the vertebral column, the cardiovascular system, and gastrointestinal tract. Bilateral CL/P is a common finding in various trisomies, particularly involving chromosome 13. Nevertheless, most cases of CL/P occur as isolated (sporadic) anomalies, they are not syndromic. Cardiac anomalies occur in approximately 8 percent of CP infants. The most common associated disorder with CP is the Robin sequence, which can be nonsyndromic or syndromic.

## Robin Sequence

*Robin sequence* is a diagnostic term that denotes mandibular micrognathia/retrognathia, glossoptosis (posterior displacement of the tongue), anterior larynx, and respiratory and feeding problems (Figure 22.3). Many infants with Robin sequence have ankyloglossia (tongue tie) which should not be severed until the infant is older and the airway is secure. Usually there is a CP but this is not an obligatory finding for Robin sequence. Most infants are either micro- or retrognathic, but not both. There are over 40 syndromes associated with Robin sequence. Stickler syndrome is the most common cause of Robin sequence (30–40 percent), followed by velocardiofacial syndrome (17 percent) (Table 22.1). In infants with nonsyndromic Robin sequence the mandible may grow to approximately normal size and a nearly normal upper/lower jaw relationship is expected so that the patients "grow out" of the airway obstruction. In infants with a syndromic Robin sequence mandibular growth potential differs depending on the particular syndrome. For example, in Stickler syndrome, mandibular growth is nearly normal. In contrast, in infants with Treacher Collins syndrome or bilateral hemifacial microsomia the mandible will remain hypoplastic

**Table 22.1** Major syndromes associated with Robin sequence

| Syndrome | Description | Anesthesia implication |
|---|---|---|
| Stickler syndrome | Arthro-ophtalmology condition: floppy infant, severe myopia, retinal detachment, glaucoma, deafness, midfacial or mandibular hypoplasia, cleft palate, hypermobile joints, spondyloepiphyseal dysplasia, CHD in 45 percent (mitral valve prolapse). | Most common cause of Robin sequence; examine neck movement; prevent damage to arthritic joints; CHD, intubation difficulty decreases with increasing age. |
| Velocardiofacial syndrome | Characteristic facies: prominent nose, vertically long face, retrognathia; cleft palate, laryngeal webs (10 percent); CHD in 40–50 percent (VSD, tetralogy of Fallot, truncus arteriosus, right-sided aortic arch, interrupted aortic arch); speech difficulties due to velopharyngeal anomalies, learning disabilities, DiGeorge syndrome (10 percent). | Second common cause of Robin sequence; orofacial deformations can make intubation very difficult; consideration for CHD; obstructive sleep apnea may occur after pharyngoplasty. |
| Treacher Collins syndrome (mandibulofacial dysostosis) | Antimongoloid slant of the eyes, coloboma of eyelids; choanal atresia; micrognathia, hypoplastic zygoma, macrostomia, high-arched palate, small cleft palate (30 percent), pharyngeal hypoplasia; low set ears with deformities; cervical vertebral malformations; often CHD. | Airway and intubation difficulties, LMA and fiberoptic scope are useful, tracheostomy might be required, intubation difficulty will persist or increase with increasing age. |
| Hemifacial microsomia (Goldenhar syndrome) | Unilateral hypoplasia of facial bones and muscles, mandibular hypoplasia, limited mouth opening, high arched palate, cleft palate, deformity of ear and eye; vertebral anomalies in 40 percent, CHD in 20 percent, renal anomalies. | Airway problems, obstructive sleep apnea; may be difficult to hold the mask; if bilateral intubation very difficult, have an LMA ready; extubate awake; consideration for CHD; airway problem will persist. |

CHD = congenital heart disease

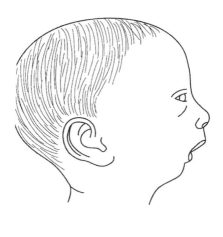
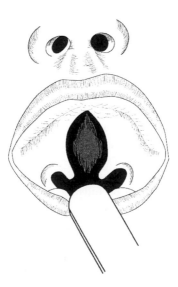

**Figure 22.3** (a) Infant with Robin sequence. (b) Intraoral view of U-shaped cleft palate. Adapted and reprinted with permission from Dr. John B. Mulliken [1]. Used with permission from the People's Medical Publishing House, USA).

and proportionally smaller and the airway problems will persist. (Figure 22.5)

A few days after birth, the severity of Robin sequence can be clinically graded: eats and breathes well with supine positioning (grade I); breathes well but obstructs when fed by mouth (grade II); cannot breathe or eat without obstruction and desaturation (grade III). Infants in the grade III group present with

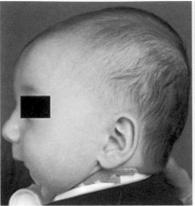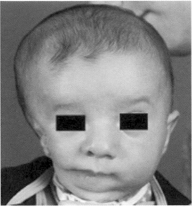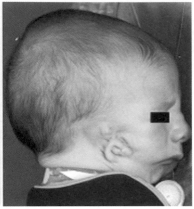

**Figure 22.4** Left lateral, frontal and right lateral view of former 33-week premature infant with Robin sequence (syndromic) and right predominant hemifacial microsomia. A tracheostomy was placed at age one month because of airway obstruction and apnea along with a gastrostomy for feeding difficulties. Note right micro-ophthalmia, right-sided soft tissue hypoplasia, bilateral mandibular deformity, retrognathia, right macrostomia (transverse oral cleft) and right microtia. He also has cervical vertebral and renal anomalies. Courtesy Dr. John B. Mulliken.

periods of cyanosis, usually with substernal and intercostal retractions. Feeding through a nasogastric tube might be a short-term solution; some infants need a gastrostomy. Initially the airway may be controlled by placing the infant in a lateral position with the head of the bed slightly raised and using a nasopharyngeal airway or a pacifier to keep the tongue forward. Prone position facilitates drainage of oral secretion and helps posture the tongue forward. Respiratory obstruction may occur combined with central and obstructive sleep apnea which can lead to cor pulmonale. If the infant desaturates despite all attempts of positioning or cannot be fed orally (many grade II and all grade III), operative intervention may include tongue–lip adhesion, mandibular distraction, and, as a last resort, tracheotomy if the tongue–lip adhesion fails (Figure 22.4) [3,4]. Airway management can be complex, with very difficult intubation, so awake techniques may be considered. In skilled hands fiberoptic intubation under general anesthesia may be used. For postoperative extubation infants should be fully awake [5].

## Preoperative Evaluation and Anesthetic Considerations

Careful *preoperative assessment*, especially of heart, lungs, and airway, is mandatory to reveal associated conditions and abnormalities related to syndromes (Table 22.1). Infants with a large cleft and acute respiratory infection tend to have a higher intra- and postoperative complication rate which should initiate a discussion with the surgeon to postpone the operation [6]. Cleft lip repair involves minimal blood loss. Cleft palate repair has more blood loss but usually does not require blood transfusion in otherwise healthy infants with hematocrit values greater than 30 percent.

In our experience, tracheal intubation is not particularly difficult in most infants with CL/P, unless concomitant defects are present. The incidence of a difficult airway in infants with CL/P ranges between 5 and 10 percent [7–9]. The incidence of difficult laryngoscopy is 7 percent in the age group of 1–6 months old infants and is greatest for infants with bilateral CL/P [8]. Midfacial anomalies, mandibular hypoplasia (retro- or micrognathia, e.g., in Robin sequence, hemifacial microsomia, Treacher Collins syndrome) or restricted cervical movement are indicators of serious airway problems. If micrognathia is present, the incidence of difficult laryngoscopy is approximately 50 percent whereas without micrognathia it is about 4 percent [8]. Intubation difficulty decreases with increasing age in infants with nonsyndromic Robin sequence; however, in syndromic Robin sequence it differs depending on the particular syndrome (Table 22.1). Given the difficulty of recognizing micrognathia and retrognathia in young infants and that the ear and mandible develop from the first and second pharyngeal arches and first branchial cleft, abnormalities of the ear should prompt a closer examination of the mandible for hypoplasia. The presence of isolated

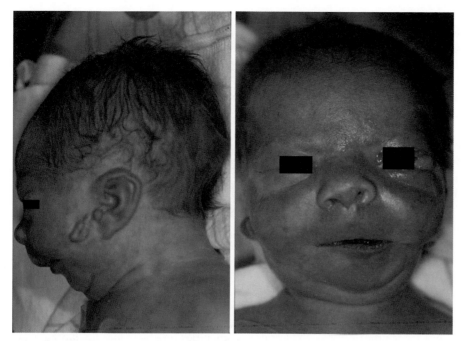

**Figure 22.5** Infant with bilateral hemifacial microsomia, predominant on left side, presented with noisy breathing and feeding difficulties requiring gastrostomy. Associated anomalies include bilateral eyelid colobomas, left limbal lipodermoid, facial asymmetry with midfacial hypoplasia, slightly elevated and rotated left nostril, small nasal airways with left-sided choanal atresia, minor bilateral macrostomia, restricted oral opening, micro-retrognathia, ankyloglossia (tongue-tie) glossoptosis, intact palate, bilateral low-set and posteriorly rotated ears with complex pretragal chondro-cutaneous remnants, and cardiac defects. During inhalational induction he did poorly with mask ventilation; two anesthesiologists were required to hold the mask, unable to pass a nasal trumpet but able to insert an oral airway. Direct laryngoscopy and intubation was difficult but possible using a video laryngoscope. Courtesy Dr. John B. Mulliken.

microtia is also an indicator for difficult intubation with an incidence of difficult laryngeal view of 42 percent in patients with bilateral microtia, and 2 percent in those with unilateral microtia [10]. A careful review of previous anesthetic records may forewarn of a difficult airway.

*Induction of anesthesia* is usually performed in a spontaneously breathing infant with a non-irritating inhalational agent and is expected to be uncomplicated in an infant presenting for closure of simple CL/P with a history of airway patency during natural sleep (no snoring or sleep apnea). In the presence of a wide cleft palate the tongue can fall into the cleft and may obstruct the nasal airway. With increased relaxation of the oropharyngeal muscles the tongue will fall further posteriorly and may obstruct the oropharynx completely, which can be prevented by placing an oropharyngeal airway. Spraying the mouth with a topical anesthetic prior to induction will allow placement of an oral airway at light depths of anesthesia. If the anesthesiologist is comfortable ventilating the infant with a mask, a nondepolarizing muscle relaxant can

be administered. Intubation of a patient with unilateral right-sided cleft is usually straightforward. Infants with left-sided complete cleft are more difficult because the laryngoscope blade will tend to fall into the cleft as the tongue gets swept to the left side and alters the line of vision. In bilateral CL/P, the premaxilla is angled anteriorly, altering the anesthesiologist's line of sight onto the entrance of the larynx and hampering the insertion of the laryngoscope blade. To prevent traumatic laryngoscopy and intubation, the wide or bilateral cleft can be packed with moist sterile gauze. Sometimes external laryngeal manipulation of the larynx is useful during direct laryngoscopy if the mandible is hypoplastic. Infants with Robin sequence and associated craniofacial syndromes have a small oral cavity because of a hypoplastic mandible (Table 22.1); the larynx is positioned cephalad and anterior under the base of the tongue, and airway management requires more planning. If the patient has a history of lack of airway patency during sleep, successful ventilation by mask might be very difficult or unlikely. Consequently, alternative techniques for securing the airway need to be considered such as sedated/awake techniques, fiberoptic intubation, intubation through a laryngeal mask airway, and in severe cases tracheostomy [11]. In severe cases an otorhinolaryngologist should be available to help with the airway management and assessment for other causes of obstruction such as anomalies of the epiglottis and laryngomalacia.

For orotracheal intubation a variety of tubes are available. The Ring–Adair–Elwyn (RAE) or the microcuff Kimberly Clark preformed tracheal tube are frequently used and can be fixed on the chin, placed over the midline of the lower lip to facilitate optimal surgical access and visualize lip and palate. In infants with micro- and retrognathia the preformed tubes can be too long, which results in one-sided intubation. The advantage of the microcuff tube is the slimmer cuff which is positioned further distal (no Murphy eye) compared to the RAE tube, which facilitates appropriate midtracheal placement. The tube and the tubing system need to be carefully arranged when the operating room table is turned 90 or 180 degrees away from the anesthesia provider to prevent inadvertent extubation. Care must be taken that bilateral ventilation of the lungs is present during all repositioning maneuvers by the surgical team and after the mouth gag and throat pack is positioned. Insertion of the gag and repositioning of the neck tends to advance the tip of the tube in the trachea, with the risk of one-sided ventilation. The eyes need to be carefully protected before incision. Monitoring should include the standard ASA monitors and ventilation parameters (compliance, ventilation pressures, tidal volume) to recognize compression of the tube caused by surgical maneuvers or obstruction (e.g., secretion).

*Maintenance of anesthesia* is achieved with low doses of inhalational agents combined with short-acting opioids (e.g., 1–2 µg kg$^{-1}$ fentanyl for induction as well as for incision and repeated doses during each consecutive surgical hour) or medium-acting opioids (e.g., 30 µg kg$^{-1}$ morphine for induction, as well as for incision and 30–40 minutes before emergence). Very short-acting opioids, like remifentanil, are avoided in our practice because of the risk of developing hyperalgesia during the immediate postoperative period. Local infiltration with local anesthetic (e.g., lidocaine 0.5 percent or bupivacaine 0.25 percent with epinephrine 1:200 000) and bilateral infraorbital blocks during CL repair may reduce the amount of opioids and risk of postoperative respiratory depression [12–15].

In neonates, Boesenberg et al. prefer a percutaneous technique instead of a perioral one, with bupivacaine 0.5 percent 0.5–0.75 ml with epinephrine 1:200 000 [16]. Communication with the surgeon and parents is recommended because even small amounts of local anesthetic can cause edema and small hematomas in the cheeks.

# Extubation, Acute Airway Obstruction and Postoperative Care

At the end of the procedure infants should wake up in an unagitated state, as hypertension and undue crying may cause bleeding or place excessive tension on the repair. After cleft repair, the minimal to moderate amount of blood in the oropharynx needs to be carefully suctioned. Extubation should be performed after airway reflexes have returned in an infant that is awake, opens the eyes, and presents with regular breathing and good muscle tone. There may be some respiratory difficulties on emergence, including acute upper airway obstruction as a result of upper airway narrowing due to the surgical reduction of the pharyngeal space, edema, and residual anesthetic effects. All infants with a nonsyndromic or syndromic Robin sequence who presented with a difficult airway management during induction should be observed in the NICU/ICU post CP repair. Rare cases are reported of massive lingual swelling in infants with Robin sequence as well as in otherwise healthy infants follow CP closure. The reasons might be prolonged procedures, head-down position, and prolonged lingual retraction [17,18]. In selected cases surgeons provide a tongue suture for traction which often proves helpful in restoring the infant's airway. In some institutions after CL repair, surgeons like to use a Logan bow to protect the operative site combined with a saline-soaked gauze over the wound (Figure 22.6). In these cases awake extubation with good airway reflexes is of special importance because mask placement and ventilation is impossible with the bow in place. The saline-soaked gauze is used for the first 24 hours to prevent crusting and the bow is temporary. Arm restraints are used in many centers to prevent trauma to the labial repair. During the *postoperative course* vigilance and monitoring is required for upper airway obstruction (48 hours), late postoperative edema, subcutaneous emphysema and negative pulmonary pressure edema. Any signs of airway obstruction and stridor require careful attention and treatment with corticosteroid

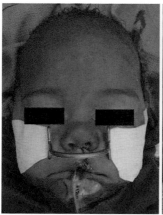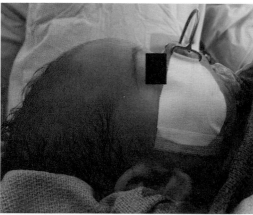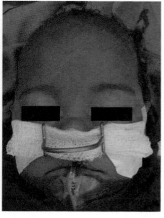

**Figure 22.6** Five-month-old infant with unilateral left incomplete cleft lip following rotation advancement repair and correction of minor nasal deformity. Xeroform gauze-wrapped tubing inserted in left nostril. Logan bow (left and center picture) holds an iced saline sponge (right picture). The infant was extubated fully awake and recovered in the postanesthesia care unit. Courtesy Dr. John B. Mulliken.

and racemic epinephrine to prevent reintubation. Postoperative bleeding is difficult to detect because the blood is usually swallowed. Postoperative analgesics should be titrated to avoid causing sedation and airway obstruction. Pain is managed with acetaminophen and IV opioids can be titrated in the PACU with conversion to oral opioids as soon as oral intake permits. Feeding is usually initiated as soon as the infant is awake.

# Craniosynostosis

The estimate of prevalence of craniosynostosis ranges from 0.4 to 1 per 1000 live births. [19] It is defined as a premature closure of one or more calvarial sutures with failure of normal growth perpendicular to the suture and compensatory overgrowth parallel to the affected suture. The abnormal cranial shape is determined by the specific sutures involved (Table 22.2). The clinical diagnosis is confirmed by plain skull roentgenogram or CT scan. Uncorrected craniosynostosis can have lifelong effects on appearance and neurocognitive development.

## Classification

**Craniosynostosis** occurs as either an isolated single fusion (80 percent) or as multiple-sutural fusion (20 percent) that can be syndromic or nonsyndromic. Sagittal craniosynostosis is the most common form (sagittal: 50–60 percent, coronal 20 percent, metopic 10 percent). Increased intracranial pressure can occur in 15–20 percent of infants with single sutural synostosis and in 40–70 percent of those with syndromic

craniosynostoses [20]. Surgical intervention is indicated to prevent complications such as cerebral compression, auditory impairment and visual loss [21–24]. The etiology of most cases is sporadic, although there is often a strong genetic component. Genetic mutations that are responsible for the syndromic craniosynostoses include mutations in the fibroblast growth factors (*FGFR* 1, *FGFR2*, *FGFR3*), *TWIST*, and *MSX2* genes.

**Progressive postnatal craniosynostosis**, a rare presentation, is characterized by a normal cranial shape and normal radiological images at birth. Later in childhood there is slow development of intracranial pressure (ICP), with signs/symptoms such as headaches, vomiting, irritability, papilledema, progressive optic atrophy, seizures, and/or bulging fontanelles [25].

**Positional plagiocephaly**, also known as deformational plagiocephaly, is extremely common and can be confused with craniosynostosis, particularly lambdoid fusion. There is characteristic unilateral occipital flattening and anterior displacement of the ipsilateral ear. This harmless condition is treated nonsurgically by an orthotic helmet if initiated early enough [26,27].

# Craniosynostotic syndromes and implications for preoperative assessment

There are important anesthetic implications in the care of infants with craniosynostoses, which can be associated with numerous syndromes. The most frequent ones are detailed in Table 22.3.

**Airway comorbidity.** Children, especially those with syndromic craniosynostosis, can present with a compromised airway. Although the incidence of

217

**Table 22.2** Nomenclature of craniosynostosis

| Affected Suture | Name (literal translation) | Clinical Description |
| --- | --- | --- |
| Sagittal | Scaphocephaly (boat-shaped cranium) | Long, narrow head, frontal and occipital bossing. |
| Metopic | Trigonocephaly (triangular-shaped cranium) | Triangular, pointed forehead, midline ridge, orbital proptosis. |
| Unilateral coronal | Frontal synostotic plagiocephaly (unilateral flat forehead) | Unilateral frontal flattening, affected orbit higher, anterior position of ear on affected side, nasal root deviated to affected side, nasal tip deviated to unaffected side, prominent brow on unaffected side. |
| Bilateral coronal | Brachycephaly (short cranium) | Broad flattened frontal bones, flattened occiput, orbital hypertelorism. |
| Lamboid | Posterior plagiocephaly (unilateral occipital flattening) | Unilateral occipital flattening, prominent ipsilateral mastoid process. |

sleep disorder and obstructive sleep apnea syndrome is high, it is often unrecognized [28,29]. Obstructive sleep apnea symptoms occur in almost half of the children during episodes of upper respiratory tract infections. Major upper airway obstruction is found more frequently in patients with Crouzon, Pfeiffer, and Apert syndromes and less often in patients with Muenke and Saethre-Chotzen syndromes [30]. Causes for severe airway obstruction include mid-facial hypoplasia, choanal atresia, and also lower airway anomalies. Tracheal cartilaginous sleeve is a rare congenital cartilage malformation reported only in children with craniosynostosis syndromes and is characterized by fusion of the tracheal arches that may be isolated to a few tracheal arches, involves the entire trachea, or extends beyond the carina into the bronchi [31]. Infants with syndromic craniosynostosis can present with difficult airway management [11,32] but rarely require tracheostomy, unless there is marked facial dysmorphism [33].

It is important to consider the effect of chronic airway obstruction on the cardiovascular system and the central nervous system. Patients who have a history of longstanding airway obstruction may have chronic hypoventilation and hypoxia that can lead to pulmonary hypertension and subsequently cor pulmonale.

**Table 22.3** Craniosynostosis and frequently associated syndromes

| Syndrome | Description | Anesthesia implications |
|---|---|---|
| Apert | Most common coronal synostosis, possible increased ICP; exorbitism, midface hypoplasia, choanal stenosis, airway anomalies (2 percent); syndactyly of hands and feet, synphalangism, partial cervical spine fusion C5/6 (70 percent); CHD (10 percent); genitourinary anomalies; cognitive impairment. | Obstructive sleep apnea; possible difficult intubation; possible increased ICP; evaluation for CHD. |
| Crouzon (craniofacial dysostosis) | Multiple suture synostosis (coronal, sagittal), possible increased ICP resulting from progressive hydrocephalus, intracranial abnormalities (Chiari); exorbitism; midface hypoplasia, choanal atresia, airway obstruction; low-set ears; rare cardiac anomaly; vertebral anomalies C2/3; mental retardation. | Difficult airway management, elective tracheostomy might be indicated; possible increased ICP; ocular protection. |
| Muenke | Most common craniosynostosis syndrome; coronal synostosis; midface hypoplasia rare. | Possible mild obstructive sleep apnea. |
| Saethre Chotzen | Unilateral or bilateral coronal suture synostosis (brachycephaly, plagiocephaly); possible increased ICP; maxillary hypoplasia; CHD; syndactyly, cervical spine abnormalities, clavicular anomalies. | Possible difficult intubation due to cervical vertebral fusion; possible increased ICP. |
| Pfeiffer | Multiple suture synostosis (brachycephaly, turricephaly, most common cause of trilobar cranial deformity (Kleeblattschädel)); possible increased ICP, Chiari malformation; ocular proptosis; midface hypoplasia; CHD; cervical vertebral fusions, mild syndactyly, short and broad thumbs and toes. | Possible difficult airway; obstructive apnea; possible seizures (interaction anticonvulsants with anesthetic drugs); evaluation for CHD. |

CHD = Congenital heart disease.

The chronic respiratory obstruction forms part of a vicious cycle with increased intracranial pressure and a subsequent decrease in cerebral perfusion pressure [34]. Recurrent episodes of intermittent reduction of cerebral perfusion pressure most likely have a negative effect on neurological and cognitive development in the long term.

**Cardiac comorbidity.** Craniosynostotic syndromes can occasionally be associated with cardiac anomalies (Table 22.3). Congenital heart disease, both repaired and unrepaired, has been shown to increase the risk for anesthesia and any surgery. Infants with patent foramen ovale or ductus arteriosus are at risk for paradoxical air emboli (coronary or cerebral air embolism) through these defects.

**Neurological Comorbidity.** Several factors contribute to the risk of developing increased ICP, including decreased intracranial volume and increased number and location of sutures involved [35]. Although it is well known that increased ICP is commonly associated with multiple suture craniosynostosis [30], ICP monitoring has demonstrated that 14–24 percent of infants with single-suture craniosynostosis also have raised ICP [24,36]. Positron emission tomography scans have shown reduced cortical blood flow in the vicinity of sagittal synostosis in 70 percent of cases, which can be corrected by early release [37]. Hydrocephalus is seen sometimes in patients with craniosynostosis. It is particularly associated with Crouzon and Pfeiffer syndrome, and Kleeblattschädel (cloverleaf skull syndrome; see Figure 22.9). Multisuture craniosynostoses, particularly with lambdoid involvement, are associated with a higher incidence of acquired Chiari deformation, require multiple operative procedures, and cause more developmental delay than isolated single-suture synostoses [38]. Evidence of jugular foraminal stenosis or atresia and dilated collateral emissary veins in children with syndromic craniosynostosis is associated with venous outflow obstruction and elevated intracranial venous hypertension [39,40]. Disruption of emissary veins during an operation can produce massive hemorrhage. Enlarged basal emissary foramina which transmit enlarged emissary veins result from stenosis or atresia of the jugular foramen. Bilateral basilar venous atresia is most common in patients with the *FGFR3* ala391glu mutation (crouzonoid features with acanthosis nigricans) but also may be found in patients with *FGFR2* mutations [39]. Preoperative assessment of patients with syndromic craniosynostosis and

**219**

enlarged emissary foramina should include skull base vascular imaging of the basilar venous drainage [39]. Significant increased intracranial bleeding is expected during craniectomy.

**Ophthalmologic Comorbidities.** Ophthalmologic examinations may show papilledema and optic atrophy with chronically raised ICP [41]. Syndromic craniosynostoses with shallow, deformed orbits, and exorbitism increases the risk of corneal abrasion and ocular trauma during an operation.

**Cervical vertebra anomalies**, particularly in Apert, Pfeiffer, and Crouzon syndromes, limit neck motion (flexion and extension) and can increase the difficulty of intubation and positioning for the operation.

## Surgical Procedures and Timing

The type and timing of the operative correction for craniosynostosis varies with age, location, and number of sutures involved, and the experience of the surgical team. Indications for repair of craniosynostosis include: increased ICP, cranial deformity, exorbitism, airway obstruction, and psychosocial reasons.

**Endoscopic-assisted strip craniectomy (ESC)** is considered for infants less than three months of age, usually for single-suture synostosis and in selected cases for multiple sutural synostosis. Endoscopic-assisted strip craniectomy is a short surgical procedure (approximately 30–45 minutes) associated with low incidence of perioperative blood transfusion (0–11 percent) [42–45], VAE (2–8 percent) [44,45], ICU admission (8 percent) [44], and expense [46]. Most infants are discharged on postoperative day one. Postoperative molding helmet therapy for approximately eight months (Figure 22.7) is an integral part of this treatment modality necessary to counteract the tendency of the cranial vault to revert to premorbid shape after strip craniectomy [43].

Patient positioning during neuroendoscopic procedures remains one of the paramount concerns in providing optimal surgical access and exposure of the suture for visualization and resection. Sagittal ESC and lambdoid ESC are usually performed in prone position, often using special headrests (e.g., Doro headrest system, PMI, Freiburg im Breisgau, Germany; Figure 22.7) and metopic and coronal ESC in supine position, commonly using the cerebellar headrest. The endotracheal tube has to be carefully placed in midtracheal position to prevent inadvertent extubation or bronchial mainstem intubation, taking into account the resultant displacement related to the head positioning (Figure 22.7).

Cranial burr holes are made through the midline of each scalp incision. An endoscope is used to visualize the fused suture, identify emissary veins, dural attachments, and assure hemostasis. The fused suture is resected as a 1 cm wide bony strip and removed through the burr hole (Figure 22.7). Bone bleeding is controlled using bone wax and thrombin-soaked absorbable gelatin (Gelfoam, Pharmacia and Upjohn, Kalamazoo, MI).

**Spring-assisted cranioplasty** involves implanted springs in the synostosed sutures that allow gradual correction of the cranial malformation over time. It is used in infants older than three months of age with single sutural craniosynostosis and in selected infants with multiple sutural synostoses [47,48]. Different surgical groups report varying mean surgical times (range 30–170 minutes for insertion and 20–60 minutes for spring removal) and need for blood transfusion ranging from no blood transfusion [49] to blood loss comparable to open strip craniectomy [48,50]. This technique involves an osteotomy and resection of the prematurely closed suture combined with the insertion of 1–3 stainless steel springs across the newly created cranial gap (Figure 22.8). The expansion of a spring is a slow process and is monitored both clinically and radiologically. The springs are surgically removed after adequate cranial expansion (2–7 months).

**Open cranial procedures** are usually performed in infants at ages 6–12 months. The surgical procedures vary in the extent of cranial elements moved, risk of dural tear, sinus injury, and blood loss (simple strip craniectomy, π cranioplasties, cranial vault remodeling). Anterior calvarial procedures and fronto-orbital advancement involve bilateral craniectomy and sometimes require also posterior cranial vault remodeling, with or without barrel stave osteotomies. These techniques are associated with major blood loss, varying between 0.2 and 4 blood volumes, lengthy operative times (3–8 hours), and hospital stay (4–7 days), and require postoperative monitoring in a pediatric intensive care unit [51–53].

## Anesthetic Considerations

### Induction, Airway Management, and Monitoring

Despite the usually obvious craniofacial deformity, the infant's underlying neurodevelopmental status and general health is frequently quite normal. An

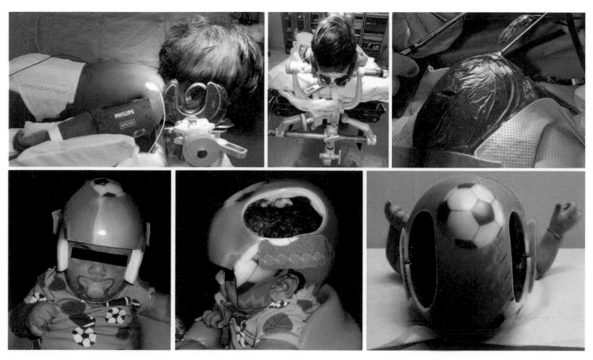

**Figure 22.7** Endoscopic-assisted strip craniectomy (ESC). Upper left and center picture: Infant in prone position for sagittal ESC on a modified prone head holder in sphinx position. It illustrates the extended head position and the significant distance between the highest point of the surgical field to the right atrium, a risk factor for venous or paradoxical air embolism. Upper right picture: Intraoperative picture of sagittal ESC with two skin incisions perpendicular to the fused sagittal suture: one posterior to the coronal sutures and the other at the junction of the lambdoid sutures. After endoscopic suturectomy, the 1–2 cm wide bone strip of the fused sagittal suture is removed. Lower pictures: Postoperative orthosis after ESC. Infant with sagittal synostosis after sagittal ESC wearing the helmet with openings at the side that allows the growing brain to push the skull out which finally results in the desired round head form. Courtesy Dr. Mark Proctor.

infant with mental retardation may not cooperate upon separation from the parents or during induction of anesthesia. *Premedication* should be cautiously considered in the presence of increased ICP, obstructive sleep apnea, and airway difficulties.

**During induction**, difficult airway management in patients with airway compromise should be expected (Table 22.3). Infants with syndromic craniosynostosis have some degree of midfacial hypoplasia with normal temporomandibular joints and normal-sized mandible (which only appears relatively prognathic), a high arched palate, small nasal passages, and some degree of choanal stenosis that causes primary mouth breathing. Management of the mask airway might be difficult because of the small, flat midface and ocular proptosis causing a problematic fit. Closure of the mouth occludes the oral airway as the tongue fills the smaller oral cavity, while the small nares and choanal stenosis cause resistance to nasal air flow. This problem can be overcome by gently holding the mouth open during induction (instead of closing it) and pressing down with the mask to obtain a good seal. Alternatively an oral airway can be used. In most cases tracheal intubation is not difficult unless there are major vertebral abnormalities and reduced cervical mobility or in the presence of craniofacial syndromes (Table 22.3). Infants with severe airway problems often have obstructive apnea and may require perioperative CPAP or tracheostomy. Abnormalities of the trachea might necessitate using a smaller-sized tube. Meticulous attention to midtracheal tube placement and secure fixation is essential because the infant's head is constantly moved during these cranial procedures, both rotated and extended. Intraoperative access to the airway is limited and the loss of the airway during the procedure is life-threatening. Most experienced surgical teams do not rely on taping the endotracheal tube to the nose or chin. A nasotracheal tube should be secured with a trans-septal suture, an orotracheal tube with a circum-mandibular wire for cranial vault remodeling procedures.

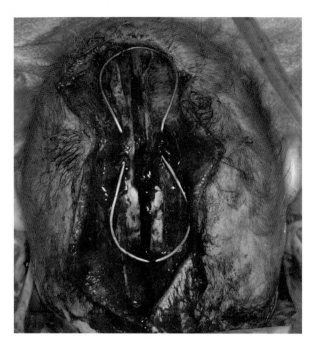

**Figure 22.8** Spring-assisted cranioplasty: After midline sagittal osteotomy, two omega-shaped springs are placed and cause a separation/distraction between the parietal bones. The two skin flaps created by the lazy-S incision are held aside with sutures. Courtesy Dr. Claes G.K. Lauritzen.

**Ventilation** should be performed with $O_2$/air and aimed at normocapnia or mild hypocapnia.

**Protection of the eyes** must be provided by the anesthesia/surgical team (i.e., lubrication, and tarsorrhaphy sutures) to prevent corneal damage, especially if there is ocular proptosis.

**Monitoring** includes the standard ASA monitors, several large-bore peripheral intravenous catheters sufficient for rapid transfusion, central line if vascular access is a problem, arterial invasive monitoring if ongoing blood loss is a concern, for hemodynamic monitoring and blood sampling. Laboratory capabilities for rapid assessment of blood gases, electrolytes, metabolic status, and coagulative status, including thromboelastography, should be available. A bladder catheter is necessary to monitor urinary output ($0.5 \text{ ml kg}^{-1}$). A variety of different monitors are used for detection of venous air embolism well before cardiovascular collapse occurs, e.g. precordial Doppler ultrasonography (characteristic change of signal, second highest sensitivity), end-tidal carbon dioxide (precipitous decrease in carbon dioxide tension), end-tidal nitrogen monitoring (sudden increase in the nitrogen concentration in the exhaled breath),

transesophageal echocardiography (presence of air in the right ventricular outflow tract, highest sensitivity) [54–59]. Insertion of central catheters for withdrawal of air is limited to a 33 percent success rate by the diminutive size of the infant and catheter because the ability to rapid aspirate air decreases with the size of the catheter.

**Maintaining normothermia** can be a major problem in infants in any lengthy procedure involving exposure of the large surface area of the head. During induction the operating room should be warmed up and warming lights and warming blankets used. Fluid warmers should be used throughout the surgical procedure. Low-flow gas anesthesia or heated humidifiers in the airway circuit minimizes evaporative heat loss from the respiratory system.

### Maintenance of Anesthesia

For maintenance of anesthesia a balanced anesthetic technique is usually used that includes inhalational agents, opioids, muscle relaxants, and antiemetics. The depth of anesthesia is titrated to maintain hemodynamics within 20 percent of baseline (heart rate, blood pressure). Opioids are titrated to the level of surgical stimulation. During fronto-orbital advancement (anterior cranial vault remodeling) oculocardiac reflex might be triggered, especially in young infants, by direct ocular pressure or ocular manipulation which most commonly leads to sinus bradycardia but also junctional rhythm, ectopic beats, atrioventricular block, or ventricular tachycardia. If notification of the surgeon to stop the stimulation does not resolve the arrhythmia/bradycardia, atropine ($20 \text{ µg kg}^{-1}$) and ephedrine should be considered. Perioperative corticosteroid reduces the postoperative edema of the eyes, which may swell shut during the first postoperative 24–48 hours, and shortens hospitalization without increasing the incidence of postoperative infection [60]. At the end of the procedure the patient should awaken comfortably, be appropriate for neurological assessment, and maintain a natural airway.

### Fluid Management, Blood Loss, and Blood Conservation

Close attention to fluid homeostasis and intravascular normovolemia is required to maintain adequate perfusion of tissue beds, kidneys, and particularly the brain in the presence of increased ICP. Maintenance should be substituted with isotonic crystalloid solutions and blood loss replaced 1:1 with blood products and blood derivatives. One study suggested that lactated Ringer's solution is the preferred crystalloid solution because it is less likely to induce metabolic acidosis than normal saline [61].

The extent of blood loss and the need for invasive monitoring are determined by the type and duration of the procedure, type of cranial malformation, number of sutures involved, and extent of osteotomies and bony movements.

**Endoscopic-assisted strip craniectomy** is a short procedure, rarely requiring blood transfusion. In healthy infants in our institution we forgo routine invasive arterial blood pressure monitoring in favor of two large-bore peripheral IV catheters, which are suitable for intraoperative venous blood sampling and rapid transfusion of blood products and derivatives. Appropriate IV access is especially important for low body weight infants (<5 kg), syndromic infants, and those with sagittal synostosis for whom there is a risk of sudden, abrupt bleeding from the sinus.

**For spring-assisted cranioplasty**, different centers report various degrees of bleeding and incidence of blood transfusion. As ESC and spring-assisted cranioplasty procedures are performed in young infants, the anesthesiologist should have always typed and crossed blood products readily available in the operating room.

**Open reconstruction procedures** have a higher comorbidity due to massive hemorrhage and potential cardiac arrest [62,63]. Blood loss occurs continuously throughout the procedure, but is especially brisk during craniectomy and if there is damage to cerebral venous sinuses. Estimation of ongoing blood loss can be difficult because of the use of large volumes of irrigation fluid and blood loss onto surgical drapes. As major blood loss has to be anticipated, at least one blood volume of blood products as well as a continuous infusion of a vasopressor (e.g. dopamine) should be available in the operating room before incision. Massive blood replacement is complicated by electrolyte and metabolic disturbances, coagulopathy, dilutional thrombocytopenia, and calcium-mediated hypotension [64,65]. High serum potassium levels, arrhythmias, and hyperkalemic cardiac arrest can occur during rapid transfusion, but also when modest amounts of old blood with high potassium concentration is transfused via a central line into the right atrium [66–69]. Administration of blood products is preferably delivered by the peripheral catheters because the central venous access delivers the more concentrated potassium load directly to the right heart through the pulmonary circulation to the left heart, where coronary circulation occurs. Discussion between the anesthesiologist and the blood bank should include (1) reservation of fresh and non-irradiated blood (less than seven days old) for infants less than one year of age undergoing a procedure necessitating rapid transfusion of blood products; or (2) use of washed blood products if those have been irradiated to diminish the possibility of graft-versus-host disease. Irradiation damages the RBC membrane and increases the erythrocyte membrane permeability, potassium leakage, and the potassium concentration in the extracellular fluid [70,71]. Therapy of a life-threatening arrhythmia includes administration of calcium gluconate, sodium bicarbonate, glucose and insulin, hyperventilation, and albuterol.

Massive blood loss requires a prompt coagulation screen and replacement therapy with platelets, fresh frozen plasma, or cryoprecipitate, as required. A *coagulopathy* should always be anticipated once the blood loss exceeds one blood volume. All intravenous fluid must be administered via a fluid warmer to prevent hypothermia. *Maintaining normothermia* helps to preserve normal coagulative indices.

**Blood conservation techniques** to reduce intraoperative blood loss have shown arguable results, have been evaluated in studies with single center design, and are based on small patient numbers. Strategies include: (1) tissue infiltration of a dilute vasoconstrictor solution (epinephrine 1:200 000 or less) to decrease blood loss upon incision through the scalp; (2) surgical technique using a Colorado needle; (3) preoperative administration of recombinant human erythropoietin to increase preoperative hematocrit [72], also used as dual therapy with cell saver [73], or combined with iron substitution [74]; (4) intraoperative antifibrinolytics; and (5) normovolemic hemodilution. Interest in the use of antifibrinolytics was generated by two randomized, double-blind, placebo-controlled studies that demonstrated the effectiveness of the antifibrinolytic agent tranexamic acid (TXA) in reducing blood loss and perioperative transfusion requirements in children with extensive craniofacial procedures [75,76]. Several dosing regimens have been described (loading dose of 15 mg kg$^{-1}$ TXA followed by an infusion of 10 mg kg$^{-1}$ h$^{-1}$ until skin closure [75]; 50 mg kg$^{-1}$ TXA loading dose followed by an infusion of 5 mg kg$^{-1}$ h$^{-1}$ until skin closure [76]), but the lowest effective intraoperative dosing regimen of TXA is uncertain, as well as the effective therapeutic plasma concentration of TXA to inhibit fibrinolysis. A combination of blood conservation techniques and an appropriately chosen surgical technique may best reduce the transfusion rate [77]. Normovolemic hemodilution and induced hypotension may compromise tissue oxygen delivery during rapid blood loss, particularly in small infants, and therefore are not suitable techniques for infants.

### Venous Air Embolism

Venous air embolism (VAE) may occur during any operative procedure in which the surgical site is above the level of the heart and non-collapsible veins are exposed to air [54]. With the operative site above the level of the heart, a pressure gradient may develop that favors air entry rather than bleeding if a vein is opened. The highest incidence of VAE during operative correction of craniosynostosis is reported by Faberowski et al. at 83 percent using precordial Doppler; Harris et al. reported an incidence of 66 percent using trans-thoracic echo [55,56]. Although hemodynamically significant VAE is rare [78], preemptive placement of a monitor for early recognition may allow for timely initiation of therapy, thereby decreasing morbidity and mortality rates. For example, a precordial Doppler ultrasound is a noninvasive, inexpensive, very sensitive (nonspecific), safe method and can detect minute VAE (0.05 ml kg$^{-1}$) [79] by a change in the character and intensity of the emitting sound (erratic, high- pitched swishing roar, "drum like" or "mill wheel" sound with greater air entrainment). The Doppler probe is best positioned on the anterior chest, usually just to the right of the sternum at the fourth intercostal space. In prone position an alternate site on the posterior thorax, between the right scapula and the spine, can be used in infants weighing approximately 6 kg or less [59]. The correct placement can be verified by rapid intravenous injection of 5–10 ml of agitated saline peripherally and the subsequent observation of characteristic Doppler tones. Other hints for VAE include sudden drops in end-tidal $CO_2$, hypotension, and dysrhythmias and/or ischemic changes in the electrocardiogram. The risk of VAE can be minimized by early detection, and maintaining euvolemia to prevent a decrease in central venous pressure caused by bleeding. The development of a pressure gradient between the surgical side and the right atrium increases the potential to entrain air via dural sinuses or bony venous sinusoids. Several therapeutic maneuvers are used simultaneously with the detection of hemodynamically significant air: (1) administration of 100 percent oxygen and fluid (often packed red blood cells); (2) application of bone wax or direct pressure to seal the sites of egress; (3) flooding the surgical field with warm saline; (4) lowering the surgical field using the Trendelenburg position; (5) positive pressure ventilation of 5 cm end-expiratory pressure; and (6) attempt to aspirate air from a right atrial catheter if a catheter is in place. These maneuvers will augment the patient's blood pressure and prevent further entrainment of intravascular air. Compression of the jugular veins increases ICP, thereby reducing cerebral perfusion, which is a severe limitation of this technique. For catastrophic VAE with cardiovascular collapse, use of inotropic support and, if necessary, cardiopulmonary resuscitation are standard measures. Extracorporeal membrane oxygenation (ECMO) might be used to clear out air in the heart. Open remodeling procedures are associated with large blood losses and frequent hypotensive episodes. Consequently, VAE might be overlooked as a possible cause of intraoperative hypotension if precordial monitoring is not utilized. During ESC a much lower incidence of VAE (2–8 percent) is reported [44,45]. This low incidence of VAE during ESC most likely relates to the low average blood loss corresponding with less decrease in central venous pressure with ESC compared to the significant amount of blood loss approaching 100 percent and more of estimated blood volume during traditional cranial vault remodeling procedures.

### Increased Intracranial Pressure

Infants with single suture and more often with syndromic craniosynostosis may have increased ICP. In these cases basic principles of neuroanesthesia to prevent further increase in ICP and prevent decreases in cerebral perfusion pressure should be followed until craniectomy is performed. Accordingly, the anesthesiologist should minimize factors that increase ICP, such as hypercapnia and hypoxia, and factors that increase venous pressure such as the patient's position and coughing. In the presence of intracranial hypertension and herniation, mild to moderate hyperventilation, appropriate use of mannitol, furosemide, and dexamethasone may be employed to reduce ICP and brain volume. Although cranial vault remodeling increases intracranial volume, infants remain at risk of increased ICP after surgery and require close follow-up.

### Postoperative Care

The majority of patients are extubated after the surgical procedure. Postoperative intubation and admission to the intensive care unit or PACU/ward depends on the duration of the operation, hemodynamic stability, preexisting comorbidities (preoperative respiratory compromise, obstructive sleep apnea, difficult intubation), and potential complications during the procedure, including hypothermia, massive fluid resuscitation, electrolyte disturbances, etc. Since the surgical procedure is focused in the cranium, the airway rarely becomes edematous except by mechanical irritation of the vocal cords caused by the tube secondary to frequent head repositioning. In selected cases, if facial morphology permits noninvasive ventilatory support, CPAP or BiPAP may be a postoperative option. The initial management centers upon airway monitoring, sedation, pain management, thermoregulation, and correction of any residual volume deficits, acidosis, or coagulopathy. Isotonic solutions are maintained until fluid shifts are complete. Of particular importance is the risk of hyponatremia. The cause of hyponatremia is likely to be related to antidiuretic syndrome or administration of hypotonic intravenous fluids. Close hemodynamic and neurologic monitoring is provided until the risk of bleeding has passed. Coagulopathy may be consumptive or dilutional in nature and requires specific correction. Continued blood loss via drains needs to be monitored and replaced appropriately and vigilance maintained for additional concealed losses.

# Congenital Hand Deformities

*Syndactyly* is one of the most common congenital hand abnormalities. It may affect fingers and/or toes. Surgical treatment is a reconstructive procedure with the purpose of separating the fingers and reconstructing a webspace to enhance hand function. The term *simple syndactyly* is used if only the soft tissues are involved and *complex syndactyly* if the bones of adjacent fingers are fused. *Complicated syndactyly* describes syndactyly with bone formation between two digital rays. For syndactylies of the first and fourth interdigital webs and syndactylies with fusion of several fingers, surgical treatment is recommended at the age of 4–9 months to provide optimal assurance of normal grip and pinch development [80]. Syndactyly can occur as an isolated anomaly, can be associated with other anomalies of the extremity, or can be part of a syndrome (Figure 22.9). The most common syndromes are: (1) Apert syndrome; (2) Poland syndrome (skeletal abnormalities, unilateral hypoplasia or aplasia of the chest wall muscles, mainly pectoralis major, gastrointestinal, and cardiac malformations); (3) amniotic band sequence (Streeter anomaly, constricting amniotic bands can lead to amputation of all or parts of a limb, one or more digits, distal limb hypoplasia, cleft lip and palate, anencephaly, encephalocele, and other internal organ anomalies); and (4) multiple craniofacial syndromes (Table 22.3).

**Precautions before anesthesia** include assessment for associated head/face, thorax, cardiac, neurological, and respiratory abnormalities. Limb defects may make vascular access difficult. In the presence of facial malformations, the potential for difficult airway management must be anticipated (Table 22.3). An association has been reported between syndactyly and prolonged QT interval with life-threatening arrhythmias and high risk of sudden death [81]. The authors recommend for infants presenting with syndactyly and any type of congenital heart disease a preoperative ECG with careful evaluation of $QT_c$. Timothy syndrome is a rare disorder characterized by the co-occurrence of both syndactyly and long QT syndrome, associated with other cardiac, facial, and neurodevelopmental features [82].

**Congenital radial deficiency** is a rare anomaly and encompasses a spectrum ranging from partial to complete absence (unilateral and bilateral) of the radius. The hand is found to be radially deviated, unstable, flexed, and pronated on the forearm as a result of varying degrees of hypoplasia or aplasia affecting the soft tissues and the skeletal elements on the radial side of the distal forearm and hand. With congenital absence of the radius, other deformities are associated, e.g., cleft lip and palate, clubfoot, hydrocephalus, absence of fusion of the ribs, aplasia, or collapse of the lung and hemivertebrae, as well as syndromes (e.g., VACTERL: vertebral, anal, cardiac, tracheal, esophageal, renal, limb anomalies) [83].

**Congenital thumb hypoplasia** is a form of radial ray deficiency and can occur as an isolated deformity or be associated with several syndromes [84]. Associations have been most commonly seen with Holt–Oram syndrome (cardiac–limb syndrome), VACTERL complex, and less commonly with Fanconi

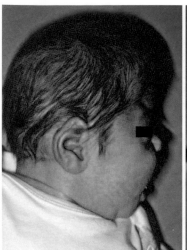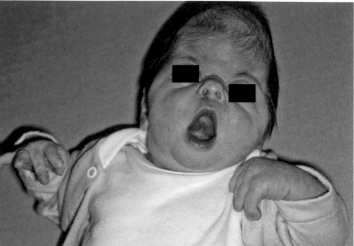

**Figure 22.9** Pfeiffer syndrome (*FGFR2* mutation) and a "cloverleaf" cranial deformity (coronal, posterior sagittal, and lambdoid synostosis), orbital hypertelorbitism, proptosis, midfacial hypopoplasia, high arched palate, choanal stenosis, Chiari I malformation, obstructive sleep apnea, scoliosis, and hand abnormalities (radial clinodactyly of both thumbs, bilateral fourth–fifth metacarpal synostosis) as well as simple syndactyly of both feet. Courtesy Dr. John B. Mulliken.

anemia (bone marrow failure), Nager syndrome (Treacher Collins mandibulofacial dysostosis type with limb anomalies), and thrombocytopenia–absent radius syndrome. *Preoperative assessment* of cardiac function and a comprehensive physical evaluation of the other organ systems are required.

## Congenital Pigmented Nevus

*Congenital pigmented or melanocytic nevi* are present at birth in approximately 1 percent of newborns and are categorized by size. They present as a dark-colored often hairy patch of skin, heterogeneous in consistency, covering any size surface area and any part of the body. *Giant congenital pigmented nevi* are rare lesions (<1:20 000 births) and occur most commonly on the posterior trunk, but may also appear on the head and extremities. These nevi are of special significance because of their association with leptomeningeal melanocytosis (neurocutaneous melanocytosis) and their predisposition for development into malignant melanoma. In the absence of neural melanosis, early excision and repair aided by tissue expanders, rotation flaps, or grafting may reduce the burden of nevus cells and thus the potential for development of melanoma. Surgical treatment often requires several expanders, serial tissue expansions, and reconstructive operations [85–89].

## Anesthetic Considerations

If the infant presents for serial procedures, premedication should be considered. The location and size determine the frequency and anesthetic technique. If the face, neck, and head are involved, airway management needs to be discussed with the surgical team. The tissue expander is implanted under general anesthesia. The expanders are usually inflated in the outpatient setting via percutaneous access using local anesthetics at the puncture site until calculated inflation volume is achieved. Some infants might also require anesthetics/sedation for the tissue expansion process. The location of the tissue expanders and their expansion can make positioning of the infant challenging for airway management and surgical exposure. It can be managed by special head rings and positioning devices (e.g., blankets) to build up the body to the level of the head. The most common complications of tissue expansion are infection, deflation, and exposure of the expander [85]. Other indications for tissue expansion include craniofacial anomalies, aplasia cutis congenital, meningomyelocele, and giant abdominal defects [90,91].

## Lymphatic Malformation

Lymphatic malformations (LMs), known in the past as "cystic hygromas," are uncommon congenital malformations that can be categorized as macrocystic, microcystic, or combined forms. Lymphatic malformation also occurs in combination with venous anomalies. Cystic lymphatic anomalies can be *diagnosed in utero by ultrasonography*. Usually an LM is obvious in the newborn nursery; cervicofacial lesions can affect breathing and swallowing. Cystic LM of the midline posterior cervical region (also called posterior nuchal translucency) is often associated with chromosomal abnormalities, particularly Turner syndrome and trisomy 13, 18, and 21. Posterior nuchal translucency has also been associated with several malformative disorders, e.g., Beckwith–Wiedemann, Brachmann–de Lange, and Noonan syndromes.

The most common *location* of LM is the cervicofacial region, followed by the extremities and the trunk. LM can be localized to the anterior tongue, presenting as intermittent lingual swelling with dorsal vesicles and intermittent bleeding. More common is microcystic involvement throughout the tongue, with extension in the oral floor, cervical region, and sometimes upper mediastinum displacing pharynx, trachea, and esophagus. Lymphatic malformation of the lingual base and oral floor is the most difficult to manage; usually adjacent structures are involved, including the neck, mandible, face, lips, pharynx, and larynx. This location is associated with major morbidity, such as chronic airway problems, recurrent infections, and functional issues related to feeding, speech, oral hygiene, and malocclusion. Frequently tracheostomy is required during infancy [92]. Lingual LM may interfere with swallowing, requiring placement of a feeding tube or gastrostomy.

The *differential diagnosis* of a cystic mass in the parotid region, cheek, or neck of a newborn includes cervical teratoma, infantile myofibromatosis, infantile fibrosarcoma, or rhabdosarcoma. Some cervical and periorbital lesions appear to be a combined lymphatico-venous malformation. Periorbital LM is usually unilateral and often associated with intracranial developmental venous anomalies. A characteristic sign of orbital LM is exacerbation of exophthalmos during an upper respiratory tract infection.

In the *clinical course*, periodic minor variations in size of a lymphatic anomaly are common, but proportionate growth with the infant's growth is the rule. Typically, LM expands coincident with a viral upper respiratory tract infection or intralesional bleeding. Often there is a history of bruising, recurrent inflammation, and bacterial infection (cellulitis), which can also cause a dramatic increase in size.

# Anesthetic Considerations

*Antenatal diagnosis* of cervicofacial LM permits planning for delivery and immediate postnatal care (Figure 22.10). If prenatal ultrasonography demonstrates a severely narrowed airway, ex utero intrapartum treatment (EXIT) can be life-saving [93–96]. After Cesarean section, the patency of the neonate's airway is assessed before clamping the umbilical cord. Intubation may be possible, but if laryngeal LM prevents insertion of the endotracheal tube, tracheostomy can be performed [97]. A cervicofacial LM is soft, allowing the neonate to breath spontaneously, whereas a large teratoma in this location is usually a firm, solid mass and more likely causes a problematic airway.

A newborn with cervicofacial LM can exhibit rapid enlargement of the tongue or floor of the mouth, leading to respiratory obstruction with stridor, dysphagea, and apnea. A *complete examination* of the airway is necessary, including fiberoptic nasopharyngoscopy and laryngoscopy to assess for potential involvement of the hypopharynx, supraglottis, and larynx. Acute airway obstruction can occur during *induction* and spontaneous ventilation should be maintained until the airway is secure. Fiberoptic intubation might be possible; however, a large cervicofacial LM usually necessitates tracheostomy due to involvement of the supraglottic airway and the risk of acute swelling secondary to intralesional hemorrhage and sepsis [92,98].

**Treatment options** for LM include sclerotherapy for macrocystic lesions, preoperative embolization to control lingual bleeding, $CO_2$ laser and radiofrequency ablation for vesicles, and well-timed staged resection to debulk the mass [99–102]. Resection of a facial LM is difficult because the lesion permeates through the soft tissue. Monitoring of the facial nerve can be helpful and requires withholding of muscle relaxation during that phase of the procedure. Corticosteroid is given intraoperatively to reduce postoperative swelling and tapered over 2–3 postoperative days.

**Postoperative complications** include: airway obstruction, laryngeal edema, nerve damage, and wound infection or delayed cellulitis. After resection of a LM, a stay in the intensive care unit is required until swelling subsides. An infant undergoing resection of LM in the tongue and oral floor usually has a tracheostomy or requires prolonged postoperative

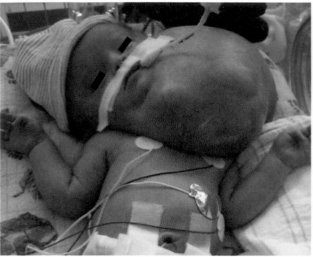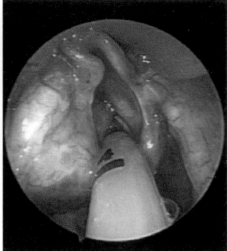

**Figure 22.10** Neonate with left cervicofacial lymphatic malformation, born at 34 weeks' gestational age. Ex utero intrapartum treatment (EXIT procedure) ensured uteroplacental gas exchange and fetal hemodynamic stability while ENT service established and secured the airway. After intubation using a Parson laryngoscope, the neonate was fully delivered and taken to the warming table and ventilated. Courtesy Dr. Reza Rahbar.

intubation because the tongue has a remarkable capacity to swell and protrude in the immediate postoperative period. A serosanguineous fluid collection may have to be tapped, often repeatedly, by ultrasonographic guidance. Partially resected LM has the potential for regeneration.

## Acknowledgments

The author thanks John B. Mulliken, MD, Department of Plastic and Oral Surgery, Boston Children's Hospital, Harvard Medical School, Boston, MA, USA for discussion, editing, and photographic images; Claes G.K. Lauritzen, MD, PhD, Department of Plastic Surgery, Sahlgrenska University Hospital, Goeteborg, Sweden; Reza Rahbar, DMD, MD, FACS, Department of Otolaryngology & Communication Enhancement; and Mark R. Proctor, MD, Department of Neurosurgery, Boston Children's Hospital, Harvard Medical School, Boston, MA, USA for providing photographs to illustrate this chapter.

## Patient's Consent

Parents or guardians provided written consent for the use of patients' images.

## References

1. Mulliken JB, MacDonald DM. Cleft lip/palate and Robin sequence. In Hansen A, Puder M, editors. *Manual of Neonatal Surgical Intensive Care*, 2nd edition. Shelton, CT: People's Medical Publishing House; 2009.

2. Milerad J, Larson O, Ph DD, Hagberg C, Ideberg M. Associated malformations in infants with cleft lip and palate: a prospective, population-based study. *Pediatrics*. 1997;100(2 Pt 1):180–6.

3. Evans AK, Rahbar R, Rogers GF, Mulliken JB, Volk MS. Robin sequence: a retrospective review of 115 patients. *Int J Pediatr Otorhinolaryngol*. 2006;70(6):973–80.

4. Butow KW, Hoogendijk CF, Zwahlen RA. Pierre Robin sequence: appearances and 25 years of experience with an innovative treatment protocol. *J Pediatr Surg*. 2009;44(11):2112–18.

5. Cladis F, Kumar A, Grunwaldt L, et al. Pierre robin sequence: a perioperative review. *Anesth Analg*. 2014;119(2):400–12.

6. Takemura H, Yasumoto K, Toi T, Hosoyamada A. Correlation of cleft type with incidence of perioperative respiratory complications in infants with cleft lip and palate. *Paediatr Anaesth*. 2002;12(7):585–8.

7. Jackson O, Basta M, Sonnad S, et al. Perioperative risk factors for adverse airway events in patients undergoing cleft palate repair. *Cleft Palate Craniofac J*. 2013;50(3):330–6.

8. Xue FS, Zhang GH, Li P, et al. The clinical observation of difficult laryngoscopy and difficult intubation in infants with cleft lip and palate. *Paediatr Anaesth*. 2006;16(3):283–9.

9. Gunawardana RH. Difficult laryngoscopy in cleft lip and palate surgery. *Br J Anaesth*. 1996;76(6):757–9.

10. Uezono S, Holzman RS, Goto T, et al. Prediction of difficult airway in school-aged patients with microtia. *Paediatr Anaesth*. 2001;11(4):409–13.

11. Nargozian C. The airway in patients with craniofacial abnormalities. *Paediatr Anaesth*. 2004;14(1):53–9.

12. Ahuja S, Datta A, Krishna A, Bhattacharya A. Infra-orbital nerve block for relief of postoperative pain following cleft lip surgery in infants. *Anaesthesia*. 1994;49(5):441–4.

13. Rajamani A, Kamat V, Rajavel VP, Murthy J, Hussain SA. A comparison of bilateral infraorbital nerve block with intravenous fentanyl for analgesia following cleft lip repair in children. *Paediatr Anaesth*. 2007;17(2):133–9.

14. Takmaz SA, Uysal HY, Uysal A, et al. Bilateral extraoral, infraorbital nerve block for postoperative pain relief after cleft lip repair in pediatric patients: a randomized, double-blind controlled study. *Ann Plast Surg*. 2009;63(1):59–62.

15. Simion C, Corcoran J, Iyer A, Suresh S. Postoperative pain control for primary cleft lip repair in infants: is there an advantage in performing peripheral nerve blocks? *Paediatr Anaesth*. 2008;18(11):1060–5.

16. Bosenberg AT, Kimble FW. Infraorbital nerve block in neonates for cleft lip repair: anatomical study and clinical application. *Br J Anaesth*. 1995;74(5):506–8.

17. Bell C, Oh TH, Loeffler JR. Massive macroglossia and airway obstruction after cleft palate repair. *Anesth Analg*. 1988;67(1):71–4.

18. Lee JT, Kingston HG. Airway obstruction due to massive lingual oedema following cleft palate surgery. *Can Anaesth Soc J*. 1985;32(3 Pt 1):265–7.

19. Cohen MM, Jr., MacLean RE. *Craniosynostosis: Diagnosis, Evaluation, and Management*, 2nd edn. New York: Oxford University Press; 2000.

20. Tamburrini G, Caldarelli M, Massimi L, Santini P, Di Rocco C. Intracranial pressure monitoring in children with single suture and complex craniosynostosis: a review. *Childs Nerv Syst*. 2005;21(10):913–21.

21. McCarthy JG, Warren SM, Bernstein JM, et al. Parameters of care for craniosynostosis. *Cleft Palate Craniofac J*. 2011;49:1S–24S.

22. Church MW, Parent-Jenkins L, Rozzelle AA, Eldis FE, Kazzi SN. Auditory brainstem response abnormalities and hearing loss in children with craniosynostosis. *Pediatrics*. 2007;119(6):e1351–60.

23. Hertle RW, Quinn GE, Minguini N, Katowitz JA. Visual loss in patients with craniofacial synostosis. *J Pediatr Ophthalmol Strabismus*. 1991;28(6):344–9.

24. Renier D, Sainte-Rose C, Marchac D, Hirsch JF. Intracranial pressure in craniostenosis. *J Neurosurg*. 1982;57(3):370–7.

25. Connolly JP, Gruss J, Seto ML, et al. Progressive postnatal craniosynostosis and increased intracranial pressure. *Plast Reconstr Surg*. 2004;113(5):1313–23.

26. Mulliken JB, Vander Woude DL, Hansen M, LaBrie RA, Scott RM. Analysis of posterior plagiocephaly: deformational versus synostotic. *Plast Reconstr Surg*. 1999;103(2):371–80.

27. Laughlin J, Luerssen TG, Dias MS. Prevention and management of positional skull deformities in infants. *Pediatrics*. 2011;128.

28. Hoeve LJ, Pijpers M, Joosten KF. OSAS in craniofacial syndromes: an unsolved problem. *Int J Pediatr Otorhinolaryngol*. 2003;67(Suppl. 1):S111–13.

29. Pijpers M, Poels PJ, Vaandrager JM, et al. Undiagnosed obstructive sleep apnea syndrome in children with syndromal craniofacial synostosis. *J Craniofac Surg*. 2004;15(4):670–4.

30. De Jong T, Bannink N, Bredero-Boelhouwer HH, et al. Long-term functional outcome in 167 patients with syndromic craniosynostosis; defining a syndrome-specific risk profile. *J Plast Reconstr Aesthet Surg*. 2010;63(10):1635–41.

31. Scheid SC, Spector AR, Luft JD. Tracheal cartilaginous sleeve in Crouzon syndrome. *Int J Pediatr Otorhinolaryngol*. 2002;65(2):147–52.

32. Nargozian C. Apert syndrome: anesthetic management. *Clin Plast Surg*. 1991;18(2):227–30.

33. Sculerati N, Gottlieb MD, Zimbler MS, Chibbaro PD, McCarthy JG. Airway management in children with major craniofacial anomalies. *Laryngoscope*. 1998;108(12):1806–12.

34. Hayward R, Gonsalez S. How low can you go? Intracranial pressure, cerebral perfusion pressure, and respiratory obstruction in children with complex craniosynostosis. *J Neurosurg*. 2005;102(Suppl. 1):16–22.

35. Bristol RE, Lekovic GP, Rekate HL. The effects of craniosynostosis on the brain with respect to intracranial pressure. *Semin Pediatr Neurol*. 2004;11(4):262–7.

36. Thompson DN, Malcolm GP, Jones BM, Harkness WJ, Hayward RD. Intracranial pressure in single-suture craniosynostosis. *Pediatr Neurosurg*. 1995;22(5):235–40.

37. David LR, Wilson JA, Watson NE, Argenta LC. Cerebral perfusion defects secondary to simple craniosynostosis. *J Craniofac Surg*. 1996;7(3):177–85.

38. Czerwinski M, Kolar JC, Fearon JA. Complex craniosynostosis. *Plast Reconstr Surg.* 2011;128(4):955–61.

39. Robson CD, Mulliken JB, Robertson RL, et al. Prominent basal emissary foramina in syndromic craniosynostosis: correlation with phenotypic and molecular diagnoses. *AJNR Am J Neuroradiol.* 2000;21(9):1707–17.

40. Rich PM, Cox TC, Hayward RD. The jugular foramen in complex and syndromic craniosynostosis and its relationship to raised intracranial pressure. *AJNR Am J Neuroradiol.* 2003;24(1):45–51.

41. Tuite GF, Chong WK, Evanson J, et al. The effectiveness of papilledema as an indicator of raised intracranial pressure in children with craniosynostosis. *Neurosurgery.* 1996;38(2):272–8.

42. Jimenez DF, Barone CM, Cartwright CC, Baker L. Early management of craniosynostosis using endoscopic-assisted strip craniectomies and cranial orthotic molding therapy. *Pediatrics.* 2002;110(1 Pt 1):97–104.

43. Berry-Candelario J, Ridgway EB, Grondin RT, Rogers GF, Proctor MR. Endoscope-assisted strip craniectomy and postoperative helmet therapy for treatment of craniosynostosis. *Neurosurg Focus.* 2011;31(2):E5.

44. Meier PM, Goobie SM, DiNardo JA, et al. Endoscopic strip craniectomy in early infancy: the initial five years of anesthesia experience. *Anesth Analg.* 2011;112(2):407–14.

45. Tobias JD, Johnson JO, Jimenez DF, Barone CM, McBride DS, Jr. Venous air embolism during endoscopic strip craniectomy for repair of craniosynostosis in infants. *Anesthesiology.* 2001;95(2):340–2.

46. Abbott MM, Rogers GF, Proctor MR, Busa K, Meara JG. Cost of treating sagittal synostosis in the first year of life. *J Craniofac Surg.* 2012;23(1):88–93.

47. Lauritzen CG, Davis C, Ivarsson A, Sanger C, Hewitt TD. The evolving role of springs in craniofacial surgery: the first 100 clinical cases. *Plast Reconstr Surg.* 2008;121(2):545–54.

48. Mackenzie KA, Davis C, Yang A, MacFarlane MR. Evolution of surgery for sagittal synostosis: the role of new technologies. *J Craniofac Surg.* 2009;20(1):129–33.

49. Ririe DG, Smith TE, Wood BC, et al. Time-dependent perioperative anesthetic management and outcomes of the first 100 consecutive cases of spring-assisted surgery for sagittal craniosynostosis. *Paediatr Anaesth.* 2011;21:1015–19.

50. Windh P, Davis C, Sanger C, Sahlin P, Lauritzen C. Spring-assisted cranioplasty vs pi-plasty for sagittal synostosis: a long term follow-up study. *J Craniofac Surg.* 2008;19(1):59–64.

51. Faberowski LW, Black S, Mickle JP. Blood loss and transfusion practice in the perioperative management of craniosynostosis repair. *J Neurosurg Anesthesiol.* 1999;11(3):167–72.

52. Meyer P, Renier D, Arnaud E, et al. Blood loss during repair of craniosynostosis. *Br J Anaesth.* 1993;71(6):854–7.

53. Stricker PA, Shaw TL, Desouza DG, et al. Blood loss, replacement, and associated morbidity in infants and children undergoing craniofacial surgery. *Paediatr Anaesth.* 2010;20(2):150–9.

54. Mirski MA, Lele AV, Fitzsimmons L, Toung TJ. Diagnosis and treatment of vascular air embolism. *Anesthesiology.* 2007;106(1):164–77.

55. Harris MM, Yemen TA, Davidson A, et al. Venous embolism during craniectomy in supine infants. *Anesthesiology.* 1987;67(5):816–19.

56. Faberowski LW, Black S, Mickle JP. Incidence of venous air embolism during craniectomy for craniosynostosis repair. *Anesthesiology.* 2000;92(1):20–3.

57. Meyer PG, Renier D, Orliaguet G, Blanot S, Carli P. Venous air embolism in craniosynostosis surgery: what do we want to detect? *Anesthesiology.* 2000;93(4):1157–8.

58. Cucchiara RF, Bowers B. Air embolism in children undergoing suboccipital craniotomy. *Anesthesiology.* 1982;57(4):338–9.

59. Soriano SG, McManus ML, Sullivan LJ, Scott RM, Rockoff MA. Doppler sensor placement during neurosurgical procedures for children in the prone position. *J Neurosurg Anesthesiol.* 1994;6(3):153–5.

60. Clune JE, Greene AK, Guo CY, et al. Perioperative corticosteroid reduces hospital stay after fronto-orbital advancement. *J Craniofac Surg.* 2010;21(2):344–8.

61. Zunini GS, Rando KA, Cox RG. Fluid replacement in craniofacial pediatric surgery: normal saline or Ringer's lactate? *J Craniofac Surg.* 2011;22(4):1370–4.

62. Czerwinski M, Hopper RA, Gruss J, Fearon JA. Major morbidity and mortality rates in craniofacial surgery: an analysis of 8101 major procedures. *Plast Reconstr Surg.* 2010;126(1):181–6.

63. Bhananker SM, Ramamoorthy C, Geiduschek JM, et al. Anesthesia-related cardiac arrest in children: update from the Pediatric Perioperative Cardiac Arrest Registry. *Anesth Analg.* 2007;105(2):344–50.

64. Cote CJ, Liu LM, Szyfelbein SK, Goudsouzian NG, Daniels AL. Changes in serial platelet counts following massive blood transfusion in pediatric patients. *Anesthesiology.* 1985;62(2):197–201.

65. Cote CJ, Drop LJ, Hoaglin DC, Daniels AL, Young ET. Ionized hypocalcemia after fresh frozen plasma administration to thermally injured children: effects

of infusion rate, duration, and treatment with calcium chloride. *Anesth Analg.* 1988;67(2):152–60.

66. Brown KA, Bissonnette B, McIntyre B. Hyperkalaemia during rapid blood transfusion and hypovolaemic cardiac arrest in children. *Can J Anaesth.* 1990;37(7):747–54.

67. Brown KA, Bissonnette B, MacDonald M, Poon AO. Hyperkalaemia during massive blood transfusion in paediatric craniofacial surgery. *Can J Anaesth.* 1990;37(4 Pt 1):401–8.

68. Flick RP, Sprung J, Harrison TE, et al. Perioperative cardiac arrests in children between 1988 and 2005 at a tertiary referral center: a study of 92,881 patients. *Anesthesiology.* 2007;106(2):226–37.

69. Mattu A, Brady WJ, Robinson DA. Electrocardiographic manifestations of hyperkalemia. *Am J Emerg Med.* 2000;18(6):721–9.

70. Weiskopf RB, Schnapp S, Rouine-Rapp K, Bostrom A, Toy P. Extracellular potassium concentrations in red blood cell suspensions after irradiation and washing. *Transfusion.* 2005;45(8):1295–301.

71. Swindell CG, Barker TA, McGuirk SP, et al. Washing of irradiated red blood cells prevents hyperkalaemia during cardiopulmonary bypass in neonates and infants undergoing surgery for complex congenital heart disease. *Eur J Cardiothorac Surg.* 2007;31(4):659–64.

72. Fearon JA, Weinthal J. The use of recombinant erythropoietin in the reduction of blood transfusion rates in craniosynostosis repair in infants and children. *Plast Reconstr Surg.* 2002;109(7):2190–6.

73. Krajewski K, Ashley RK, Pung N, et al. Successful blood conservation during craniosynostotic correction with dual therapy using procrit and cell saver. *J Craniofac Surg.* 2008;19(1):101–5.

74. Helfaer MA, Carson BS, James CS, et al. Increased hematocrit and decreased transfusion requirements in children given erythropoietin before undergoing craniofacial surgery. *J Neurosurg.* 1998;88(4):704–8.

75. Dadure C, Sauter M, Bringuier S, et al. Intraoperative tranexamic acid reduces blood transfusion in children undergoing craniosynostosis surgery: a randomized double-blind study. *Anesthesiology.* 2011;114(4):856–61.

76. Goobie SM, Meier PM, Pereira LM, et al. Efficacy of tranexamic acid in pediatric craniosynostosis surgery: a double-blind, placebo-controlled trial. *Anesthesiology.* 2011;114(4):862–71.

77. Di Rocco C, Tamburrini G, Pietrini D. Blood sparing in craniosynostosis surgery. *Semin Pediatr Neurol.* 2004;11(4):278–87.

78. Phillips RJ, Mulliken JB. Venous air embolism during a craniofacial procedure. *Plast Reconstr Surg.* 1988;82(1):155–9.

79. Chang JL, Albin MS, Bunegin L, Hung TK. Analysis and comparison of venous air embolism detection methods. *Neurosurgery.* 1980;7(2):135–41.

80. Kvernmo HD, Haugstvedt JR. Treatment of congenital syndactyly of the fingers. *Tidsskr Nor Laegeforen.* 2013;133(15):1591–5.

81. Joseph-Reynolds AM, Auden SM, Sobczyzk WL. Perioperative considerations in a newly described subtype of congenital long QT syndrome. *Paediatr Anaesth.* 1997;7(3):237–41.

82. Napolitano C, Splawski I, Timothy KW, et al. GeneReviews® (Internet). Seattle, WA: University of Washington, Seattle; 1993–2017.

83. Khalid S, Faizan M, Alam MM, et al. Congenital longitudinal radial deficiency in infants: spectrum of isolated cases to VACTERL syndrome. *J Clin Neonatol.* 2013;2(4):193–5.

84. Ashbaugh H, Gellman H. Congenital thumb deformities and associated syndromes. *J Craniofac Surg.* 2009;20(4):1039–44.

85. Gibstein LA, Abramson DL, Bartlett RA, et al. Tissue expansion in children: a retrospective study of complications. *Ann Plast Surg.* 1997;38(4):358–64.

86. Bauer BS, Few JW, Chavez CD, Galiano RD. The role of tissue expansion in the management of large congenital pigmented nevi of the forehead in the pediatric patient. *Plast Reconstr Surg.* 2001;107(3):668–75.

87. Gosain AK, Santoro TD, Larson DL, Gingrass RP. Giant congenital nevi: a 20-year experience and an algorithm for their management. *Plast Reconstr Surg.* 2001;108(3):622–36.

88. Vaienti L, Masetto L, Davanzo D, Marchesi A, Ravasio G. Giant congenital nevi of the scalp and forehead treated by skin expansion. *Pediatr Med Chir.* 2011;33(2):98–101.

89. Rasmussen BS, Henriksen TF, Kolle SF, Schmidt G. Giant congenital melanocytic nevus: report from 30 years of experience in a single department. *Ann Plast Surg.* 2013;74(2):223–9.

90. Clifton MS, Heiss KF, Keating JJ, Mackay G, Ricketts RR. Use of tissue expanders in the repair of complex abdominal wall defects. *J Pediatr Surg.* 2011;46(2):372–7.

91. Mhamane R, Dave N, Garasia M. Delayed primary repair of giant omphalocele: anesthesia challenges. *Paediatr Anaesth.* 2012;22(9):935–6.

disease and cardiac abnormalities. Gastrointestinal dysfunction may also lead to prolonged ileus, feeding delay or feeding intolerance and prolonged hospitalization [14]. Gastroschisis originally was associated with 100 percent mortality, but now with a staged closure has a 90 percent survival rate with specialist care. There is an overall good prognosis, although the risk of long-term disability associated with prematurity and gastrointestinal dysfunction exists [15]. A small cohort of over 60 neonates born with gastroschisis followed to 36 months had long-term problems with bowel motility, reflux, short gut syndrome and tube-feed or dependence on total parenteral nutrition [16].

Most cases of gastroschisis are diagnosed with prenatal ultrasound, and the diagnosis is supported with elevated maternal serum alpha-fetoprotein [17,18]. Once diagnosed, arrangements should be made for delivery at a facility capable of resuscitating the neonate with gastroschisis. The goals of resuscitation immediately after birth include airway protection, rapid assessment and support of adequate ventilation and oxygenation, protection of exposed bowel, and minimization of insensible fluid and heat losses [2]. The baby should be actively dried and warmed, with exposed bowel and the lower half of the body covered with a sterile transparent plastic bowel bag as a temporizing measure. The baby should be placed in the right lateral decubitus position to reduce the risk of compromised blood flow to the gastrointestinal tract while further assessment and resuscitation continues. A nasogastric tube for bowel decompression should be placed to reduce the risk of aspiration and regurgitation. Intravenous access should be established for targeted resuscitation with intravenous isotonic fluids and administration of broad-spectrum antibiotics. Catheterization of umbilical vessels is contraindicated in gastroschisis [1].

The high degree of third space losses with gastroschisis should not be underestimated. The neonate should be actively resuscitated with isotonic fluids, with regular assessment of volume status by exam, vital signs, urine output, and laboratory measurements of acid–base status [19]. Invasive monitoring with a peripheral arterial line should be considered. Care should be taken to keep the bowel covered with sterile plastic wrap to reduce the risk of profound hypothermia and dehydration, and the viscera should be physically supported to ensure that no twisting or impingement occurs at the herniation site leading to ischemia, particularly during times of transport [2,5].

Urgent reduction of abdominal contents is necessary due to the risk of ischemia and infection. The size of the abdominal wall defect determines surgical approach. Small defects may be managed with primary closure in the operating room or at bedside in the neonatal intensive care unit. Large defects may be managed in one of several ways, with many practitioners favoring a staged reduction using a pre-formed spring-loaded silo or a formal silastic silo, which is then suspended [20,21]. Gravity will allow the exposed bowel to gradually return to the abdominal cavity, with the silo concomitantly reduced in size daily. Physiologic neonatal diuresis will also lead to a decrease in bowel edema, enhancing reduction. The abdominal defect is closed in the operating room once the viscera have been completely reduced.

Preoperative preparation includes evaluation of volume status and adequacy of resuscitation, as well as screening for any comorbidities. These patients are at risk for infection, dehydration, hypothermia, acidosis, hypoproteinemia with decreased plasma oncotic pressure, and obstruction with vomiting and abdominal distention. The operating room should be warmed, with forced-air warming blankets, external heat lamps, heat-moisture exchangers and other devices to combat hypothermia [22,23]. Blood products should be cross-matched and available.

Prior to anesthetic induction, the nasogastric tube should be aspirated to drain gastric contents. A rapid-sequence or modified rapid-sequence induction is suggested after adequate preoxygenation. A difficult airway may necessitate advanced airway techniques including video laryngoscopy or fiberoptic intubation. Anesthesia may be maintained with volatile inhaled anesthetic, narcotic techniques, or supplemented with a caudal/epidural [24]. Neuraxial techniques are not contraindicated and can be particularly useful in cases of early extubation. Both ropivacaine 0.2 percent and chloroprocaine 3 percent infusions have been described and used successfully as adjuncts for major abdominal wall repair in the neonate [25]. Nitrous oxide should be avoided due to the propensity for bowel distention. Intravenous dextrose solution administration is recommended for maintenance of serum glucose, and additional intravenous isotonic fluids should be given to maintain euvolemia. A bladder catheter is often placed to monitor urine output. Standard monitors as well as arterial pressure monitoring may be necessary for larger defects. Both core and peripheral temperatures should be monitored.

A central venous catheter may be placed for additional access or if total parenteral nutrition will be required postoperatively [23].

Intragastric or bladder pressures may also be monitored during primary closure of a large defect to assess for abdominal compartment syndrome [26]. Herniated viscera reduced into a relatively small abdominal cavity will raise intra-abdominal pressure, compressing the inferior vena cava, decreasing venous return and cardiac output [27]. In severe cases, this may lead to compromised renal and splanchnic circulation, leading to end-organ ischemia with resultant metabolic acidosis, renal failure, bowel perforation, and/or necrotizing enterocolitis. A tight closure may also lead to high wound tension and dehiscence, as well as compromised respiratory function, necessitating higher pulmonary inflation pressures. Peak inspiratory pressure prior to reduction should be noted to assist in evaluation of increased abdominal pressure [3,28]. Ventilation may become problematic with an endotracheal tube with a large leak after a tight reduction.

**Omphalocele**, or exomphalos, is a midline herniation of the gastrointestinal tract through the umbilical ring into the base of the umbilical cord, and can consist of any amount of intestine as well as liver, spleen, or other abdominal organs. The viscera are housed in a gelatinous-appearing membranous sac consisting of peritoneum, Wharton's jelly, and amnion. The umbilical vessels themselves insert into the membrane, and the bowel is normal [7,29].

Most cases of omphalocele are sporadic. Unlike gastroschisis, the overall incidence has remained stable at approximately 1:5000 live births [30,31]. The exact mechanisms are unknown, but omphalocele is thought to result from the failure of the midgut to return to the developing abdominal cavity after the tenth week of gestation, with incomplete closure of the anterior abdominal wall at the umbilicus [32]. The size of the defect can be variable, ranging from 2–5 cm (small) in diameter to greater than 10 cm (large), with organ herniation and pulmonary hypoplasia from poorly developed abdominal and thoracic cavities. Greater than 60 percent of cases have associated congenital abnormalities, including cardiac (30–40 percent) defects such as Tetralogy of Fallot, chromosomal disorders (trisomy 13, 18, 21), cloacal or bladder extrophy, Beckwith–Wiedemann syndrome, congenital diaphragmatic hernia, malrotation of the gut, microcephaly, meningocele, and rarely, pentalogy of Cantrell (Table 23.1) [11]. Outcomes are affected by the severity of associated congenital defects, surgical complications, low birth weight, membrane rupture, bowel obstruction, and sepsis [33,34].

As with gastroschisis, most cases of omphalocele are detected on prenatal ultrasound, and associated with elevated levels of maternal serum alpha-fetoprotein, although values are generally not as high as with gastroschisis. Once omphalocele is suspected, amniocentesis and chorionic villus sampling should be pursued for karyotype analysis to screen for chromosomal abnormalities, along with fetal echocardiogram to evaluate for congenital heart disease

**Table 23.1** Characteristics of omphalocele and gastroschisis

|  | Omphalocele | Gastroschisis |
|---|---|---|
| Incidence | 1:5000; stable | 1:3000 – 1:8000; increasing worldwide |
| Position | Midline | Right of umbilicus |
| Size of defect | Variable size, small (2–5 cm), large (>10 cm) | Full thickness; variable, usually <5 cm |
| Presence of sac | Yes, although sac may rupture | No; bowel completely exposed pre- and postnatally |
| Associated defects | Greater than 60 percent cases<br>– cardiac (30 – 40 percent), i.e., Tetralogy of Fallot<br>– chromosomal disorders, i.e., trisomy 13, 18, or 21<br>– urologic, i.e., bladder extrophy, cloacal defect<br>– metabolic, i.e., Beckwith–Wiedemann<br>– neurologic, i.e., microcephaly, meningocele<br>– congenital diaphragmatic hernia<br>– Pentalogy of Cantrell | Uncommon; usually isolated lesion |

[18,35]. There is associated high risk for intrauterine growth restriction, preterm labor and fetal demise [11]. Babies with a large omphalocele defect should be delivered by Cesarean section to decrease the risk of sac rupture [35]. The sac may rupture prior to, during or after delivery, leaving the bowel unprotected.

The goals of resuscitation immediately after birth include airway protection, rapid assessment and support of adequate ventilation and oxygenation, protection of exposed bowel and minimization of insensible fluid and heat losses [2]. Third-space losses, however, are not as profound as with gastroschisis, and there is less immediate urgency for surgical repair unless the sac has ruptured, although the risks of ischemia, bowel obstruction and sepsis are still present. A nasogastric tube for bowel decompression should be placed. The baby may be placed in the left lateral decubitus position to reduce the risk of compression of the inferior vena cava and compromised venous return. Intravenous access should be established for targeted resuscitation with intravenous isotonic fluids, administration of broad-spectrum antibiotics and dextrose solution. Catheterization of umbilical vessels is contraindicated [36]. Infants with Beckwith–Wiedemann syndrome have macroglossia so intubation may be difficult. Intraoperatively, they can develop hypoglycemia so a means of measuring serum glucose should be available.

Reduction of abdominal contents is necessary due to the risk of ischemia and infection. As with gastroschisis, care should be taken to keep the bowel covered with sterile wrap to reduce hypothermia and dehydration, and the viscera should be physically supported to ensure that no twisting or impingement occurs at the herniation site leading to ischemia, particularly during times of transport. Given the known association between omphalocele and other congenital defects, preoperative preparation should include a thorough medical screening, including chest radiograph, echocardiogram, renal ultrasound and laboratory panel [2].

Intraoperative management concerns are similar to those for gastroschisis repair, with the size of the abdominal wall defect determining the surgical approach. Primary closure may be used for small defects. Staged repair using a silo over days to weeks, mesh closure, and tissue expanders have all been described [20,21,37]. Large unruptured, stable defects may be allowed to epithelialize using escharotic topical agents (i.e., silver sulfadiazine), with later repair of the

abdominal wall defect. If the liver is herniated, hepatic vein compression or damage to the liver itself during reduction may lead to hemodynamic instability.

Both term and premature neonates are thermogenically active. In order to maintain constant temperature, infants exposed to a cold environment increase their metabolic activity and heat production without shivering. This, however, has high energy and oxygen costs. Heat loss is favored due to the neonatal body habitus of reduced subcutaneous fat and large surface area to body ratio. Neonates have limited shivering and non-shivering thermogenesis (brown fat) and are at high risk for temperature losses in the perioperative period. Survival of premature neonates is directly related to ambient temperature. Perioperative goals of care should include maintenance of a neutral thermal environment. This is facilitated by use of heated transport, warmed solutions, warmed blood products, heated mattress, radiant warmer, and forced-air warmer [23].

## Umbilical Hernia

Residual patency of the umbilical ring and the omphalomesenteric duct may lead to other, less severe forms of ventral abdominal wall defects, including umbilical hernia, Meckel's diverticulum, umbilical polyp, or fistula [38].

All neonates have an umbilical defect for the umbilical vessels and cord. The umbilical ring closes naturally during the first few weeks of life, but in 10–30 percent of patients the ring fails to close. Certain ethnic groups have a higher incidence, with African Americans 6–10 times more likely than Caucasians to present with an umbilical hernia [39]. Those with low birth weight (less than 1200 g) are four times more likely to have umbilical ring defect than those with a birth weight greater than 2500 g. Other risk factors include trisomy 21 and Beckwith–Wiedemann syndrome [40]. Umbilical hernias are covered by skin and peritoneum. Most umbilical hernias will close spontaneously in the first few years of life, depending on the size of the defect and the age of the child at presentation. Most repairs are performed after three years of age. Incarceration is uncommon at less than 5 percent of cases, with a less than 2 percent rate of recurrence [41,42].

Preoperative preparation includes an assessment of any residual comorbidities of prematurity, associated syndromes, and evidence of incarceration or obstruction. Anesthetic techniques include general anesthesia supplemented with truncal (rectus sheath, paraumbilical) blocks [43] or caudal injection of local anesthetic, and regional anesthesia such as spinal or caudal injection of local anesthetic. Umbilical hernia repairs may be scheduled as ambulatory or day surgery cases for older patients that do not require postoperative apnea monitoring [44]. Recent studies have shown superior analgesia from ultrasound-guided rectus sheath blocks compared with peri-incisional infiltration of local anesthetic [45,46].

# Inguinal Hernia

Indirect inguinal hernia results in a protrusion of intestine through a congenitally patent processus vaginalis, while a direct hernia is due to a defect in the transversalis fascia. The incidence is 0.8–4 percent of the population, and is approximately 5–10 times more common in boys than girls. It is quite common in premature infants and infants of low birth weight, affecting 10–30 percent of premature infants as opposed to 3–5 percent of term infants, with an incidence of 13 percent in babies born at less than 32 weeks' gestation, and 30 percent in babies weighing less than 1000 g. It is found more commonly on the right (75 percent) than the left side (25 percent), reflecting the later descent of the right testicle in development. Bilateral hernias occur in 15–20 percent of cases, and risk factors for bilateral hernias include female gender, presentation with a left-sided hernia, prematurity, age less than one year and undescended testicle [47,48].

During development, the gonads descend from the urogenital ridge in the upper abdomen to the inguinal ring at three months' gestation. The processus vaginalis develops from the peritoneal lining. At 6–7 months' gestation, the testes descend through the inguinal canal, following the gubernaculum, and come to lie in the scrotum. The processus vaginalis is gradually obliterated, leaving behind the tunica vaginalis, with closure occurring earlier on the left than the right side during development [49]. There is greater likelihood of incomplete obliteration with decreasing age, and higher chance of indirect inguinal hernia formation. In females, the round ligament is analogous to the processus vaginalis, and inguinal hernias occur frequently at the canal of Nuck, anterior to the round ligament.

Hernias may be asymptomatic or minimally symptomatic, with intermittent presentation of a bulge at the internal or external inguinal ring. The bulge can disappear with rest or sleep, and may reappear with Valsalva maneuvers such as crying or straining. The differential diagnosis includes hydrocele, lymphadenopathy, neoplasm, torsion, and retractable testis. Ultrasound may reveal a patent processus vaginalis.

An easily reducible, asymptomatic hernia may be repaired electively. An incarcerated hernia is one that is not reducible, and may be associated with pain, tenderness, abdominal distention, emesis, and anorexia. Attempts should be made to reduce an incarcerated hernia at presentation, which may require the use of pain medication, sedation, or repositioning, with subsequent repair after reduction in 1–2 days to prevent recurrence of incarceration. If the hernia is irreducible or is causing obstruction, it should be repaired urgently due to the risk of strangulation. A strangulated hernia is an incarcerated hernia with compromised blood flow to the bowel or testes, and is a surgical emergency. Presentation includes emesis, pain, fever, leukocytosis, erythema, tachycardia, and history of a prolonged bulge. The patient may require a bowel resection for ischemic or infarcted bowel. Premature infants and those less than six months old are more likely to have incarceration [50,51].

Timing of inguinal hernia repair depends upon the age of the patient and existing comorbidities. The risk of incarceration is balanced with the risk of undergoing surgery, particularly amid evolving concerns about anesthetic neurotoxicity in the young and premature [52]. Factors affecting postoperative apnea and respiratory complications include young postconceptual age, existing lung disease, oxygen requirement, anemia, home apnea monitoring, and administration of sedatives, general anesthetics, and opioids [53]. The risk for postoperative apnea decreases with increasing postconceptual age, and many centers have in place institutional policies requiring postoperative admission for apnea monitoring for those patients whose postconceptual age is less than 52–60 weeks in the former premature infant and less than 45 weeks in the former term infant [44,54]. Hernia repair is often scheduled prior to planned discharge home for the former premature infant, or alternatively, the patient may be discharged home and scheduled to return for elective repair at a later time [55].

Inguinal hernia repair may be performed either open or laparoscopically, and opinion is divided regarding superiority of one approach over the other [56]. Surgical complications include infection, bleeding, infarction, and atrophy of the testis, injury to the vas deferens, bowel perforation, and hernia recurrence (less than 5 percent). Some practitioners will perform laparoscopic evaluation of the contralateral side for patent processus vaginalis and hernia, but whether to do so routinely remains controversial [57]. Fifty percent of children less than two years old will have a patent processus vaginalis on the contralateral side, but it is unclear how many of them will eventually present with hernia, with variable reported rates of 8–20 percent [50,58].

Preoperative preparation includes an assessment of residual comorbidities of prematurity, the nature of the hernia, and the planned surgical approach [53]. Administration of caffeine 10 mg kg$^{-1}$ IV may be considered for those patients at risk of postoperative apnea [59]. Anesthetic techniques include general anesthesia supplemented with truncal (ilioinguinal, iliohypogastric, transversus abdominis plane) blocks [60,61] or caudal injection of local anesthetic, and regional anesthesia such as spinal or caudal injection of local anesthetic with or without placement of a caudal catheter [62]. The advantage of a spinal anesthetic is its quick onset, and the benefit of avoiding the effects of systemic sedation and postoperative apnea, but drawbacks include limited duration of action and variable reported failure rates [63]. Supplemental sedatives or opioids will eliminate the advantages of awake regional anesthesia on postoperative apnea [44]. Intraoperative restlessness can be soothed with a pacifier dipped in sucrose solution [64]. Caudal anesthesia may be more reliable but has a slower onset [65]. Large, bilateral, and complicated repairs may necessitate general anesthesia. Laparoscopic evaluation of the contralateral side for hernia is not an absolute contraindication for awake regional anesthesia, but can pose specific challenges during insufflation and pneumoperitoneum [63].

## Hydrocele

Hydrocele is a fluid collection in the tunica vaginalis around the testicle. A communicating hydrocele is essentially a hernia, with a connection to the abdominal cavity via a patent processus vaginalis, whereas a noncommunicating hydrocele does not maintain such a connection [66].

During development, incomplete obliteration of the processus vaginalis will lead to either hernia or hydrocele. An open processus vaginalis with complete failure of obliteration leads to an inguinal or scrotal hernia. Distal obliteration of the processus vaginalis with a patent proximal portion will lead to inguinal hernia. Narrowing of the proximal processus creates a communicating hydrocele, and partial patency of the processus with obliteration of the proximal portion leads to a noncommunicating hydrocele [47].

Communicating hydroceles fluctuate in size during the day, enlarging especially in the dependent position, and are easily compressible. They are treated like inguinal hernias and generally require surgical repair [67]. Noncommunicating hydroceles do not fluctuate in size daily, but can gradually change in size over the course of weeks and are non-compressible. They are quite common after birth, with most resolving spontaneously by the first two years of life. If they have not resolved in the first 12–24 months of life, noncommunicating hydroceles should undergo surgical repair [50,68].

Like hernias, hydroceles are more common on the right than the left side. Those found at birth do not increase the chance of hernia later, although hydroceles that develop later in life imply the presence of a patent processus vaginalis with a chance of hernia formation. Repair is via an inguinal approach to evaluate for a patent processus [69]. A high ligation is performed, the distal sac is opened and the hydrocele is evacuated but is not completely excised due to potential risk of injury to the testicle.

Preoperative preparation includes screening for any residual comorbidities of prematurity or from the neonatal period, and the type of hydrocele and the surgical approach. Older infants and toddlers may benefit from premedication with an anxiolytic prior to parental separation and induction [70]. Anesthetic techniques include general anesthesia with or without caudal injection of a local anesthetic or ilioinguinal and iliohypogastric nerve blocks [71]. Either inhalational or intravenous induction may be performed. Regional anesthesia options include caudal or spinal anesthesia.

## References

1. Christison-Lagay ER, Kelleher CM, Langer JC. Neonatal abdominal wall defects. *Semin Fetal Neonatal Med.* 2011;16(3):164–72.

2. Brusseau R, McCann ME. Anaesthesia for urgent and emergency surgery. *Early Hum Dev.* 2010;86(11):703–14.

3. Banieghbal B, Gouws M, Davies M. Respiratory pressure monitoring as an indirect method of intra-abdominal pressure measurement in gastroschisis closure. *Eur J Pediatr Surg.* 2006;16(2):79–83.

4. Mutoh T, Lamm WJ, Embree LJ, Hildebrandt J, Albert RK. Abdominal distension alters regional pleural pressures and chest wall mechanics in pigs in vivo. *J Appl Physiol.* 1991;70(6):2611–18.

5. Ledbetter DJ. Congenital abdominal wall defects and reconstruction in pediatric surgery: gastroschisis and omphalocele. *Surg Clin North Am.* 2012;92(3):713–27.

6. Hoyme HE, Higginbottom MC, Jones KL. The vascular pathogenesis of gastroschisis: intrauterine interruption of the omphalomesenteric artery. *J Pediatr.* 1981;98(2):228–31.

7. deVries PA. The pathogenesis of gastroschisis and omphalocele. *J Pediatr Surg.* 1980;15(3):245–51.

8. Arnold MA, Chang DC, Nabaweesi R, et al. Risk stratification of 4344 patients with gastroschisis into simple and complex categories. *J Pediatr Surg.* 2007;42(9):1520–5.

9. Kilby MD. The incidence of gastroschisis. *BMJ.* 2006;332(7536):250–1.

10. Loane M, Dolk H, Bradbury I. EUROCAT Working Group. Increasing prevalence of gastroschisis in Europe 1980–2002: a phenomenon restricted to younger mothers? *Paediatr Perinat Epidemiol.* 2007;21(4):363–9.

11. Frolov P, Alali J, Klein MD. Clinical risk factors for gastroschisis and omphalocele in humans: a review of the literature. *Pediatr Surg Int.* 2010;26(12):1135–48.

12. Fratelli N, Papageorghiou AT, Bhide A, et al. Outcome of antenatally diagnosed abdominal wall defects. *Ultrasound Obstet Gynecol.* 2007;30(3):266–70.

13. Juhasz-Böss I, Goelz R, Solomayer E-F, Fuchs J, Meyberg-Solomayer G. Fetal and neonatal outcome in patients with anterior abdominal wall defects (gastroschisis and omphalocele). *J Perinat Med.* 2012;40(1):85–90.

14. Aljahdali A, Mohajerani N, Skarsgard ED. Effect of timing of enteral feeding on outcome in gastroschisis. *J Pediatr Surg.* 2013;48(5):971–6.

15. Minutillo C, Rao SC, Pirie S, McMichael J, Dickinson JE. Growth and developmental outcomes of infants with gastroschisis at one year of age: a retrospective study. *J Pediatr Surg.* 2013;48(8):1688–96.

16. Van Manen M, Hendson L, Wiley M, et al. Early childhood outcomes of infants born with gastroschisis. *J Pediatr Surg.* 2013;48(8):1682–7.

17. David AL, Tan A, Curry J. Gastroschisis: sonographic diagnosis, associations, management and outcome. *Prenat Diagn.* 2008;28(7):633–44.

18. Tucker JM, Brumfield CG, Davis RO, et al. Prenatal differentiation of ventral abdominal wall defects: are amniotic fluid markers useful adjuncts? *J Reprod Med.* 1992;37(5):445–8.

19. Murat I, Humblot A, Girault L, Piana F. Neonatal fluid management. *Best Pract Res Clin Anaesthesiol.* 2010;24(3):365–74.

20. Mortellaro VE, Peter SDS, Fike FB, Islam S. Review of the evidence on the closure of abdominal wall defects. *Pediatr Surg Int.* 2011;27(4):391–7.

21. Marven S, Owen A. Contemporary postnatal surgical management strategies for congenital abdominal wall defects. *Semin Pediatr Surg.* 2008;17(4):222–35.

22. Daily WJR, Klaus M, Belton H, Meyer P. Apnea in premature infants: monitoring, incidence, heart rate changes, and an effect of environmental temperature. *Pediatrics.* 1969;43(4):510–18.

23. Mellor DJ, Lerman J. Anesthesia for neonatal surgical emergencies. *Semin Perinatol.* 1998;22(5):363–79.

24. Goeller JK, Bhalla T, Tobias JD. Combined use of neuraxial and general anesthesia during major abdominal procedures in neonates and infants. *Paediatr Anaesth.* 2014; doi: 10.1111/pan.12384.

25. Tobias JD, Rasmussen GE, Holcomb GW, Brock JW, Morgan WM. Continuous caudal anaesthesia with chloroprocaine as an adjunct to general anaesthesia in neonates. *Can J Anaesth.* 1996;43(1):69–72.

26. Yaster M, Scherer TLR, Stone MM, et al. Prediction of successful primary closure of congenital abdominal wall defects using intraoperative measurements. *J Pediatr Surg.* 1989;24(12):1217–20.

27. Yaster M, Buck JR, Dudgeon DL, et al. Hemodynamic effects of primary closure of omphalocele/gastroschisis in human newborns. *Anesthesiology.* 1988;69(1):84–8.

28. Pelosi P, Vargas M. Mechanical ventilation and intra-abdominal hypertension: "Beyond Good and Evil." *Crit Care.* 2012;16(6):187.

29. Sadler TW. The embryologic origin of ventral body wall defects. *Semin Pediatr Surg.* 2010;19(3):209–14.

30. Calzolari E, Bianchi F, Dolk H, Milan M. Omphalocele and gastroschisis in Europe: a survey of 3 million births 1980–1990. *Am J Med Genet.* 1995;58(2):187–94.

31. Tan KH, Kilby MD, Whittle MJ, et al. Congenital anterior abdominal wall defects in England and Wales 1987–93: retrospective analysis of OPCS data. *BMJ.* 1996;313(7062):903–6.

32. Vermeij-Keers C, Hartwig NG, van der Werff JF. Embryonic development of the ventral body wall and its congenital malformations. *Semin Pediatr Surg.* 1996;5(2):82–9.

33. Islam S. Clinical care outcomes in abdominal wall defects. *Curr Opin Pediatr*. 2008;20(3):305–10.

34. Mitanchez D, Walter-Nicolet E, Humblot A, et al. Neonatal care in patients with giant ompholocele: arduous management but favorable outcomes. *J Pediatr Surg*. 2010;45(8):1727–33.

35. Mann S, Blinman TA, Douglas Wilson R. Prenatal and postnatal management of omphalocele. *Prenat Diagn*. 2008;28(7):626–32.

36. Liu LMP, Mei Pang L. Neonatal surgical emergencies. *Anesthesiol Clin N Am*. 2001;19(2):265–86.

37. Clifton MS, Heiss KF, Keating JJ, Mackay G, Ricketts RR. Use of tissue expanders in the repair of complex abdominal wall defects. *J Pediatr Surg*. 2011;46(2):372–7.

38. Moore TC. Omphalomesenteric duct malformations. *Semin Pediatr Surg*. 1996;5(2):116–23.

39. Meier DE, OlaOlorun DA, Omodele RA, Nkor SK, Tarpley JL. Incidence of umbilical hernia in African children: redefinition of "normal" and reevaluation of indications for repair. *World J Surg*. 2001;25(5):645–8.

40. Kelly KB, Ponsky TA. Pediatric abdominal wall defects. *Surg Clin North Am*. 2013;93(5):1255–67.

41. Zendejas B, Zarroug AE, Erben YM, Holley CT, Farley DR. Impact of childhood inguinal hernia repair in adulthood: 50 years of follow-up. *J Am Coll Surg*. 2010;211(6):762–8.

42. Snyder CL. Current management of umbilical abnormalities and related anomalies. *Semin Pediatr Surg*. 2007;16(1):41–9.

43. Willschke H, Bösenberg A, Marhofer P, et al. Ultrasonography-guided rectus sheath block in paediatric anaesthesia: a new approach to an old technique. *Br J Anaesth*. 2006;97(2):244–9.

44. Coté CJ, Zaslavsky A, Downes JJ, et al. Postoperative apnea in former preterm infants after inguinal herniorrhaphy: a combined analysis. *Anesthesiology*. 1995;82(4):809–22.

45. Dingeman R, Barus LM, Chung H, et al. Ultrasonography-guided bilateral rectus sheath block vs local anesthetic infiltration after pediatric umbilical hernia repair: a prospective randomized clinical trial. *JAMA Surg*. 2013;148(8):707–13.

46. Gurnaney HG, Maxwell LG, Kraemer FW, et al. Prospective randomized observer-blinded study comparing the analgesic efficacy of ultrasound-guided rectus sheath block and local anaesthetic infiltration for umbilical hernia repair. *Br J Anaesth*. 2011;107(5):790–5.

47. Lao OB, Fitzgibbons RJ Jr., Cusick RA. Pediatric inguinal hernias, hydroceles, and undescended testicles. *Surg Clin North Am*. 2012;92(3):487–504.

48. Ein SH, Njere I, Ein A. Six thousand three hundred sixty-one pediatric inguinal hernias: a 35-year review. *J Pediatr Surg*. 2006;41(5):980–6.

49. Sadler TW Urogenital system. In *Langman's Medical Embryology*, 12th edn. Philadelphia, PA: Lippincott Williams & Wilkins; 2011.

50. Lau ST, Lee Y-H, Caty MG. Current management of hernias and hydroceles. *Semin Pediatr Surg*. 2007;16(1):50–7.

51. Wang KS, Committee on Fetus and Newborn, American Academy of Pediatrics, Section on Surgery, American Academy of Pediatrics. Assessment and management of inguinal hernia in infants. *Pediatrics*. 2012;130(4):768–73.

52. Olsen EA, Brambrink AM. Anesthetic neurotoxicity in the newborn and infant. *Curr Opin Anaesthesiol*. 2013;26(5):535–42.

53. Welborn LG, Greenspun JC. Anesthesia and apnea: perioperative considerations in the former preterm infant. *Pediatr Clin North Am*. 1994;41(1):181–98.

54. Murphy JJ, Swanson T, Ansermino M, Milner R. The frequency of apneas in premature infants after inguinal hernia repair: do they need overnight monitoring in the intensive care unit? *J Pediatr Surg*. 2008;43(5):865–8.

55. Lee SL, Gleason JM, Sydorak RM. A critical review of premature infants with inguinal hernias: optimal timing of repair, incarceration risk, and postoperative apnea. *J Pediatr Surg*. 2011;46(1):217–20.

56. Yang C, Zhang H, Pu J, et al. Laparoscopic vs open herniorrhaphy in the management of pediatric inguinal hernia: a systemic review and meta-analysis. *J Pediatr Surg*. 2011;46(9):1824–34.

57. Lazar DA, Lee TC, Almulhim SI, et al. Transinguinal laparoscopic exploration for identification of contralateral inguinal hernias in pediatric patients. *J Pediatr Surg*. 2011;46(12):2349–52.

58. Matthews RD, Neumayer L. Inguinal hernia in the 21st century: an evidence-based review. *Curr Probl Surg*. 2008;45(4):261–312.

59. Henderson-Smart DJ, Steer PA. Prophylactic caffeine to prevent postoperative apnoea following general anaesthesia in preterm infants. *Cochrane Database Syst Rev*. 2001;4:CD000048.

60. Disma N, Tuo P, Pellegrino S, Astuto M. Three concentrations of levobupivacaine for ilioinguinal/iliohypogastric nerve block in ambulatory pediatric surgery. *J Clin Anesth*. 2009;21(6):389–93.

61. Mai CL, Young MJ, Quraishi SA. Clinical implications of the transversus abdominis plane block in pediatric anesthesia. *Pediatr Anesth*. 2012;22(9):831–40.

62. Jagannathan N, Sohn L, Sawardekar A, et al. Unilateral groin surgery in children: will the addition of an ultrasound-guided ilioinguinal nerve block enhance the duration of analgesia of a single-shot caudal block? *Pediatr Anesth*. 2009;19(9):892–8.

63. Frawley G, Ingelmo P. Spinal anaesthesia in the neonate. *Best Pract Res Clin Anaesthesiol*. 2010;24(3):337–51.

64. Harrison D, Beggs S, Stevens B. Sucrose for procedural pain management in infants. *Pediatrics*. 2012;130(5):918–25.

65. Hoelzle M, Weiss M, Dillier C, Gerber A. Comparison of awake spinal with awake caudal anesthesia in preterm and ex-preterm infants for herniotomy. *Pediatr Anesth*. 2010;20(7):620–4.

66. Palmer LS. Hernias and hydroceles. *Pediatr Rev Am Acad Pediatr*. 2013;34(10):457–464; quiz 464.

67. Cozzi DA, Mele E, Ceccanti S, et al. Infantile abdominoscrotal hydrocele: a not so benign condition. *J Urol*. 2008;180(6):2611–15.

68. Koski ME, Makari JH, Adams MC, et al. Infant communicating hydroceles: do they need immediate repair or might some clinically resolve? *J Pediatr Surg*. 2010;45(3):590–3.

68. Wilson JM, Aaronson DS, Schrader R, Baskin LS. Hydrocele in the pediatric patient: inguinal or scrotal approach? *J Urol*. 2008;180(Suppl. 4):1724–8.

70. Banchs RJ, Lerman J. Preoperative anxiety management, emergence delirium, and postoperative behavior. *Anesthesiol Clin*. 2014;32(1):1–23.

71. Bhalla T, Sawardekar A, Dewhirst E, Jagannathan N, Tobias JD. Ultrasound-guided trunk and core blocks in infants and children. *J Anesth*. 2013;27(1):109–23.

# 24

# Anesthesia for Intra-Abdominal Procedures

Raymond Park and Edward Cooper

## Introduction

Abdominal procedures constitute a large percentage of operating room cases in the neonatal and infant population. Therefore, it is vital for anesthesiologists caring for pediatric patients to be knowledgeable regarding general surgical conditions common to this specific patient population, as well as their typical presentation, associated comorbidities and perioperative management strategies. Patients presenting for surgery often have associated syndromes or genetic abnormalities that predispose them to abdominal complications, and the anesthesiologist should be cognizant of the other associated systemic manifestations of the underlying disease.

Foremost among the considerations in evaluating patients presenting for intra-abdominal surgery is the potential for either altered or frankly obstructed gastrointestinal emptying. In children, there are currently no noninvasive methods to reliably discriminate patients with full stomachs from those with relatively intact gastric emptying. Therefore, common practice is to assume that the patient is at high risk for aspiration during induction and emergence, unless actively tolerating oral feeding without complications. Rapid sequence induction should be considered, though with this approach neonates and infants may develop hypoxemia during the time period needed for adequate muscle relaxation due to their higher baseline oxygen consumption ($>5$ ml kg$^{-1}$ min$^{-1}$ vs. $2$–$3$ ml kg$^{-1}$ min$^{-1}$ in adults) and decreased apneic functional residual capacity compared with adults [1,2]. Due to these considerations, many practitioners choose to utilize a modified rapid sequence induction with cricoid pressure and low-pressure mask ventilation prior to intubation. Though use of a modified rapid sequence technique can mitigate risk of hypoxia during induction, application of cricoid pressure can potentially obscure airway anatomy and hinder mask ventilation. Despite these precautions, judicious mask

ventilation with pressures as low as 10 cmH$_2$O has still been shown to result in gastric insufflation, though applying cricoid pressure can increase this threshold [3–5]. Additionally, use of a nasogastric tube, placed prior to induction, can be used to decompress the stomach. The potential benefit of this maneuver must be weighed against the possibility that the stomach may still not be fully empty and the possibility of additional patient agitation. Though studies in infant and adult cadavers demonstrated effective esophageal occlusion with cricoid pressure of up to 100 cmH$_2$O in the presence of a nasogastric tube, concerns with leaving a nasogastric tube in place during induction include potentially interfering with esophageal sphincter function and serving as a "wick" for regurgitant contents [6,7]. Consequently, if a nasogastric tube is placed for gastric evacuation, whether it should be removed prior to induction is not clear.

In addition to addressing the direct anatomical and surgical concerns of intra-abdominal injury, the pediatric anesthesiologist must be acutely aware of and thoroughly investigate the potential systemic manifestations of abdominal pathology. Patients will often have signs consistent with sepsis and capillary leak syndrome pre-, post-, and intraoperatively secondary to underlying bowel ischemia or perforation. These patients will often require aggressive fluid resuscitation and will occasionally require the use of vasoactive medications when vasoplegia is present. Perioperative management can also be complicated by florid intra-abdominal inflammation and fluid retention, leading to abdominal compartment syndrome. Depending on the degree of abdominal swelling and concerns for postoperative abdominal compartment syndrome, abdominal closure may not be immediately possible or advisable at the end of the procedure. Airway edema secondary to rapid fluid administration, ongoing hemodynamic instability, and unfavorable acid–base status may preclude safe extubation and result in subsequent difficulty with ventilation. These concerns coupled with increased relative evaporative losses in the neonate with an open abdomen can make these cases particularly challenging from a fluid management perspective. Regional anesthetics for postoperative analgesia such as epidural, caudal, and transversus abdominis plane catheters can be considered, but expected duration of postoperative ventilation, future and present coagulation status, and risk of postoperative infection should be considered prior to placement.

Increasingly, many intra-abdominal procedures are being performed laparoscopically, and understanding the physiological changes that occur with abdominal insufflation is important. Carbon dioxide is the preferred gas for laparoscopy due to the fact that it is not readily flammable, clears quickly from the peritoneum, and does not expand within closed spaces. Carbon dioxide is readily absorbed across the peritoneum and necessitates an increase in minute ventilation to maintain normocapnia. The insufflated abdomen can lead to cephalad displacement of the diaphragmatic, to compression of dependent lung areas and to subsequent V/Q mismatch and hypoxemia. Higher airway driving pressures may be needed to compensate for reduced pulmonary and thoracic compliance with laparoscopy [8]. Hemodynamically, higher insufflation pressures can lead to reduction in cardiac output [9,10]. If insufflation pressures exceed venous pressure in the setting of open abdominal venous channels, clinically significant carbon dioxide embolism can occur [11]. Intracranial pressure can be increased by a combination of increased abdominal pressure, hypercarbia, and head-down positioning, and therefore the risks and benefits of laparoscopy should be carefully considered in patients with elevated intracranial pressure or an existing ventriculoperitoneal shunt [12,13].

## Specific Conditions

### Gastrointestinal Duplications

Gastrointestinal duplications are rare congenital lesions that occur in approximately 1 in 4500 live births [14]. Duplications have been described at all points along the gastrointestinal tract as proximally as the mouth and as distal as the anus. The etiology of gastrointestinal duplications is unclear, but they are thought to occur between four and eight weeks during embryonic development. Existing theories to explain their occurrence include errors in recanalization of the primitive intestine, failure of regression of embryonic diverticuli, and errors of notochord splitting [15,16]. Gastrointestinal duplications can either occur as an isolated occurrence or involve multiple locations. Duplications generally do not communicate with adjacent gastrointestinal structures, though this is not universally the case. Similar to the case of many congenital malformations, there are often associated systemic abnormalities that should be identified and evaluated [17,18].

With the advent of and improvements in prenatal imaging, most gastrointestinal duplications are detected in utero and have in only rare instances required fetal intervention. Most pediatric surgeons advocate resection of the duplication, though for asymptomatic patients the optimal timing of surgery remains unclear, and presently there are no concrete data to aid in guiding practice [14]. Patients who develop sequelae of duplications usually do so in the context of secretions that accumulate in noncommunicating and closed space duplications, leading to pain and compression of adjacent structures. Such developments are of particular concern when the compression of adjacent vasculature leads to bowel ischemia. The duplication can also serve as a lead point for the bowel to telescope around surrounding intestinal segments, leading to intussusception. Ulcerations resulting in bleeding can occur in the duplication itself secondary to ectopic gastric tissue or in adjacent tissue [19].

Anesthetic considerations for gastrointestinal duplications include localization of the duplication, identification of any associated abnormalities, and the clinical manifestations of the duplication. Potential for airway obstruction may require the use of rigid bronchoscopy, and bowel obstruction will mandate full stomach precautions.

### Pyloric Stenosis

Pyloric stenosis is a relatively common condition requiring surgical intervention in infants and occurring in approximately 2–5 out of 1000 live births [20]. The etiology of pyloric stenosis is not entirely clear, though likely multifactorial. The condition occurs four times more commonly in males than in females and has a higher prevalence in first-born children [21]. Unlike many other gastrointestinal abnormalities, patients with pyloric stenosis are otherwise generally healthy, though a familial genetic predisposition is observed.

The pathological finding in pyloric stenosis is hypertrophy of the muscularis layer of the pyloric sphincter, leading to gastric outlet obstruction. Patients typically present with immediate, nonbilious, nonbloody, postprandial projectile vomiting at the age of 3–12 weeks [22] that often increases with intensity over time. The severity of dehydration and electrolyte abnormalities generally correlates with the degree and duration of symptoms prior to presentation [23]. In general, patients will present with a chloride-sensitive, hypochloremic, hypokalemic, metabolic alkalosis with some degree of hyponatremia secondary to volume depletion and paradoxical aciduria. However, if there is longstanding volume loss without correction, patients can present with metabolic acidosis as a result of both lactic acidosis and renal dysfunction.

Pyloric stenosis can often be diagnosed by history alone, but supporting physical exam findings include an olive-shaped mass in the right upper quadrant. Diagnosis is typically confirmed with an abdominal ultrasound, though barium studies have also been utilized [24].

Pyloric stenosis is not a surgical emergency, though definitive treatment is surgical pyloromyotomy, which can often be performed laparoscopically. Prior to surgical intervention, acid–base status and electrolyte abnormalities should be corrected. Patients with persistent or untreated metabolic alkalosis are at increased risk of postoperative apnea [25]. Metabolic alkalosis is often corrected after hospital admission and preoperatively with saline administration that corrects volume status, replenishes total-body sodium and chloride, and promotes excretion of urine bicarbonate. Secondary to dehydration, patients may present with renal insufficiency, and potassium repletion should be initiated only with the establishment of urine output. Serum chloride concentration can be followed to gauge the adequacy of rehydration and correction of the underlying metabolic alkalosis. Studies by Goh et al. and Shanbhogue et al. demonstrated that a serum chloride concentration greater than 106 meq $L^{-1}$ predicts correction of alkalosis in the majority of patients with pyloric stenosis [26,27].

Due to functional gastric outlet obstruction, patients with pyloric stenosis are at high risk for aspiration during induction. The stomach should be emptied with a large-bore orogastric tube, sometimes with several passes, prior to induction. This does not necessarily guarantee an empty stomach. The airway should be secured by means of a (modified or standard) rapid sequence induction or awake intubation. Anesthesia can be maintained with nondepolarizing neuromuscular blockade and volatile anesthetics, though Davis et al. showed decreased postoperative respiratory events with the use of a remifentanil-based anesthetic [28]. For longer cases, a dextrose infusion should be started. Surgeons may ask that an orogastric tube be used to insufflate the stomach to rule-out luminal perforation following repair. Adequate analgesia can generally be obtained with rectal or intravenous acetaminophen combined with local anesthetic via caudal block or local infiltration by the surgeon. Sparing use of intermediate and long-acting opioids is advocated. The patient should be awake and vigorous at the end of the case prior to extubation. In addition to remaining metabolic alkalosis, hypothermia, hypoglycemia, residual neuromuscular blockade, and previous opioid administration can all further increase the risk of postoperative apnea, and every attempt should be made to avoid these conditions [21,29].

## Necrotizing Enterocolitis

Necrotizing enterocolitis (NEC) is characterized by ischemic necrosis of the intestinal mucosa, leading to gut translocation of enteric organisms and to potential local and systemic complications. Necrotizing enterocolitis occurs in approximately 1 out of 1000 live births, is inversely related to birth weight and rarely occurs spontaneously in full-term neonates unless associated with predisposing conditions, such as congenital heart disease, sepsis, or hypotension, that lead to compromise of intestinal blood flow [30,31]. Mortality from NEC is 15–30 percent, and survivors often suffer from long-term sequelae such as short-gut syndrome, parenteral nutrition dependence, and growth and neurodevelopment deficits [30,32].

Necrotizing enterocolitis classically develops in the second to third week of life after the initiation of feeding, though it can develop in patients prior to initiation of feeding and has been rarely observed in patients who have tolerated feeding for a significant length of time. NEC often initially presents with constitutional symptoms such as lethargy, temperature instability, hypotension, and apnea in conjunction with or followed by gastrointestinal symptoms such as feeding intolerance, emesis, abdominal distention, or bloody stool. As the disease progresses, worsening abdominal distention, increased abdominal tympany, palpable bowel loops, and periumbilical abdominal wall erythema and ecchymosis can develop. Imaging studies can help to confirm diagnosis, although NEC is a clinical diagnosis and radiographic findings are not always appreciated. Findings that are highly suspicious for NEC include pneumatosis intestinalis, pneumoperitoneum, and evidence of air within the portal system. Patients may concurrently experience deterioration of other organ systems by avenues such as hematologic abnormalities (disseminated intravascular coagulation, thrombocytopenia, coagulopathy), metabolic acidosis, respiratory failure, and septic shock.

Initial management includes supportive measures such as bowel rest, nasogastric tube decompression, broad-spectrum antibiotics, and hemodynamic and respiratory support if necessary. Medical management is continued with serial monitoring of abdominal exam and radiographic studies. If there is high suspicion or frank evidence of intestinal perforation, surgical intervention is indicated and includes laparotomy with resection of affected bowel segments and/or bedside peritoneal drainage. Between 20 and 40 percent of NEC cases require surgical intervention [31,33], with Guthrie et al. showing a mortality rate of 23 percent for surgical NEC patients compared with 4 percent for medically managed NEC patients [33].

Patients who present requiring surgical treatment will often have multi-organ dysfunction that will complicate perioperative management. Existing hematologic abnormalities may require ongoing treatment with appropriate blood component therapy. Hypotension secondary to intravascular volume depletion and septic vasoplegia is common in the presence of intra-abdominal fluid sequestration and distributive shock. Consequently, the patient may require additional or initiation of vasoactive infusions and continued fluid administration to maintain blood pressure. A primarily narcotic-based anesthetic may be better tolerated from a hemodynamic perspective than one that utilizes higher concentrations of volatile anesthetics. In addition, delivery of volatile agents may be limited if an ICU ventilator is utilized for transport and better control and monitoring of respiratory parameters. If the airway is not already secured, consideration should be given to a rapid sequence induction or to an awake intubation. Venous access should take into account the likely need for administration of large amounts of volume and vasopressor

therapy. Obtaining arterial access for hemodynamic monitoring and blood sampling is optimal but should not unduly delay definitive surgical treatment in a clinically deteriorating patient.

## Meconium Ileus

Meconium ileus (MI) is characterized by bowel obstruction, generally at the level of the terminal ileum and ileocecal valve secondary to accumulation and failure of passage of thick, desiccated meconium. Patients with cystic fibrosis (CF) in particular have a propensity to develop MI due to secretion of highly viscous meconium that adheres to the intestinal lumen. Twenty percent of CF patients who develop MI represent 80–90 percent of the total MI cases [34,35]. Meconium ileus is categorized as simple or complex. Simple MI presents clinically with abdominal distention, failure to pass meconium and, in some cases, emesis. Roughly 50 percent of cases of MI are classified as complex. Meconium ileus is classified as complex if there is associated gastrointestinal pathology such as perforation, peritonitis, atresia, or volvulus. Volvulus and other ischemic insults that occur in utero may manifest postnatally as bowel atresia. Simple MI is treated with nasogastric decompression, correction of any fluid or electrolyte abnormalities, and administration of serial hyperosmolar enemas [36]. Repeat enema administration is common but increases the risk of perforation and other complications with each additional attempt [37,38]. Simple MI that is refractory to more conservative medical management requires surgical intervention.

Preparation for the operating room should identify and initiate correction of electrolyte abnormalities and volume depletion as a result of potential dehydration, hyperosmolar enema therapy, or fluid shifts associated with bowel injury or obstruction. In CF patients, the lung pathology is generally not a concern until after several years of life [39], unless the clinical presentation is associated with previous aspiration or secondary lung injury due to sepsis or systemic inflammatory response syndrome. Stomach contents should be decompressed with an orogastric tube prior to induction to minimize the risk of aspiration during anesthetic induction. Rapid sequence induction or awake intubation with local anesthetic should be employed to secure the airway. Anesthetic can be maintained with neuromuscular blockade and, depending on hemodynamic status, with volatile versus an opioid-based anesthetic. Vasoactive infusions should be readily available to treat potential hypotension.

# Malrotation

Malrotation results from in utero arrest of normal rotation of the embryonic gut, leading to narrowing of the mesenteric base and to a predisposition to mesenteric twisting and consequent volvulus. With malrotation, there can also be abnormal attachments, known as Ladd's bands, that form in the process of attempting to affix the bowel in the peritoneal cavity and that can lead to duodenal obstruction. Symptomatic malrotation occurs in approximately 1 in 5000 live births [40], and 50–70 percent of cases are associated with other congenital abnormalities. Gastrointestinal anomalies are most common, though cardiac, orthopedic, and central nervous system anomalies also frequently occur [41,42]. Intestinal atresia can be seen in cases in which malrotation occurs in utero during bowel development. In children with malrotation requiring surgery, up to 65 percent present during the first month of life [42].

Patients with malrotation can clinically present with either volvulus or nonischemic intestinal obstruction due to Ladd's bands or atretic bowel. Patients with volvulus present with bilious emesis, symptoms of bowel obstruction, and potentially an acute abdomen. Grossly bloody stool can also be seen and usually indicates a more severe presentation with significant bowel ischemia. Diagnosis of malrotation in a clinically stable patient can be made radiographically with plain film or fluoroscopic upper gastrointestinal series with small-bowel follow-through or an abdominal ultrasound to determine the relative orientation of mesenteric vessels [43].

A patient with suspected or confirmed volvulus requires prompt surgical treatment to salvage affected bowel segments. Because volvulus is a surgical emergency, every effort should be made to safely proceed as quickly as possible to surgery with the goal of saving any viable bowel. The airway should be secured using full-stomach precautions. Arterial access can be obtained as needed, though doing so should not delay surgery and relief of ischemic bowel. As with many other ischemic abdominal pathologies, patients may present with a combination of intravascular depletion due to intra-abdominal inflammation and swelling along with vasodilation from sepsis. Treatment

for hypotension may therefore require both fluid and blood component therapy in addition to vasoactive infusions. In cases in which abdominal compartment syndrome is present, concern should be exercised upon surgical decompression of the peritoneal cavity. With the relief of elevated abdominal pressures, subsequent systemic washout of lactate and products of cell ischemia, such as potassium, can result in rapid clinical deterioration.

# Intestinal Atresia

Intestinal atresia is the complete congenital obstruction of the lumen of a hollow viscus. Intestinal atresia can occur at any point of the intestinal tract, with the small intestine being the most common site of pathology. Of the cases of small-bowel atresia, the majority occur within the jejunum and ileum. The atresia can also be present in the large bowel, though these cases constitute only 7–10 percent of all cases of intestinal atresia [44].

Intestinal atresia is classified into types I–IV using the following definitions:

Type I: Intact muscularis and serosa, with the lumen obstructed by an intact diaphragm or membrane.
Type II: Obvious gap in bowel with the proximal and distal segments connected by a fibrous band.
Type III:
  a. Obvious gap in bowel with no connection between proximal and distal segments.
  b. Proximal small-bowel atresia, absence of mid-small bowel that would normally be supplied by the superior mesenteric artery and a large gap in small-bowel mesentery.
Type IV: Multiple II or IIIA atresias.

In many cases, intestinal atresia can be diagnosed prenatally and is often accompanied by polyhydramnios. Patients with intestinal atresia present with abdominal distention, emesis, and failure to pass meconium. With bowel obstruction, there can be increased enterohepatic circulation of bilirubin and resultant jaundice. Patients with partial obstruction or stenosis will often present later than those with complete intestinal atresia. Diagnosis should exclude other intra-abdominal pathologies, and additional radiographic studies can help to confirm the diagnosis, particularly plain film or fluoroscopy with and without contrast imaging.

Patients with duodenal atresia should be screened for other associated abnormalities, with particular attention to the heart, kidneys, spine, and hepato-biliary system. There are associated chromosomal abnormalities in approximately 30 percent of cases of duodenal atresia, most often trisomy 21 [45]. Though the majority of patients with jejunal and ileal atresia are otherwise healthy, it can be associated with coexisting disease such as CF, gastroschisis, and, less commonly, omphalocele [44]. Patients with CF are predisposed to develop in utero bowel ischemia due to volvulus or perforation; the resultant necrotic bowel is resorbed, leaving behind an atretic segment of gut. Patients with colonic atresia are generally healthy, though they can also be affected with pathology such as gastroschisis and Hirschsprung's disease (HD) [44].

Initial management of intestinal atresia involves discontinuation of feeding, decompression with a nasogastric tube, and correction of fluid and electrolyte abnormalities. Patients with duodenal atresia should be evaluated for possible comorbidities, while those with jejunal or ileal atresia should be tested for CF.

Emergent surgery for intestinal atresia is generally not indicated, and clinical stability should be established and further evaluation of potential associated abnormalities should be completed prior to bringing the patient to the operating room. Patients with intestinal atresia by definition have a full stomach, and appropriate measures should be taken during anesthetic induction to minimize risk of aspiration. Adequate peripheral intravenous access should be obtained and an arterial line placed if needed in the setting of associated cardiac abnormalities.

## Hirschsprung's Disease and Anorectal Malformations

Hirschsprung's disease results from failure of neural crest cells to migrate during intestinal development, leading to a segment of aganglionic colon and, in approximately 7–10 percent of cases, to complete involvement of the colon, resulting in depressed gut motility [46,47]. In rare cases of HD, the entire colon and a portion of the small bowel may also be affected. Males are disproportionately affected, with a male:female gender ratio of 3–4:1 cases [48]. Multiple specific genetic mutations are associated with HD. Furthermore, HD is often associated with chromosomal abnormalities and monogenic syndromes [49].

The majority of cases of HD are diagnosed in the neonatal period when affected individuals develop symptoms of distal intestinal obstruction such as vomiting, abdominal distention, and the failure to pass meconium and stool within the first 48 hours of life. Older patients typically present with symptoms of chronic constipation, failure to thrive, and abdominal distention. Hirschsprung's disease patients can also present acutely with enterocolitis, toxic megacolon, and associated sepsis, fever, and abdominal distention [50]. Rarely, volvulus can also occur in patients with HD due to twisting of feces or meconium-filled, enlarged bowel segments.

Patients with enterocolitis may require immediate surgical intervention, though it is preferable to stabilize the patient and obtain a definitive diagnosis of HD prior to surgery and then proceed with a single-stage definitive surgery rather than with a diverting colostomy and the need for a later pull-through procedure. Stable patients with suspected HD should undergo an appropriate diagnostic workup consisting of a rectal suction biopsy, though abdominal radiographs, contrast enemas, and anorectal manometry have all been used to provide supportive diagnostic information. Definitive treatment for HD involves surgical resection of affected bowel segments with an anal sphincter-preserving re-anastomosis of normal ganglionic bowel. Even after definitive surgical treatment for HD, patients can present later with enterocolitis [39,49].

Patients with HD presenting for surgery should be carefully evaluated for comorbid disease and syndromes that could potentially impact anesthetic management. Anesthetic induction should take into account the degree of abdominal obstruction. Patients with HD enterocolitis may require aggressive fluid resuscitation, vasoconstrictive drug infusions such as dopamine, and arterial access for monitoring of hemodynamics and metabolic status. Pull-through procedures may require lithotomy positioning, which can limit placement of intravenous catheters to the upper extremities and in rare cases has been associated with complications such as lower extremity compartment syndrome.

A similar surgical condition that the pediatric anesthesiologist may need to treat is anorectal malformations. Anorectal anomalies manifest with a wide spectrum of severity and have an incidence rate of 1 in 2500–4000 live births [51,52]. These anomalies arise from failure of normal development of the cloaca into the urogenital and rectal structures [53]. Consequently, the correction of these congenital defects will often require a multidisciplinary surgical approach.

Presurgical planning is centered on definitively defining the anatomy and identifying associated defects that may require more immediate treatment. Pre-procedure studies should include evaluation of the heart, kidney, urinary collection system, spine, and remainder of the GI tract [54]. Surgical approach will be dependent on the nature of the anomaly and on whether it is amenable to repair via a simple anoplasty, pull-through, or temporizing staged colostomy. Given the often elective nature of these procedures, anesthetic concerns similar to those entertained in HD should be considered. After corrective surgery, postoperative course often requires serial dilations that may also require the services of an anesthesiologist.

## Intussusception

Intussusception is the invagination of one segment of intestine into another, leading to compromised lymphatic and venous drainage. Eighty-five percent of patients with intussusception are under three years of age [55] and are generally otherwise healthy. Intussusception is the most common cause of intestinal obstruction in the pediatric population. The site of intussusception is often in close proximity to the ileocecal junction, though bowel segments in both the large and small intestines can be affected. If left untreated, intussusception results in progressive bowel edema, ischemia, and possible perforation. Though the majority of cases of intussusception have no clear etiology, commonly associated predispositions include viral illness, viral or bacterial enteritis, and identifiable "lead points" for intussusception such as Meckel's diverticulum, lymphoma, duplication cysts, inflamed Peyer's patches with concurrent Henoch–Schonlein purpura, and vascular malformations [39].

Patients with intussusception present with sudden intermittent cramps, severe paraoxysmal colicky abdominal pain, and progressive lethargy often out of proportion to abdominal exam. The classic presentation of pain, a palpable sausage-shaped mass, and currant jelly stool is observed only in a minority of patients [56]. Abdominal plain film can be suggestive of intussusception, but abdominal ultrasound is generally the preferred modality of diagnosis [56], though computed tomography (CT) can be helpful if prior workup has been unrevealing.

Surgical intervention is indicated for patients with evidence of perforation. Otherwise, patients should be stabilized with intravenous fluids and decompression with a nasogastric tube and reduction attempted with hydrostatic or pneumatic enema. Nonoperative reduction has a success rate of 80–95 percent and can be repeated, but does carry a 1 percent risk of perforation [57] and a recurrence rate of 5–7 percent [58]. Surgical intervention is necessary if nonoperative intervention is not successful or results in perforation.

Anesthesiologists may be asked to provide anesthesia or sedation during nonoperative or surgical reduction. Patient with intussusception should be considered to have full stomachs, and appropriate precautions should be taken during anesthetic induction. Similar to considerations for other intra-abdominal surgical emergencies, intravenous access, hemodynamic monitoring, and need for vasoactive medications and fluid resuscitation will be contingent on the severity of clinical presentation.

## Biliary Atresia

Infants born with biliary atresia (BA) are most often treated with a hepatoportoenterostomy or Kasai procedure that allows for bile drainage from small bile ducts into the small intestine. There are three common types of BA: type 1 – atresia restricted to the common bile duct; type 2 – atresia of the common hepatic duct; type 3 – atresia of the right and left hepatic duct. If the Kasai procedure is performed in the first two months of life, greater than 80 percent of infants will achieve some bile drainage, although a majority of these eventually will require a liver transplant.

A **hepatoportoenterostomy** or **Kasai portoenterostomy** is a surgical treatment performed on infants with biliary atresia to allow for bile drainage. In these infants, the bile is not able to drain normally from the small bile ducts within the liver into the larger bile ducts that connect to the gall bladder and small intestine.

The surgery involves exposing the porta hepatis (the area of the liver from which bile should drain) and attaching part of the small intestine to the exposed liver surface. The rationale for this approach is that minute residual bile duct remnants may be present in the fibrous tissue of the porta hepatis and thus provide direct connection with the intrahepatic ductule system to allow bile drainage [1].

# Prognosis

- If performed before 60 days of age, 80 percent of children achieve some bile drainage.
- Prognosis is progressively worse the later surgery is done.
- Postoperatively, cholangitis and malabsorption are common.
- Many children with biliary atresia will require liver transplantation despite the attempted surgical repair.
- In type I, atresia is limited to the common bile duct, and the gallbladder and hepatic ducts are patent (i.e., "distal" BA). In type II, atresia affects the hepatic duct, but the proximal intrahepatic ducts are patent (i.e., "proximal" BA). Type II is subgrouped in type IIa, where a patent gallbladder and patent common bile duct are present (sometimes with a cyst in the hilum, i.e., "cystic BA"), and in type IIb, where the gallbladder as well as the cystic duct and common bile duct are also obliterated. In type III, there is discontinuity of not only the right and left intrahepatic hepatic ducts, but also of the entire extrahepatic biliary tree (i.e., "complete" BA). The French classification is similar, but the designation of the above types IIa and IIb as types 2 and 3 results in a total of four types [3].
- Most often, BA is complete (Japanese/Anglo-Saxon type III, 73 percent) or subcomplete (type IIb, 18 percent), with "cystic" BA and "distal" BA being infrequent (types IIa and I, 6 percent and 3 percent, respectively) [4].

# References

1. Adamson K Jr., Gandy GM, James LS. The influence of thermal factors upon oxygen consumption of the newborn human infant. *J Pediatr.* 1965;66:495–508.

2. Kliegman RM, Stanton BMD, Geme JS, Schor NF, Behrman RE. Respiratory system. In Kliegman RM, Stanton BMD, Geme JS, Schor NF, Behrman RE, editors. *Nelson Textbook of Pediatrics.* Philadelphia, PA: Elsevier; 2011; 2680.

3. Walker RWM, Ravi R, Haylett K Effect of cricoid force on airway calibre in children: a bronchoscopic assessment. *Br J Anaesth.* 2009; 104(1):71–4.

4. Bouvet L, Albert ML, Augris C. Real-time detection of gastric insufflation related to facemask pressure-controlled ventilation using ultrasonography of the antrum and epigastric auscultation in nonparalyzed patients. *Anesthesiology.* 2014;120(2):326–34.

5. Moynihan RJ, Brock-Utne JG, Archer JH, Feld LH, Kreitzman TR. The effect of cricoid pressure on preventing gastric insufflation in infants and children. *Anesthesiology.* 1993;78(4):652–6.

6. Biebuyck JF, Benumof JL. Management of the difficult adult airway with special emphasis on awake tracheal intubation. *Anesthesiology.* 1991;75(6):1087.

7. Salem MR, Wong AY, Mani M, Sellick BA. Efficacy of cricoid pressure in preventing gastric inflation during bag-mask ventilation in pediatric patients. *Anesthesiology.* 1974;40(1):96–8.

8. Bannister CF, Brosius KK, Wulkan M. The effect of insufflation pressure on pulmonary mechanics in infants during laparoscopic surgical procedures. *Pediatr Anesth.* 2003;13(9):785–9.

9. Gueugniaud P-Y, Abisseror M, Moussa M, et al. The hemodynamic effects of pneumoperitoneum during laparoscopic surgery in healthy infants: assessment by continuous esophageal aortic blood flow echo-Doppler. *Anesth Analg.* 1998;86(2):290–3.

10. Sakka SG, Huettemann E, Petrat G, et al. Transoesophageal echocardiographic assessment of haemodynamic changes during laparoscopic herniorrhaphy in small children. *Br J Anaesth.* 2000;84(3):330–4.

11. Yacoub OF, Cardona IJ, Coveler LA, Dodson MG. Carbon dioxide embolism during laparoscopy. *Anesthesiology.* 1982;57(6):533.

12. Irgau I, Koyfman Y, Tikellis JI. Elective intraoperative intracranial pressure monitoring during laparoscopic cholecystectomy. *Arch Surg Am Med Assoc.* 1995;130(9):1011–13.

13. Schöb OM, Allen DC, Benzel E, et al. A comparison of the pathophysiologic effects of carbon dioxide, nitrous oxide, and helium pneumoperitoneum on intracranial pressure. *Am J Surg.* 1996;172(3):248–53.

14. Puligandla PS, Nguyen LT, St-Vil D, Flageole H Gastrointestinal duplications. *J Pediatr Surg.* 2003;38(5):740–4.

15. Gross RE, Holcomb GW Jr., Farber S. Duplications of the alimentary tract. *Pediatrics.* 1952;9(4):449–68.

16. Faris JC, Crowe JE. The split notochord syndrome. *J Pediatr Surg.* 1975;10(4):467–72.

17. Laje P, Flake AW, Adzick NS. Prenatal diagnosis and postnatal resection of intraabdominal enteric duplications. *J Pediatr Surg.* 2010;45(7):1554–8.

18. Stringer MD, Spitz L, Abel R, et al. Management of alimentary tract duplication in children. *Br J Surg.* 1995;82(1):74–8.

19. Iyer CP, Mahour GH. Duplications of the alimentary tract in infants and children. *J Pediatr Surg.* 1995;30(9):1267–70.

20. MacMahon B. The continuing enigma of pyloric stenosis of infancy. *Epidemiology*. 2006;17(2):195–201.

21. Bissonnette B, Sullivan PJ. Pyloric stenosis. *Can J Anesth*. 1991;38(5):668–76.

22. Schechter R, Torfs CP, Bateson TF. The epidemiology of infantile hypertrophic pyloric stenosis. *Paediatr Perinat Epidemiol*. 1997;11(4):407–27.

23. Breaux CW, Hood JS, Georgeson KE. The significance of alkalosis and hypochloremia in hypertrophic pyloric stenosis. *J Pediatr Surg*. 1989;24(12):1250–2.

24. Pandya S, Heiss K. Pyloric stenosis in pediatric surgery. *Surg Clin North Am*. 2012;92(3):527–39.

25. Ein SH, Masiakos PT, Ein A The ins and outs of pyloromyotomy: what we have learned in 35 years. *Pediatr Surg Int*. 2014;30(5):467–80.

26. Goh DW, Hall SK, Gornall P, et al. Plasma chloride and alkalaemia in pyloric stenosis. *Br J Surg*. 1990;77(8):922–3.

27. Shanbhogue LKR, Sikdar T, Jackson M, Lloyd DA. Serum electrolytes and capillary blood gases in the management of hypertrophic pyloric stenosis. *Br J Surg*. 1992;79(3):251–3.

28. Davis PJ, Galinkin J, McGowan FX, et al. A randomized multicenter study of remifentanil compared with halothane in neonates and infants undergoing pyloromyotomy: I. Emergence and recovery profiles. *Anesth Analg*. 2001;93(6):1380–6.

29. Carlo W Respiratory Tract Disorders. In Kliegman RM, Stanton BMD, Geme JS, Schor NF, Behrman RE, editors. *Nelson Textbook of Pediatrics*. Philadelphia, PA: Elsevier; 2011.

30. Berman L, Moss RL. Necrotizing enterocolitis: an update. *Semin Fetal Neonat Med*. 2011;16(3):145–50.

31. Lambert DK, Christensen RD, Henry E, et al. Necrotizing enterocolitis in term neonates: data from a multihospital health-care system. *J Perinatol*. 2007;27(7):437–43.

32. Rees CM, Pierro A, Eaton S. Neurodevelopmental outcomes of neonates with medically and surgically treated necrotizing enterocolitis. *Arch Dis Child FetalNeonatal Ed*. 2007;92(3):F193–8.

33. Guthrie SO, Gordon PV, Thomas V, et al. Necrotizing enterocolitis among neonates in the United States. *J Perinatol*. 2003;23(4):278–85.

34. Dicken BJ, Ziegler MM. Surgical management of pulmonary and gastrointestinal complications in children with cystic fibrosis. *Curr Op Pediatr*. 2006;18(3):321–9.

35. Fakhoury K, Durie PR, Levison H, Canny GJ. Meconium ileus in the absence of cystic fibrosis. *Arch Dis Child*. 1992;67(10):1204–6.

36. Carlyle BE, Borowitz DS, Glick PL A review of pathophysiology and management of fetuses and neonates with meconium ileus for the pediatric surgeon. *J Pediatr Surg*. 2012;47(4):772–81.

37. Leonidas JC, Burry VF, Fellows RA, Beatty EC. Possible adverse effect of methylglucamine diatrizoate compounds on the bowel of newborn infants with meconium ileus. *Radiology*. 1976;121(3 Pt. 1):693–6.

38. Burke MS, Ragi JM, Karamanoukian HL, et al. New strategies in nonoperative management of meconium ileus. *J Pediatr Surg*. 2002;37(5):760–4.

39. Gourlay DM. Colorectal considerations in pediatric patients. *Surg Clin North Am*. 2013; 93(1):251–72.

40. Shew SB. Surgical concerns in malrotation and midgut volvulus. *Pediatr Radiol*. 2009; 39(Suppl 2):S167–71.

41. Powell DM, Othersen HB, Smith CD. Malrotation of the intestines in children: the effect of age on presentation and therapy. *J Pediatr Surg*. 1989;24(8):777–80.

42. Ford EG, Senac MO, Srikanth MS, Weitzman JJ. Malrotation of the intestine in children. *Annals of Surgery*. 1992;215(2):172–8.

43. Dilley AV, Pereira J, Shi ECP, et al. The radiologist says malrotation: does the surgeon operate? *Pediatr Surg Int*. 2000;16(1–2):45–9.

44. Vecchia LKD, Grosfeld JL, West KW, et al. Intestinal atresia and stenosis: a 25-year experience with 277 cases. *Arch Surg Am Med Assoc*. 1998;133(5):490–7.

45. Best KE, Tennant PWG, Addor M-C, et al. Epidemiology of small intestinal atresia in Europe: a register-based study. *Arch Dis Child Fetal Neonatal Ed*. 2012;97(5):F353–8.

46. N-Fek C. Total colonic aganglionosis (with or without ileal involvement): a review of 27 cases. *J Pediatr Surg*. 1986;21(3):251–4.

47. Suita S, Taguchi T, Kamimura T, Yanai K. Total colonic aganglionosis with or without small bowel involvement: a changing profile. *J Pediatr Surg*. 1997;32(11):1537–41.

48. Badner JA, Sieber WK, Garver KL, Chakravarti A. A genetic study of Hirschsprung disease. *Am J Hum Genet*.1990;46(3):568–80.

49. Amiel J, Sproat-Emison E, Garcia-Barcelo M Hirschsprung disease, associated syndromes and genetics: a review. *J Med Genet*. 2008;45(1):1–14.

50. Shah S. An update on common gastrointestinal emergencies. *Emerg Med Clin North Am*. 2013;31(3):775–93.

51. Cuschieri A. Descriptive epidemiology of isolated anal anomalies: a survey of 4.6 million births in Europe. *Am J Med Genet*. 2001;103(3):207–15.

52. Levitt MA, Peña A. Outcomes from the correction of anorectal malformations. *Curr Op Pediatr.* 2005;17(3):394–401.

53. Levitt MA, Peña A. Anorectal malformations. *Pediatr Surg.* 2012: 1–21. doi: 10.1186/1750-1172-2-33.

54. Stoll C, Alembik Y, Dott B, Roth MP. Associated malformations in patients with anorectal anomalies. *Eur J Med Genet.* 2007;50(4):281–90.

55. Mandeville K, Chien M, Willyerd FA, et al. Intussusception: clinical presentations and imaging characteristics. *Pediatr Emerg Care.* 2012;28(9):842–4.

56. Kuppermann N, O'Dea T, Pinckney L, Hoecker C. Predictors of intussusception in young children. *Arch Pediatr Adolesc Med Am Med Assoc.* 2000;154(3):250–5.

57. Daneman A, Navarro O. Intussusception. *Pediatr Radiol.* 2004;34(2):97–108.

58. Whitehouse JS, Gourlay DM, Winthrop AL Is it safe to discharge intussusception patients after successful hydrostatic reduction? *J Pediatr Surg.* 2010;45(6):1182–6.

Chapter

# 25

# Anesthesia for Urologic Surgery

Deepa Kattail, Jessica A. George, and Myron Yaster

## Introduction

In most instances, the perioperative anesthetic management plan for pediatric genitourinary patients depends more on the patient's age, on the site and emergent nature of surgery, and on the need for perioperative analgesia and sedation than it does on the underlying disease or the specifics of the surgical procedure. In fact, regardless of the underlying condition, almost all genitourinary surgical procedures have recurring anesthetic concerns, including presence or absence of associated anomalies, airway management, blood loss and fluid replacement, positioning, conservation of body temperature, and postoperative pain and sedation management. Indeed, in our experience, it is pain and sedation management that most determines the perioperative anesthetic plan. In our practice, we use a multimodal approach to pain management [1,2]. In this analgesic method, opioid-induced adverse side-effects are minimized by maximizing pain control with smaller doses of opioids supplemented with neural blockade and nonopioid analgesics, such as nonsteroidal anti-inflammatory drugs, N-methyl-D-aspartate antagonists, and α2-adrenergic agonists. Neural blockade, be it topical, central, or peripheral, is ubiquitous. How to administer local anesthetics and other adjuvant analgesics in neural blockade is discussed in Chapter 36. How to safely administer analgesics and sedatives in the perioperative period is discussed in Chapter 13. The purpose of this chapter is to provide an overview of common genitourinary diseases and the surgical and perioperative anesthetic management plans that guide therapy.

## Posterior Urethral Valves

The incidence of posterior urethral valves (PUVs) is approximately 1 in 5000 to 8000 male births [3], making it among the most common congenital anomalies of the genitourinary system. Indeed, the true incidence may be even higher, as fetal demise can occur secondary to pulmonary hypoplasia and renal failure [4]. Not only are PUVs the most common cause of end-stage renal disease, they are also the underlying pathology for 35 percent of children who eventually need renal transplantation [3].

Most cases of PUV are diagnosed prenatally with ultrasound, which exposes bilateral hydronephrosis, distended bladder, and a dilated prostatic urethra ("keyhole sign") (Figure 25.1). Oligohydramnios is highly suggestive of significant obstruction, with associated pulmonary hypoplasia. In neonates who have not been diagnosed prenatally, presentation will include delayed voiding or poor urinary stream, abdominal mass, failure to thrive, poor feeding, lethargy, urosepsis, and, in the most severe forms, pulmonary hypoplasia causing respiratory distress. Less frequently, children may present at five years of age or older with recurrent urinary tract infection (UTI), diurnal enuresis, voiding pain or dysfunction, and decreased urinary stream [5].

Definitive diagnosis of PUV is made by voiding cystourethrography (VCUG). VCUG involves catheterization of the bladder followed by instillation of contrast material and visualization of voiding under fluoroscopy. The valves will be seen as a defined lucency in the distal prostatic urethra, and the posterior urethra will be dilated and elongated (Figure 25.2). Voiding cystourethrography is usually well tolerated without sedation or anesthesia. Posterior urethral valves may also be associated with vesicoureteral reflux (VUR). Twenty-five percent of cases are associated with unilateral VUR and 25 percent with bilateral VUR.

Management of PUV may begin prenatally, although morbidity from the procedure makes such intervention rare. Prenatal interventions include vesicoamniotic shunt, vesicostomy, and fetal endoscopic

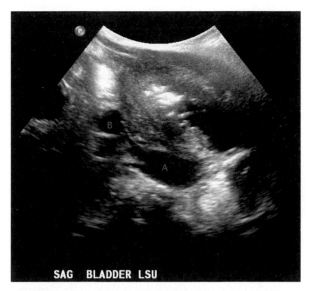

**Figure 25.1** Ultrasound of kidneys and bladder demonstrating "keyhole sign." Often seen in prenatal ultrasound and is diagnostic for posterior urethral valves. The thickened distended bladder (A) with an elongated, dilated posterior urethra (B) resembles a keyhole.

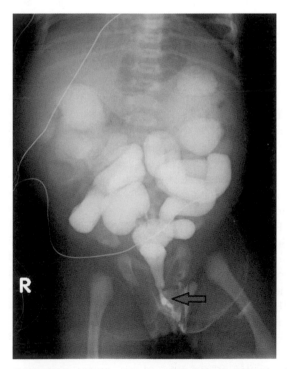

**Figure 25.2** Voiding cystourethrography (VCUG) of a child with congenital posterior urethral valves. The posterior urethral valve is indicated by the arrow. The image is significant for markedly dilated and tortuous bilateral ureters and markedly dilated intrarenal collecting systems secondary to posterior urethral valves.

valve ablation. One indication to intervene prenatally is oligohydramnios associated with a decrease in renal function (based on laboratory studies). Initially, serial bladder taps are performed. An improvement in renal function studies indicates salvageability of kidneys [5]. All fetal interventions are associated with risk of preterm labor and fetal loss and are performed only if the likelihood of benefit to the child is high.

Neonatal management of PUV is primarily medical, with the initial goal of relieving the bladder obstruction via catheterization (either urethral or suprapubic) and correcting dehydration, electrolyte imbalances, and infection. In severe cases, the neonate may have pulmonary hypoplasia that requires mechanical ventilation. Once the neonate has been stabilized and bladder decompression shows improvement in renal function, surgical intervention can be considered. A temporary vesicostomy will be performed if the neonate is premature, has insufficient urethral diameter to allow for surgical instrumentation, and/or has persistently high serum creatinine levels.

Primary surgical management of PUV involves ablation of the obstructive valves. Endoscopic transurethral ablation is the treatment of choice and requires general anesthesia. Most neonates with PUV will require inpatient hospitalization for medical stabilization before surgical intervention. Therefore, anesthesiologists can expect patients to enter the operating room with a previously established intravenous line. If they do not have an intravenous line, mask induction may be performed safely if no other contraindications exist. Choice of airway device is left to the discretion of the anesthesiologist; in our practice, endotracheal intubation is generally preferred in all neonates. Endotracheal intubation may be further indicated for this procedure because it involves placing the child in the lithotomy position at the end of the operating table. Other surgical techniques include hook method, laser ablation, and Mohan's valvotome.

After valve ablation, the child will be monitored by VCUG and may return to the operating room for cystoscopy if ablation of valves was incomplete. Bladder management later in life may include bladder augmentation and is guided by close monitoring of renal function and urodynamics. Unfortunately, one-third of children will develop end-stage renal disease despite therapy, and may eventually require renal transplantation [5].

# Hydronephrosis

Hydronephrosis is the distention and dilation of the renal pelvis and calyces. It is usually caused by an obstruction between the kidney and bladder. A urinary obstruction signifies "any restriction to urinary outflow that, if left untreated, will cause progressive renal deterioration" [6]. The causes of obstructive uropathy include congenital urogenital obstructive lesions, functional obstructive disease states, and acquired lesions that result in damage to the nephrons. The most common etiologies of prenatal hydronephrosis are transient/physiologic (50–70 percent), ureteropelvic junction obstruction (10–30 percent), vesicoureteral reflux (10–40 percent), and ureterovesical junction obstruction (5–15 percent). Transient, physiologic hydronephrosis is self-limited without significant clinical manifestations [7].

Upper urinary tract obstruction is more common in males than in females. A proximal obstruction at the ureteropelvic junction is the leading cause of hydronephrosis. A distal obstruction at the ureterovesical junction causes megaureter. The diagnosis of upper urinary tract dilation caused by obstruction is based on the results of prenatal and postnatal ultrasounds, VCUG, or diuretic renography [6,8]. Depending on the cause and severity of the obstruction, it is managed either medically or surgically.

Hydronephrosis is diagnosed prenatally in 1–3 percent of all pregnancies, making it one of the most commonly detected birth defects [9]. Ultrasonography is the diagnostic modality of choice. Prenatal ultrasonography is now performed in over 90 percent of pregnancies, compared to only 33 percent in 1980 [7]. Higher vigilance has resulted in increased detection of prenatal anomalies of the renal system. However, many cases will not benefit from further investigation or intervention and will resolve spontaneously. Although diagnosis by ultrasonography is quite reliable, no method can determine whether a case of hydronephrosis will self-resolve.

Prenatal intervention is used only in rare cases when it will result in preservation of renal and pulmonary function. The goal for fetal intervention is to relieve urinary tract obstruction, thus allowing the kidneys to develop normally. Preservation of normal renal development will then facilitate normal lung development by enabling restoration of amniotic fluid levels. Fetal intervention includes open fetal surgery, vesicocentesis/renal pelvis aspiration, and vesicoamniotic shunt. Fetal intervention of any type is associated with significant morbidity and mortality to both mother and fetus; therefore, it is infrequently performed [7].

Indication, timing, and method of surgical intervention for hydronephrosis remain controversial issues without a clear consensus. For symptomatic ureteropelvic junction obstruction, such as that accompanied by recurrent UTIs, a pyeloplasty is recommended. Surgical intervention is also indicated for a decline in split renal function of more than 10 percent, increased anteroposterior diameter on ultrasound, and grade III or IV dilation, as defined by the Society for Fetal Urology [10]. Because of the high rate of recurrence, surgical treatment of megaureters is indicated only in cases of recurrent UTIs, declining split renal function, and significant obstruction [11].

Pyeloplasty may be performed open, by laparoscopy, or by robot-assisted laparoscopy. Historically, neonates and infants with ureteropelvic obstruction were not candidates for an endourological repair because of their physical size, radiation exposure, and the need for multiple procedures under general anesthesia [8,12]; however, the times are gradually changing. Laparoscopic pyeloplasty is "minimally invasive, safe, and effective for treating ureteropelvic junction obstruction in children" [13]. Now, in some institutions, it is being utilized for infants as well [14]. Laparoscopic procedures offer the advantage of improved cosmesis, shorter hospitalization, and decreased incidence of postoperative ileus and pain, without any increase in postoperative complication rate [13]. During laparoscopic surgery, it is important for the anesthesiologist to be aware of potential physiologic changes caused by positioning and insufflation (see Table 25.1).

Pyeloplasty, regardless of surgical approach, requires general anesthesia with endotracheal intubation in order to control ventilation and provide muscle paralysis as needed. Nitrous oxide should be avoided to prevent intestinal expansion. Positioning of the patient should be discussed with the surgeon before the procedure, because pyeloplasty may be approached anteriorly, posteriorly, or from the lateral flanks. Positioning is even more challenging for the anesthesiologist if a robotic approach is used, especially in smaller pediatric patients. Postoperative analgesia can be achieved with intravenous opioids or neuraxial anesthesia, specifically either a caudal or epidural blockade, depending on the patient's age and

**Table 25.1** Physiologic changes associated with laparoscopy in the pediatric population [15,16]

| System | Physiologic change |
|---|---|
| Cardiovascular | Bradycardia/asystole (secondary to the increased vagal tone in children) |
| | Dysrhythmias |
| | Decreased venous return |
| | Hypercapnia ($CO_2$ insufflation) |
| | Hypovolemia |
| | Venous air embolism |
| Respiratory | Increased airway pressures |
| | Atelectasis |
| | Cephalad shifting of the diaphragm |
| | Relative reduction in functional residual capacity |
| | Intrapulmonary shunting |
| | Hypoxemia |
| | Pneumothorax or pneumomediastinum |
| Neurologic | Increased intracranial pressure (secondary to hypercapnia and trendelenburg positioning) |
| Endocrine | Increased stress hormone levels |

**Table 25.2** Classification of genitourinary tumors

| |
|---|
| Renal tumors |
|   Wilms tumor |
|   Clear cell sarcoma |
|   Malignant rhabdoid tumor |
|   Renal cell carcinoma |
| Testicular tumors |
|   Malignant |
|     Mixed germ cell tumors |
|     Seminomas |
|     Yolk sac tumor |
|   Benign |
|     Teratoma |
|     Epidermoid cyst |
|     Juvenile cell of granulosa |
| Adrenal tumors |
|   Neuroblastoma |
|   Adrenocortical carcinoma |
|   Pheochromocytoma |

lumbosacral anatomy. Please refer to the chapter on regional anesthesia for specifics regarding neuraxial techniques.

# Genitourinary Tumors

## Renal Tumors

Tumors of the genitourinary system differ vastly in the adult and pediatric populations in respect to natural history, incidence, and treatment (Table 25.2). Fortunately, tumors of renal, testicular, and adrenal origin are less prevalent in children than in adults. Regardless of the specific cancer, all require general anesthesia for surgical removal. Virtually any anesthetic technique can be used, but almost all are performed with general endotracheal anesthesia. Because postoperative pain is universal, all patients are treated with a multimodal analgesic approach. In our practice, most patients receive a continuous caudal or lumbar epidural catheter that is used both intra- and postoperatively.

### Wilms Tumor

Wilms tumor, or nephroblastoma, is a common, but highly treatable, malignant cancer of childhood. Of all pediatric malignancies, it is the fifth most common and represents approximately 6 percent of all pediatric cancers [17]. It is the most common pediatric tumor of the genitourinary system, with peak incidence at 2–3 years of age.

Wilms tumors occur most often in otherwise healthy children; however, approximately 8 percent of such tumors are associated with specific syndromes such as WAGR syndrome (Wilms tumor, Aniridia, Genitourinary anomaly, Retardation), Beckwith–Wiedemann, and Denys–Drash. Tumor risk varies among the different syndromes, with the most significant tumor risk being 90 percent in Denys–Drash. These syndromes are associated with gene mutations, and additional investigation of the chromosomal abnormality offers information such as risk and prognosis for the tumor. Genetic studies are used to tailor specific therapy because treatment may range from a minimal regimen to more intensive treatment for high-risk tumors [12].

In 90 percent of cases, the patient will be asymptomatic with a palpable abdominal mass, usually detected by the caregivers. Other symptoms may include hematuria, fever, and malaise. A ruptured tumor may cause pain and hypotension and clinically may resemble an acute abdomen. Additional signs and symptoms, such as respiratory, cardiac, or hepatic symptoms, occur secondary to metastasis of the tumor.

Initial mainstay treatment is radical nephrectomy to ensure removal of the primary tumor and to stratify staging based on anatomy of the tumor. Radical nephrectomy is usually performed via laparotomy, although recent studies have described a laparoscopic approach. Anesthetic management includes general anesthesia with endotracheal intubation, often with muscle paralytic for relaxation of abdominal musculature. For perioperative pain management, neuraxial techniques should be considered; a lumbar epidural should provide excellent analgesia.

Additional treatment is tailored to the patient's prognostic factors to limit therapy for low-risk tumors and maximize treatment for children who are at risk for relapse or failure [12]. Prognostic factors include staging based on anatomical extent of the tumor, histology, patient age, and genetic factors. Surgical resection may be supplemented with adjuvant therapy, including chemotherapy and radiation. Survival rates for Wilms tumor are more than 90 percent [17].

## Clear Cell Sarcoma

Clear cell sarcoma is the second most common malignant renal tumor after Wilms tumor. It presents most commonly between the ages of 1 and 4 years and more often in boys. It is not associated with any syndrome and is usually unilateral in presentation. Clinical presentation includes a palpable abdominal mass, with pain secondary to bony metastases. The tumor is difficult to differentiate based on imaging, and the presence of bony metastases is the only factor that differentiates it from Wilms tumor [18]. Treatment includes radical nephrectomy followed by chemotherapy. Survival rates after treatment are greater than 75 percent [19].

## Rhabdoid Tumor

Though rhabdoid tumors are extremely rare, 80 percent occur in children less than two years of age, and incidence is higher in boys than in girls. One-third of patients have an underlying genetic mutation that may also cause associated brain lesions. Patients commonly present with hematuria as well as signs and symptoms of metastatic spread. Radical nephrectomy is indicated for curative treatment, although it is pre-empted by diagnostic biopsy [18]. It is an aggressive tumor with poor response to chemotherapy and radiation. The survival rate is less than 50 percent, even for those with localized disease [12].

## Renal Cell Carcinoma

Renal cell carcinoma (RCC) is uncommon in the pediatric population, with only 0.5–2 percent incidence in patients under the age of 21 years. The mean age at diagnosis is 8–11 years [19]. RCC in the adult population has been linked to environmental factors, but no contributing factors have been identified for the pediatric population. Pediatric RCC also differs from adult RCC in histology, as most tumors occur in papillary form. RCC has been linked as a second malignancy in children with other primary malignancies, specifically neuroblastoma. The secondary malignancy has been shown to occur at an average of 14.7 years after primary malignancy diagnosis [20].

Clinical presentation includes painless hematuria, palpable mass, and flank pain. More than two-thirds of patients have localized disease at presentation and are treated by radical nephrectomy, which can be performed open or laparoscopically. Survival rates are relatively good with surgical resection alone. Adjuvant therapy is added only if metastases are present. Metastatic disease is generally nonresponsive to chemotherapy and radiation, thus making it difficult to treat.

# Testicular Tumors

The characteristics of testicular tumors in the pediatric population are also distinct from those in adults. Pediatric testicular tumors are mostly benign in nature, whereas adult tumors tend to be malignant. Testicular tumors account for 2 percent of all pediatric tumors, with two-thirds being benign [19].

Patients will present with palpable, painless testicular mass and noticeable increase in scrotal size. Often, these findings may be attributed to hydrocele or hernia and acute processes. In particular, testicular torsion must be excluded. Diagnosis can be made by Doppler ultrasonography, and metastases should be ruled out with computed tomography (CT) imaging. Elevated alpha-fetoprotein (AFP) is an indicator of malignancy and is taken into account when devising the treatment plan.

The mainstay of treatment is radical orchiectomy, which is especially recommended if AFP is elevated. Orchiectomy is performed through an inguinal incision. General anesthesia is necessary and may be supplemented with an ilioinguinal nerve block, which is highly efficacious if guided by ultrasonography. Treatment of malignant tumors is highly efficacious.

Recurrent cases usually respond well to chemotherapy. Testicular masses with normal AFP are presumed to be benign tumors, such as a teratoma. Benign tumors are managed based on histology but in general are treated surgically with either partial or simple orchiectomy.

## Adrenal Tumors

Tumors originating from the adrenal gland can be benign or malignant, primary or metastatic. Tumors most commonly seen in children are neuroblastomas and cortical adenomas. Clinical diagnosis is usually based on hormonal abnormalities and confirmed by ultrasound imaging. Additional imaging, including CT and/or magnetic resonance imaging (MRI), is used to investigate whether the tumor has spread.

Neuroblastoma is a malignant tumor and is the most common extracranial solid tumor in children. Eighty percent of these tumors occur in children under the age of five. Diagnosis may be made prenatally or upon investigation of a palpable abdominal mass in the first year of life. Symptoms are related to mass effect, such as pain and abdominal distention, as well as abnormal catecholamine production. Patients appear very ill and with an almost malignant malaise. In infants and young children, neuroblastomas may spontaneously regress. Tumors in older children are resected by adrenalectomy, which is performed either in open fashion or laparoscopically. Prognosis is very poor in children older than 18 months who have metastatic progression.

Pheochromocytoma is very rare in children and occurs at a mean age of 11 years. It may be associated with syndromes such as multiple endocrine neoplasia type 2 [19]. Anesthetic management during surgical removal of pheochromocytoma can be complex because excess catecholamines may cause manifestations such as tachycardia and hypertension. Surgical resection may cause acute crisis from additional release of catecholamines. Patients should have heart rate and blood pressure optimized first with alpha blockers and then only with beta blockers. Anesthesiologists should use the drugs in that sequence to prevent hypertension from unopposed alpha-adrenergic action, which can occur if beta blockers are given first.

Because patients undergoing pheochromocytoma resection may have hemodynamic instability, large-bore intravenous access is essential, preferably central access and an arterial line. Hypertension may require titration of vasodilators and very close blood pressure monitoring. After resection, hypotension may occur with sudden loss of catecholamines. Such patients will require significant fluid resuscitation and therefore adequate intravenous access.

## Bladder and Cloaca Exstrophy

Bladder exstrophy is a congenital malformation that occurs in approximately one per 50 000 live births; the incidence is higher in boys than in girls. It is an anatomical defect of the abdomen that causes separation of the pubic symphysis and an open bladder and urethra. It is a disease complex that ranges from cloacal exstrophy, in its most severe form, to a milder presentation with a normal bladder position and isolated epispadias. Most patients with classical bladder exstrophy present with an open bladder. Cloacal (Latin for cesspool or sewer) exstrophy is associated with other malformations of the abdomen, skeleton, and nervous system. It is distinguished by an imperforate anus that results in common drainage of both stool and urine. Diagnosis can occur prenatally, as early as 15 weeks' gestation, allowing for parental counseling and planning for early, postnatal surgical intervention. Despite widespread prenatal ultrasonography, only 25 percent of malformations are detected before birth [21].

Surgical repair is complex and multistaged for children with this deformity. Ideally, primary closure of the abdominal wall and bladder is performed in the newborn. The procedure requires primary urological repair as well as involvement of orthopedic surgeons to perform iliac and pelvic osteotomies. Repair and healing require lengthy inpatient hospitalization with management by a multidisciplinary team composed of urologists, anesthesiologists, pain physicians, pediatricians, nutritionists, and nurses.

Intraoperatively, patients require general anesthesia with endotracheal intubation. The anesthesiologist should secure adequate intravenous access and bear in mind that patients, especially neonates, may lose substantial amounts of blood when the osteotomies are performed. Unless otherwise indicated, an arterial line is not required. Epidural anesthesia is extremely beneficial for intraoperative and postoperative management. Owing to the high risk of bladder extrusion, immobilization and sedation is of great importance for several weeks after surgery. Epidural catheters are tunneled subcutaneously to decrease catheter colonization, and infusions containing local anesthetic and opioid are delivered continuously [22].

Sedation regimens often include long-acting opioids, benzodiazepines, and alpha agonists such as dexmedotomadine and clonidine. These cases are very challenging for members of a pediatric pain service because they must achieve immobilization and sedation while maintaining spontaneous ventilation, often in toddlers who are uncooperative and active [22]. Long-term use of opioids and benzodiazepines will likely lead to tolerance. Therefore patients will require formal weaning from medications [23–25].

## Disorders of Sexual Development

Disorders of sexual development (DSDs) were previously known as "intersex disorders." The "term disorders of sexual development is proposed to indicate congenital conditions with atypical development of chromosomal, gonadal, or anatomical sex" [6]. Disorders of sexual development occur when there is a defect in one of the four stages of sexual differentiation. The four stages described by Jost [26] include chromosomal sex determination at fertilization, undifferentiated gonad formation, gonadal differentiation into either testes or ovaries, and lastly the development of internal and external genitalia.

When an infant presents with ambiguous genitalia, it is considered a medical emergency. A thorough history is taken and physical examination performed. The medical history will include questions regarding prior DSD, parental consanguinity, neonatal deaths, familial infertility, and maternal exposure to androgens [6]. On physical examination, the physician may notice a micropenis, hypospadias, or pigmentation of the genital or areolar region. Physicians should also be suspicious in cases of phenotypic females with palpable gonads or clitoral enlargement. Conversely, physicians should investigate phenotypic males without palpable gonads or those with a diagnosis of hypospadias [27]. Regardless of the actual chromosomal abnormality, a multidisciplinary team of neonatologists, geneticists, endocrinologists, pediatric urologists, gynecologists, psychologists, ethicists, and social workers should manage all pediatric patients with ambiguous genitalia [28].

The initial laboratory workup includes a karyotype, steroid precursors, serum electrolytes, gonadotropins, anti-Müllerian hormone, androgen-binding studies, and plasma 17-hydroxyprogesterone assay.

Ultrasound and MRI provide additional specific anatomical information. Patients with congenital adrenal hyperplasia, caused by 21-hydroxylase or 11β-hydroxylase deficiency, have a karyotype of 46, XX, and are SRY-negative with increased 17-hydroxyprogesterone levels. Congenital adrenal hyperplasia is the most commonly occurring DSD.

Once the laboratory workup is complete, the multidisciplinary team will begin the complex task of assigning a gender. Standardized protocols have supported corrective surgery during infancy, thereby allowing the patient to be raised as either a girl or a boy [29]. However, other parents, patient advocates, and ethicists consider cosmetic surgery mutilating and debate whether children should be old enough to give informed consent, which would enable them the opportunity to verbalize whether they identify with being a male or a female [30]. Gender assignment is usually based on age, fertility, penile size, presence of a vagina, endocrine function, general appearance, psychosocial well-being, sociocultural influences, and parental preference [6].

In reality, the question of when a child with ambiguous genitalia should undergo corrective surgery is controversial. Therefore, each family should decide what is best for them on an individual basis with the medical information provided. Children with ambiguous genitalia may come for multiple anesthetic procedures, such as for cystoscopy to evaluate the vagina, laparoscopy to determine gonadal presence or absence, and potentially a reconstructive repair, such as feminizing surgery, vaginoplasty, gonadectomy, or masculinizing surgery. All of the procedures are performed under general anesthesia. For the reconstructive procedures, patients are encouraged to have a neuraxial block for postoperative pain management (see Chapter 36 for specific information regarding neuraxial blocks).

In cases of ambiguous genitalia, it is important to consider the long-term physical and psychological effects. Postoperatively, patients may struggle with gender identity and later with sexual function. It is imperative that the anesthesiologist be an integral part of the child's multidisciplinary team preoperatively, intraoperatively, and postoperatively.

## Circumcision Phimosis

Circumcision is one of the most common pediatric surgical procedures performed. Circumcision can be performed for religious, cosmetic, or medical reasons (i.e., recurrent UTIs) or to reduce the risk of contracting human immunodeficiency virus through penile–vaginal intercourse. Regardless of when or why circumcision is performed, regional anesthesia, primarily in combination with general anesthesia, is required. One specific reason to perform a circumcision is phimosis.

Phimosis is a narrowing of the foreskin that prevents complete retraction of the foreskin over the glans. At birth, phimosis is normal because of adhesions between the prepuce and the glans [31]. By three years of age, 89 percent of children can retract the foreskin over the glans; however, phimosis persists in 8 percent of six-year-olds and 1 percent of teenagers 16–18 years of age [6]. Phimosis may be physiologic or pathologic owing to scarring of the foreskin [32] (Figure 25.3).

Hayashi et al. [31] described four alternatives to circumcision for the treatment of phimosis. These four treatments include manual retraction therapy, topical steroid therapy, dorsal slit, or preputioplasty. Manual retraction therapy is performed under general anesthesia. Postoperatively, parents continue to retract the child's foreskin daily. After manual retraction therapy, 82 percent of children have resolution of symptoms and 62 percent report the ability to fully retract the foreskin. The topical application of potent steroid creams, such as betamethazone, clobetasol propionate, monometasonefuroate, or triamucinolone acetonide, have been reported to have a success rate of 67–95 percent [33–35].

The dorsal slit and preputioplasty can be performed for either paraphimosis or severe balanitis. The dorsal slit procedure is typically performed with a longitudinal incision in the dorsal preputial skin. The preputioplasty attempts to preserve the foreskin. Preputioplasty can either be a modified dorsal slit procedure, with or without a ventral slit, or a longitudinal incision proximal to the preputial meatus [36].

Circumcision is indicated in children with recurrent balanoposthitis, recurrent UTI and abnormal urinary tract, vesicoureteral reflux, secondary phimosis, and paraphimosis [6]. Circumcision is also recommended for children with congenital spinal anomalies who require intermittent catheterization [37]. Contraindications to circumcision include parental refusal, micropenis, ambiguous genitalia, coagulopathy, local or systemic infection, and penile congenital abnormalities, such as hypospadias [37].

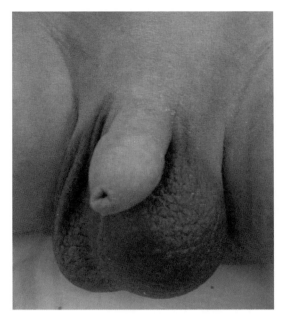

**Figure 25.3** Phimosis is a narrowing of the foreskin that prevents complete retraction of the foreskin over the glans.

Circumcisions, even in the newborn period, are painful. Fetuses begin to perceive pain mid to late gestation [38] therefore, pain management for circumcisions is essential. Local anesthetics are only partially effective at relieving pain associated with the procedure. Combination interventions have been proven to be more effective than a single intervention. The American Academy of Pediatrics recommends the administration of local anesthesia via a local block with 2.5 percent lidocaine after using 2.5 percent prilocaine to numb the skin at the injection site [39]. In 2000, a study performed by Taddio et al. [40] compared two groups undergoing circumcision. One group of infants was anesthetized with a eutectic mixture of local anesthetic (EMLA) and the other with EMLA cream, a lidocaine dorsal penile nerve block, acetaminophen, and sugar-coated gauze. Infants given the combined analgesic regimen cried less during the procedure and for a shorter period of time, reinforcing the importance of a multimodal approach.

When possible, circumcision should be delayed until the child is over one year of age, and then performed under general anesthesia. Once the child is anesthetized, there are four potential options for intraoperative and postoperative pain management: penile block, caudal block, acetaminophen, and intravenous opioids. In 2013, Haliloglu et al. [41] compared the postoperative analgesic efficacy of a penile block, caudal block, and paracetamol in 159 randomized children with a mean age of 5.7 years. Postoperatively, the children in the penile and caudal block groups had similar and significantly lower pain scores, measured by Children's Hospital of Eastern Ontario Pain Scale, than the children who received only intravenous paracetamol.

Opioids are another analgesic option; however, to minimize the side-effects, including pruritis, nausea, vomiting, and somnolence, anesthesia providers should administer opioids in combination with a regional technique. In 2012, Kaya et al. [42] conducted a study to compare caudally administered levobupivacaine 0.25 percent to bupivacaine 0.25 percent in children undergoing circumcisions. This study revealed that bupivacaine provided a longer duration of action than levobupivacaine; however, neither group required additional analgesia until discharge.

Children undergoing a circumcision for phimosis should receive adequate pain management postoperatively. The past medical history of the child will help dictate the appropriate pain management options, and the plan should be discussed with the parents preoperatively. If there is no contraindication to regional anesthesia, then general anesthesia with a regional technique is the recommended approach.

## Hypospadias

Hypospadias is defined as "hypoplasia of the tissues forming the ventral aspect of the penis beyond the division of the corpus spongiosum" [6]. It affects 4–6 per 1000 male births. Hypospadias is a congenital malformation that is classified by the anatomical location of the urethral orifice: mild (urethral meatus distal to the coronal sulcus), moderate (urethral meatus on the penile shaft), or severe (urethral meatus in the penoscrotal area) [43]. In addition to the ectopic opening of the urethral meatus, hypospadias is associated with a ventral curvature of the penis and a hooded foreskin [12]. Hypospadias is diagnosed at birth by physical examination. The urologist examines the appearance, size, and curvature of the penis and scrotum and describes the orifice location, urethra quality, and corpus spongiosum division. If a child presents with severe hypospadias and impalpable testis or ambiguous genitalia, a genetic and endocrine workup should be requested to exclude another disorder of sexual development (Figure 25.4) [44].

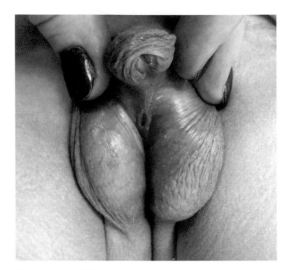

**Figure 25.4** Child presenting with severe hypospadias with the urethral meatus in the penoscrotal area.

Genetic, developmental, and environmental factors have been implicated in the development of hypospadias [45]. Genetic polymorphisms affect single or multiple genes, resulting in syndromic presentations. Isolated single-gene mutations include *SRY*, *DAX1*, *WNT4*, *DMRT1*, *DMRT2*, and chromosome deletions [12]. Syndromic gene mutations include *SF1*, *WT1*, Denys–Drash syndrome, WAGE syndrome, Frasier syndrome, *SOX9*, and *HOXA13* [12]. Hormone defects that affect testosterone synthesis may also play a role in the development of hypospadias, specifically defects in 3β-hydroxysteroid, 17α-hydroxylase, 17,20-lyase, and 5α-reductase deficiency [12,45–47]. Environmental factors include low birth weight, maternal hypertension, and preeclampsia, which could impact placental blood flow.

In 1996, a report from the American Academy of Pediatrics suggested that surgery to correct hypospadias be completed between 6 and 12 months of age [48]. A tubularized incised plate technique has become the most popular procedure for anterior hypospadias repair [46]. Bracka repair is the gold standard for salvage hypospadias repair, but over 200 different subvariants of hypospadias repair technique exist [49]. Even with advances in tissue transfer and surgically refined repair techniques, no definitive consensus has been reached regarding the best surgical repair [49]. All of the different repair techniques have similar outcomes. Risks after the repair include sexual dysfunction and psychosocial difficulties.

For pediatric patients undergoing a hypospadias repair, general anesthesia with a regional technique for postoperative pain management is recommended. Caudal blockade is the most popular regional technique for children undergoing lower abdominal, perineal, or lower extremity procedures; however, a pudendal nerve block is another potential option for postoperative analgesia [50]. To prolong the effect of caudal blockade, anesthesia providers may co-administer epinephrine, morphine, clonidine, ketamine, midazolam, tramadol, and neostigmine with the local anesthetic.

In 2005, Gunduz et al. [51] studied 62 children undergoing hypospadias surgery and discovered superior analgesia with a caudally administered mixture of ketamine and lidocaine. Abdulatif and El-Sanabary [52] conducted a study combining neostigmine with bupivacaine and found a substantially longer period of postoperative analgesia. In fact, the recovery to first rescue analgesic in this group was 22.8 hours compared to 8.1 hours with bupivacaine alone. Turan et al. [53] also recommended co-administration of caudal local anesthetic with neostigmine to prolong analgesia in children undergoing genitourinary surgery. The time to first rescue analgesic in their study was 19.2 hours when neostigmine was co-administered with ropivacaine, compared to 7.1 hours without neostigmine. Apiliogullari et al. [54] recommended spinal anesthesia with hyperbaric bupivacaine and intrathecal morphine for distal hypospadias repair. The published literature on potential neuraxial medication combinations is vast, and each anesthesiologist will have to weigh the risks and benefits of each regimen to determine the most appropriate combination for his/her practice.

# Regional Anesthesia in Urological Procedures

Regional anesthesia as a supplement to general anesthesia is a standard of care for several urological procedures. Regional anesthesia encompasses neuraxial techniques as well as nerve blocks such as penile blocks, transversus abdominis planus (TAP) blocks, and ilioinguinal/iliohypogastric blocks. Effective nerve blockade decreases perioperative opioid usage and opioid-related side-effects, such as postoperative nausea and vomiting and respiratory depression.

Caudal anesthesia provides excellent anesthesia for short outpatient procedures such as hypospadias repair or circumcision. It is a low-risk, cost-effective procedure that may be performed very quickly by an experienced anesthesiologist. Although temporary lower extremity weakness may not be well tolerated in older children, caudal anesthesia is very effective in infants.

More complex procedures such as bladder exstrophy or epispadias repair are almost absolute indications for the placement of epidural catheters. Along with providing excellent analgesia, the added benefit of immobilization prevents disruption to the surgical repair. Sedation is also effectively provided when adjuvant medications, such as opioids or alpha agonists, are added to the epidural solution.

With the popularity of ultrasonography use, other nerve blocks have become more common. TAP blocks provide excellent anesthesia for a variety of procedures. When the ilioinguinal nerve is identified and anesthetized in the transversus abdominis plane, complete anesthesia of the inguinal region may be achieved. This block is efficacious for hernia repairs and orchiopexies.

Regional techniques should be incorporated whenever possible to decrease opioid usage, particularly in the vulnerable pediatric population. Please refer to Chapter 36 for further details.

# References

1. Yaster M. Multimodal analgesia in children. *Eur J Anaesthesiol*. 2010;27(10):851–7.

2. Monitto CL, Kost-Byerly S, Yaster M Pain management. In Davis PJ, Cladis FP, Motoyama EK, editors. *Smith's Anesthesia for Infants and Children*, 8th edn. Philadelphia, PA: Elsevier; 2006.

3. Elder JS, Shapiro E. Posterior urethral valves. In Holcomb GW, Murphy JP, Ostlie DJ, editors. *Ashcraft's Pediatric Surgery*, 6th edn. Philadelphia, PA: Elsevier; 2014; 762–72.

4. Krishnan A, de Souza A, Konijeti R, Baskin L. The anatomy and embryology of posterior urethral valves. *J Urol*. 2006;175(4):1214–20.

5. Nasir AA, Ameh EA, Abdur-Rahman LO, Adeniran JO, Abraham MK. Posterior urethral valve. *World J Pediatr*. 2011;7(3):205–16.

6. Tekgul S, Riedmiller H, Dogan HS, et al. *Guidelines on Paediatric Urology*. n.p.: European Society for Paediatric Urology; 2013.

7. Yamaçake KGR, Nguyen HT. Current management of antenatal hydronephrosis. *Pediatr Nephrol*. 2013;28(2):237–43.

8. Figenshau RS, Clayman RV. Endourologic options for management of ureteropelvic junction obstruction in the pediatric patient. *Urol Clin North Am.* 1998;25:199–209.

9. Lee RS, Borer JG. *Perinatal urology.* In Wein AJ, Kavoussi LR, Novick AC, Partin AW, Peters CA, editors. *Campbell-Walsh Urology,* 10th edn. Philadelphia, PA: Elsevier Saunders; 2014.

10. Brandström P, Nevéus T, Sixt R, et al. The Swedish reflux trial in children: IV. Renal damage. *J Urol.* 2010;184(1):292–7.

11. Esbjörner E, Hansson S, Jakobsson B. Management of children with dilating vesico-ureteric reflux in Sweden. *Acta Paediatr.* 2004;93:37–42.

12. Gundeti M. Wilms tumor. In Gearhart JP, Rink RC, Mouriquand PDE, editors. *Pediatric Urology.* 2nd edn. Philadelphia, PA: Elsevier; 2014.

13. Mei H, Pu J, Yang C, et al. Laparoscopic versus open pyeloplasty for ureteropelvic junction obstruction in children: a systematic review and meta-analysis. *J Endourol.* 2011;25:727–36.

14. Turner RM, Fox JA, Tomaszewski JJ, et al. Laparoscopic pyeloplasty for ureteropelvic junction obstruction in infants. *J Urol.* 2013;189:1503–6.

15. Cunningham AJ. Anesthetic implications of laparoscopic surgery. *Yale J Biol Med.* 1998;71:551–78.

16. Goel S. Anesthesia for pediatric laparoscopy . *Pediatric OnCall.* 2005. Available at: www.pediatriconcall.com/Journal/Article/FullText.aspx?artid=748&type=J&tid=&imgid=&reportid=392&tbltype=.

17. Davidoff AM. Wilms tumor. *Adv Pediatr.* 2012;59(1):247–67.

18. Ross JH. Genitourinary tumors. In Palmer JS, editor. *Pediatric Urology.* Totowa, NJ: Humana Press; 2011.

19. Dénes FT, Duarte RJ, Cristófani LM, Lopes RI. Pediatric genitourinary oncology. *Front Pediatr.* 2013;1:48.

20. Sausville JE, Hernandez DJ, Argani P, Gearhart JP. Pediatric renal cell carcinoma. *J Pediatr Urol.* 2009;5(4):308–14.

21. Massanyi EZ, Gearhart JP, Kost-Byerly S. Perioperative management of classic bladder exstrophy. *Res Reports Urol.* 2013;5:67–75.

22. Kost-Byerly S, Jackson E. Perioperative anesthetic and analgesic management of newborn bladder exstrophy repair. *J Pediatr.* 2008;4(4):280–5.

23. Yaster M, Kost-Byerly S, Berde C, Billet C. The management of opioid and benzodiazepine dependence in infants, children, and adolescents. *Pediatrics.* 1996;98(1):135–40.

24. Tobias JD, Schleien CL, Haun SE. Methadone as treatment for iatrogenic narcotic dependency in pediatric intensive care unit patients. *Crit Care Med.* 1990;18(11):1292–3.

25. Tobias JD, Deshpande JK, Gregory DF. Outpatient therapy of iatrogenic drug dependency following prolonged sedation in the pediatric intensive care unit. *Intensive Care Med.* 1994;20(7):504–7.

26. Jost A. Becoming a male. *Adv Biosci.* 1973;10:3–13.

27. Woodhouse CJ. Ambiguous genitalia in male adolescents. In Gearhart JP, Rink RC, Mouriquand PDE, editors, *Pediatric Urology.* 2nd edn. Philadelphia, PA: Elsevier; 2014.

28. Vidal I, Gorduza DB, Haraux E, et al. Surgical options in disorders of sex development (DSD) with ambiguous genitalia. *Best Pract Res Clin Endocrinol Metab.* 2010;24(2):311–24.

29. Rangecroft L. Surgical management of ambiguous genitalia. *Arch Dis Child.* 2003;88:799–801.

30. Kipnis K, Diamond M. Pediatric ethics and the surgical assignment of sex. *J Clin Ethics.* 1998;9:398–410.

31. Hayashi Y, Kojima Y, Mizuno K, Kohri K. Prepuce: phimosis, paraphimosis, and circumcision. *Scientific World J.* 2011;11:289–301.

32. Drake T, Rustom J. Phimosis in childhood. *BMJ.* 2013;3678:1–4.

33. Monsour MA, Rabinovitch HH, Dean GE. Medical management of phimosis in children: our experience with topical steroids. *J Urol.* 1999.162:1162–4.

34. Palmer LS, Palmer JS. The efficacy of topical betamethasone for treating phimosis: a comparison of two treatment regimens. *Urology.* 2008;72:68–71.

35. Golubovic Z, Milanovic D, Vukadinovic V, Rakic I, Perovic S. The conservative treatment of phimosis in boys. *Br J Urol.* 1996;78:786–8.

36. De Castella H. Prepuceplasty: an alternative to circumcision. *Ann R Coll Surg Engl.* 1994;76:257–8.

37. Steadman B, Ellsworth P. To circ or not to circ: indications, risks, and alternatives to circumcision in the pediatric population with phimosis. *Urol Nurs Off J Am Urol Assoc Allied.* 2006;26:181–94.

38. Stevens B. *Pain: Clinical Manual,* 2nd edn. St. Louis, MO: Mosby; 1999.

39. Pasero C. Circumcision requires anesthesia and analgesia. *Am J Nurs.* 2001;101(9):22–3.

40. Taddio A, Pollock N, Gilbert-MacLeod C, Ohlsson K, Koren G. Combined analgesia and local anesthesia to minimize pain during circumcision. *Arch Pediatr Adolesc Med.* 2000;154(6):620–3.

41. Haliloglu AH, Gokce MI, Tangal S, et al. Comparison of postoperative analgesic efficacy of penile block,

caudal block and intravenous paracetamol for circumcision: a prospective randomized study. *Int Braz J Urol.* 2013;39:551–7.

42. Kaya Z, Süren M, Arici S, et al. Prospective, randomized, double-blinded comparison of the effects of caudally administered levobupivacaine 0.25% and bupivacaine 0.25% on pain and motor block in children undergoing circumcision surgery. *Eur Rev Med Pharmacol Sci.* 2012;16:2014–20.

43. Carmichael SL, Shaw GM, Lammer EJ. Environmental and genetic contributors to hypospadias: a review of the epidemiologic evidence. *Birth Defects Res A Clin Mol Teratol.* 2012;94:499–510.

44. Hayashi Y, Kojima Y. Current concepts in hypospadias surgery. *Int J Urol.* 2008;15:651–64.

45. Kalfa N, Philibert P, Baskin LS, Sultan C. Hypospadias: interactions between environment and genetics. *Molec Cell Endocrinol.* 2011;335:89–95.

46. Roberts J. Hypospadias surgery past, present and future. *Curr Opin Urol.* 2010;20:483–9.

47. Shukla AR, Patel RP, Canning DA. Hypospadias. *Urol Clin North Am.* 2004;31:445–60.

48. American Academy of Pediatrics. Timing of elective surgery on the genitalia of male children with particular reference to the risks, benefits, and psychological effects of surgery and anesthesia. *Pediatrics.* 1996;97(4):590–4.

49. Macedo A, Rondon A, Ortiz V. Hypospadias. *Curr Op Urol.* 2012;22:447–52.

50. Naja ZM, Ziade FM, Kamel R, et al. The effectiveness of pudendal nerve block versus caudal block anesthesia for hypospadias in children. *Anesth Analg.* 2013;117:1401–7.

51. Gunduz M, Ozalevli M, Ozbek H, Ozcengiz D. Comparison of caudal ketamine with lidocaine or tramadol administration for postoperative analgesia of hypospadias surgery in children. *Paediatr Anaesth.* 2006;16:158–63.

52. Abdulatif M, El-Sanabary M. Caudal neostigmine, bupivacaine, and their combination for postoperative pain management after hypospadias surgery in children. *Anesth Analg.* 2002;95:1215–18.

53. Turan A, Memiş D, Başaran UN, Karamanlioğlu B, Süt N. Caudal ropivacaine and neostigmine in pediatric surgery. *Anesthesiology.* 2003;98:719–22.

54. Apiliogullari S, Duman A, Gok F, Akillioglu I, Ciftci I. Efficacy of a low-dose spinal morphine with bupivacaine for postoperative analgesia in children undergoing hypospadias repair. *Paediatr Anaesth.* 2009;19:1078–83.

## Chapter 26

# Anesthesia for Thoracic Surgery

Cornelius A. Sullivan

The care of the neonate or infant undergoing thoracic surgery presents the anesthesiologist with a unique set of challenges. Here, the disparate goals of mitigating the physiologic stress to patients who often have limited cardiopulmonary reserve confront the need for surgical exposure and highlight the limitations of our available equipment and technique.

An understanding of the fundamental physiology of ventilation and perfusion balance, both normal and in illness, is essential if the iatrogenic disease that is single lung ventilation is to be managed with minimal morbidity. The physiologic disturbances that result from lung isolation are, or course, superimposed on the pathophysiology that necessitated the surgery. Both open and minimally invasive approaches to the thoracic cavity have their own advantages and risks, familiarity with which can allow anticipation and avoidance of many intraoperative complications related to the anesthetic. Finally, no discussion of this topic would be complete without a survey of the surgical pathology of the chest in this vulnerable age group.

## Respiratory Development and Physiology

The pulmonary system develops as a ventral outpouching of the foregut during the first postconceptual weeks. Subsequent stages of development are pseudoglandular (5–17 weeks), canalicular (16–25 weeks), saccular (24–36 weeks), and alveolar (>36 weeks) [1]. Of note, penetration of pulmonary capillary networks into terminal air sacs begins in the saccular stage, permitting some degree of gas exchange in the extremely premature neonate. Type II pneumocytes appear at about 24 weeks' gestation and produce surfactant [2]. Surfactant is a mixture of phospholipids, primarily phosphatidylcholine, and proteins called SP-a through SP-d, that reduces surface tension

of the alveolar wall. This reduced surface tension in smaller alveoli prevents complete collapse at functional residual capacity (FRC). Prenatal administration of steroids to the mother prior to delivery has been demonstrated to accelerate fetal lung maturity and reduce the incidence of respiratory distress syndrome, but a Cochrane review concluded that the optimal drug, dose, and regimen are still unclear [3]. Postnatal development largely consists of a gradual increase in the number of alveoli, from about 10–50 million to approximately 200–300 million during the first decade of life.

At birth, the dramatic changes involved in transition to extrauterine life center on the replacement of liquid-filled airways and placental gas exchange, by gas-filled airways and pulmonary capillary/alveolar gas exchange. Extrinsic chest compression during vaginal birth is thought to expel some of this fluid. Neonates born via Cesarean section, by comparison, have increased parenchymal lung water, and a higher incidence of transient tachypnea of the newborn (TTN). Recent data suggest that active transepithelial absorption via amiloride-sensitive sodium channels actually accounts for most of this difference [4]. The first breaths, with the generation of highly negative intrapleural pressure, help move intra-alveolar fluid into the lymphatic drainage of the lung. Mechanical compression and hypoxic vasoconstriction of the small intraparenchymal vessels are diminished. Pulmonary vascular resistance falls and pulmonary blood flow increases in response to the increasing alveolar and arterial $pO_2$. The resulting increase in left atrial volume and pressure functionally closes the foramen ovale, usually within days. While anatomic closure follows in some weeks, up to 30 percent of adults will still be probe-patent. The ductus arteriosus similarly constricts in response to oxygen and falling levels of prostaglandins. In the term newborn, functional closure of the patent ductus arteriosus (PDA) usually occurs by day 2 of life, and anatomic closure within 2–3 weeks. Because all of these changes are physiologic rather than anatomic for several weeks, the neonate is particularly vulnerable to their reversal by hypoxemia, hypercarbia, acidosis, and hypothermia. Progressive systemic hypoxemia with elevated pulmonary artery pressures and subsequent right ventricular failure rapidly ensue and can quickly become unrecoverable.

Respiratory effort is seen in utero during the second trimester, and plays an essential role in normal lung development [5]. Nuclei in the medulla generate rhythmic stimulation modulated by baroreceptors located at the carotid body, and chemoreceptors at the brainstem level, as well as a host of other inputs. These signals can originate from the respiratory epithelium, the muscles of respiration, the limbic system or the cerebral cortex. Efferents flow via the phrenic nerve to the diaphragm, and through spinal nerves to the intercostals and strap muscles of the neck.

The mechanics of respiration are fundamentally different in the infant and neonate, primarily because of the markedly increased compliance of the chest wall. The ribs are cartilaginous and the accessory muscles of respiration are incompletely developed, and the cross-section of the thorax tends more toward the square than the rectangle, with a proportionally smaller AP diameter. In combination, these factors mean that the FRC is disproportionately smaller in the newborn than in older children. The chest wall offers less resistance to the elastic recoil of the lung, hence small airways can close even in normal tidal breathing. The diaphragm is normally a complete membrane by eight weeks' gestation, but in the newborn has only 10–30 percent type 1, slow-twitch fibers compared to about 55 percent in the adult, rendering it more susceptible to fatigue. Type 2 fibers are now described as either fast-oxidative or fast-glycolytic based on myosin isoforms, and are recruited during tachypnea and respiratory distress. These fibers are also responsible for responsiveness to caffeine, based on the presence of RyR3, which is expressed only in diaphragmatic muscle [6]. The upper airway is also dependent on cyclic activation of the pharyngeal and supraglottic musculature to maintain patency; all of the mechanisms described are negatively impacted by most anesthetics. Oxygen consumption in the neonate (6–8 ml $kg^{-1}$ $min^{-1}$) is about twice that of the adult

(3–4 ml $kg^{-1}$ $min^{-1}$) and further reduces the respiratory reserve of these patients. The inverse fourth relationship of Poiselle's law also means that the work of breathing is increased disproportionately by the high resistance of the smaller airways throughout the tracheobronchial tree.

Since the classic work of West, ventilation and perfusion have been understood to each increase across gravitational gradients, minimizing mismatch [7]. Perfusion increases at a greater rate, hence V/Q ratio declines across the same gradient, whether it's cranial/caudad in the upright patient, or "toward the floor" in the lateral decubitus position. In a surgical setting, this implies that the dependent, presumably "good" lung is functionally more important. This is indeed true in the adult. Under spontaneous breathing, the diaphragm also functions more efficiently under Starling's law, because it is "loaded" or under stretch from the locally increased pressure of the abdominal contents. In the infant or child, in contrast, chest compressibility opposes the diaphragmatic loading, and the higher compliance of the chest wall reduces expiratory reserve and pushes FRC closer to residual volume. Even the awake patient may experience small airway closure during normal tidal breathing, promoting atelectasis of the dependent lung. General anesthesia, neuromuscular blockade and mechanical ventilation each have additive effects on decreasing FRC and impairing oxygenation.

The primary homeostatic mechanism that minimizes V/Q mismatch is hypoxic pulmonary vasoconstriction (HPV). While still poorly understood, this refers to the calcium-mediated, eNOS-modulated increase in regional pulmonary vascular resistance triggered by alveolar hypoxia, thus relatively diverting flow away from the nonventilated areas [8]. In comparison, systemic arterioles respond to hypoxia with dilatation; this is a major distinction between the two parallel circulations. Although its precise mechanism remains unclear, hypoxia triggers via several pathways a small rise in intracellular ionized calcium in pulmonary arterial smooth muscle cells. When persistent, animal models suggest that altered gene expression leads to myocyte hypersensitivity to endothelial thromboxane, which may be relevant in persistent pulmonary hypertension of the newborn [9]. This mechanism is believed to be inhibited by volatile agents, nitrates, and calcium channel blockers, although some studies have shown no effect of clinically relevant concentrations of isoflurane.

## Thoracotomy

The first recorded chest operation dates to the Ebers papyrus, roughly 3600 years ago, while the modern era of thoracic surgery can be dated to 1909, when Lillienthal performed the first thoracotomy under positive pressure ventilation with a tracheal tube [10]. The epidemic of post-pneumonic empyema accompanying the 1917 influenza pandemic led to the first wave of rapid development in thoracic surgery by Graham and others [11]. Entry into the chest can be through an intercostal space, or through the bed of a subperiostially resected rib, and is typically described anatomically as anterior, lateral, axillary, or posterolateral [12]. The latter affords the widest exposure and operative flexibility, not surprisingly at the cost of greatest morbidity as it sections both the serratus anterior and the latissimus dorsi. Particularly in infants and children, this can lead to long-term problems with scoliosis and other deformities; muscle-sparing incisions are an effort to limit these [13]. Postoperative pain control can be challenging, even with effective regional or neuraxial techniques, and can lead to secondary complications from poor coughing and atelectasis. The incidence of chronic pain after thoracotomy approaches 60 percent at one year [14].

## Thoracoscopy/VATS (Video-Assisted Thoracic Surgery)

Thoracoscopy was first performed in 1910 by Jacobeus in Sweden (using a cystoscope), and proved useful in the diagnosis and treatment of pleural disease, which at the time usually meant tuberculous effusion [15]. It took the technological explosion of instrumentation and imaging systems that was spurred by laparoscopic cholecystectomy to bring this into the mainstream, and allow its extension to parenchymal disease. As more complicated procedures were undertaken, including anatomic resections, the term VATS (for video-assisted thoracic surgery) was introduced, to replace the implication that "thoracoscopy" was a noninvasive medical procedure. As with laparoscopic surgery, the promise of smaller incisions, less postoperative pain, and faster recovery seemed self-evident, and led to widespread enthusiasm and adoption, more often than not without randomized controlled trials demonstrating superiority. In fact, a recent pilot randomized controlled trial from Great Ormond Street showed that compared to open surgery, VATS repair of congenital diaphragmatic hernia (CDH) and

tracheoesophageal fistula (TEF) were associated with severe and prolonged hypercapnia and acidosis, raising questions about the safety of the practice [16]. Other reviews caution that the improved cosmetic and musculoskeletal benefits must be balanced against a potentially higher risk of complications, especially in young infants [17,18].

## Single Lung Ventilation

From a surgical perspective, all intrapleural procedures would ideally be conducted with the operative lung collapsed and unmoving; that is, under single lung ventilation of the contralateral side. Prior to the mid-1990s almost all chest operations, especially in children, were performed through open thoracotomy. In patients under about ten years of age, this involved conventional tracheal intubation/ventilation with the surgeon retracting the inflated lung as necessary for exposure. As the trend toward minimally invasive surgery has moved forward, an increasing percentage of interventions are performed using VATS techniques. While conventional ventilation/retraction aided by $CO_2$ insufflation is sometimes unavoidable, the technical performance of any procedure is vastly simplified by single lung ventilation. Similarly, the risk of lung injury (tear, intraparenchymal hemorrhage, or postoperative air leak) and uncontrolled bleeding is lessened. But single lung ventilation is an iatrogenic pneumothorax, hence by definition a pathologic state. The ability of an individual to tolerate this depends on the health of the nonoperative (dependent) lung, and their capacity to mitigate the V/Q mismatch triggered by the sudden increase in shunt.

Single lung ventilation is typically carried out with an $FiO_2$ of 1, some degree of permissive hypercapnia, smaller tidal volumes, and higher respiratory rates. With a double lumen tube, the operative side is opened to atmosphere and/or a suction catheter can be passed to facilitate collapse. In VATS procedures, gentle $CO_2$ insufflation can expedite this. If lung isolation is accomplished using a bronchial blocker as opposed to a double lumen endotracheal tube, effective collapse is more dependent on insufflation and absorption atelectasis.

If unexpected hypoxemia develops during single lung ventilation, bronchoscopy should be performed quickly to determine correct placement of the double lumen endotracheal tube or bronchial blocker. In particular, the complication of herniation of a bronchial cuff into the trachea must be immediately recognized and corrected. Continuous positive airway pressure (CPAP) to the nondependent lung is generally agreed to be the most effective next step, but cannot be accomplished if a bronchial blocker is in use since these typically have no functional internal lumen. The application of positive end-expiratory pressure (PEEP) to the dependent lung can also be effective, and is often added empirically. Communication with the surgical team should be ongoing. Isolation and occlusion of the main pulmonary artery either by digital pressure or temporary clamping can rapidly correct hypoxemia and may avoid the need for reinflation of the operative lung, but this is only easily performed in open procedures.

## Techniques for Single Lung Ventilation

### Mainstem Intubation

The earliest technique for single lung ventilation, still often used, is to selectively intubate the mainstem bronchus of the nonoperative side. Several techniques have been described. This can usually be accomplished by turning the head toward and elevating the shoulder of the opposite side after passing a conventional tube through the vocal cords. Use of a stylet precurved similarly to a double lumen tube shape, and placed with the same technique (see below), has also been reported. Since the standard endotracheal tube bevel faces left, when placing a conventional oral endotracheal tube into the right mainstem bronchus, ventilation of the right upper lobe bronchus is often not possible. Two proposed solutions are to cut the tip to a right-facing bevel, or leaving the original bevel and cutting a Murphy eye. To place the endotracheal tube into the left mainstem bronchus, some clinicians rotate the tube 180° to gain a favorable bevel orientation to promote left-sided advancement, and then rotate back when at depth to minimize risk of covering the left upper lobe orifice. Perhaps the simplest method is to place the tube in the trachea in the usual fashion, advance a bronchoscope into the mainstem of interest, and then advance the tube over the scope. Whatever method or device is used, position must be confirmed with auscultation and fiberoptic bronchoscopy, both immediately and after turning lateral. Finally, in an attempt to regain some of the distinct advantages of a double lumen tube, passing two smaller endotracheal tubes and directing one into each mainstem bronchus has been described, but has the disadvantage of the extra bulk at the glottis potentially causing pressure damage, and is not recommended. Additionally, the smaller diameter conventional tubes required for bronchial as opposed to tracheal placement in this method are of proportionately shorter length, leaving little tube length available at the mouth to secure.

### Double Lumen Tubes

Conventional double lumen endotracheal tubes (e.g., Rusch Robert Shaw, Teleflex, Triangle Park, NC) are available down to size 26. While their use has been described in a six-year-old, it is more commonly avoided in patients less than 8–10 years or about 30 kg. These are almost always left-sided tubes; the very short right mainstem bronchus and correspondingly smaller tolerances make right-sided double lumen tubes difficult to use in pediatrics. Unlike in adults in whom pneumonectomy for malignancy may require stapling across the origin of a mainstem bronchus, this seldom presents a technical challenge to the surgeon, even operating on the left lung. They are placed similarly to adults: the tip of the tube is passed just through the vocal cords, the stylet is removed, the tube rotated 90° and then advanced. Usually this results in correct placement of the bronchial lumen in the left mainstem bronchus. The tracheal cuff is inflated and both lungs ventilated, after which the bronchial cuff can be inflated and each side tested clinically for chest rise and auscultation. Fiberoptic bronchoscopy should then be performed for confirmation. With the scope through the tracheal lumen, the blue bronchial cuff should be seen just at the origin of the left mainstem bronchus. Inspection should then be made through the bronchial lumen to be sure that the left upper lobe bronchus has access to the airway; i.e., that it has not been covered by the length of the tube between the bronchial cuff and the tip of the bronchial lumen. Double lumen tubes must be exchanged at the end of the case for conventional devices when continuation of ventilation postoperatively is planned. Newer designs include silicone DLTs (e.g., Sil-Broncho, Teleflex, Triangle Park, NC), which on insertion may be less traumatic and more resistant to balloon tears, but not yet available in smaller than 33 Fr.

### Bronchial Blockers

In patients too small for double lumen tubes, an appealing alternative is the bronchial blocker. This was first described using a Fogarty embolectomy catheter (Edwards Life Sciences, Irvine, CA) passed through the cords outside of (and usually prior to) the endotracheal tube (ETT), advanced under bronchoscopic guidance into the operative mainstem [19]. Still used by some, they are manufactured with inflated balloon diameters of 4, 5, and 9 mm. Alternatively, in larger patients passing a guidewire through the scope and then exchanging the scope for a catheter, with or without fluoroscopy, has been described; the Fogarty Thru-Lumen (over-the-wire) embolectomy catheter is available with balloon sizes of 5, 9, and 11 mm diameter. While balloon-tipped PA catheters and atrial septostomy balloons have been used, neither has as small a catheter diameter or is as guidable as the Fogarty.

Released in 1999, the Arndt bronchial blocker (Cook Medical, Bloomington, IN) has gained popularity for its improved ease of use [20]. This device is available in 5, 7, and 9 Fr sizes, which can be placed through ETTs of at least 4.5, 6.5, and 7.5 mm respectively (using a 2.2 mm bronchoscope). A multiport adapter has a 15 mm connector on its side for the anesthesia circuit, an in-line diaphragm for a flexible scope, and an angled Tuohy-Borst adapter through which the catheter itself is passed. The tip of the catheter holds a wire guide loop, which can be cinched around the tip of the bronchoscope, either before connecting the adapter (preferred, if scope plus catheter fit together through the tube) or in the airway. This system has the distinct advantage of being able to continuously ventilate during the process, and giving more control over the direction taken by the catheter. After placement, the guide loop assembly is removed, leaving a small central lumen to which suction can be applied to expedite collapse.

The UniBlocker is a 5 Fr and the Fuggiano Blocker a 9 Fr device by LMA North America (San Diego, CA). These are conceptually similar to the Arndt Blocker described above.

Another device recently available is the Rusch EZ Blocker (Teleflex Medical, Research Triangle Park, NC), essentially a single catheter which bifurcates to short bronchial lengths, each with its own, independently inflatable balloon. Placed straddling the carina, the lung is allowed to passively deflate with exhalation, and the balloon is inflated on the surgical side prior to resuming ventilation. Particularly advantageous for bilateral procedures, it is manufactured in a single size, 7 Fr.

With any bronchial blocker, one of the main challenges is dislodgement. Balloon herniation into the distal trachea can acutely impede all ventilation, and can often be precipitated by surgical manipulation. The immediate response is to deflate the balloon and to assess and reposition as necessary under bronchoscopic guidance. Using saline rather than air to fill the blocker balloon makes it somewhat less likely to dislodge.

## Univent

A Japanese product, the Univent (LMA North America, Inc., San Diego, CA) consists of a single lumen ETT with an integral balloon-tipped catheter that can be advanced independently into a mainstem bronchus using a malleable shaft for torque control. It is available in sizes 3.5–9 mm. Its main disadvantage is a comparatively large overall external diameter for a given internal tracheal lumen size. The blocking catheter does have a central lumen to allow aspiration of, as well as PEEP application to, the nonoperative lung.

## Bronchoscopes

As essential to these procedures as the anesthesia workstation itself is the flexible fiberoptic bronchoscope. First developed in the 1970s, the smallest currently available instruments are 2.2 mm in diameter (e.g., BF-N20, Olympus, Tokyo, Japan). The smallest scopes available with a suction channel (of 1.2 mm) has a 2.8 mm outer diameter (e.g., BF-XP60, Olympus, Tokyo, Japan). While the increased number of optical fibers delivers a marginally better image, the suction channel is not surprisingly overwhelmed by anything beyond the smallest drops of fluid.

One important limitation of these devices is their inherent fragility and the associated expense of maintenance and replacement, especially in a teaching hospital.

## Preoperative Assessment

Unlike in the adult or older child, where spirometry, peak flows, and flow-volume loops are routine and provide an objective assessment of many aspects of pulmonary function, no such testing is possible in the neonate and infant. History, physical exam, and selective imaging still provide the compass with which to navigate safely through a thoracic intervention in this population.

Gestational age and perinatal history should be considered, with particular regard to intubation, surfactant therapy, length of NICU stay if any, or apnea events. The timing of symptom onset, or prenatal diagnosis, as well as any prior interventions, especially previous thoracotomy, should be considered. In addition to review of chest radiographs, a cardiac echo is often a necessary part of pre-anesthetic assessment in these patients, particularly in the infant with airway anomalies or VACTERL association. In the older infant, the usual concern over possible recent upper respiratory tract infection or exposure to second-hand smoke is always present. While having blood available is advisable for all but the most minor thoracic procedures, sending a type and cross after line placement can avoid a difficult venipuncture in an awake infant. Some centers use type-specific irradiated blood without crossmatch in neonates when necessary. Prior to going to the OR, a thorough discussion must be held with the surgical team regarding the operative plan, extent of pulmonary resection anticipated, likelihood of major blood loss, and the degree to which single lung ventilation is important. The plan for post-op disposition must be understood but flexible.

## General Considerations

Following standard inhalational induction of general anesthesia, with parental presence or premedication as indicated in older infants, and taking care to keep the infant warm, IV access adequate for resuscitation is obtained. This usually includes both upper and lower extremity sites. Arterial catheterization is indicated for most thoracotomies, particularly in longer and more complex procedures or in patients in whom postoperative ventilation is anticipated, where its availability for arterial blood gas sampling is invaluable. Central venous access is obtained if peripheral access is inadequate, inotrope use is considered likely, or if any other considerations make determination of mixed venous $O_2$ saturation desirable. For any of these access procedures, ultrasound can be significantly time-saving, especially in the smallest patients, and is becoming the standard of care for placement of CVLs. Bladder and orogastric catheters are placed, and the patient is usually placed on an under-body forced-air warmer. Caution must be exercised and the device typically not operated at its high (43 °C) setting on these smallest patients, particularly if in direct contact with skin. The patient is then moved to the lateral decubitus position with appropriate padding and protection of the axilla, extremities, and ear; new-generation fluidized positioners (e.g., Z-FLOW, Sundance Solutions, White Plains, NY) can be extremely useful in this regard. The position of the airway management device is then rechecked with bronchoscopy.

If epidural placement has been planned, it is now undertaken, and used as an intraoperative adjunct as well as for post-op analgesia. In these vulnerable patients it is imperative that a second provider be present to assist in positioning and attend to the details of the anesthetic during placement of the epidural. In contrast, if a paravertebral catheter has been selected, it is often best placed at the end of the procedure, as it is practically impossible to keep out of the surgical field.

A balanced anesthetic is maintained with oxygen, opioid, and low-dose volatile anesthetics with muscle relaxation. The transition to single lung ventilation requires particular vigilance of both respiratory parameters and attention to the surgical field to assess efficacy. End-tidal $CO_2$ values are known to be sometimes inaccurate in neonates due to circuit volume/Vt ratio and sampling rate factors; transcutaneous $CO_2$ sensors have been developed and are under investigation (TCM CombiM, Radiometer Medical, Copenhagen, Denmark), but measurement of arterial blood gases is the gold standard to assess the adequacy of ventilation. Patients who arrive intubated, have significant comorbidities, or are less than a few months old are rarely extubated in the operating room.

## Regional Anesthesia/Analgesia

Surgical breach of the thoracic cavity unavoidably results in tissue injury, which in turn leads to a local inflammatory response as well as activation of a systemic neurohumeral cascade. Nocioceptive afferents to the central nervous system trigger efferent autonomic activation and catecholamine release from the adrenal medulla. Alterations in hemodynamics, metabolism, and immune function follow, which have been associated with less favorable outcomes. Regional anesthesia combined with general anesthesia has been shown to more completely suppress this stress response compared to general anesthesia with opioids [21]. Neuraxial anesthesia has been shown to essentially eliminate the hyperglycemic response and relative insulin resistance following thoracic procedures in children. There are other potential advantages to the addition of a regional technique to the general anesthesia for these patients. Diminished NK cell activity is a marker for downregulated cellular immunity, and is associated with increased risk for metastasis in several human tumors. In animal models this has been directly observed following exposure to both opioids as well as volatile anesthetics. The latter have also been observed to increase hypoxia-induced factor (HIF-1alpha) in tumor cells, stimulating angiogenesis [22]. Effective regional anesthesia/analgesia allows the administration of lower dose opioid and inhaled anesthetic agents, potentially mitigating these untoward effects. In the pediatric population, perhaps most relevant is the growing body of literature concerning apoptosis and neurocognitive development risk. In a recent consensus conference, a panel of experts stressed the importance of developing strategies to limit potential brain injury from general anesthetics [23].

A recent study of 40 patients has shown that infants undergoing thoracic procedures have superior analgesia, earlier return to full feeds, and shorter ICU stays with perioperative regional analgesia [24]. Although complications from epidural placement in small babies are infrequent, the seriousness of the potential neurologic deficit is leading toward increasing use of paravertebral as opposed to epidural catheters in these patients.

## Cystic Lesions of the Chest

### Congenital Cystic Adenomatoid Malformation

Failure of normal embryologic development of the tracheobronchial budding from the primitive foregut can lead to a constellation of cystic lesions that have overlapping clinical and histologic findings. The term bronchopulmonary-foregut malformation has been proposed to encompass many of these.

The most common of these is the congenital cystic adenomatoid malformation (CCAM), with an incidence of about 1:30 000 births. First described by Ch'in and Tang in 1949, the term "congenital pulmonary airway malformation" has been used more recently [25,26]. Increasingly diagnosed by prenatal ultrasound, these are believed to represent the disorderly proliferation of terminal bronchioles without distal alveoli. Although some lesions are seen to involute on serial ultrasounds, postnatal CT scans will usually demonstrate their persistence, even with a normal chest radiograph. Congenital cystic adenomatoid

malformations are more common on the left, are usually confined to a single lobe, and have an 18 percent rate of associated abnormalities such as cardiac anomalies and renal agenesis. Prenatally the differentiation between CCAM and pulmonary sequestration can be difficult, and indeed hybrid lesions have been confirmed at operation, where the typical histology of CCAM is accompanied by a systemic arterial supply. Other prenatal ultrasound findings suggestive of CCAM include polyhydramnios, pleural effusion, or hydrops fetalis. The X-ray or sonographic finding of multiple air/fluid levels in the inferior left chest can generate confusion with congenital diaphragmatic hernia.

Patients with CCAM can have a range of presentations, from being entirely asymptomatic at birth to having severe fetal compromise. Case reports exist of fetal lobectomy using EXIT, as well as thoracoamniotic shunting. Those born with minimal symptomatology will inevitably develop cough, respiratory distress, recurrent infection, or pneumothorax. Tube thoracostomy can be life-saving in extreme cases. Malignant degeneration can occur, with poorly differentiated blastoma in the younger cohort, and bronchoalveolar carcinoma in adolescents and adults. Surgical resection is most commonly performed between 3 and 12 months, with a trend toward earlier definitive treatment as infectious complications become more frequent after about seven months, and earlier removal offers greater potential for compensatory growth of the remaining pulmonary parenchyma. Anatomic lobectomy is the standard of care and provides excellent long-term results; lesser resections have significant rates of recurrence.

### Pulmonary Sequestration

Another lesion of disordered pulmonary embryogenesis, the hallmark of pulmonary sequestration is the absence of a clear connection with the airway, and the presence of a systemic arterial supply. Whereas in normal development, more distal generations of bronchioles are closely coupled with development of the pulmonary arterial tree, sequestrations are felt to arise from continued alveolar development caudally, somehow stimulating a systemic arterial inflow [27]. This is consistent with the observation that they occur most commonly in the medial lower lobes, the left involved more than the right. Arterial supply is usually from a branch directly arising from the aorta and can be infradiaphragmatic in up to 20 percent of cases; venous drainage is much more variable and can be systemic, pulmonary, or both.

Sequestrations are described as intralobar (75 percent) or extralobar (25 percent) based on whether the lesion lies within the visceral pleura of the adjacent lung, or are covered by its own visceral pleura, respectively. Intralobar sequestrations usually present with recurrent respiratory infection or failure to thrive. While associated anomalies are uncommon, a small percentage will have a connection to the esophagus. In contrast, about 40 percent of extralobar sequestrations will have other anomalies, including cardiac, chest wall, and vertebral defects. They have even been described entirely below the diaphragm, especially in the left suprarenal area. Extralobar sequestrations have a lower incidence of infection, but can present with feeding difficulties, pain from torsion, or congestive failure.

Most authors recommend that all pulmonary sequestrations be surgically treated in the first year of life, once any infections complication has been controlled. Intralobar lesions are resected by wedge resection or lobectomy as appropriate. Extralobar sequestrations are usually resectable with minimal if any loss of normal lung tissue; the challenge is control of the systemic vascular supply. Magnetic resonance has replaced conventional angiography, but imaging is essential to preoperative planning. Gaining proximal arterial control in the abdomen can prevent exsanguination, should one of these typically thin-walled, tortuous, and high-flow vessels be injured. Patients presenting with heart failure are best served by preoperative angiography with embolization.

## Bronchogenic and Dermoid Cysts

Conceptually, perhaps the simplest of these lesions is the bronchogenic cyst, which might be thought of as resulting from "exocytosis" from the bronchial tree. More common on the right, and in males, these are lined with respiratory epithelium and often show cartilage, goblet cells, and smooth muscle. In infants they usually present as mass lesions causing airway compromise with stridor, retractions, wheezing, or cyanosis. Older children more often develop infection as their initial symptom. These lesions should be resected when diagnosed because of the risk of infection as well as malignant degeneration. While not communicating with the airways, they are often densely adherent and

technically challenging. If complete resection is not feasible, any residual mucosa should be cauterized in situ. Dermoid cysts are clinically indistinguishable, but show squamous rather than ciliated columnar epithelium [28].

For this and all of the congenital lesions, the primary anesthetic consideration is whether positive pressure ventilation is likely to exacerbate air trapping in the anomaly, leading to mediastinal shift, tension physiology, and resultant hemodynamic compromise. In general, CCAM, sequestrations, and duplication cysts do not significantly communicate with the airway and controlled ventilation presents no undue risk. If, however, the precise anatomic relationships of the anomaly are unknown, maintaining spontaneous respiration until the chest is open or single lung ventilation of the normal side is achieved is the most prudent course.

## Congenital Lobar Emphysema

Congenital lobar emphysema (CLE) is an uncommon entity, first described by Nelson in 1932; it is characterized by the abnormal hyperinflation of otherwise normal lung parenchyma, classically in a lobar distribution [29]. CT angiography typically shows absence of arterial flow to the involved segments. The left upper lobe is the most common site, followed by the right upper and middle lobes. Involvement of the lower lobes is rare; this can be a useful distinction from CCAM. Its pathophysiology is produced by a functional one-way valve effect, which can be either extrinsic, usually thought to be from an abnormal vascular structure, or intrinsic due to bronchomalacia. Because of this, positive pressure ventilation can precipitate acute decompensation. Maintaining spontaneous breathing until the chest is open is preferred. Despite the "lobar" nomenclature, a recent series demonstrated that among 24 left upper lobe lesions, all but one in fact showed sparing of the two lingular segments; the authors advocated lung-sparing surgery and saw no recurrences in long-term follow-up [30].

## Congenital Diaphragmatic Hernia

Congenital diaphragmatic hernia (CDH) is among the more common life-threatening thoracic anomalies, occurring in about 1:2500 live births. Progress in its management has been frustratingly slow, the discussion of which could occupy an entire chapter if not textbook. The first successful repair is credited to Heidenhain in Germany in 1905 [31]. Congenital diaphragmatic hernia is usually diagnosed with prenatal ultrasound in developed countries. Whether or not there is a prenatal diagnosis, the presentation at delivery usually includes respiratory distress, a scaphoid abdomen with absent breath sounds, and often the presence of bowel sounds on the left. The diaphragm, a uniquely mammalian structure, consists of a central tendon and peripheral muscular elements, now believed to be derived solely from the embryologic pleuroperitoneal fold. Normal development requires a complex interplay of differentiation, migration, and integration of neural and vascular elements. A defect in the amuscular mesenchymal component occurring as early as 3–4 weeks appears to inhibit normal migration of muscle cell precursors. Roughly one-third of cases will have other major anomalies, and over 70 genetic syndromes include CDH as part of their clinical criteria. Associated anomalies, especially cardiac, have been clearly associated with poorer outcomes. The vast majority of defects occur at the left-sided posterolateral foramen of Bochdalek, allowing herniation of abdominal contents into the chest after 10–12 weeks and subsequent mechanical interference with lung development. The resulting pulmonary hypoplasia and pulmonary hypertension are the most difficult physiologic insults to manage. While some reports have demonstrated improvement in mortality since the application of newer technologies such as extracorporeal membrane oxygenation (ECMO), high-frequency oscillatory ventilation (HFOV), inhaled nitric oxide (iNO), and PDE5 inhibitors, population-based studies still show roughly 50 percent mortality because of what has been termed the "hidden mortality" of selection bias and prenatal diagnosis leading to termination [32]. While right-sided Bochdalek hernias do occur, they tend to have less severe pulmonary disease as the liver relatively impedes bowel translocation into the thorax [33]. Bilateral hernias occur in <1 percent, are more frequently associated with other anomalies, and have a very high mortality. Defects can also occur in the anterior (retrosternal) foramen of Morgagni or rarely in the central tendon; these tend to present later, even into adult life, and often with bowel obstruction. Work with rodent models has revealed a critical role of the retinoic acid pathway and its genetic control early in gestation interfering with normal development of the pleuroperitoneal fold and its muscular mesenchymal component [34]. Curiously, the timing of teratogen exposure seems to affect laterality of the condition [35].

Because the defect occurs early in gestation, and overall treatment results are suboptimal, prenatal intervention is intuitively appealing. Progressive models in rats, rabbits, and sheep showed that tracheal occlusion appears to induce lung growth and decrease the resulting degree of hypoplasia, because the lung is a net producer of amniotic fluid. These efforts have evolved to a percutaneous balloon technique called FETO (fetal endoscopic tracheal occlusion) [36]. While several studies have shown no clear improvement, Ruano et al. have published a prospective randomized controlled trial of FETO vs. conventional therapy for fetuses with severe isolated CDH, in which mortality was 4.8 percent in the treatment group vs. 50 percent with standard therapy [37]. While some experts still consider it an option in the most severe cases, its use has declined. It has been increasingly appreciated that the pathophysiology of this condition involves not only the grossly hypoplastic lung, but the contralateral "normal" lung as well. The more global nature of this anomaly is also reinforced by reports indicating that survivors have a higher incidence of recurrent respiratory infections, GI reflux disease, skeletal anomalies, hearing loss, and neurocognitive delay [38].

Although described in postmortem exams by Riverius in 1679, surgical treatment did not become commonplace until 1940, when Ladd and Gross reported 16 operated cases with 9 survivors [39]. Gross went on to report a successful repair on the first day of life in 1946, and the concept that early relief of pressure on the lung and heart by the abdominal viscera would improve outcomes stimulated the trend toward immediate postnatal repair. Only since the late 1980s, with a growing understanding that the pulmonary hypoplasia and hypertension are the critical physiologic derangements, has surgical repair of CDH evolved from an emergency procedure to a delayed, often scheduled one, today. After intubation and nasogastric decompression in the delivery room, invasive lines are placed for monitoring acid–base status and nutritional support. Strategies for lung protective ventilation and permissive hypercapnia are employed in the NICU. Even with lung protective ventilation, the occurrence of a pneumothorax is still a possibility. In addition to the ventilation strategy, PGE-1 is commonly employed to maintain ductal patency and unload the right ventricle.

Echocardiography is obtained early to rule out cardiac anomalies and repeated often to assess the right ventricular/systemic pressure relationship. After a period of stabilization sometimes lasting up to weeks (for infants on ECMO), repair is undertaken either transabdominally (more commonly open) or thoracoscopically. The patient is brought to and returned from the operating room intubated. Continuing the use of the NICU-type ventilator for both transport and surgery is considered advantageous over bag-mask ventilating and use of the anesthesia machine, even if the child is not on HFOV. This approach mandates an intravenous anesthetic technique. Primary repair is preferred, while prosthetic patch repair is required for larger defects. Prostanoids and iNO are continued if in use, with inotropic support immediately available if needed. Use of a chest drain is controversial, but often employed.

## Tracheoesophageal Fistula/ Esophageal Atresia

After CDH, the next most common major intrathoracic anomaly presenting in the neonate is tracheoesophageal fistula with esophageal atresia (TEF/EA), with an incidence of about 1:3500. Five anatomical subtypes are well known, based on the site of origin of the fistula relative to the atretic or complete esophagus. Almost 80 percent of cases are Type C, with the fistula communicating with the esophagus distal to an atretic segment. Sometimes causing polyhydramnios in utero, the diagnosis is suggested in a newborn with copious salivation, gastric distention, and respiratory distress upon feeding. Chest radiograph after gently attempting to pass a gastric tube until the first hint of resistance is perceived is diagnostic. The tube is secured in place and kept on gentle suction to continuously evacuate the upper pouch contents, and the infant is kept in reverse Trendelenberg to minimize aspiration risk. More than half of patients have associated anomalies of which congenital heart disease has the most relevance to anesthetic management and long-term outcome. VACTERL (Vertebral, Anal, Cardiac, TE fistula, Renal and Limb) association anomalies are present in 30 percent; other related syndromes include CHARGE, Feingold, Fanconi's anemia, DiGeorge, and right-sided aortic arch. Iatrogenic fistulas have occurred in infants with long-term endotracheal and nasogastric tubes, presumably from pressure-related changes.

After echocardiography, repair is undertaken most often through an extrapleural dissection in the right chest, assuming a left aortic arch. The goal is fistula division, repair of the posterior tracheal wall, careful mobilization of the esophageal segments, and primary tension-free anastomosis if possible. When this is not achievable due to a long gap, one technique involves placing the buttressed esophageal ends under traction sutures brought through the chest wall, where they are thought to stimulate longitudinal growth [40]. The tension on the sutures is adjusted daily and the infant is kept paralyzed and ventilated for several days. When imaging suggests adequate growth has been achieved, primary anastomosis is then performed. After 1–2 weeks, gaps of almost 7 cm have become amenable to anastomosis. Regardless of the length, gastrostomy is performed to allow early enteral nutrition. Occasionally, neonates present with respiratory compromise from massive gastric distention from air passing preferentially from the trachea to the GI tract. Emergency decompression can be life-saving in this event.

Anesthesia for the repair can be managed in multiple ways, with the principle that further inflating the stomach with positive pressure ventilation is to be avoided. Flexibility is required because, although the vast majority are Type C, the precise anatomy may be unknown at induction. Often the procedure will begin with laryngoscopy and rigid bronchoscopy by the surgeon under spontaneous ventilation to evaluate potential tracheomalacia or signs of a vascular ring, as well as to identify the fistula site. Following this, the traditional technique is to intubate the trachea with the tip distal to the fistula and keeping inflation pressures low until a gastrostomy is opened or the fistula controlled. Alternatively, prior to the procedure a Fogarty catheter can be passed through the fistula at the time of bronchoscopy. Another option to isolate the esophagus from the trachea is to pass the occlusion catheter retrograde through the gastrostomy. Muscle relaxation and intubation can follow, again with attention to avoid distending the stomach. One-lung ventilation is typically neither practical (given the size of these patients), nor necessary (since the dissection is usually extrapleural). Some centers are advancing VATS repair, but there are no randomized trials showing superior safety or efficacy. Mid-term complications include stricture with need for frequent dilatation, and anastomotic leak or dehiscence. Associated significant trachea- or bronchomalacia can be improved by aortopexy through a partial sternotomy, or by posterior tracheopexy at the time of thoracotomy. Many of these infants will require anti-reflux surgery and a few will require esophageal replacement.

## Mediastinal Mass

Although more common in children and young adults, mediastinal masses do occur in infants. Regardless of age, the same concerns and management principles apply: compression by tumor of the trachea and bronchi, heart, and great vessels can result in cardiovascular collapse with loss of spontaneous respiration and the normal awake transpleural pressure relationships. While initiating treatment without tissue diagnosis is an option, this is clearly suboptimal from an oncologic viewpoint. Biopsy under local anesthesia alone is impractical in this population, but its use along with regional and neuraxial techniques should always be considered. Presence of symptoms at rest (supine dyspnea, stridor, SVC syndrome) is particularly concerning, and observing changes with lateral or prone positioning preoperatively is useful. Imaging may be challenging to accomplish in an uncooperative infant, but a cardiac echo is a very important diagnostic test that does not require sedation and can help elucidate whether the mass impairs filling of the right atrium. Maintenance of spontaneous ventilation and having rigid bronchoscopy immediately available until it is clear that positive pressure ventilation will be successful is essential. Cardiopulmonary bypass is sometimes required for the largest lesions. CT imaging showing cross-sectional area trachea to be greater than 50 percent predicted for age has been associated with successful positive pressure ventilation [41].

## Summary

Providing anesthesia for neonates and infants undergoing thoracic surgery remains a proposition requiring detailed preoperative assessment, methodical planning, and meticulous conduct. While these vulnerable patients present with some unique pathologic lesions as well as associated anomalies, the first principles of maintaining homeostasis and minimizing the stress response to surgical trauma remain universally applicable. Integral to this is providing adequate postoperative analgesia incorporating regional or neuraxial adjuncts. Single lung ventilation presents its own unique set of technical and physiologic challenges. While no single anesthetic technique has been shown to provide superior outcomes, maintaining a global view of the individual patient at hand, with his or her unique position on the spectrum of history, anatomy, and physiology, will be the surest way to return that infant safely to its parents.

## References

1. Guidry C, McGahren ED. Pediatric chest I: developmental and physiologic conditions for the surgeon. *Surg Clin North Am.* 2012;92(3):615–43. doi: 10.1016/j.suc.2012.03.013.

2. Griese M. Pulmonary surfactant in health and human lung diseases: state of the art. *Eur Respir J.* 1999;13(6):1455–76.

3. Brownfoot FC, Gagliardi DI, Bain E, Middleton P, Crowther CA. Different corticosteroids and regimens for accelerating fetal lung maturation for women at risk of preterm birth. *Cochrane Database Syst Rev.* 2013;29(8): CD006764.

4. Ramachandrappa A, Jain L. Elective cesarean section: its impact on neonatal respiratory outcome. *Clin Perinatol.* 2008;35(2):373–93. doi: 10.1016/j.clp.2008.03.006.

5. Blanco CE. Maturation of fetal breathing activity. *Biol Neonate.* 1994;65(3–4):182–8.

6. Polla B, D'Antona G, Bottinelli R, Reggiani C. Respiratory muscle fibres: specialization and plasticity. *Thorax.* 2004;59:808–17. doi:10.1136/thx.2003.009894

7. West J. *Respiratory Physiology: The Essentials*, 8th edn. Philadelphia, PA: Lippincott Williams & Wilkins; 2008.

8. Aaronson PI, Robertson TP, Knock GA, et al. Hypoxic pulmonary vasoconstriction: mechanisms and controversies. *J Physiol.* 2006;570(Pt 1):53–8.

9. Hinton M, Mellow L, Halayko AJ, Gutsol A, Dakshinamurti S. Hypoxia induces hypersensitivity and hyperreactivity to thromboxane receptor agonist in neonatal pulmonary arterial myocytes. *Am J Physiol Lung Cell Mol Physiol.* 2006;290(2):L375–84.

10. Fell SC. Special article: a brief history of pneumonectomy. *Chest Surg Clin North Am.* 2002;12(3):541–63.

11. Graham EA. The first pneumonectomy. *Cancer Bull.* 1949;2:2.

12. Fry WA. Thoracic incisions. *Chest Surg Clin North Am.* 1995;5(2):177–88.

13. Elshiekh MA, Lo TT, Shipolini AR, McCormack DJ. Does muscle-sparing thoracotomy as opposed to posterolateral thoractomy result in better recovery? *Interact Cardiovasc Thorac Surg.* 2013;16(1):60–7.

14. Wildgaard K, Ravn J, Kehlet H. Chronic post-thoracotomy pain: a critical review of pathogenic

mechanisms and strategies for prevention. *Eur J Cardiothorac Surg*. 2009;36(1):170–80.

15. Rodriguez-Panadero F, Janssen JP, Astoul P. Thoracoscopy: general overview and place in the diagnosis and management of pleural effusion. *ERJ*. 2006;28(2):409–22.

16. Bishay MI, Giacomello L, Retrosi G, M et al. Hypercapnia and acidosis during open and thoracoscopic repair of congenital diaphragmatic hernia and esophageal atresia: results of a pilot randomized controlled trial. *Ann Surg*. 2013; 258(6):895–900. doi: 10.1097/SLA.0b013e31828fab55.

17. Kunisaki SM, Powelson IA, Haydar B, et al. Thoracoscopic vs open lobectomy in infants and young children with congenital lung malformations. *J Am Coll Surg*. 2014;218(2):261–70. doi: 10.1016/j.jamcollsurg.2013.10.010

18. Seong YW, Kang CH, Kim JT, et al. Video-assisted thoracoscopic lobectomy in children: safety, efficacy, and risk factors for conversion to thoracotomy. *Ann Thorac Surg*. 2013;95(4):1236–42. doi: 10.1016/j.athoracsur.2013.01.013.

19. Vale R. Selective bronchial blocking in a small child. *Br J Anaesth*. 1969;41:453–4.

20. Hammer GB, Harrison TK, Vricella LA et al. Single-lung ventilation in children using a new paediatric bronchial blocker. *Paediatr Anaesth*. 2002;12:69–72.

21. Wolf AR. Effects of regional analgesia on stress responses to pediatric surgery. *Paediatr Anaesth*. 2012;22(1):19–24.

22. Heaney A, Buggy DJ. Can anaesthetic and analgesic techniques affect cancer recurrence or metastasis? *Br J Anaesth*. 2012;109 (S1): i17–i28.

23. Jevtovic-Todorovic V, Absalom AR, Blomgren K, et al. Anaesthetic neurotoxicity and neuroplasticity: an expert group report and statement based on the BJA Salzburg Seminar. *Br J Anaesth*. 2013;111(2):143–51. doi: 10.1093/bja/aet177.

24. Di Pede A, Morini F, Lombardi MH, et al. Comparison of regional vs. systemic analgesia for post-thoracotomy care in infants. *Paediatr Anaesth*. 2014;24(6):569–73.

25. Ch'in KY, Tang MY. Congenital adenomatoid malformation of one lobe of a lung with general anasarca. *Arch Pathol Lab Med*. 1949;48:221–9.

26. Stocker JT. Congenital pulmonary airway malformation: a new name for and an expanded classification of congenital cystic adenomatoid malformation of the lung. *Histopathology*. 2002;41(Suppl. 2): 424–31.

27. Hammer GB. Pediatric thoracic anesthesia. *Anesthesiol Clin North Am*. 2002;20:153–80.

28. Petroze R, McGahren ED. Pediatric chest II: benign tumors and cysts. *Surg Clin North Am*. 2012;92(3):645–58. doi: 10.1016/j.suc.2012.03.014.

29. Nelson RL. Congenital cystic disease of the lung. *J Pediatr*. 1932;1:233.

30. Krivchenya DU, Rudenko EO, Dubrovin AG. Congenital emphysema in children: segmental lung resection as an alternative to lobectomy. *J Pediatr Surg*. 2013;48:309–14.

31. Irish MS, Holm BA, Glick PL. Congenital diaphragmatic hernia: a historical review. *Clin Perinatol*. 1996;23(4):625–53.

32. Mah. VK, Zamakhshary, M, Mah, DY, et al. Absolute vs relative improvements in congenital diaphragmatic hernia survival: what happened to "hidden mortality". *J Pediatr Surg*. 2009; 44(5):877–82. doi: 10.1016/j.jpedsurg.2009.01.046.

33. Jani P, Bidarkar SS, Walker K, et al. Right-sided congenital diaphragmatic hernia: a tertiary centre's experience over 25 years. *J Neonatal Perinatal Med*. 2014;7(1):39–45.

34. Ruttenstock EM, Doi T, Dingemann J, Puri P. Prenatal retinoic acid upregulates connexin 43 (*Cx43*) gene expression in pulmonary hypoplasia in the nitrofen-induced congenital diaphragmatic hernia rat model. *J Pediatr Surg*. 2012;47(2):336–40.

35. Snowise S, Johnson A. Tracheal occlusion for fetal diaphragmatic hernia. *Am J Perinatol*. 2014;31(7):605–16. doi: 10.1055/s-0034-1373842.

36. Kitano Y. Prenatal intervention for congenital diaphragmatic hernia. *Semin Pediatr Surg*. 2007;16(2):101–8.

37. Ruano R, Yoshisaki CT, da Silva MM, et al. A randomized controlled trial of fetal endoscopic tracheal occlusion versus postnatal management of severe isolated congenital diaphragmatic hernia. *Ultrasound Obstet Gynecol*. 2012;39:20–7.

38. Hidaka N, Ishii K, Mabuchi A. Associated anomalies in congenital diaphragmatic hernia: perinatal characteristics and impact on postnatal survival. *J Perinat Med*. 2014;43(2):245–52 doi: 10.1515/jpm-2014-0110.

39. Ladd WE, Gross RE. Congenital diaphragmatic hernia. *N Engl J Med*. 1940;223:917–25.

40. Kkunisaki SM, Foker JE. Surgical advances in the fetus and neonate: esophageal atresia. *Clin Perinatol*. 2012;39(2):349–61. doi: 10.1016/j.clp.2012.04.007.

41. Shamberger RC. Preanesthetic evaluation of children with anterior mediastinal masses. *Semin Pediatr Surg*. 1999;8(2):61–8.

# Congenital Diaphragmatic Hernia

Elizabeth C. Eastburn and Bridget L. Muldowney

## Introduction

The diaphragm begins to form at four weeks gestation and is completely formed by the eighth to tenth week. The diaphragm is made up of four embryonic structures: the septum transversum, dorsal esophageal mesentery, the pleuroperitoneal membrane, and muscular ingrowth from the body wall [1]. When these components do not develop properly a defect occurs which permits the abdominal contents to enter the thorax, causing a congenital diaphragmatic hernia (CDH). The most common location of a defect is posterolateral through the foramen of Bochdalek, and occurs more frequently on the left side. Defects in an anterior parasternal location through the foramen of Morgagni and at the esophageal hiatus are less common [2]. The diaphragmatic defect allows abdominal contents to herniate into the thorax, compressing the developing lung. This compression results in irreversible pulmonary hypoplasia on the side of the defect. If the defect is so large that bowel contents shift the mediastinum toward the contralateral side, lung compression and hypoplasia can also occur on the contralateral side. Compression from the bowel has deleterious effects on the pulmonary vasculature as well. Pulmonary arterial remodeling may occur and can lead to persistent pulmonary hypertension, a major cause of morbidity and mortality in patients with a CDH.

## Epidemiology

The incidence of CDH is 1 in 2500–3000 live births [3]. Approximately 40 percent of patients with a CDH have concurrent congenital anomalies including congenital heart disease, neural tube defects, and chromosomal abnormalities [4]. Pregestational diabetes and maternal alcohol use may be associated with CDH occurrence [5]. There is significant morbidity and mortality associated with CDH [6]. Survival rates for patients with CDH range from 60 to 90 percent

[7]. Current ongoing research suggests that retinoid-regulated genes may play a role in the development of CDH [8].

## Diagnosis and Clinical Presentation

The diagnosis of CDH is often made through routine prenatal ultrasonography. Once the diagnosis is made, further imaging can help diagnose other congenital abnormalities, delineate the contents of the hernia, and approximate the severity. Either ultrasound or MRI can aid in determining the ratio of lung area to head circumference, known as the lung-to-head-ratio. MRI can further be used to measure fetal lung volume (FLV). Both of these tests can grade the severity of the hernia and are beneficial in determining prognosis [9].

A neonate with a CDH typically presents with severe respiratory distress at birth, although smaller defects with less hypoplastic lung tissue can present with gradual onset of symptoms during the first days to weeks of life. On physical exam, the patient may have a scaphoid abdomen due to the abdominal contents residing in the chest. Breath sounds are often diminished or absent on the side of the hernia. A left-sided hernia may displace the heart to the right, with heart sounds best auscultated on the right chest. A chest radiograph will show bowel contents in the chest and subsequent decreased lung aeration on the affected side. It may also reveal the aberrant course of a nasogastric or orogastric tube, if present. In large defects, particularly on the right, the liver may also herniate into the chest.

## Preoperative Care and Management

Initial management of a neonate with CDH focuses on respiratory symptoms. An endotracheal tube is placed to support oxygenation and ventilation while an orogastric tube is passed to decompress the stomach and intestines. Bag-mask ventilation should be avoided, as distention of the abdominal contents in the chest can impair already compromised oxygenation and ventilation. Distention of the thoracic abdominal contents can also decrease cardiac preload and compress the heart, causing hemodynamic instability. Furthermore, bag-mask ventilation can cause barotrauma to the hypoplastic and noncompliant lungs.

A CDH was once treated as a surgical emergency and carried a very high mortality rate. Patients are now medically managed prior to undergoing repair. Both cardiac and pulmonary functions are optimized prior to proceeding to the operating room. Lung protective ventilation with low inspiratory pressures, low tidal volumes, adequate positive end-expiratory pressure (PEEP), and permissive hypercapnia protects the hypoplastic lung from barotrauma. Surfactant is only useful in preterm neonates with surfactant deficiency [10]. High-frequency oscillatory ventilation (HFOV) may be necessary to ensure adequate oxygenation and ventilation while preventing barotrauma. Cardiac management focuses on prevention and treatment of pulmonary hypertension. Narcotics are used to blunt sympathetic stimulation while ventilation strategies limit hypoxia and severe hypercarbia. Inhaled nitric oxide (iNO), a selective pulmonary vasodilator, can be used in cases of refractory pulmonary hypertension. Inotropic support is often needed to maintain ventricular function and systemic perfusion. Arterial access is necessary for both hemodynamic monitoring and frequent blood gas sampling. An echocardiogram is necessary to measure ventricular function and pulmonary artery pressure while diagnosing any other congenital cardiac anomalies.

A neonate not stabilized on the above-mentioned therapies may require extracorporeal membrane oxygenation (ECMO) support. A head ultrasound is included in the diagnostic workup as intracranial hemorrhage is a contraindication to extracorporeal membrane oxygenation (ECMO) support.

## Extracorporeal membrane oxygenation

Extracorporeal membrane oxygenation is an important therapy in the management of a subset of patients with CDH. Neonates known to have very low estimated lung volumes, those failing escalation of respiratory and hemodynamic support, and those who acutely decompensate may require ECMO support.

Many medical centers have specific inclusion and exclusion criteria for placing critically ill neonates on ECMO support. Respiratory indications for ECMO support include a high oxygen index (OI) (OI = MAP × $FiO_2$ × 100 / $PaO_2$), high peak inspiratory pressures, and refractory hypercarbia. Cardiac indications include a rising or persistently elevated lactate, long-term need for high-dose inotropic support, low mixed venous oxygen saturation, persistent arrhythmias, and severe cardiac dysfunction. Contraindications to ECMO include conditions in which systemic anticoagulation must be avoided, such as intracerebral hemorrhage, irreversible cardiac or respiratory failure where transplant or ventricular assist device (VAD) is not possible, extreme prematurity, and other significant comorbid conditions with a poor prognosis [11,12]. Extracorporeal membrane oxygenation can be achieved with either two venous cannulas (veno-venous) or with one arterial and one venous cannula (veno-arterial). Veno-venous ECMO only supports gas exchange while veno-arterial ECMO supports both gas exchange and systemic perfusion. Veno-arterial ECMO is often used in patients with CDH to support both ventricular dysfunction due to pulmonary hypertension and oxygen exchange due to hypoplastic lungs. In a neonate on ECMO, the surgical repair of the CDH is often completed while the patient is supported by ECMO.

## Operative Repair of CDH

A primary repair, in which the native diaphragm is approximated and sewn together, is done when the defect in the diaphragm is small. The majority of large defects are repaired via an open subcostal abdominal approach. Some centers do minimally invasive laparoscopic CDH repairs through either a thoracoscopic or abdominal approach [13]. Minimally invasive repair is associated with a higher recurrence rate [14]. Large defects often require a patch of synthetic material to close the defect, as the existing diaphragm segments are unable to be approximated. Synthetic patch closure is associated with higher rates of hernia recurrence compared to primary closure [15]. In patients with good pulmonary function and small defects, a minimally invasive thoracoscopic technique can be used for primary repair. Thoracic insufflation may be poorly tolerated with this technique [14].

Although not currently a standard therapy nor shown to improve mortality, fetal interventions exist to modulate the degree of lung hypoplasia [16]. Fetal endoluminal tracheal occlusion (FETO) may be done in cases of very low lung to head ratio that carry a very poor prognosis. In this procedure a fetoscope is inserted percutaneously through the uterus into the trachea of the fetus, and a balloon is deployed. The balloon causes the amniotic fluid in the lungs to buildup pressure and distend the airways, encouraging alveolar growth. The balloon must be removed prior to or at birth, as it would prevent adequate oxygenation after delivery [17].

## Anesthetic Management of CDH

Preoperative evaluation of a neonate prior to repair of a CDH should include assessment of current hemodynamic status and echographic assessment of ventricular function and pulmonary artery pressure. Review of current medications and inotropic infusions is imperative. It is important to evaluate if the patient is a candidate for ECMO and have the ECMO team on standby should intraoperative deterioration occur.

Lung protective ventilation strategies used in the ICU and described previously should be continued in the perioperative period. Intraoperative monitoring should include invasive blood pressure monitoring and pre- and postductal oxygen saturation measurement. Venous access should be sufficient for large-volume resuscitation and transfusion, as well as inotrope infusion. Central venous access may be helpful in this regard. Temperature must be meticulously controlled with forced-air warmers, fluid warmers, heating lamps, and elevated operating room temperature. Hypothermia can exacerbate pulmonary hypertension, worsen coagulopathy, and lead to poor enzymatic function. Normal intravascular fluid volume should be targeted. Blood product transfusion is common. Frequent arterial blood gas measurements will help guide intraoperative management to maintain acid–base balance. It is helpful to have iNO readily available should the patient decompensate.

Anesthesia can be maintained with muscle relaxants, narcotics, and potent inhalational agents. Nitrous oxide is avoided as it can distend bowel in both the abdomen and chest. Furthermore, it limits the ability to use a high inspired oxygen concentration. Oxygenation and ventilation are strictly monitored during closure of the abdomen, as patients are at risk of developing abdominal compartment syndrome. Elevated peak inspiratory pressures may be the first sign of abdominal tension that may require a staged closure of the abdomen. Controlled mechanical ventilation is usually continued postoperatively as impaired lung function is not corrected with the CDH repair.

In patients on ECMO, a narcotic-based anesthetic is often performed with use of muscle relaxants. Temperature can be carefully regulated by the ECMO machine. Medications, fluid, and blood products can be administered through the ECMO circuit or intravenously. The ECMO circuit increases the volume of distribution of drugs while the synthetic material of the circuit can absorb medications, making the dosing of lipophilic drugs, such as midazolam and fentanyl, unpredictable [17].

Neuraxial or regional analgesia is a reasonable option in very select patients with excellent pulmonary function and minimal comorbidities in order to facilitate early extubation. Thoracic epidural or paravertebral catheters can provide postoperative analgesia. Prior to placement of any neuraxial catheter, coagulation studies should be performed to evaluate for coagulopathy. In patients who will require multiple days of postoperative mechanical ventilation the risks of neuraxial catheter placement may outweigh the benefit. Extracorporeal membrane oxygenation is a contraindication to neuraxial anesthesia owing to the systemic anticoagulation required.

## Outcomes

Factors associated with poor long-term prognosis and decreased survival to discharge include prenatal diagnosis, prematurity, patch repair, need for ECMO, low birth weight, liver herniation, and major postoperative complication such as infection or abdominal compartment syndrome. Patients with coexisting complex congenital heart disease and/or a genetic syndrome have a worse prognosis [18].

Patients that survive into childhood often develop chronic conditions that require long-term follow-up. The most common comorbidities seen in these patients with repaired CDH include chronic lung disease, persistent pulmonary hypertension, recurrent CDH, synthetic patch infection or failure, developmental delay, feeding difficulties, and gastroesophageal reflux [19]. Many of these patients require multiple general anesthetics over their lifetime and careful preoperative assessment should be performed in all children and adults with a history of CDH repair.

# References

1. Clugston RD, Greer JJ. Diaphragm development and congenital diaphragmatic hernia. *Semin Pediatr Surg.* 2007;16(2):94–100.

2. Veenma DC, de Klein A, Tibboel D. Development and genetic aspects of congenital diaphragmatic hernia. *Pediatr Pulmonol.* 2012;47:534–45.

3. Langham Jr. MR, Kays DW, Ledbetter DJ, et al. Congenital diaphragmatic hernia: epidemiology and outcome. *Clin Perinatol.* 1996;23:671–88.

4. Pober BR. Genetic aspects of human congenital diaphragmatic hernia. *Clin Genet.* 2008;74:1–15.

5. McAteer JP, Hecht A, De Roos AJ, Goldin AB. Maternal medical and behavioral risk factors for congenital diaphragmatic hernia. *J Pediatr Surg.* 2014;49:34–8.

6. Colvin, J, Bower, C,Dickinson, JE, Sokol, J. Outcomes of congenital diaphragmatic hernia: a population-based study in Western Australia. *Pediatrics.* 2005;117:356–63.

7. Skari H, Bjornland K, Haugen G, et al. Congenital diaphragmatic hernia: a meta-analysis of mortality factors. *J Pediatr Surg.* 2000;35:1187–97.

8. Green JJ, Babiuk RP, Thebaud B, et al. Etiology of congenital diaphragmatic hernia: the retinoid hypothesis. *Pediatr Res.* 2003;53 726–30.

9. Zamora IJ, Olutoye OO. Prenatal MRI fetal lung volumes and percent liver herniation predict pulmonary morbidity in congenital diaphragmatic hernia (CDH). *J Pediatr Surg.* 2014;49(5):688–93.

10. Lally KP, Lally PA, Langham MR, et al. Surfactant does not improve survival rate in preterm infants with congenital diaphragmatic hernia. *J Pediatr Surg.* 2004;39(6):829–33.

11. Kim ES, Stolar CJ. ECMO in the newborn. *Am J Perinatol.* 2000;17(7):345–56.

12. Clark RH, Hardin WD Jr., Hirschl RB, et al. Current surgical management of congenital diaphragmatic hernia: a report from the Congenital Diaphragmatic Hernia Study Group. *J Pediatr Surg.* 1998;33:1004–9.

13. Tsao K, Lally PA, Lally KP, Congenital Diaphragmatic Hernia Study Group. Minimally invasive repair of congenital diaphragmatic hernia. *J Pediatr Surg.* 2011;46(6):1158–64.

14. Moss RL, Chen CM, Harrison MR. Prosthetic patch durability in congenital diaphragmatic hernia: a long-term follow-up study. *J Pediatr Surg.* 2001;36(1):152–4.

15. Yang EY, Allmendinger N, Johnson SM, et al. Neonatal thoracoscopic repair of congenital diaphragmatic hernia: selection criteria for successful outcome. *J Pediatr Surg.* 2005;40(9):1369–75.

16. Harrison MR, Keller RL, Hawgood SB, et al. A randomized trial of fetal endoscopic tracheal occlusion for severe fetal congenital diaphragmatic hernia. *N Engl J Med.* 2003;349(20):1916–24.

17. Vrecenak JD, Flake AW. Fetal surgical intervention: progress and perspectives. *Pediatri Surg Int.* 2013;29 407–17.

18. Wildschut ED, Ahsman MJ. Determinants of drug absorption in different ECMO circuits. *Intensive Care Med.* 2010;36:2109–16.

19. Wynn J, Krishnan U, Aspelund G, et al. Outcomes of congenital diaphragmatic hernia in the modern era of management. *J Pediatr.* 2013;163(1):114–19.

**Chapter**

# 28
# Congenital Heart Disease in the Neonate and Infant
## Cardiac Catheterization and Cardiac Surgery

Morgan L. Brown, James A. DiNardo, and Kirsten C. Odegard

## Prenatal and Neonatal Diagnosis

With the improvement in echocardiographic technology, many children with congenital heart disease (CHD) can be diagnosed prenatally. In general, an anatomic ultrasound is performed at 18–20 weeks' gestation. In the United States, prenatal detection rates of >50 percent have been reported for single ventricle lesions [1]. However, for two-ventricle lesions, the detection rate is usually less than 30 percent due to variations in quality of prenatal ultrasounds and access to prenatal care. Maternal and fetal risk factors such as first-degree relatives with CHD; in vitro fertilization; and chromosomal anomalies, extracardiac anomalies, or severe polyhydramnios may trigger fetal echocardiography to prenatally diagnose CHD [2].

Physical examination and pulse oximetry may be used to screen for CHD in the neonatal period [1]. In a recent meta-analysis, the overall sensitivity of pulse oximetry for detection of a critical heart defect was 76.5 percent (95 percent CI 57.7–83.5 percent) [3]. Despite advances in technology, some children will still present with new murmur, respiratory distress, decreased or absent peripheral pulses, or shock in the days and weeks following birth.

Neonates or infants who have been diagnosed with CHD should be reviewed with other tests, including an electrocardiogram for rhythm and a chest radiograph for the size and shape of the heart and the presence of pulmonary edema. Echocardiography is often performed in an unsedated neonate or infant; however, anesthesiologists may also be asked to provide sedation for a more thorough or complete transthoracic evaluation or for a transesophageal echocardiogram (TEE). Cardiac catheterization may be needed for diagnostic or therapeutic indications. A computed topography (CT) scan is often performed in infants in whom vascular anomalies may be present and

may be contributing to airway compression. Cardiac magnetic resonance imaging (CMRI) is becoming more common, as it provides important information regarding vascular anomalies, as well as precise measurements of left ventricular and right ventricular size. Several of these diagnostic tests will require anesthesia, and many will require intubation due to one or more of patient factors, the length of the procedure, or the requirement for breath holds to attain adequate images.

## Basic Principles of Management

It is important to recognize that despite the complexity of many congenital cardiac lesions, basic anesthetic principles remain a priority. Experienced congenital cardiac anesthesiologists are very much aware that the loss of an airway is still a major cause of morbidity or mortality in these infants. There are some general principles of anesthesia for neonates and infants with CHD that should be considered, although the specifics of the anesthetic plan are dictated by both the specific type of CHD and the severity of the disease. The patient's condition should be optimized as much as possible prior to proceeding with anesthesia. In general, diuretics are held on the morning of operation, while beta blockade, antiarrhythmics, and pulmonary antihypertensive agents are continued. The risks and benefits of continuing or stopping anticoagulation such as warfarin or aspirin should be discussed with cardiology and cardiac surgery services, as both thrombosis and bleeding can be life-threatening. Prevention of endocarditis is also an important aspect of anesthesia for CHD. These issues are discussed in more detail in Chapter 29.

All patients with intracardiac shunts are at risk of systemic air emboli. Even if shunting patterns are reported as left-to-right, transient right-to-left shunting may occur during the normal cardiac cycle and also during periods of anesthesia, such as intubation or extubation, when the pulmonary vascular resistance (PVR) might be elevated. Air traps or intravenous lines are advisable, although careful attention to detail and constant vigilance to purge air bubbles is the most important intervention to avoid a devastating systemic air embolus.

The preoperative period is an anxious time for parents and adequate preoperative discussion about anesthesia and the induction plan is essential. This discussion may take place in the preoperative clinic or in the hospital when the children are admitted. Clear fluids such as Pedialyte may be given up to two hours prior to operation. Breast milk may be given up to four hours prior to induction. Cyanotic or small infants may be admitted preoperatively for intravenous placement and hydration prior to cardiac catheterization or surgery.

In the majority of neonates, premedications are not administered until the patient is safely placed in the operating room or cardiac catheterization laboratory. A small dose of intravenous midazolam or fentanyl may facilitate monitor placement and avoid periods of extreme cyanosis due to agitation. Infants may receive premedication based on anticipation of a difficult separation from parents in the preoperative area or in patients who have limited hemodynamic reserve and who are unsuited for an inhalational induction. Oral premedication, such as midazolam, can act as an anxiolytic and may be combined with oral ketamine. Intramuscular premedication with midazolam and ketamine is very effective and is often more reliable due to difficulties some children have taking a premedication. Patients who receive a premedication should be carefully monitored, as the effect can be quite variable, especially in cyanotic patients who might have a decreased hypoxic drive to breath [4] and in children with decreased reserve.

Careful attention must be paid to detail at all times when giving anesthesia to patients with CHD. The cardiovascular system in the neonate and infant is primarily dependent on heart rate and preload for adequate cardiac output. While an intravenous induction is preferable, many neonates and infants may present without intravenous access or have very difficult intravenous access. The younger the patient, the more desirable is an intravenous induction. Neonates should be induced intravenously, but in older infants

some cardiac lesions may tolerate a low-dose inhalational anesthetic for intravenous placement, but care should be taken with aggressive inhalational inductions in all but the most straightforward of cardiac lesions. Other strategies such as intramuscular induction may need to be considered in order to be able to fully manage the airway, which may be necessary to avoid issues with prolonged inhalational induction. Following intravenous placement, consideration should be given to a fluid bolus with either crystalloid or a colloid such as albumin, prior to proceeding with induction, especially in patients who have a large fluid deficit, those on multiple diuretics, and children with left ventricular or right ventricular outflow tract obstructive lesions. Some patients may require low-dose inotropic support such as dopamine infusions or boluses of ephedrine, phenylephrine, or calcium gluconate in order to maintain adequate blood pressure and cardiac output during induction and the transition to positive pressure ventilation.

## Concomitant Issues

Chromosomal abnormalities have been reported with various frequencies in patients with CHD. DiGeorge syndrome, which has now been identified as a deletion in 22q11.2, deserves specific mention due to its prevalence in patients with CHD, specifically interrupted aortic arch and conotruncal defects such as truncus arteriosus, transposition of the great arteries, double outlet of the right ventricle, and Tetralogy of Fallot. 22q11.2 syndrome is also known as velocardiofacial syndrome. Patients who have DiGeorge syndrome have a small or absent thymus and need irradiated blood products to prevent graft-versus-host disease. These patients have hypoparathyroidism with resultant hypocalcemia. Also important for the anesthesiologist are the associated dysmorphic features of the head and oropharynx, which may make either bag-mask ventilation or intubation challenging.

Children with heterotaxy can have abnormal situs and the majority will have congenital cardiac anomalies. It is important to understand that these patients have many different cardiac anomalies, including single ventricles and complex venous anatomy [5]. When taking care of these patients, the anesthesiologist should also be aware of the multiple systemic manifestations of heterotaxy, including midline defects such as: cleft lip or palate; abnormal ciliary function which may result in impaired pulmonary function; and asplenia or polysplenia, which may result in abnormal immune function.

## Technical Procedures

For cardiac surgical procedures, including many cardiac catheterization or other diagnostic procedures required in neonates and infants, the anesthesiologist will be required to place an endotracheal tube. These endotracheal tubes may be placed either nasally, with potential benefits of decreased sedation requirements in the ICU and more stability; or orally, which are generally more easily placed.

Ventilation is critical to the successful management of children with CHD. Reductions or increases in PVR caused by mechanical ventilation should be appropriately managed with careful attention to the administration of oxygen and the degree of hyper- or hypocarbia in relation to the specific cardiac anatomy and physiology. In general, we aim for a slower respiratory rate and ventilate at tidal volumes of 8–10 ml kg$^{-1}$. Small endotracheal tubes may be susceptible to mucous plugging. However, suctioning of the airway should be done carefully in any patient who has systemic or suprasystemic right ventricular pressures, and it is often best to ensure adequate sedation and/or paralysis prior to doing so.

Venous and arterial access in neonates and infants can be a challenge. Many patients will be on prostaglandin infusion, or admitted for prehydration, and will have intravenous access in place before the procedure. It is important to distinguish patients who may not tolerate either any inhalational induction or a prolonged inhalational induction. Patients who present to the operating room without intravenous access, an oral or intramuscular premedication might be considered. If the child is insufficiently calm for placement of intravenous access, an intramuscular induction may be performed as long as the anesthesiologist feels comfortable about the ability to bag-mask ventilate and intubate without an intravenous line in place. There is much variation across different centers in terms of central venous access. Because of previous procedures, some vessels may be occluded. With ultrasound, the internal jugular vein is often the preferred location, although others prefer subclavian or femoral venous access. Some neonates may have an umbilical venous catheter, but these are usually removed after surgery due to the risk of infection. Patients who undergo primary sternotomy may not need central access if the surgeon provides a right or common atrial line prior to separation from bypass. Arterial access may be obtained in the radial or femoral arteries.

## Blood Products and Cardiopulmonary Bypass

The majority of neonates and infants with CHD will need blood or blood products at some point during their hospitalization. The risks of transfusion must be balanced with concerns related to systemic oxygen delivery in the setting of patients who may have cyanotic lesions or have poor cardiac output.

The bypass temperature, use of deep hypothermic circulatory arrest versus low-flow antegrade perfusion, the acceptable degree of hemodilution, the use of antifibrinolytics, the use of steroids, the choice of myocardial cardioplegic solution, the ideal arterial oygenation, and the flow on cardiopulmonary bypass remain controversial [6]. Some centers use miniaturized bypass circuits to reduce hemodilution and many use ultrafiltration to achieve the highest possible hematocrit following cardiopulmonary bypass. However, the vast majority of infants and neonatal patients will still require blood on cardiopulmonary bypass. In addition, many patients will require platelets and/or cryoprecipitate following cardiopulmonary bypass. Some institutions practice blood product administration algorithms, while others do not. It is beyond the scope of this chapter to discuss all the pertinent issues of bypass and blood products, as there is much variability between centers.

## Disposition

The majority of neonates undergoing cardiac catheterization or cardiac surgery will return to the intensive care unit postoperatively. In some cases, neonates or infants may be extubated in the cardiac catheterization laboratory or, less commonly, in the operating room. However, this practice should be based on multiple factors, including the comfort level of the intensivists and support staff in managing neonatal or infant airways.

## Neurodevelopmental Outcomes

There has been much interest in the last decade regarding the neurodevelopmental outcomes of patients with CHD. Of specific interest are those patients who had surgery in the neonatal period requiring deep hypothermic circulatory arrest. Variations in practice between surgical sites include duration of circulatory arrest, use of selective antegrade cerebral perfusion, cooling strategy, acid–base management during cardiopulmonary bypass (alpha versus pH stat), and hematocrit levels on cardiopulmonary bypass [7]. The effects of anesthetics on the neurodevelopmental outcome of patients with CHD are unknown, but are a subject of interest and research [8].

## Lesion Types

Congenital cardiac disease is a very complex topic and can be thought of in many different ways. We have chosen to classify cardiac lesions into six major categories; these are not mutually exclusive and patients may have combinations of these various lesions (Table 28.1). An understanding of the anatomy and physiology, along with the anesthetic implications of each type of lesion, will allow the anesthesiologist to safely care for any neonate or infant with CHD. However, this chapter should not be considered to be an exhaustive review.

## Left-to-Right Shunts

The degree of left-to-right shunt depends on the size of the defect, the compliance of the right and left ventricles, and the vascular resistance in the pulmonary and systemic circulations. Thus, as PVR begins to fall in the neonatal period, these lesions may present with heart failure symptoms due to an increase in the left-to-right shunt, excessive pulmonary blood flow, and the volume load imposed on the left side of the heart. If unrepaired, these patients may eventually develop pulmonary hypertension. Initial medical therapy consists of standard heart failure management including diuretic therapy. However, surgical repair may be required due to failure to thrive. Surgical treatment of a left-to-right shunt may include complete repair of the defect, or palliation with a pulmonary artery band to control pulmonary blood flow.

### Atrial Septal Defect

Atrial septal defects (ASDs) are divided into four standard types. The most common is the ostium secundum or fossa ovalis defect. The second most common is the ostium primum, which occurs with an atrioventricular septal defect (AVSD) or endocardial cushion defect. This type of ASD will be discussed more in detail under AVSD. The third type of ASD is a sinus venosus type which is associated with partial anomalous pulmonary venous drainage. Superior sinus venosus defects often involve communication between the upper and/or middle pulmonary veins and the superior vena cava, and inferior sinus venosus defects involve the right lower pulmonary vein and inferior vena cava. The fourth is the coronary sinus defect type which is a defect of the wall between the coronary sinus and the left atrium. There is often a persistent superior vena cava draining into the coronary sinus in these patients.

Patients with ASDs tend to be asymptomatic at birth. The degree of left-to-right shunting is determined by the relative right and left ventricular compliances. Patients are generally asymptomatic and the lesion is usually incidentally discovered. If left untreated, these patients will develop right atrial and right ventricular dilation due to volume overload on

**Table 28.1** Cardiac lesion divided by physiologic effect

Left-to-right shunts
  Atrial septal defects (ASDs)
  Ventricular septal defects (VSDs)
  Atrioventricular septal defect (AVSDs)
  Truncus arteriosus and aortopulmonary window
  Patent ductus arteriosus (PDA)
  Anomalous left coronary artery from the pulmonary artery

Left ventricular or systemic outflow obstruction
  Aortic coarctation
  Critical aortic stenosis
  Interrupted aortic arch
  Mitral stenosis

Inadequate pulmonary blood flow
  Critical pulmonary stenosis
  Pulmonary atresia, intact ventricular system
  Pulmonary atresia, ventricular septal defect
  Tetralogy of Fallot
  Ebstein's anomaly

Mixing lesions and single ventricles
  Transposition of the great arteries
  Hypoplastic left heart syndrome
  Tricuspid atresia
  Other single ventricles

Pulmonary venous obstruction
  Total anomalous pulmonary venous return
  Pulmonary venous obstruction

Airway obstructive lesions
  Tetralogy of Fallot with absent pulmonary artery
  Vascular rings
  Pulmonary slings

the right cardiac chambers. Longstanding atrial-level shunts can result in the development of atrial arrhythmias and pulmonary hypertension. Isolated secundum ASDs rarely need to be closed in infancy. Repair is undertaken when there is evidence of right ventricular volume overload, and usually at preschool age.

Surgical closure remains the gold standard for large secundum ASDs, sinus venosus ASDs, and coronary sinus ASDs. This is generally performed through a sternotomy with cardiopulmonary bypass. Considerations for anesthesia include potential for residual defects, atrial arrhythmias, and pulmonary hypertension. Pulmonary venous obstruction may occur with repair of venosus defects. Redirection of the IVC flow to the LA may occur with repair of secundum defects. Careful post-bypass assessment should be made using TEE.

Percutaneous closure of secundum ASD in infancy has been reported. This procedure generally requires general anesthesia. Transesophageal echocardiography in conjunction with cardiac catheterization imaging techniques are required to both size and place these devices. In a recent series of 128 patients with a mean age of 1.9 years (range 3 months to 4.9 years) there were five major complications, including stroke/seizure, complete heart block, mitral regurgitation, emergency surgery, and cardiac arrest [9].

### Ventricular Septal Defects

Ventricular septal defects (VSDs) are classified based on their anatomic location and have various nomenclatures. There are four types. Perimembranous is the most common VSD and is in the membranous region of the septum, under the aortic valve, closely associated with the tricuspid valve. These types of VSD rarely close when they are large, and do not restrict flow. The aortic valve leaflet may prolapse into the defect and result in aortic regurgitation. Muscular VSDs are located in the muscular septum. They may be multiple and can be Swiss-cheese-like. Small muscular VSDs may spontaneously close. An atrioventricular canal VSD is associated with an atrioventricular canal defect and is located in the inlet septum. The AVSD will be discussed more below. Lastly, the doubly committed subarterial VSD, is found between and just under the aortic and pulmonary valves. Subarterial VSDs do not close and the aortic valve may prolapse into the defect, leading to aortic insufficiency.

Children with large and unrestrictive VSD will present in infancy with congestive heart failure (CHF) and failure to thrive. There is evidence of left ventricular volume overload on echocardiography. Diuretics are usually prescribed and enteral tube feeding may be needed. Repair is recommended in the first year of life to prevent the development of pulmonary vascular disease. In patients without heart failure, and prolapse of the aortic valve into the VSD, developing aortic insufficiency will be an indication for surgery. Endocarditis is an uncommon indication. In a subarterial VSD, the presence generally indicates surgical repair.

Anesthetic considerations of nonrestrictive VSDs include the potential for excessive flow to the pulmonary vasculature. After induction, a significant drop on PVR should be avoided by decreasing inspired oxygen to room air and avoiding hypocarbia. Patients will generally have good ventricular function and if complete repair is planned, the ventricle postoperatively will have a decreased volume load. Rarely, inotropic support will be needed unless a ventriculotomy was required to close the VSD.

Ventricular septal defects are usually closed through a sternotomy on cardiopulmonary bypass. The approach to a VSD depends on location. Most perimembranous VSDs can be adequately accessed through an incision in the right atrium and visualized through the tricuspid valve. In some instances, the tricuspid valve may need to be detached to allow for adequate inspection. Other VSDs may require an incision in the right ventricle itself. Subarterial VSDs may be repaired through an incision in the right ventricle, but more commonly through an incision in the pulmonary artery. Occasionally an aortotomy may be required to repair both a subarterial VSD, as well as the aortic valve, depending on the degree of insufficiency.

Muscular VSDs may be closed in the cardiac catheterization laboratory. A combination of transesophageal imaging and cardiac angiography is required to adequately delineate anatomy and the relationship between the VSD and cardiac valves. If possible, the device is delivered from the venous side, but this requires a large sheath. VSDs are often technically easier to cross from the left side due to the presence of trabeculations in the right ventricle, which make wire placement difficult. Thus, the wire path can be either from femoral vein to right atrium to left atrium across the atrial septum. The wire then courses from the left ventricle through the VSD to the right ventricle, then through the tricuspid valve to the right atrium to the femoral vein or internal jugular vein. Alternatively, the wire can course from the aorta through the aortic valve, into the left ventricle, across the VSD, into the right ventricle, through the tricuspid valve and into the right atrium, where it can either exit to the femoral vein or internal jugular vein. A large sheath is then placed over the wire from the right ventricle to the left ventricle across the VSD and a device is deployed. Anesthetic concerns in this procedure include multiple access sites, arrhythmias, and low cardiac output caused by multiple wires and sheaths stenting valves open, necessitating inotropic support. There is also a high incidence of blood transfusion due to bleeding. Devices can also be embolized and can impinge on other cardiac structures, including valves [10].

In cases with multiple VSDs or in very small neonates, a pulmonary arterial band may be placed to control pulmonary blood flow. Banding of the pulmonary artery to reduce pulmonary blood flow is a difficult palliative procedure. If the band is too tight, severe cyanosis may occur; if the band is too loose, the increase in pulmonary blood flow will contribute to CHF and possibly increased PVR. Distortion, stenosis, and migration of the band may complicate later surgery, cause right ventricular hypertrophy, subaortic stenosis, and pulmonary valve stenosis. Determining the correct size of a band at the time of surgery is difficult and there are no accurate formulae for band size. Echocardiographic or direct pressure measurements may be used to adjust the band. At a subsequent operation to repair the VSD, the band will be taken down.

Transesophageal echocardiography is often used intraoperatively to assess the adequacy of repair. Epicardial echocardiography may also be used when TEE is contraindicated. Intraoperative calculation of any residual shunt is performed by identifying a "step-up" in the saturation measured from the superior vena cava and the main pulmonary artery. A shunt fraction (Qp:Qs) of greater than 1.5 is generally considered significant. Residual shunts are more commonly encountered when tackling multiple muscular VSDs. There is also a risk to the conduction system with perimembranous VSD repairs, with a risk of up to 2 percent requiring a permanent pacemaker [11].

## Atrioventricular Septal Defects

A common atrioventricular (AV) canal, complete ASD, or endocardial cushion defect consists of inlet atrial and ventricular septal defects and a common AV valve. There is shunting at both the atrial and ventricular levels. The ventricular defect may be large

and nonrestrictive. Clinically, the patients present in infancy with symptoms of CHF, as the physiology is determined by the degree of shunting at the ventricular level. In the spectrum of AVSD, the VSD may be restrictive or absent, making the primum ASD determine the clinical presentation. These are the transitional or partial AVSDs.

Patients with complete AVSDs may be medically managed with diuretic therapy and repaired at 3–6 months of age, prior to the development of pulmonary vascular disease. The surgical approach to this includes both closure of the ASD and VSD, but also division of the common AV valve into right- and left-sided valves. This may be accomplished with several different techniques, including a single patch, a modified single patch (Australian technique), or a two-patch technique. Closure of a cleft in the left AV valve is a routine part of the operation [12].

Anesthetic concerns in patients with AVSD include a large left-to-right shunt that may result in CHF and/or pulmonary hypertension. Maneuvers such as induction of anesthesia and mechanical ventilation, which further decrease PVR, or agents which act as myocardial depressants, may be poorly tolerated in these patients. These patients are at risk for residual ASDs or VSDs, and AV valve stenosis or regurgitation. Left ventricular outflow tract obstruction may also occur. Patients with trisomy 21 have an increased association with endocardial cushion defects and anesthetic concerns in these patients should include potential large tongues and c-spine instability, among others [13].

## Truncus Arteriosus

Truncus arteriosus is a relatively rare cardiac anomaly and is defined as a single arterial vessel arising from the heart, receiving blood from both ventricles, and supplying blood to the aorta, lung, and coronary arteries. The embryonic truncus fails to develop into two great arteries and straddles a large VSD. There is complete mixing of blood in the single great artery. One or two pulmonary arteries may arise from the single truncus. There is a single truncal valve which may be regurgitant or stenotic. As the PVR drops in the neonatal period, blood flow increases to the pulmonary circulation, which may result in increased arterial oxygen saturation and symptoms of CHF. Increasing pulmonary blood flow may create a steal phenomenon resulting in decreased systemic blood flow and cardiac output associated with low diastolic pressure causing insufficient blood flow to the coronary circulation, resulting in ischemia and ventricular fibrillation.

In a neonate or infant with truncus arteriosus, anesthetic management must be done carefully with attention paid to balancing the systemic and pulmonary circulation. Induction, specifically preoxygenation and hyperventilation, will decrease PVR, causing excessive pulmonary blood flow, systemic hypotension, and myocardial ischemia. In general, the patient is maintained on room air to increase the PVR and a narcotic-based technique is employed; agents that may cause myocardial depression should be avoided or administered very carefully, especially in those patients with truncal valve regurgitation or preexisting ventricular dysfunction. If measures to increase PVR do not decrease pulmonary blood flow, the cardiac surgeon may need to occlude a branch pulmonary artery to restore systemic perfusion pressures until cardiopulmonary bypass can be instituted. Repair of this lesion involves VSD closure, establishing right ventricle to pulmonary artery continuity with a homograft conduit, and repair of truncal valve regurgitation.

Following the repair of truncus arteriosus, measures should be taken to avoid any further pulmonary arterial hypertension and right ventricular dysfunction. Pulmonary hypertension can be anticipated in infants who present beyond the neonatal period and have preoperative elevation of pulmonary arterial pressures. Precautions against pulmonary arterial hypertensive crises should be taken, including hypoxia, hypercarbia, acidosis, pain, airway stimulation, and left ventricular failure. Any residual VSD will result in a volume and pressure load on the right ventricle, which may be a significant problem in the postoperative period. The majority of patients will require inotropic support for the right ventricle in the early postoperative period. Truncal valve stenosis or regurgitation may significantly impair left ventricular function and may necessitate re-repair or replacement with a homograft. Neonates with a right ventricle to pulmonary artery conduit are at risk for conduit compression and often undergo delayed sternal closure.

## Aortopulmonary Window

Aortopulmonary (AP) windows are caused by failure of fusion of separation of the truncus arteriosus in the developing fetus. This results in a connection between the aorta and pulmonary artery. These patients may be diagnosed after birth with a left-to-right shunt that increases as the PVR drops. The connection between the aorta and pulmonary artery can be small and restrictive, or can be large and result in tachypnea, poor feeding, and diaphoresis. If decreased systemic perfusion develops, one should consider measures to attempt to control shunting, including increasing PVR. If the connection is very large, bidirectional shunting can result in systemic desaturation. In the vast majority of cases, surgical closure remains the procedure of choice in which the aorta and pulmonary artery are divided and a patch placed between to eliminate the shunt. There are case reports of closure of anatomically favorable AP windows, closed in the cardiac catheterization laboratory using devices usually used for PDA or ASD closure [14]. Like most patients with large left-to-right shunts, they should do very well postoperatively [15].

## Patent Ductus Arteriosus

A PDA may be found in both the premature neonate, as well as in older infants. The PDA is a fetal vascular communication between the descending, usually just below the origin of the left subclavian artery, and the main pulmonary artery. During fetal circulation the ductus arteriosus is a conduit of blood for lower body systemic perfusion. As the PVR increases immediately at birth with the first breath, blood flow through the ductus may reverse right-to-left. The degree of shunting through the PDA is determined by both the resistance of the pulmonary and systemic vasculatures, as well as the diameter of the duct itself. Normally, the ductus will close shortly after birth. However, it may remain patent. As PVR falls in the neonate, a left-to-right shunt will ensue. If the PDA is large and nonrestrictive there will be excessive pulmonary blood flow, causing a volume load on the left ventricle and CHF. In addition, the left-to-right shunt will result in a low diastolic blood pressure due to the flow of blood to the pulmonary circulation in diastole. These "steal" effects of blood flow in systole and diastole may result in decreased end-organ perfusion.

The management of PDAs remains somewhat controversial, especially in premature neonates [16]. Indications to close a PDA include prolonged ventilation, evidence of left ventricular dilation suggesting volume overload, and gastrointestinal complications felt related to the left-to-right shunt. Indomethacin or ibuprofen may be used to medically close the duct. However, the use of nonsteroidal anti-inflammatory medications may be associated with risks including renal dysfunction, intracranial hypertension, and gastrointestinal complications [17].

When an isolated PDA is surgically closed, it usually consists of a left thoracotomy with ligation of the duct using clips. Cardiopulmonary bypass is not required. A PDA may also be ligated through a sternotomy when other procedures are necessary. In infants, a video-assisted thoracoscopic surgical (VATS) approach may be used to decrease pain postoperatively and improve cosmesis [18].

Some institutions prefer to perform this procedure in the neonatal intensive care unit, while others prefer to perform this in the operating room due to better lighting and suction in the event of any disastrous bleeding or inadvertent ligation of the descending aorta or left pulmonary artery. Anesthetic issues in the very premature infant include those of severe lung disease and the surgical requirement for lung retraction to identify and ligate the PDA. A decrease in lung volume, as well as an increase in lung compliance, often increases oxygen and ventilatory requirements. In general, a combination of narcotic and a paralytic are all that are required. Arterial pressure monitoring is rarely required. However, ligation of a significant PDA will often cause an immediate increase in the diastolic blood pressures and the sudden increase in afterload may cause some left ventricular dysfunction [19]. There is also the potential for transient or permanent injury to the recurrent laryngeal nerve, and this should always be considered in any patient who has stridor postoperatively [20].

In the interventional suite, PDAs may be percutaneously closed using a coil or other occlusion device [21]. This may be done under sedation or general anesthesia based on concomitant comorbidities and the preference of the interventional cardiologist.

### Anomalous Left Coronary Artery from the Pulmonary Artery (ALCAPA)

The left (or right) coronary artery arises anomalously from the pulmonary artery. In infant cases there is little to no development of coronary collaterals [22]. Due to the low diastolic pressures in the pulmonary arteries, these patients will have early onset of myocardial ischemia, which leads to left ventricular dysfunction and dilation, and is associated with mitral valve regurgitation. Any infant with left ventricular dysfunction should undergo diagnostic imaging to rule out ALCAPA. These patients may present incidentally and be profoundly ill and in shock, needing intubation and high-dose inotropic support. If these children are not intubated, induction should proceed very carefully with inotropic support readily available and often prophylactically initiated to avoid further cardiac ischemia. Repair usually involves transfer of the anomalous coronary artery to the aorta. Ventricular function will not improve immediately and these patients may require temporary mechanical circulatory support (ECMO). If patients with this anomaly present late, and ventricular function does not recover, they may be considered for longer-term mechanical support or cardiac transplantation.

## Decreased Systemic Blood flow

### Aortic Coarctation

Aortic coarctation occurs as a narrowing of the descending aorta near the insertion of the ductus arteriosus. Patients may have a concomitant hypoplastic aortic arch, aortic and mitral valve abnormalities, or VSDs. In the neonate who has severe aortic coarctation, the increased left ventricular afterload, and therefore left ventricular end-diastolic pressure, is not well tolerated in the noncompliant neonatal heart and will result in pulmonary hypertension. This increase in pulmonary arterial pressure will permit flow to the lower body through a patent ductus arteriosus. As the PDA closes, the lower limb pulses will become weak and may disappear. The baby may present with shock as the PDA closes. In neonates who present with this diagnosis, prostaglandins are usually started to maintain ductal perfusion to the lower body. In the most ill patients, left ventricular function may be depressed, but will likely recover with opening of the ductus by a reduction in the left ventricular end-diastolic pressure.

In general, neonates are operated on soon after the diagnosis is made. The optimal treatment is felt to be complete excision of all ductal tissue and an end-to-end or extended end-to-end repair. Alternatively, in extremely small children or long segment coarctation, the subclavian artery can be used as a flap to augment the aorta. This is well tolerated, but will result in decreased or absent pulses in the left arm. In general, patches, including Dacron, are avoided when possible, as patch material has been associated with late aneurysm formation [23].

Repair of isolated aortic coarctation is usually performed through a left thoracotomy incision, off-bypass. In these cases, there is a 10–25 minute period of aortic cross-clamping while the coarctation is excised and the repair is performed; during this period, the spinal cord is at risk of ischemic injury. Although the time of cross-clamp is probably the most important factor, it is extremely important to have careful anesthetic management, including maintenance of blood pressure through monitoring of right radial arterial pressures. Invasive monitoring of arterial pressures in the lower extremities may be helpful, but it is impractical in the neonate or infant with aortic coarctation, as they do not usually have sufficient collateral development. Patients who present with preoperative left ventricular dysfunction may require inotropic support during the repair. Hyperthermia is to be avoided, but mild hypothermia (33–35 °C) may be beneficial for spinal cord protection.

After aortic cross-clamp, hypertension proximal to the area of coarctation may develop. This can cause an abrupt increase in the left ventricular end-diastolic pressure and result in left ventricular dysfunction. Younger patients may not have collateral blood flow to the lower body, and in these patients care must be taken to avoid excessive vasodilation prior to repair, as it may result in decreased lower body perfusion.

Following repair and after removal of the cross-clamp, rebound hypertension may be a problem. Patients are also at risk for bowel ischemia due to insufficient flow in the mesenteric artery if hypertension is poorly controlled. Sodium nitroprusside, along with beta blockade, may be required in the early postoperative period until patients can be started on oral afterload-reducing agents such as an ace inhibitor.

Neonates or infants who present with coarctation may undergo balloon dilation of the descending aorta. Sometimes this may be done in the sickest neonates or those with other comorbidities, in order to palliate before surgical repair. However, neonates and infants have a high rate of reocclusion [24]. These procedures are generally performed under a general anesthetic as the balloon dilation can be very stimulating. It is important in these patients to monitor blood pressures in the right arm, and to pay careful attention to blood pressure control during and after the procedure.

## Critical Aortic Stenosis

Neonates with critical aortic stenosis will generally have fusion of various valvular commissures and it is often associated with left ventricular endocardial fibroelastosis. In addition, some of these patients may have associated mitral valve dysplasia or other types of left ventricular outflow tract obstruction. This lesion is poorly tolerated, and neonates will develop left ventricular dysfunction, which may even result in a right-to-left shunt at the PDA level and left-to-right shunting through an interatrial communication.

Medical management of these patients includes initiation of prostaglandin infusion to try to improve systemic perfusion and therefore decrease acidosis. Percutaneous balloon angioplasty is often the preferred treatment strategy, but may result in multiple complications, including residual aortic stenosis, persistence of left ventricular dysfunction, or aortic regurgitation. Aortic insufficiency is poorly tolerated [25].

Surgical management for these patients may include a surgical valvotomy, which must be performed on cardiopulmonary bypass. The risks of valvotomy are similar to those performed in the catheterization laboratory. In those cases where the left ventricle is small or if the mitral valve is sufficiently dysplastic, a decision may be made to proceed with a single ventricle palliation.

Anesthetic considerations in these patients are those of a neonate who has little myocardial reserve. A high-dose narcotic-based anesthetic is advantageous to maintain hemodynamic stability. If the child is not on inotropic support, it is advisable to initiate it prior to proceeding with induction of anesthesia. These patients may be dependent on ductal flow, and as such significant reductions in PVR will result in poor systemic perfusion and acidosis (avoid hyperventilation, hyperoxia, alkalosis, and hyperthermia). These patients will generally have a prolonged ICU course with need for inotropic support initially following even successful procedures.

## Interrupted Aortic Arch

In patients with an interrupted aortic arch (IAA), the aorta is completely interrupted at one or more points in the aortic arch. The most common site of interruption is between the left common carotid and the left subclavian artery, but the interruption may occur after the subclavian artery or, more rarely, between the innominate and carotid arteries. A nonrestrictive VSD, which is almost always present, and the PDA supply systemic blood flow below the interruption. Patients with interruption may have concomitant left ventricular outflow tract obstruction [26].

Patients with IAA at birth will appear well perfused due to the presence of a PDA and the high PVR of the newborn. If the diagnosis has not been made prenatally, the patient may present in shock as the PDA closes. A prostaglandin infusion is necessary to maintain lower body perfusion. If prostaglandins are not initiated, these neonates will begin to develop sequelae of inadequate lower body perfusion including lactic acidosis, hepatic and renal dysfunction, and gut ischemia. Patients presenting in shock are stabilized prior to surgical repair. Operative repair consists of a patch closure of the VSD and a direct anastomosis of the descending and the underside of the transverse arch.

A prostaglandin infusion should be continued in the operating room until the onset of cardiopulmonary bypass. Upper and lower body perfusion is monitored by cerebral and flank near-infrared spectroscopy (NIRS) and by nasopharyngeal and rectal temperature probes. If the flank NIRS is low and the rectal temperature does not decrease after cooling on cardiopulmonary bypass, these are indications of poor lower body perfusion. The surgeon may elect to additionally cannulate and perfuse through the PDA. This procedure requires a period of deep hypothermic circulatory arrest or antegrade cerebral perfusion. Anesthetic management is the same as in patients with critical aortic stenosis.

Residual lesions after repair include residual VSD, subaortic obstruction, or aortic arch gradient. These patients may later develop recurrent arch obstruction necessitating cardiac catheterization in later infancy or childhood.

### Mitral Stenosis

Mitral stenosis can occur at multiple levels, including supravalvular, valvular, and/or subvalvular. Supramitral rings are part of the Shone's complex (supravalvular mitral membrane, parachute mitral valve, subaortic stenosis, and coarctation of the aorta). Parachute mitral valves may have subvalvular obstruction.

In neonates or infants with severe congenital mitral stenosis, balloon dilation of the mitral valve may be an effective palliation, but there are risks for mitral regurgitation, arrhythmia, and stroke. Mitral stenosis will result in left atrial hypertension and associated pulmonary artery hypertension; if there is no ASD or PFO present decompression with an atrial septostomy may be required. The objective is to palliate the child to allow somatic growth, as there are no durable valve replacement options in neonates and infants.

There are few good options for surgical management of mitral stenosis. Repairs are possible, but difficult in neonates and infants due to the delicate valve tissue. Repairs must address all valvular levels of obstruction, but may not be durable. In general, prostheses are too large for these small patients. There has been some success in implanting an externally stented bovine jugular vein graft (Melody valve) in the mitral position, as it can be progressively dilated in the catheterization laboratory as the patient grows [27].

Anesthetic considerations of mitral valve stenosis include avoidance of tachycardia and reductions in afterload, as in any patient with left-sided obstruction. These patients may be at risk for atrial arrhythmias due to enlarged left atriums. Some patients with mitral stenosis will not tolerate any loss of atrioventricular synchrony and care should be taken when placing central venous access. In addition, these patients may have developed pulmonary hypertension associated with right ventricular hypertension and dysfunction, and avoidance of further precipitants is important. Inotropic support is often necessary from induction of anesthesia. After intervention on the mitral valve, there may be residual mitral stenosis and/or regurgitation. Implantation of a mitral prosthesis may lead to heart block or ischemia due to compression of the circumflex coronary artery. Sometimes, the prosthesis may need to be placed in the supra-annular position, within the left atrium.

## Decreased Pulmonary Blood flow

### Critical Pulmonary Stenosis

Infants with critical pulmonary stenosis have only a very small orifice across the pulmonary valve. In these patients pulmonary blood flow is dependent on an atrial-level right-to-left shunt and pulmonary blood flow with left-to-right flow through a PDA. Therefore, if the PDA closes after birth, they will become very cyanotic due to the absence of any other source of pulmonary blood flow. A prostaglandin infusion is used to maintain PDA patency. In general, these patients are reasonably stable and are taken for percutaneous pulmonary balloon dilation in the catheterization laboratory the first few days of life. Following the balloon dilation, it may take some time for improvement in the right ventricular hypertrophy to allow for antegrade flow through the right ventricular outflow tract.

Anesthetic considerations of critical pulmonary stenosis include those of a patient who has a ductal-dependent lesion including continuation of prostaglandins. The right ventricle may require inotropic support during the catheterization procedure. Pulmonary valve balloon dilation may result in regurgitation, which is generally well tolerated.

Those patients who fail percutaneous balloon dilation may undergo surgical valvotomy. Alternatively, the right ventricular outflow tract may be reconstructed with a transannular patch or a right ventricle-to-pulmonary artery homograft conduit. If there is a contraindication, a modified Blalock–Taussig (BT) shunt can be placed to maintain pulmonary blood flow. Considerations of a modified BT shunt are discussed below.

### Pulmonary Atresia, Intact Ventricular System

Neonates born with pulmonary atresia and intact ventricular septum (PA, IVS) often have a very small right ventricle and tricuspid valve. There is generally a plate-like obstruction between the right ventricle and the pulmonary arteries. These neonates are cyanotic and dependent on an adequate atrial-level shunt and pulmonary blood flow across a PDA. The size of the right ventricle and tricuspid valve will determine whether the patient is eligible for a two-ventricle repair, or needs single-ventricle palliation.

After prostaglandin initiation, these patients will undergo echocardiography and cardiac catheterization in order to assess the size of the tricuspid valve (TV), right ventricle, and the coronary anatomy. Some patients will have fistulous connections between the small hypertensive right ventricle and the coronary arteries. The coronary circulation may be dependent on these fistulous connections, so-called right ventricle-dependent coronary circulation. If the right ventricle is decompressed, with resultant decrease in pressures, flow through these fistulae will be impaired. The resultant myocardial ischemia can lead to cardiac arrest.

In the cardiac catheterization laboratory, attempts can be made to open the right ventricular outflow tract (RVOT). This may be done by either a stiff wire or a radiofrequency ablation catheter, followed by balloon dilation of the RVOT. In patients in whom the right ventricle and TV are clearly too small, the PDA may be stented to allow a reliable source of pulmonary blood flow. Alternatively, these patients may undergo a modified BT shunt in the operating room [27].

If the right ventricle and TV appear adequate for a two-ventricle repair and attempts to open the RVOT in the catheterization laboratory are unsuccessful, patients may go to the operating room for a transannular patch across the RVOT. A modified BT shunt may be added if there is concern for adequacy of pulmonary blood flow. Alternatively, a right ventricle to pulmonary artery conduit may be used for reconstruction of the RVOT.

These neonates are often intubated and in the intensive care unit. Like any patient with a patent PDA, there must be care taken to not cause excessive pulmonary blood flow. Most patients will be on room air and should remain on it, especially those patients with a patent PDA when a secondary source of pulmonary blood flow is created through the RVOT. The right ventricle is hypertrophied and may have resultant systolic and diastolic dysfunction. In patients with right ventricle-dependent coronary fistulae, right ventricular pressures must be maintained, as any drop will lead to resultant myocardial ischemia. These patients are especially at high risk during angiography, because, for several cardiac cycles there will be contrast medium, rather than blood, returning to the myocardium. If there is a suspicion of right ventricle-dependent coronaries on transthoracic echocardiography, the anesthesiologist should be adequately prepared with resuscitation medications, as well as plans for potential extracorporeal mechanical oxygenation (ECMO).

### Pulmonary Atresia With Ventricular Septal Defect

Pulmonary atresia with VSD is a spectrum of conditions in which there can be confluent, well-sized, central pulmonary arteries supplied by a PDA, with a single conoventricular VSD. These patients will present with cyanosis and require prostaglandins to secure pulmonary blood flow. Their repair involves VSD closure with reconstruction of the RVOT, usually with a homograft conduit. If there are contraindications to cardiopulmonary bypass, then a modified BT shunt can be used to palliate the patient.

At the other end of the spectrum, the central pulmonary arteries may be absent and the pulmonary vasculature is diffusely hypoplastic. These patients have major aortopulmonary collaterals (MAPCAs), which are fibromuscular collateral arteries that supply multiple or all segments of the lungs. These patients may present with only very mild cyanosis. There is usually no PDA present, or pulmonary blood flow may not be PDA-dependent. If the MAPCAs are significant in number and size, there may be CHF.

There are generally two repair strategies for these patients. The strategy chosen will depend on the size of any existing central pulmonary arteries and the institutional philosophy. In the staged approach, if there are accessible central hypoplastic pulmonary arteries, an aortopulmonary shunt can be constructed to promote pulmonary arterial growth. The same can be achieved with a right ventricle to pulmonary artery conduit. The right ventricle to pulmonary artery conduit has the advantage of allowing catheter-based imaging and interventions on the distal pulmonary vasculature. This will prevent systemic pressure in the pulmonary vasculature. This intermediate stage can require multiple operations through thoracotomies or sternotomies. The final stage will bring together the MAPCAs to the central pulmonary vasculature, so-called unifocalization, and reconstitute the right ventricle to the centrally reconstructed pulmonary artery using a conduit. Depending on the anatomic state of the distal pulmonary vasculature and the pulmonary artery pressures, the VSD may or may not be closed at this time.

Alternatively, the single-stage approach involves bringing together all the MAPCAs, and using existing pulmonary arteries to create a central pulmonary arterial confluence. A right ventricle to pulmonary artery conduit is used to reconstruct the RVOT. The VSD is closed, if pulmonary artery pressures permit. This single stage unifocalization has been advocated by Hanley at Stanford [29].

During unifocalization the anesthesiologist will be challenged during the dissection of the MAPCAs, as these are in the posterior mediastinum. The dissection is done prior to cardiopulmonary bypass. If the MAPCAs are not controlled, there will be a low perfusion pressure on bypass. After complete repair, the condition of the right ventricle should be carefully followed. VSD closure in the face of significant pulmonary vascular disease can precipitate right ventricular failure and right-to-left shunting at the atrial level. Single-stage unifocalizations can be long and complex procedures, followed by low cardiac output and bleeding from multiple suture lines.

Anesthesiologists may encounter these patients at different stages of their disease. It is important to know the details of the repair, the right ventricular function, source of pulmonary blood flow, and presence of ASDs or VSDs to formulate a detailed anesthetic plan.

## Tetralogy of Fallot

Tetralogy of Fallot (ToF) consists of right ventricular outflow tract obstruction (subvalvar, valvar or supravalvar obstruction), right ventricular hypertrophy, a perimembranous VSD, and an overriding aorta (Figure 28.1). In patients with ToF, there is resistance to pulmonary blood flow, encouraging desaturated blood from the right ventricle to the left ventricle through the VSD. The degree of shunting through the VSD is a dynamic process and is dependent on right ventricular outflow obstruction, resistance to pulmonary blood flow, and the systemic vascular resistance. The classic hypercyanotic "tet spell" is a process in which a combination of systemic vasodilation and dynamic right ventricular infundibular stenosis increases the right-to-left shunting. There is a subset of patients who do not have significant right-sided obstruction, and may behave more like a VSD ("pink tets") (see VSDs).

Neonates or infants with a history of cyanosis are generally treated with beta blockade, specifically propranolol. Beta blockade both decreases heart rate and also may decrease the degree of spasm of the right ventricular infundibulum. This medical management hopes to decrease the number and severity of hypercyanotic spells, to avoid repair until the child is older

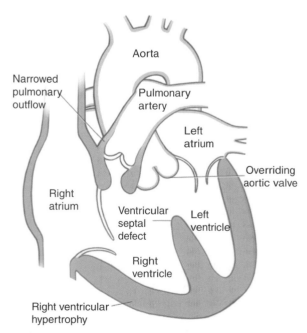

**Figure 28.1** Tetralogy of Fallot. The classic description of Tetralogy of Fallot includes right ventricular outflow tract obstruction, right ventricular hypertrophy, a VSD, and an overriding aorta. Source: [30].

and larger, usually more than three months. However, some children will continue to have significant problems with hypercyanotic spells despite adequate medical management, and may need intervention in the neonatal period.

Traditionally, neonates and infants with ToF have undergone only surgical repair due to difficult and unpredictable results with catheter-based interventions. However, a recent report from Birmingham Children's Hospital of pulmonary balloon valvotomy and stent placement in the RVOT in neonates and young infants with ToF demonstrated a procedural mortality of 1.9 percent and an early surgical reintervention rate of 5.7 percent [31].

Neonates or young infants who remain symptomatic (prostaglandin infusion dependent, frequent hypercyanotic spells, or progressive cyanosis) despite medical management, may undergo either a staged repair or a complete repair. A staged repair consists of a systemic to pulmonary artery shunt and may be chosen due to the size of the baby and technical issues such as abnormal coronary artery distribution. A complete repair is then performed, usually after three months. This includes taking down of the systemic-pulmonary shunt, closure of the VSD, and relief of the RVOT obstruction. Alternatively, a complete repair may be done as the initial operation in the symptomatic neonate. The differences in approach will depend on experience of the operator and the institutional philosophy. Advantages of an early anatomic correction include decreased stimulus for continued right ventricular hypertrophy, avoidance of cyanosis, and preservation of myocardial function. It also avoids the risks of a systemic-pulmonary shunt including shunt thrombosis, pulmonary artery distortion, and pulmonary vascular disease due to systemic pressures in the low-resistance pulmonary vasculature [32].

Closure of the VSD and relief of RVOT obstruction can be performed via the transatrial approach, through the right ventricle, or a combination. Relief of RVOT obstruction may involve resection of outflow tract muscle, outflow tract patch reconstruction, transannular patch reconstruction, pulmonary valvotomy, and/or pulmonary patch arterioplasty. Sometimes, an attempt is made to spare the pulmonary valve by a combination of valvotomy and intraoperative balloon dilation.

Anomalous coronary artery distribution occurs in fewer than 5 percent of patients, in which the right coronary artery arises from the left coronary artery and crosses the right ventricular outflow tract. In these cases, a right ventricle to pulmonary artery conduit may be required in order to successfully relieve the RVOT obstruction.

In patients with ToF who have not yet undergone complete repair, anesthetic management should consist of maintaining preload, avoid decrease in systemic vascular resistance, and avoiding increasing the dynamic right ventricular obstruction (avoid tachycardia, avoid hypovolemia, and catecholamine release such as pain). Traditional management of patients with hypercyanotic spells in awake children consists of oxygen, a knee-to-chest position, and morphine sulfate. This treatment allows for relaxation of the dynamic right ventricular infundibular stenosis and maintains systemic vascular resistance. If the patient remains cyanotic, IV fluids, as well as treatment with a vasopressor such as phenylephrine may be required. Additional treatment may include beta blockade such as propranolol or esmolol. If the hypercyanotic spell does not improve, anesthetizing the patients with further IV narcotics and careful administration of inhalational agents may help to relax the right ventricular infundibular stenosis. Careful attention to ventilation should include avoidance of high inspiratory pressures and short expiratory times to avoid further decreases in pulmonary blood flow. Ultimately, urgent surgical correction may be required in select cases. In the operating room, generally adequate anesthetic administration, volume administration, and/or phenylephrine administration will relieve the majority of hypercyanotic spells.

After surgical repair, the right ventricle must be supported when weaning from cardiopulmonary bypass by minimizing the afterload on the right ventricle. Immediately after repair, the right ventricle may have diastolic dysfunction caused by the ventriculotomy, pulmonary, and cardiac edema from bypass, and ischemia caused by inadequate myocardial protection of a hypertrophied right ventricle. One must be cognizant of the potential of coronary artery injury; residual outflow tract obstruction; residual VSD; and pulmonary regurgitation. Complete heart block and accelerated junctional rhythm may be problematic. In some patients the distal pulmonary arteries may be hypoplastic and stenotic. Systemic or suprasystemic right ventricular pressures should prompt a search for residual lesions. There may be right-to-left shunting across a residual interatrial communication, in the face of a compromised right ventricle. Desaturation may be traded for adequate cardiac output.

## Ebstein's Anomaly

Ebstein's anomaly consists of adherence of the tricuspid valve leaflets to the underlying myocardium ("failure of delamination"), downward or apical displacement of the functional tricuspid valve annulus, and dilation of the atrialized portion of the right ventricle. As a result of atrial dilation, atrial tachyarrhythmias are common, including Wolff–Parkinson–White syndrome and atrioventricular nodal reentrant tachycardia [33]. Ventricular arrhythmias may also occur due to profound right ventricular dilation and failure.

In the neonate, the elevated pulmonary arterial resistance accentuates the degree of tricuspid regurgitation, and results in right-sided heart failure and cyanosis. The severe tricuspid regurgitation can result in elevated right atrial pressures and cause a right-to-left atrial shunt across the patent foramen ovale (PFO) or ASD. The reduction in antegrade flow across the right ventricular outflow tract, which is termed "functional" pulmonary atresia, must be distinguished from true anatomic obstruction of the right ventricular outflow tract.

If the neonate survives, the degree of cyanosis and degree of heart failure may diminish as pulmonary pressures decrease. During this time period, pulmonary vasodilators such as nitric oxide may be used to unload the right ventricle and promote antegrade blood flow into the lungs. This may allow for improvement in right ventricular function.

In neonates who remain in CHF or are profoundly cyanotic with appropriate medical therapy, operation is required. There are three potential treatment pathways that can be considered in the neonate: the biventricular repair (Knott–Craig approach) [34], single ventricle repair, i.e., right ventricular exclusion technique (Starnes approach) [35], or cardiac transplantation. The biventricular repair includes subtotal closure of the ASD and repair of the tricuspid valve, which may be done in different fashions, including the Knott–Craig technique or the Cone repair [36]. The residual ASD is left to allow for right-to-left shunting in the presence of right ventricular dysfunction and high PVR. In the single ventricle approach, the tricuspid valve is patch-closed, the interatrial communication is enlarged to allow for complete mixing, and a systemic to pulmonary artery shunt is placed. A small fenestration may be placed in the tricuspid valve patch to allow for right ventricular decompression. If the right ventricular outflow tract is patent, the main

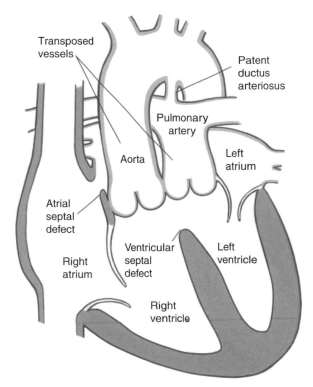

**Figure 28.2** D-transposition of the great arteries with a VSD. Many of these patients will have subpulmonary stenosis or left ventricular outflow tract obstruction, although not pictured here. There is mixing in this lesion at the PDA, ASD, and VSD levels. Source: [30].

pulmonary artery is often ligated to avoid persistent dilation of the right ventricle, which may eventually cause compression of the left ventricle. Rarely, cardiac transplant may be required.

Anesthetic concerns in Ebstein anomaly are primarily related to the profound degree of right ventricular dysfunction. In addition, patients who undergo tricuspid valve repair may have resultant tricuspid valve stenosis or regurgitation. Residual right-to-left shunt allows for the continued risk of paradoxical embolism. Arrhythmias can also be a significant problem and patients may require preoperative, intraoperative, or postoperative electrophysiologic procedures. In any patient who develops arrhythmias, early consultation with a congenital electrophysiologist is advised, as they can be very difficult to treat.

# Mixing Lesions and Single Ventricles

## Transposition of the Great Arteries

In patients born with transposition of the great arteries (d-TGA), the aorta originates from the right ventricle and the pulmonary artery originates from the left ventricle (Figure 28.2). Approximately half of these patients have a VSD and some will have sub-pulmonary stenosis, i.e., left ventricular outflow tract obstruction. Some patients will also have subaortic stenosis, i.e., right ventricular outflow tract obstruction. The latter group may also have aortic coarctation. In patients with d-TGA, pulmonary venous return is to the left atrium and is recirculated to the pulmonary vasculature without ever going to the systemic circulation. Systemic venous return is to the right atrium and right ventricle and goes to the body without passing the lungs, remaining unoxygenated. These are two circuits in parallel. The oxygen saturation is therefore higher in the pulmonary artery than the aorta, defining transposition physiology. For any oxygenated blood to reach the systemic circulation, mixing must occur through a PDA, an ASD, or a VSD. Inadequate mixing in the neonatal period will manifest as hypoxemia and metabolic acidosis. To temporize, an infusion of prostaglandin can be started to keep the PDA open, or an emergent balloon atrial septostomy may be required. The degree and direction of shunting through a PDA will be dependent on the underlying PVR and the degree of restriction in the atrial septum, as left atrial hypertension will cause an increase in pulmonary pressures.

When balloon atrial septostomy is performed emergently in the intensive care unit or more electively in the cardiac catheterization laboratory, neonates will usually be intubated due to cyanosis and will require sedation for the procedure. Echocardiography will establish the diagnosis and is usually sufficient to determine the coronary anatomy. Cardiac catheterization may be needed if the coronary anatomy is in question. In delayed presentations, catheterization is needed to assess PVR. High PVR should be suspected in the presence of reverse differential cyanosis, in which the saturations in the right hand are lower than those in the feet, suggesting significant shunting from right-to-left across the PDA.

Anesthetic management, maintenance of heart rate, contractility, and preload is needed to maintain cardiac output and mixing. A decrease in cardiac output causes decreased systemic venous saturation, which results in decreased arterial saturation. Prostaglandins need to be continued to maintain shunting at the PDA level. A decrease in SVR relative to PVR should also be avoided, because this could cause increases in systemic venous blood which could cause increasing cyanosis. A high-dose narcotic-based anesthetic will provide hemodynamic stability, without affecting the intercirculatory mixing.

In order to return an in-series circulation in a corrective procedure, there must be a "switch" at either the atrial or arterial level. The original atrial-level switches were the Mustard and Senning operations. These are baffles created in the atria to direct systemic venous return (SVC and IVC flow) to the left ventricle, which is the pulmonary ventricle. Long term, these patients have problems with baffle obstructions or leaks, atrial arrhythmias, and right ventricular failure, as the morphologic right ventricle remains the systemic ventricle. Since the 1980s, the majority of patients with d-TGA have undergone an arterial switch procedure. In this operation, the aorta and pulmonary arteries are switched. The pulmonary valve becomes the neoaortic valve. The coronary arteries must be transferred to the neoaortic root, which was originally the pulmonary root. The ASD is closed during a brief period of hypothermic circulatory arrest. If present, the VSD is closed. The long-term results of the arterial switch operation are excellent [37].

Intraoperative issues with the arterial switch procedure include bleeding due to multiple suture lines and coagulopathy from the use of hypothermic circulatory arrest. Coronary ischemia from problems with the coronary transfer may lead to ventricular dysfunction. Coronary problems may be more prevalent with some of the anatomic variations of coronary artery anatomy in d-TGA. In the rare circumstances when the patient without VSD presents after a few weeks, the left ventricle may be unprepared to handle systemic afterload, and may require temporary mechanical support after arterial switch.

In patients with significant subpulmonary stenosis and a VSD, an aortic root translocation procedure (Nikaidoh operation) may be needed, in which the entire aortic root is moved over the left ventricle. The RVOT is reconstructed with a conduit. The Nikaidoh operation is also an option in double outlet right ventricle, VSD, and significant pulmonary stenosis.

### Hypoplastic Left Heart Syndrome

Hypoplastic left heart syndrome (HLHS) is the most common example of single ventricle physiology (Figure 28.3). In these patients there is severe stenosis or atresia of the mitral and aortic valves. In the most extreme cases, the left ventricle is almost absent, with atretic mitral and aortic valves and a diminutive

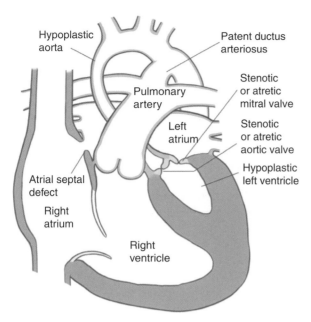

Figure 28.3 Hypoplastic left heart syndrome. This lesion is characterized by small left-sided structures including mitral stenosis or atresia and aortic stenosis or atresia. There is also a very small ascending aorta and hypoplastic aortic arch. Source: [30].

ascending aorta, giving rise to the coronary arteries. The aortic arch is also small, with a significant coarctation. Pulmonary venous return enters the small left atrium and is then shunted across the atrial septum, where complete mixing of the venous return occurs. The right ventricle pumps blood to the pulmonary artery, providing systemic blood flow through a PDA (right-to-left flow).

Most commonly these patients are diagnosed prenatally and are placed on prostaglandins to maintain the PDA soon after birth. In an undiagnosed patient with HLHS, the neonate will become acidotic as the PDA begins to close and insufficient cardiac output reaches the body. The arterial oxygenation may remain high. Once the PDA reopens, with the improvement in systemic perfusion, the metabolic acidosis should resolve and a corresponding drop in the arterial oxygenation is observed. Some patients will have associated poor right ventricular function or tricuspid regurgitation and will require inotropic support. These patients will require a period of stabilization before repair.

The first step in the palliation on HLHS involves using the single right ventricle as the systemic ventricle and providing a reliable source of pulmonary blood flow. Depending on institutional preferences

and results, the options include the hybrid stage 1 operation or the operative stage 1 (modified Norwood procedure). The hybrid procedure is usually performed in the cardiac catheterization laboratory in combination with the operating room team. To ensure systemic circulation from the right ventricle, the PDA is stented. The stented PDA provides pulmonary blood flow, so bilateral PA bands are placed to protect the pulmonary vascular bed. A median sternotomy is usually required. If necessary, a balloon atrial septostomy is done to ensure complete mixing of the circulations. These interventions can occur simultaneously or be staged.

The operative stage 1 or modified Norwood operation involves a Damus–Kaye–Stansel (DKS) anastomosis between the pulmonary artery and aorta with patch augmentation of the ascending aorta and arch. An atrial septectomy is performed for complete mixing. To establish pulmonary blood flow a modified BT shunt or a Sano shunt are used. The modified BT shunt is a systemic to pulmonary shunt created from the right subclavian artery or the innominate artery to the right pulmonary artery using a Gortex tube. The Sano shunt is a right ventricle to pulmonary artery conduit, using a ringed Gortex tube.

Because the right ventricle provides both systemic and pulmonary blood flow, the relative flows through each bed will be determined by the resistances in each. The objective of care is to "balance" pulmonary and systemic circulations to achieve adequate systemic perfusion. This usually means a Qp/Qs of 1–2 and a systemic saturation of 80–85 percent (assuming fully saturated pulmonary venous return and a mixed venous oxygen saturation of 60–65 percent). It is very easy to "unbalance" the circulation, which results in pulmonary overcirculation and systemic hypoperfusion. Pre-procedure management of neonates involves maneuvers that preserve systemic perfusion while avoiding excessive pulmonary blood flow. A high-dose narcotic-based anesthetic is advantageous in these patients too, to maintain hemodynamic stability. Excessive pulmonary blood flow will volume-load the systemic right ventricle, and decrease the systemic flow, so PVR needs to be kept high to avoid acidosis and hypotension. Other maneuvers include: avoiding hyperthermia; judicious use of oxygen; avoidance of hypocarbia and alkalosis. Patients will often require inotropic support before induction and intubation due to the decrease in PVR caused by intubation and mechanical ventilation. It can be very difficult to manage these patients, so careful attention must be paid to avoid further reduction in PVR. Increased pulmonary blood flow and decreased systemic blood pressure will cause a drop in diastolic blood pressure and decreased coronary blood flow. Runoff and decreased diastolic pressure is the reason there is a high incidence of coronary ischemia and ventricular fibrillation in neonates undergoing the stage 1 operation.

After a stage 1 procedure, neonates will often require inotropic support, bleed from multiple suture lines, and develop coagulopathy from hypothermia and a long bypass time. The sternum is often left open and closed after a few days; in the meantime the patient will remain sedated and chemically paralyzed. Events such as arrhythmias or impaired ventilation causing increasing PVR and increased right ventricular afterload, can result in cardiac arrest, often rescued with ECMO support.

After 3–6 months, patients who have had the hybrid stage 1 procedure will undergo a comprehensive stage 2 operation, involving reconstruction of the arch, a DKS procedure anastomosis, removal of PDA stent, takedown of pulmonary artery bands, and a bidirectional Glenn shunt. If the patient had an operative stage 1 or modified Norwood operation, these infants will undergo a bidirectional Glenn procedure in which the superior vena cava is connected to the pulmonary artery. At this time the Sano or modified BT shunt will be taken down. In patients who have had a modified BT shunt, care must be taken to maintain SVR during induction, since pulmonary blood flow is dependent on blood pressure to force blood through a now often small, restrictive BT shunt. Patients after a BT shunt might still have a low diastolic pressure predisposing them for coronary ischemia due to runoff. Care should also be taken to ensure that noninvasive and invasive blood pressure measurements are taken on the opposite side of the BT shunt, or at least compared with the operative side to determine if there is any gradient. Patients who have had a Sano shunt as part of the stage 1 procedure are thought to be at decreased risk of coronary ischemia. However, due to the need for an incision in the right ventricle, there is potential for right ventricular dysfunction. The bidirectional Glenn procedure is generally well tolerated and many patients can be extubated the same day or the next day. Patients following a bidirectional Glenn procedure may be quite irritable and hypertensive, likely secondary to the increase in intracranial pressure due to the higher venous pressures. As the body accommodates to the new circulation, central venous pressures will fall and the irritability will resolve.

Patients who are scheduled for a bidirectional Glenn are often cyanotic. The cyanosis may have multiple causes, including that the child has "outgrown" the shunt, obstruction of the shunt, pulmonary artery stenosis, or severe ventricular failure with a low systemic mixed venous oxygenation. Underlying pulmonary disease with pulmonary hypertension, or systemic-pulmonary venous collaterals can also contribute to cyanosis. Patients may undergo either a cardiac MRI or a cardiac catheterization prior to a bidirectional Glenn procedure to delineate causes of cyanosis.

In patients who require anesthesia who have a bidirectional Glenn procedure, most will accommodate a careful inhalational induction. However, as soon as IV access is obtained, a fluid bolus is generally warranted, since patients with bidirectional Glenn physiology are preload dependent. The anesthesiologist should note that fluids from the lower half of the body will directly return to the heart, while fluid from the upper extremity, must first traverse the pulmonary circulation.

## Tricuspid Atresia

In neonates born with tricuspid atresia there will be an imperforate tricuspid valve, as well as a hypoplastic right ventricle. These patients often have a concomitant VSD and some degree of pulmonary stenosis. The great arteries may be transposed. An ASD or PFO is necessary for systemic and pulmonary venous return to mix completely and reach the left ventricle. If the great vessels are not transposed, the extent of cyanosis is determined by the degree of subpulmonary obstruction and/or by restriction of the VSD, as the blood from the left ventricle must cross to the right side of the heart through a VSD to provide pulmonary blood flow.

Medical management of patients with tricuspid atresia will often include initiation of prostaglandins to maintain ductal patency if there is no VSD, to provide adequate pulmonary blood flow. A surgical or balloon atrial septostomy may be needed if there is a restrictive ASD for right-to-left shunt at the atrial level. Neonates and infants with tricuspid atresia may require early operation in the form of a BT shunt if they are excessively cyanotic. A PDA stent is another option to ensure reliable pulmonary blood flow. A pulmonary artery band might be needed if the child has excessive pulmonary blood flow from a VSD and no pulmonary outflow gradient. Others may remain well balanced and avoid operation in the neonatal period. These patients will generally proceed down a "single ventricle pathway" that will include eventual bidirectional Glenn and Fontan operations.

The anesthetic considerations of a neonate or infant with tricuspid atresia are those of any child with single ventricle physiology (balance PVR versus SVR). Over time, patients with a left ventricle as the systemic ventricle will fare better than those whose primary ventricle is a morphologically right ventricle [38].

### Single Ventricles With Impaired Pulmonary Blood flow

There are many other types of single ventricle lesions, although the classic descriptions are HLHS and tricuspid atresia. Patients who have adequate mixing, with an unrestrictive atrial septum, and have a reliable source of pulmonary blood flow (i.e., not ductal-dependent, with restricted antegrade pulmonary blood flow from the heart), might not need an intervention in the neonatal period. Sometimes the patient's first intervention is a bidirectional Glenn procedure. However, if the patient becomes cyanotic, there may be need for an early systemic to pulmonary artery shunt. This can be in the form of a PDA stent in the cardiac catheterization laboratory or a BT shunt in the operating room.

Patients who go to the cardiac catheterization lab will generally have the prostaglandins turned off prior to the procedure if the PDA is large. If the PDA is too large, there is a risk of stent embolization into either the pulmonary arteries or the aorta. As in many patients with single ventricles, inotropic support may be required during induction and the procedure. When crossing the PDA, there is risk of spasm and resulting cyanosis. During this portion of the procedure, additional oxygen may be administered. Careful management must be undertaken to ensure appropriate balance between systemic and pulmonary circulations.

Many patients will need to go to the operating room for placement of a modified BT shunt. This is performed through a sternotomy or thoracotomy, depending on the underlying anatomy of the aortic arch and its branches and preference of the surgeon. Sternotomy allows for easy access to the right and main left pulmonary arteries and allows for the use of cardiopulmonary bypass in those children who

will not tolerate clamping of the pulmonary artery for placement of the shunt.

Opening of the shunt results in immediate flow into the pulmonary arteries. This flow is continuous and occurs both in systole and diastole. As a result, there is generally a lower diastolic pressure, which might result in inadequate flow to the coronary arteries. These shunts have a propensity to thrombose, particularly if there are competing sources of pulmonary blood flow. Desaturation should raise suspicion for shunt thrombosis. Absence of a continuous murmur can aid in the diagnosis. In patients whose only source of pulmonary blood flow is the shunt, hypotension will ensue. Temporizing measures include increase systemic blood pressure to drive blood through the shunt and bolus administration of heparin. Immediate reopening of the sternum and "milking" of the shunt is required. Cardiopulmonary bypass or ECMO may need to be instituted. Due to this risk of thrombosis, surgeons may avoid antifibrinolytics or other procoagulant blood products or agents during the shunt procedure unless absolutely required for bleeding. In addition, these patients will receive postoperative anticoagulation.

In patients with large shunts, systemic perfusion may be compromised due to excessive pulmonary blood flow (sometimes referred to as "pulmonary overcirculation"). This can result in progressive lactic acidosis. The volume loaded single ventricle may become dysfunctional, with impaired cardiac output and further compromise systemic perfusion. It is important to adjust ventilation to avoid hypocapnea and respiratory alkalosis. Room air should be used as much as possible. The first manifestation of "overcirculation" may be systemic saturations above 90 percent. Systemic desaturation may be a result of reduced mixed venous saturation from low cardiac output, which is still a manifestation of "overcirculation." Systemic saturation alone is an unreliable indicator of "pulmonary overcirculation." One must carefully follow the indicators of adequate systemic oxygen delivery, including lactate levels, mixed venous saturation, urine output, and cerebral oxygenation values.

## Pulmonary Venous Obstruction

### Total Anomalous Pulmonary Venous Return

Obstructed total anomalous pulmonary venous return (TAPVR) is one of the only true surgical emergencies in congenital cardiac surgery. Neonates who are born with TAPVR are cyanotic because all of the pulmonary veins connect to a systemic vein. This results in both oxygenated and unoxygenated blood returning to the right atrium. A PFO or ASD must be present to allow for a right-to-left shunt, to allow for systemic blood delivery. If there is no pulmonary venous obstruction, this extra volume load will cause progressive right ventricular dilation. However, in those patients with pulmonary venous obstruction, pulmonary edema will develop with low cardiac output and progressive cyanosis in the neonatal period. This subset of patients require an emergent operation to relieve the pulmonary venous obstruction and return the pulmonary venous return to the left atrium.

There are four types of TAPVR based on the location of the venous connection. Supracardiac type involves a connection to the superior vena cava, innominate, or azygous vein. The cardiac type drains directly to the right atrium or into the coronary sinus. The infracardiac type drains infradiaphragmatically. Lastly, there is a mixed type of TAPVR, which is any combination of the others as described above. The infracardiac type is the most likely to develop obstruction.

Patients with obstructed TAPVR may be critically ill due to severe pulmonary edema and pulmonary hypertension. Resuscitation may be required, including mechanical ventilation and inotropic support. Agents that increase pulmonary blood flow, such as prostaglandins or nitric oxide, are best avoided, as in the setting of obstruction it will simply worsen pulmonary edema. Medical therapy is limited and these patients require urgent intervention. There are some reports of catheter-based interventions with stenting of the obstruction [39]. This is only palliative, but may be preferred in extremely small neonates or children with multiple other major congenital anomalies or contraindications to cardiopulmonary bypass.

Current therapy for TAPVR is a sutureless pulmonary vein repair in which the left atrium is sutured to the pericardium around where the pulmonary vein enters the confluence, so as to avoid sutures in the pulmonary veins and confluence themselves. This is usually performed under circulatory arrest or a low-flow state, for optimal visualization when suturing behind the heart. The interatrial communication is closed with a fenestrated patch. Complications from sutureless repair include bleeding, coagulopathy, pulmonary venous obstruction, and a highly reactive pulmonary vascular bed with right ventricular failure.

Pre-repair anesthetic considerations in these patients include those of a large right-to-left shunt preoperatively in unobstructed patients. In those with obstructed TAPVR, neonates may be very ill, cyanotic, and require ongoing resuscitation until they can be placed on cardiopulmonary bypass. Post-bypass, aggressive treatment of coagulopathy is necessary. In addition, treatments for pulmonary hypertension should be considered, including oxygen, avoidance of hypercarbia, suppression of catecholamines, muscular paralysis, and nitric oxide. Inotropic support will likely be needed to support the right ventricle. The sternum will often be left open.

### Pulmonary Vein Stenosis

Neonates and infants can be diagnosed with primary or secondary pulmonary vein stenosis. Stenoses can involve a single vein or multiple veins. Primary pulmonary vein stenosis is associated with prematurity and there is no associated CHD. Secondary pulmonary vein stenosis is associated with CHD and may occur in patients with previous TAPVR repair, whether sutureless or not. The consequence of multivessel pulmonary vein stenosis is right ventricular hypertension.

In this condition, there are few options. Primary or repeat sutureless repair may be attempted, or intervention such as balloon dilation and/or stenting may be done in the catheterization laboratory. There are also multiple investigational medical therapies. However, the prognosis for these patients is guarded [40]. Lung transplantation can be offered, but donor lungs are a limited resource, especially for young patients.

Anesthetic implications of pulmonary vein stenosis include careful induction in the presence of right ventricular hypertension. Systemic hypotension should be avoided and aggressively treated. Patients who have extensive reopening of obstructed pulmonary veins in the operating room or in the cardiac catheterization laboratory are at risk of pulmonary edema, which may manifest as pulmonary hemorrhage. Attention to the endotracheal tube and administration of diuretics is often required. Many of these patients will return to the ICU intubated and will undergo repeated interventions on one or several pulmonary veins.

# Lesions With Airway Involvement

### Tetrology of Fallot with Absent Pulmonary Valve

Tetrology of Fallot with absent pulmonary valve is an unusual condition. Due to the lack of a pulmonary valve in utero, the severe pulmonary regurgitation can cause severe pulmonary artery dilation resulting in airway compression, severe obstructive lung disease, and a decrease in the number of alveoli [41].

Management of these patients includes closure of a VSD and plication of enlarged pulmonary arteries. It is generally advisable to consider these patients to be similar to those with an anterior mediastinal mass, and to carefully undertake the transition to positive pressure ventilation and paralysis. These patients may be challenging to ventilate postoperatively, with some infants requiring ventilation due to an inability to wean from mechanical ventilation.

### Vascular Rings

Vascular rings include a double aortic arch; a right aortic arch with either an aberrant left subclavian artery with a left ligamentum arteriosum or mirror-image branching with right ligamentum arteriosum; a left aortic arch with an aberrant right subclavian artery or a right descending aorta and right ligamentum arteriosum; or an anomalous innominate artery. In all of these anatomic variations there is a vascular structure surrounding or compressing the trachea and esophagus. Compression of the airway for even a short period of time can lead to significant tracheomalacia. Airway compression will cause stridor or respiratory distress [42]. Many patients will be mislabeled as asthmatic until the correct diagnosis of vascular compression is made. It is unusual to have symptoms related to esophageal compression early in life.

Computed tomography or magnetic resonance imaging will diagnose the vascular ring. The CT scan can delineate the airway anatomy, including tracheomalacia. Fiberoptic or rigid bronchoscopy is also performed to assess the airway. In the symptomatic patient, there is no medical or percutaneous management of a vascular ring.

The surgical approach will vary depending on the anatomy. Most lesions can be approached through a left thoracotomy, especially the most common ones (double aortic arch and right arch with left ductal ligament). In neonates and infants, lung isolation is generally not required, as the surgeon can retract the lung effectively. A VATS approach has been described. Vascular rings can also be repaired through a sternotomy if there are concomitant procedures required. A combination of upper and lower limb arterial lines, blood pressure cuffs, and pulse oximetry should be used, aiding the surgeon to correctly identify the appropriate vascular structures. Significant bleeding is rare, but can be catastrophic, so appropriate intravenous access is required.

### PA Slings

In a pulmonary artery sling, the left pulmonary artery (LPA) arises from the right pulmonary artery (RPA), coursing between the trachea and the esophagus. The ligamentum arteriosus runs anteriorly from the RPA to the aorta, creating a vascular ring that surrounds the trachea, but not the esophagus.

These patients are often identified by feeding or respiratory difficulties. Anterior compression of the esophagus on a swallowing study is characteristic of this lesion. Almost 50 percent of these patients will have concomitant CHD and 50 percent of patients have associated complete tracheal rings. In general, surgical repair is only done if the child demonstrates significant respiratory symptoms. The abnormal take-off of the LPA rarely has any hemodynamic consequence and is not an indication for operation.

The approach to a pulmonary artery sling is determined by the presence of concomitant CHD and/or abnormal tracheal findings. Simple tracheal compression caused by the abnormal pulmonary artery can be relieved by translocation of the left pulmonary artery from its origin on the right to the left side. However, pulmonary artery slings are associated with stenosis of the trachea, especially with complete rings, and may require tracheal reconstruction with a slide tracheoplasty.

Anesthetic concerns relate to the presence of tracheomalacia or tracheal stenosis with complete tracheal rings. This requires careful airway management with appropriate selection and positioning of the endotracheal tube. The concomitant heart lesions will also dictate the anesthetic plan.

## References

1.  Mahle WT, Newburger JW, Matherne GP, et al. Role of pulse oximetry in examining newborns for congenital heart disease: a scientific statement from the American Heart Association and American Academy of Pediatrics. *Circulation*. 2009;120:447–58.

2. Fetal Echocardiography Task Force, American Institute of Ultrasound in Medicine Clinical Standards Committee, American College of Obstetricians and Gynecologists, Society for Maternal-Fetal Medicine. AIUM practice guideline for the performance of fetal echocardiography. *J Ultrasound Med.* 2011;30:127–36.

3. Thangaratinam S, Brown K, Zamora J, et al. Pulse oximetry screening for critical congenital heart defects in asymptomatic newborn babies: a systemic review and meta-analysis. *Lancet.* 2012;379:2459–64.

4. Edelman NH, Lahiri S, Braudo L, et al. The blunted ventilatory response to hypoxia in cyanotic congenital heart disease. *N England J Med.* 1970:282;405–11.

5. Williams GD, Feng A. Heterotaxy syndrome: implications for anesthesia management. *J Cardiothorac Vasc Anesth.* 2010;24:834–44.

6. Prouard P, Bojan M. Neonatal cardiopulmonary bypass. *Semin Thorac Cardiovasc Surg Pediatr Card Surg Annu.* 2013;15:59–61.

7. Tabutt S, Gaynor JW, Newburger JW. Neurodevelopmental outcomes after congenital heart surgery and strategies for improvement. *Curr Opin Cardiol.* 2012:27:82–91.

8. Olsen EA, Brambrink AM. Anesthetic neurotoxicity in the newborn and infant. *Curr Opin Anaesthesiol.* 2013;26:677–84.

9. Bartakian S, Fagan TE, Schaffer MS, et al. Device closure of secundum atrial septal defects in children <15 kg: complication rates and indications for referral. *JACC Cardiovasc Interv.* 2012;5:1178–84.

10. Laussen PC, Hansen DD, Perry SB, et al. Transcatheter closure of ventricular septal defects: hemodynamic instability and anesthetic management. *Anesth Analg.* 1995;80:1076–82.

11. Anderson BR, Stevens KN, Nicolson SC, et al. Contemporary outcomes of surgical ventricular septal defect closure. *J Thorac Cardiovasc Surg.* 2013:145:641–7.

12. Karl TR, Provenzano SC, Nunn GR, et al. The current surgical perspective to repair of atrioventricular septal defect with common atrioventricular junction. *Cardiol Young.* 2010;20:120–7.

13. Mitchell V, Howard R, Facer E. Down's syndrome and anaesthesia. *Paediatr Anaesth.* 1995;5:379–84.

14. Noonan PM, Desai T, Degiovanni JV. Closure of an aortopulmonary window using the Amplatzer Duct Occluder II. *Pediatr Cardiol.* 2013;34:712–14.

15. Barnes ME, Mitchell ME, Tweddell JS. Aortopulmonary window. *Semin Thorac Cardiovasc Surg: Pediatr Card Surg Annu.* 2011:14:67–74.

16. Noori S. Patent ductus arteriosus in the preterm infant: to treat or not to treat? *J Perinatol.* 2010;30:S31–7.

17. Ramagnoli C, Bersani I, Rubortone SA, et al. Current evidence on the safety profile of NSAIDs for the treatment of PDA. *J Matern Fetal Neonatal Med.* 2011;24:10–13.

18. Chen H, Weng G, Chen Z, et al. Comparison of posterolateral thoracotomy and video-assisted thocoscopic clipping for the treatment of patent ductus arteriosus in neonates and infants. *Pediatr Cardiol.* 2011;32:386–90.

19. Nagata H, Ihara K, Yamamura K, et al. Left ventricular efficiency after ligation of patent ductus arteriosus for premature infants. *J Thorac Cardiovasc Surg.* 2013;146:1353–8.

20. Clement WA, El-Hakim H, Phillipos EZ, et al. Unilateral vocal cord paralysis following patent ductus arteriosus ligation in extremely low-birth-weight infants. *Arch Otolaryngol.* 2008;134:28–33.

21. El-Said HG, Bratincsak A, Foerster SR, et al. Safety of percutaneous patent ductus arteriosus closure: an unselected multicenter population experience. *J Am Heart Assoc.* 2013;27:e000424.

22. Dodge-Khatami A, Mavroudis C, Backer CL. Anomalous origin of the left coronary artery from the pulmonary artery: collective review of surgical therapy. *Ann of Thorac Surg.* 2002;74:946–55.

23. Walhout RJ, Lekkerkerker JC, Oron GH, et al. Comparison of polytetrafluroethylene patch aortoplasty and end-to-end anastomosis for coarctation of the aorta. *J Thorac Cardiovasc Surg.* 2003;126:521–8.

24. Rao PS, Galal O, Smith PA, et al. Five-to nine-year follow-up results of balloon angioplasty of native aortic coarctation in infants and children. *J Am Coll Cardiol.* 1996;27:462–70.

25. McElhinney DB, Lock JE, Keane JG, et al. Left heart growth, function, and reintervention after balloon aortic valvuloplasty for neonatal aortic stenosis. *Circulation.* 2005;111:451–8.

26. Moulaert AJ, Bruins CC, Oppenheimer-Dekker A. Anomalies of the aortic arch and ventricular septal defects. *Circulation.* 1976;53:1011–15.

27. Quinonez LG, Breitbart R, Tworetsky W, et al. Stented bovine jugular vein graft (melody valve) for surgical mitral valve replacement in infants and children. *J Thorac Cardiovasc Surg.* 2013;148(4):1443–9.

28. Alwi M, Geetha K, Bilkis AA, et al. Pulmonary atresia with intact ventricular septum percutaneous radiofrequency-assisted valvotomy and balloon dilation versus surgical valvotomy and Blalock Taussing shunt. *J Am Coll Cardiol.* 2000;35:468–76.

29. Reddy VM, Liddicoat JR, Hanley FL. Midline one stage completes unifocalization and repair of pulmonary atresia with ventricular septal defect and major aorto

pulmonary collaterals. *J Thorac Cardiovasc Surg.* 1995;109:832–45.

30. Vacanti C, Segal S, Sikka P, Urman R, editors. *Essential Clinical Anesthesia.* Cambridge: Cambridge University Press; 2011.

31. Stumper O, Ramchandani B, Noonan P, et al. Stenting of the right ventricular outflow tract. *Heart.* 2013;99:1603–8.

32. Pigula FA, Khalil PN, Mayer JE, et al. Repair of tetralogy of Fallot in neonates and young infants. *Circulation.* 1999;100:II157–61.

33. Delhaas T, Sarvaas GJ, Rijlaarsdam ME, et al. A multicenter, long-term study on arrhythmias in children with Ebstein anomaly. *Pediatr Cardiol.* 2010;31:229–33.

34. Knott-Craig CJ, Overhold ED, Ward KE, et al. Neonatal repair of Ebstein's anomaly: indications, surgical technique, and medium-term follow-up. *Ann Thorac Surg.* 2000;69:1505–10.

35. Starnes VA, Pitlick PT, Bernstein D, et al. Ebstein's anomaly appearing in the neonate: a new surgical approach. *J Thorac Cardiovasc Surg.* 1991:101;1082–7.

36. daSilva JP, Baumgratz JF, da Fonseca L, et al. The cone reconstruction of the tricuspid valve in Ebstein's anomaly: the operation. Early and midterm results. *J Thorac Cardiovasc Surg.* 2007;133:215–23.

37. Fricke TA, d'Udekem Y, Richardson M, et al. Outcomes of the arterial switch operation for transposition of the great arteries: 25 years of experience. *Ann Thorac Surg.* 2012;94:139–45.

38. D'Udekem Y, Xu MY, Galati JC, et al. Predictors of survival after single-ventricle palliation: the impact of right ventricular dominance. *J Am Coll Cardiol.* 2012;13:1178–85.

39. Kobayashi D, Forbes TJ, Aggarwal S. Palliative stent placement in vertical vein in a 1.4 kg infant with obstructed supracardiac total anomalous pulmonary venous connection. *Catheter Cardiovasc Interv.* 2013;82:574–80.

40. Yoshimura N, Fukahara K, Yamashita A, et al. Management of pulmonary venous obstruction. *Gen Thorac Cardiovasc Surg.* 2012;60:785–91.

41. Rabinovitch M, Grady S, David I, et al. Compression of intrapulmonary bronchi by abnormally branching pulmonary arteries associated with absent pulmonary valves. *Am J Cardiol.* 1982;50:804–13.

42. Kussman BD, Geva T, McGowan FX. Cardiovascular causes of airway compression. *Paediatr Anaesth.* 2004;14:60–74.

**Chapter**

# 29

# Noncardiac Surgery in Neonates and Infants With Cardiac Disease

Annette Y. Schure

## Introduction

The incidence of congenital heart disease (CHD) is about 4–9 per 1000 live-born full-term infants. Recent advances in pediatric cardiology, surgery, and critical care have significantly improved the survival rates of even the most complex defects. Many children will require multiple cardiac surgeries or interventional procedures, starting in the neonatal period and continuing into adulthood. In addition, CHD is often (30 percent) associated with extracardiac anomalies, syndromes or significant comorbidities, potentially requiring further imaging studies and surgical interventions, especially in the first year of life. Given the current trend for early diagnosis and intervention, with increasingly sophisticated imaging and treatment modalities, all pediatric anesthesiologists, with or without specific cardiac training, will encounter more and more patients with repaired or unrepaired CHD and other cardiac diseases in their daily practice.

Several recent studies demonstrated an increased risk for patients with cardiac disease undergoing noncardiac surgery, notably for the younger age group (<2 years), complex lesions, and patients with preexisting pulmonary hypertension, congestive heart failure (CHF), or significantly decreased ventricular function [1–4].

This chapter introduces the pediatric anesthesiologist to a systematic approach for the preoperative assessment and preparation of neonates and infants with cardiac disease; discusses anesthetic considerations for the most common repaired and unrepaired defects; and also reviews the anesthetic management for specific procedures that are frequently performed within the first year of life.

## Evaluation and Preparation of the Neonate and Infant With Cardiac Disease

It is beyond the scope of this chapter to discuss an anesthetic plan for all possible cardiac defects and their repairs or interventions. Every child must be evaluated on an individual basis, often a very demanding task that can be greatly facilitated by a systematic approach:

(1) preoperative assessment;
(2) endocarditis prophylaxis;
(3) prevention of paradoxical embolization;
(4) special considerations for monitoring and intravenous access;
(5) management of fluid status;
(6) risks and goals for hemodynamic and respiratory management;
(7) preoperative planning.

## Preoperative Assessment

A thorough preoperative assessment includes an understanding of the anatomy and pathophysiology of the underlying defect or disease, the type and outcome of repairs, palliations or interventions, a review of potential extracardiac malformations or coexisting syndromes, as well as the evaluation of the current functional status and medications.

### Anatomy and Pathophysiology of the Underlying Defect or Disease

Table 29.1 shows a simplified classification of the most common congenital heart defects according to appearance (cyanotic versus acyanotic) and basic pathophysiology (please refer to Chapter 28 for more details). For complex cases it is advisable to contact the primary cardiologist or cardiac surgeon and discuss specific details and implications for the upcoming procedure. Pediatric cardiologists are very involved in the care of their patients but may be unaware of the potential effects of anesthesia or certain surgical requirements (immobility, positioning, abdominal insufflation, etc.).

### Type and Outcome of Repairs, Palliations, and Interventions

In the past, surgical repairs were often differentiated into definitive and palliative procedures. Definitive

**Table 29.1** Classification of CHD (incidence of lesion as percentage of all CHD)

| Cyanotic | Acyanotic |
|---|---|
| **Right-to-left shunts** | **Left-to-right shunts** |
| Tetralogy of Fallot (10 percent) | Ventricular septal defect (20–25 percent) |
| Pulmonary atresia (1 percent) | Atrial septal defect (5–10 percent) |
| Tricuspid atresia (< 1 percent) | Endocardial cushion defect (AV canal) (4–5 percent) |
|  | Patent ductus arteriosus (5–10 percent) |
| **Complex "mixing" lesions** |  |
| Transposition of the great vessels (5 percent) |  |
| Total anomalous pulmonary venous return (1 percent) |  |
| Truncus arteriosus (1 percent) |  |
| Hypoplastic left heart syndrome (1 percent) |  |
| Double outlet right ventricle (< 1 percent) |  |
| **Obstructive lesions (right-sided)** | **Obstructive lesions (left-sided)** |
| Pulmonary stenosis (5–8 percent) | Coarctation of the aorta (8–10 percent) |
|  | Aortic stenosis (5 percent) |

Source: [5].

procedures are intended to correct the defect and can either be anatomic, leading to a "normal" acyanotic serial circulation where the blood flows through two separate sequential circulations with the right ventricle supporting the pulmonary circulation and the left ventricle the systemic one, or "non-anatomic or functional" repairs where a serial circulation is established but the right ventricle or a single ventricle is supporting the systemic circulation (e.g., Mustard or Senning repair of transposition of the great arteries [d-TGA], Fontan). There are simple surgeries like patch repairs of ASDs, VSDs, or PDA ligations with an otherwise normal heart and a low likelihood of long-term complications, but also complex reconstructions with conduits and valves that will obstruct and calcify over time and often require lifelong follow-up and multiple interventions. Some of these repairs are therefore not so "definitive."

Palliative procedures like arterio-pulmonary shunts or pulmonary artery banding are used to temporarily improve severe cyanosis or pulmonary overcirculation if the baby is premature, too small, or too sick for a complete neonatal repair.

Many cardiac defects are corrected or palliated during interventions in the cardiac catheterization suite: device closures of ASDs, VSDs, or PDAs, balloon dilations and stent placements for obstructions, or coil embolization of aortopulmonary collaterals or shunts are just a few examples (see also Chapter 28). Parents should be specifically asked about recent cardiac catheterizations. These can be an indication of residual postoperative problems but are often "downplayed" as diagnostic tests and not mentioned during the initial interview.

Obviously, the outcome after a surgical procedure or an intervention is another important question. Classic complications like complete heartblock after a VSD patch repair or coronary injury and ventricular dysfunction after an outflow tract reconstruction have to be distinguished from residual defects (subvalvular obstruction, valve regurgitation, residual VSDs, pulmonary hypertension, etc.) or altered physiology (single ventricle or systemic right ventricle).

## Extracardiac Malformations and Genetic Syndromes Associated With Congenital Heart Disease

Approximately 25–30 percent of neonates with CHDs have additional extracardiac malformations or associated syndromes that may require further workup or interventions prior to the cardiac repair.

Moreover, they can have significant implications for the anesthetic management: difficult airway or tracheoesophageal fistulas, metabolic and endocrine problems, immunodeficiency (requiring irradiated blood products), or limb abnormalities with limited intravenous access. Table 29.2 is a short list of the most common syndromes associated with CHD. Unfamiliar syndromes should be carefully reviewed in major pediatric or cardiology textbooks.

## Current Functional Status and Medications

A detailed history, physical examination, and review of recent imaging studies are important to assess the

303

**Table 29.2** Syndromes frequently associated with CHD

| Syndrome | Commonly associated CHD | Other anesthetic implications |
| --- | --- | --- |
| CHARGE association (**C**oloboma, congenital **H**eart defects, choanal **A**tresia, **R**enal abnormalities, **G**enital hypoplasia, **E**ar deformities) | 65 percent conotruncal anomalies, aortic arch anomalies | Difficult airway and intubation, renal dysfunction |
| DiGeorge syndrome (chromosome 22 deletion, CATCH 22) | Interrupted aortic arch, truncus arteriosus, VSD, PDA, ToF | Hypocalcemia, immunodeficiency, need for irradiated blood products |
| Duchenne muscular dystrophy | Cardiomyopathy | Hyperkalemic cardiac arrest with succinylcholine, rhabdomyolysis with inhalational agents |
| Ehler–Danlos syndrome | Aneurysm of aorta and carotid vessels | Difficult IV, increased bleeding |
| Ellis–van Creveld syndrome (chondro-ectodermal dysplasia) | 50 percent common atrium | Possible difficult intubation |
| Fetal alcohol syndrome | 25–30 percent VSD, PDA, ASD, ToF | Difficult airway, renal disease |
| Friedreich's ataxia | Cardiomyopathy | Progressive neurological degeneration, glucose intolerance |
| Glycogen storage disease II (Pompe) | Cardiomyopathy | |
| Holt–Oram syndrome | ASD, VSD | Upper limb abnormalities |
| Leopard syndrome (cardio-cutaneous syndrome) | PS, long PR interval, cardiomyopathy | Growth retardation, possible difficult intubation |
| Long QT syndromes:<br>– Jervell and Lange Nielsen<br>– Romano–Ward | Long QT interval, ventricular tachyarrhythmia | Congenital deafness |
| Marfan syndrome | Aortic aneurysm, AR and/or MR | Spontaneous pneumothorax, cervical spine instability |
| Mucopolysaccharidosis:<br>– Hurler (type I)<br>– Hunter (type II)<br>– Morquio (type III) | AR and/or MR, coronary artery disease, cardiomyopathy | Difficult airway, atlantoaxial instability, kyphoscoliosis |
| Noonan syndrome | PS (dystrophic valve), LVH, septal hypertrophy | Possible difficult intubation, platelet dysfunction, renal dysfunction |
| Tuberous sclerosis | Myocardial rhabdomyoma | Seizure disorder, renal dysfunction |
| Shprintzen syndrome (velocardiofacial, 22q11.2 deletion) | Conotruncal anomalies, ToF | Difficult airway |
| VACTERL association | VSD, conotruncal anomalies (ToF, truncus arteriosus, etc.) | **V**ertebral anomalies, **A**nal atresia, **C**ardiac defects, **T**racheoesophageal fistula, **E**sophageal atresia, **R**enal anomalies, **L**imb defects |
| Williams syndrome | Supravalvular AS, PA stenosis | Developmental delay, occasional difficult airway, renal dysfunction |
| Zellweger syndrome (cerebrohepatorenal syndrome) | PDA, VSD, ASD | Neonatal jaundice, kidney and liver dysfunction, coagulopathy, hypotonia |

current functional status. Specific questions regarding signs and symptoms of CHF, pulmonary hypertension, or severe ventricular dysfunction, episodes of syncope or palpitations, cyanotic "spells" with or without agitation, feeding difficulties, recurrent infections, and recent changes in medications will help to stratify the risk for anesthesia. In addition to a careful airway, cardiac and pulmonary examination, the physical examination should include the assessment of peripheral pulse quality, capillary refill, clubbing, hepatomegaly,

**Table 29.3** Important aspects for the preoperative evaluation

| | |
|---|---|
| History | • Signs and symptoms of CHF:<br>  – Failure to thrive, poor feeding, tachypnea, sweating<br>  – Recurrent pulmonary infections (secondary to congestion)<br>  – Decreased activity level and fatigue in older patients<br>• Palpitations or syncope<br>• Additional congenital anomalies (e.g., airway, genitourinary)<br>• Recent and current medications (e.g., diuretics, digoxin, ACE inhibitors)<br>• Review of previous surgeries and interventional procedures<br>• Last follow-up with the patient's pediatric cardiologist |
| Physical examination | • Characteristic heart murmur, precordial thrill, arrhythmias<br>• Tachypnea, increased work of breathing, rales<br>• Poor peripheral perfusion, delayed capillary refill<br>• Bounding or diminished pulses<br>• Cool extremities, mottled skin, sweating<br>• Hepatomegaly<br>• Peripheral edema, puffy eye lids |
| Laboratory studies | • CBC: polycythemia (secondary to cyanosis), anemia (secondary to malnutrition)<br>• Electrolytes: hypokalemia, hyponatremia (secondary to diuretic therapy)<br>• Coagulation profile |
| Additional tests | • Echocardiography: cardiac function and intracardiac anatomy<br>• EKG: rhythm, signs of atrial or ventricular hypertrophy<br>• CXR: cardiomegaly, pulmonary edema, or infiltrates |
| Specific studies | • Cardiac catheterization: anatomy, pressure gradients, saturations, shunts<br>• Cardiac MRI: anatomy, pulmonary blood flow, right and left ventricular function |

Source: [5].

potential blood pressure gradients between the extremities, and access sites for intravenous or arterial lines. All available recent cardiac studies or diagnostic tests should be reviewed and if necessary discussed with the cardiologist. Many cardiac medications can have significant implications for anesthetic management and may warrant preoperative laboratory studies. For example, diuretics can be associated with intravascular volume depletion and electrolyte disturbances, ACE inhibitors with severe hypotension after induction of anesthesia, digoxin with increased toxicity triggered by electrolyte and fluid shifts, beta blockers can mask the heart rate response to pain and stress, and platelet inhibitors increase the risk for bleeding. A complete list of current medications should be compiled during the preoperative evaluation and the perioperative continuation or discontinuation decided on an individual basis. All cyanotic patients will need a complete blood count to assess for polycythemia and the need for preoperative hydration or admission to prevent spontaneous thromboembolism due to severely elevated hematocrit levels (>55–60 percent). A normal hematocrit in a cyanotic patient is usually a sign of anemia, often caused by iron deficiency. Coagulation tests can be helpful to evaluate platelet and factor deficiencies that are often associated with severe cyanosis. Table 29.3 summarizes the important aspects of the preoperative evaluation.

# Endocarditis Prophylaxis

In 2007, the American Heart Association [6] published their latest update of the guidelines for endocarditis prophylaxis. The focus was shifted toward cardiac conditions that are associated with the highest risk for adverse outcomes from endocarditis. Currently, endocarditis prophylaxis is only recommended for all dental procedures involving manipulations of gingival tissue or oral mucosa and the following conditions:

• prosthetic cardiac valve or prosthetic material used for cardiac valve repair;
• previous endocarditis;
• Congenital heart disease:
  – unrepaired cyanotic CHD, including palliative shunts and conduits;

- completely repaired CHD with prosthetic material or device, whether placed by surgery or catheter intervention, during first six months after the repair;
- repaired CHD with residual defects in the site or adjacent to the site of a prosthetic patch or prosthetic device (which inhibits endothelialization);
- cardiac transplantation recipients who develop cardiac valvulopathy.

Endocarditis prophylaxis is no longer recommended for routine gastrointestinal or genitourinary procedures.

## Prevention of Paradoxical Embolization

All newborns and many cardiac patients, especially those with single ventricle lesions, complete atrioventricular canals, or preexisting right-to-left shunts, are at risk for paradoxical embolization and sudden or worsening cyanosis. Changes in pulmonary vascular resistance or loading conditions can lead to increased pressures in the right side of the heart and open the only functionally closed fetal shunt connections (PFO and PDA), which can worsen existing right-to-left shunting or reverse preexisting left-to-right shunts. Air or thrombotic material from the venous circulation can directly enter the arterial system and cause limb ischemia or ischemic infarcts in the brain or intestinal organs. Many neonatal cardiac repairs involve fenestrated patch closures to allow for decompression of the right ventricle during the initial recovery period. Decreased right ventricle function, perioperative episodes of pulmonary hypertension, or increased right ventricle afterload with breath holding and coughing during emergence from anesthesia can result in severe cyanosis. Careful evaluation of all cardiac patients for potential intracardiac shunt connections and appropriate anesthetic management including prophylactic use of air filters whenever possible and meticulous avoidance of air entrapment in stopcocks and injection ports are important measures to decrease the risk for paradoxical embolization.

## Special Considerations for Monitoring and Intravenous Access

A five-lead ECG with ST segment analysis is recommended for all cardiac patients at risk for ischemia, especially before and after stage 1 palliation and for hypertrophied ventricles. Patients with modified Blalock–Taussig (BT) shunts (steal effect) or known vascular occlusions can have decreased blood pressure readings on the respective extremities and the noninvasive BP cuff should be placed accordingly. Depending on the procedure, the complexity of the cardiac defect and the functional status of the patient, invasive monitoring with an arterial line and central venous access might be indicated. Capnography is well known to be inaccurate to assess the adequacy of ventilation in defects with right-to-left shunting, compromised pulmonary blood flow or "unbalanced" single ventricle physiology [7]. Direct blood pressure monitoring will not only allow for close monitoring of hemodynamic changes, but also ventilator adjustments based on arterial blood gases. Anticipation of hemodynamic instability and the need for inotropic support or monitoring of mixed venous saturations may warrant placement of a central venous line. After a long hospitalization peripheral intravenous access can be very difficult and limited to small cannulas. Central venous access is often the only reliable choice. A careful preoperative evaluation and examination of all potential access sites, including blood pressure measurements on all four extremities to assess for gradients as well as a review of previous surgeries and catheterization reports for known occlusions, shunts, subclavian flaps, or surgical cut-downs, is very important. For "frequent flyers," such as patients with Tetralogy of Fallot and pulmonary atresia (ToF/PA), if at all possible, the femoral vessels should be spared for future access in the catheterization lab.

## Management of Fluid Status

Many cardiac patients will benefit from a small fluid bolus ($5–10\,\mathrm{ml\,kg^{-1}}$) prior to or shortly after induction. Intravascular volume depletion due to chronic diuretic therapy, loss of sympathetic tone, and vasodilation, as well as decreased preload with onset of positive pressure ventilation, can lead to significant hypotension. Some patients are especially preload dependent, such as patients with right ventricle hypertrophy and pulmonary hypertension (PH), bidirectional Glenn physiology, or hypertrophic cardiomyopathy. Cyanotic patients with polycythemia are at risk for spontaneous thrombosis. NPO times should be either kept to a minimum or, alternatively patients can be admitted the day before for adequate hydration.

On the other hand, there are a group of cardiac patients who will not tolerate rapid fluid administration, like the 25 ml kg$^{-1}$ usually given during short day surgery cases. Patients with pulmonary vein stenosis (for example after TAPVR repair), mitral stenosis, or diastolic dysfunction can easily decompensate with rapid fluid administration and develop severe pulmonary edema.

## Risks and Goals for Hemodynamic and Respiratory Management

Depending on the underlying pathophysiology, the goals and potential risks of alterations in the hemodynamic or respiratory status have to be carefully assessed. Patients with severe CHF from pulmonary overcirculation, pulmonary hypertension, restricted pulmonary blood flow, obstructive or regurgitant valvular defects, or single ventricle physiology will require very different hemodynamic and ventilatory strategies. Optimization of the current status and avoidance of detrimental changes with induction of anesthesia, positioning, fluid shifts, or surgical instrumentation/stimulation are important and can often be facilitated by a preoperative team discussion between anesthesiologist, surgeon, and cardiologist. A quick review of the individual arrhythmia risk for the specific defect or procedure will help with preparing appropriate antiarrhythmic medications and equipment (defibrillator, pacing devices). In complex cases, a preoperative consultation with an electrophysiology specialist can be very valuable. Specific goals and potential problems for individual congenital heart defects will be discussed in the section "Considerations for specific cardiac diseases."

## Preoperative Planning

Anesthesiologists play an important role in perioperative care. Evaluating the need for preoperative consultations with cardiology, new updated imaging studies (echo, chest X-ray) as well as timing of the procedure (e.g., first case of the day) and possible coordination with other procedures are important tasks. In preparation for the case, the appropriate location (satellite facility versus main campus), staffing, and level of support has to be selected and all necessary material and equipment organized such as additional syringe pumps for inotropic agents, difficult airway cart, defibrillator, or antiarrhythmic medications. Finally, the right venue for the initial postoperative recovery and

further observation has to be chosen. Depending on the complexity of the cardiac disease and/or the surgical procedure, this can range from a specialized cardiac intensive care unit to the recovery room, followed by admission to a regular floor or cardiac ward, or even a day surgery unit. Once again, a preoperative team discussion can be a valuable tool to make timely arrangements and avoid unnecessary waiting periods in the operating or recovery room.

## Considerations for Specific Cardiac Diseases

It is beyond the scope of this chapter to describe the detailed management of all cardiac defects and cardiac diseases for potential procedures and interventions in the first year of life, so the following section will highlight the most important anesthetic considerations for common CHD and diseases. Various anesthetic agents and techniques have been used successfully. More details can be found in recent review articles and Chapter 28 [8–10].

## Ventricular Septal Defect

Ventricular septal defects (VSDs) are the most common form of CHD, affecting 20–25 percent of CHD patients. Thirty to forty percent of VSDs will close spontaneously within the first year of life.

### Pathophysiology

The resulting left-to-right shunt is dependent on the size of the defect and the pressure gradient across the septum, which is determined by left and right ventricle pressures, pulmonary vascular resistance (PVR), and systemic vascular resistance (SVR). Large left-to right shunts lead to pulmonary overcirculation, CHF, and poor cardiac output.

### Associated Anomalies

Less than 5 percent of VSDs are associated with chromosomal abnormalities such as trisomy 13, 18, and 21.

### Anesthetic Considerations

- Small VSD with no obvious CHF:
  - Careful inhalation induction possible; be aware of reduced cardiac reserve
  - "Bubble" precautions
  - Risk of shunt reversal (see below)

- Large VSD with significant CHF:
  - "Bubble" precautions
  - Careful intravenous induction aiming for a stable PVR/SVR ratio and normoventilation
  - Avoidance of hyperventilation and high FiO$_2$: a high PaO$_2$ and low PaCO$_2$ can decrease PVR, which will increase left-to-right shunting and decrease systemic cardiac output
  - Avoidance of potent negative inotropic anesthetic agents in the volume overloaded, failing ventricle with poor reserve and compliance; low-dose inotropic support often beneficial
  - Risk of shunt reversal (right-to-left) with severe hypotension or increases in PVR due to loss of airway during induction, bronchospasm, hypoxia or acidosis, coughing, or breath holding during emergence.

### Considerations for Patients With Repaired VSDs

- Dysrhythmias and conduction defects such as right bundle branch block (RBBB), ventricular arrhythmias, and heart block
- Residual ventricular dysfunction, especially after severe CHF or repairs requiring ventriculotomy.
- Residual pulmonary hypertension or exaggerated pulmonary vascular reactivity, which is sometimes associated with a late repair, high altitude, or syndromes like trisomy 21.

## Patent Ductus Arteriosus

The ductus arteriosus is a normal fetal structure that connects the main pulmonary artery and the upper descending aorta. In utero, approximately 60 percent of right ventricular output bypasses the lungs via the ductus arteriosus.

In full-term infants, functional closure (i.e., smooth muscle contraction) usually occurs 10–15 hours after birth, but can be delayed by many factors. Permanent closure (fibrosis) is usually completed by the first 2–3 weeks of life. Patent ductus arteriosus (PDA) represents about 10 percent of congenital heart defects. In preterm infants, the overall incidence is 20–30 percent.

### Pathophysiology

The degree of shunting via the PDA depends on the size of the PDA and the ratio of PVR to SVR.

With declining PVR, large PDAs can result in significant left-to-right shunting, left ventricle volume overload, CHF, and pulmonary hypertension.

### Associated Anomalies

A PDA is often essential for pulmonary or systemic blood flow in patients with complex cardiac lesions. In preterm infants, the cardiovascular changes associated with a PDA can exacerbate conditions like necrotizing enterocolitis, intracranial hemorrhage, or respiratory distress syndrome.

### Anesthetic Considerations

**Ductal Dependent Lesions** (e.g., hypoplastic left heart, transposition of the great arteries with intact ventricular septum, critical aortic stenosis, and interrupted aortic arch). Usually maintenance of ductal patency with prostaglandin E$_1$ infusion (PGE$_1$).

- Second IV access for medication and fluid bolus, potentially difficult access ("doughy" tissue)
- Side-effects of PGE$_1$ therapy: dose-dependent apnea, platelet dysfunction, gastric mucosal hyperplasia, etc.
- Ratio of PVR to SVR will determine adequacy of pulmonary or systemic blood flow
- ICU admission for apnea monitoring.

**Isolated PDA.** Shunt direction and degree of shunting dependent on size of PDA and ratio of PVR to SVR. Presentation can range from very sick neonates or infants in CHF and on inotropic support to completely asymptomatic infants awaiting cardiac intervention or surgery.

- "Bubble" precautions
- Potential episode of cyanosis during emergence if coughing or breath holding, etc.

For symptomatic patients in CHF, please see recommendations for "large VSD" above.

### Considerations for Patients With Repaired PDAs

- Recurrent laryngeal nerve injury
- Pulmonary hypertension and ventricular dysfunction if late repair

## Coarctation of the Aorta

Coarctation of the aorta is present in 5–10 percent of patients with CHD. Most patients have a discrete stenosis of the upper thoracic aorta, opposite the insertion of the ductus arteriosus, but the anatomic spectrum can range from a long tubular hypoplasia of the transverse arch to band-like strictures in the descending aorta.

## Pathophysiology

The hemodynamic picture is highly dependent on the severity of the stenosis and the presence of associated cardiac defects and collateral circulation. For instance, a newborn with critical stenosis may decompensate acutely when the ductus arteriosus closes. Or the patient may develop severe CHF and pulmonary over-circulation within the first 1–2 weeks of life if associated with a large VSD.

## Associated Anomalies

Coarctation of the aorta is often associated with other congenital anomalies: 50 percent of patients have an additional intracardiac lesion, such as a large VSD, aortic stenosis, or hypoplastic left ventricle; 85 percent have a bicommissural aortic valve. In addition, variations of the brachiocephalic vessels with an abnormal origin of the subclavian arteries may occur, and 3–5 percent of patients have berry aneurysms of the circle of Willis. Patients with Turner syndrome have a high incidence of coarctation; other congenital malformations are present in 25 percent of patients.

## Anesthetic Considerations

- Maintain ductal patency with prostaglandin infusion, use second intravenous access for other drugs and bolus administration
- Newborns and infants in CHF: Usually careful IV induction and narcotic-based maintenance
- Patients with large VSD, at risk for pulmonary overcirculation: Avoid hyperventilation and high $FiO_2$.
- Consider inotropic support if severe CHF
- Invasive BP monitoring in the right radial artery (preductal, unless there are arch anomalies like an anomalous right subclavian artery)
- Consider additional BP monitoring and pulse oximetry in lower extremities

## Considerations for Patients With Repaired Coarctation

- Risk of residual or recoarctation and exercise-induced pressure gradient
- Preferred blood pressure monitoring on right upper extremity

- Associated berry aneurysms in cerebral circulation
- Persistent hypertension and myocardial hypertrophy (diastolic dysfunction)

# Atrial Septal Defect

In its isolated form, atrial septal defect (ASD) comprises 5–10 percent of congenital heart defects, but is part of more complex cardiac defects in 30–50 percent of CHD patients.

## Pathophysiology

Left-to-right shunt with slowly progressive right atrium and right ventricle dilation, and eventually development of pulmonary hypertension late in life. Eighty percent of all ASDs, especially those <8 mm, will close spontaneously within the first two years of life.

## Associated Anomalies

Atrial septal defects may be associated with virtually any congenital anomaly. The most commonly associated cardiovascular defects include pulmonary stenosis, partial anomalous venous return, and VSD. There is a higher incidence of secundum ASDs in patients with Holt–Oram, Noonan, Marfan, and Turner syndromes.

## Anesthetic Considerations

- Careful removal of all air bubbles from lines to prevent paradoxical air embolus
- Higher incidence of perioperative dysrhythmias
- Inhalation induction is usually well tolerated (except in sick infants with CHF).

## Consideration for Patients With Repaired ASDs

- Perioperative dysrhythmias
- Occasionally persistent right ventricle dilation or pulmonary hypertension (associated syndromes).

# Tetralogy of Fallot

Between 5 and 10 percent of all CHDs are classified as ToF. It is by far the most common cyanotic lesion. There is a wide anatomic spectrum ranging from the classical form with pulmonary stenosis to pulmonary atresia and variations without evidence of right ventricular outflow obstruction ("pink Tet").

## Pathophysiology

The most important pathophysiological aspect of ToF is the obstruction to pulmonary blood flow; this leads to a right-to-left shunt via the VSD and subsequent hypoxemia and cyanosis. The obstruction can be an anatomically fixed stenosis at the level of the valve or pulmonary artery and/or a dynamic narrowing of the infundibular area due to thickened muscle bundles and septal malalignment.

## Associated Anomalies

Tetralogy of Fallot is often associated with other cardiac anomalies. Some of these are of special concern for the surgical approach:

- Right-sided aortic arch (20–25 percent): Affects surgical approach for shunts and repair of tracheoesophageal fistula
- Coronary anomalies (5–8 percent): Abnormal origin or coronary branch crossing the right ventricular outflow tract (RVOT).

There is also an important association with noncardiac anomalies; only 68 percent of ToF are isolated cardiac lesions:

- Chromosomal abnormalities (11.9 percent): Trisomy 13, 18, and 21.
- Genetic syndromes (7.2 percent):
  - DiGeorge Syndrome/velocardiofacial or Shprintzen syndrome (22q deletion syndromes)
  - CHARGE association
  - VATER/VACTERL

## Anesthetic Considerations

- Dehydration and long fasting periods should be avoided due to polycythemia
- Consider admission and hydration overnight if severely polycythemic (Hct > 55 percent)
- Preinduction fluid bolus is often beneficial
- Careful removal of all air bubbles from lines to avoid systemic air embolism
- Medications for treatment of "hypercyanotic spells" should be immediately available (see Table 29.4)
- If previously shunted, note site of previous shunt as pressure monitoring may provide an unreliable reading
- Generally, an IV induction using ketamine is used to maintain SVR and preload; in mild forms,

**Table 29.4** Treatment of hypercyanotic spells

- "Knee–chest position" or abdominal compression
- Supplemental oxygen
- Sedation
  - Morphine: 0.1 mg kg$^{-1}$ IM/SC or ketamine 1–2 mg kg$^{-1}$ IV/IM
- Volume expansion: 10–20 ml kg$^{-1}$ crystalloid
- Phenylephrine IV
  - 0.5–1–2 µg kg$^{-1}$ bolus, 0.1–0.5 µg kg$^{-1}$ min$^{-1}$ infusion
- Propranolol 0.1 mg kg$^{-1}$ IV
- Esmolol: 50–300 µg kg$^{-1}$ min$^{-1}$ ± loading dose 100–500 µg kg$^{-1}$ IV
- Bicarbonate IV

careful inhalation induction is possible (watch for delayed induction with right-to-left shunt).

## Considerations for Patients With Repaired Tetralogy of Fallot

- Residual VSD
- Residual RVOT obstruction – mostly mild, but severe in 10 percent of cases
- Pulmonic regurgitation and right ventricle dilation after transannular patch repair
- Arrhythmias and right ventricle dysfunction may occur after ventriculotomy and infundibular patch repair due to scarring and fibrosis
- Left ventricle dysfunction (anomalous coronaries and ischemic injury)
- Aortopulmonary collaterals, especially with ToF/PA.

# Atrioventricular Septal Defect

Between 4 and 5 percent of CHD are endocardial cushion defects, which can be divided into several types: partial, transitional, and complete atrioventricular (AV) canals. The most extensive form, the complete AV canal (CAVC), consists of a primum ASD with a common AV valve orifice, bridging leaflets, and a moderate to large inlet VSD.

## Pathophysiology

Large left-to right shunt with AV regurgitation leading to pulmonary overcirculation, CHF, and early onset of pulmonary hypertension. Increasing cyanosis is often the first sign of pulmonary hypertension.

## Associated Anomalies

- Trisomy 21: Often isolated CAVC
- Cardiac anomalies: ToF ("Tet canal") 6 percent, double outlet right ventricle (DORV) 6 percent
- DiGeorge syndrome.

## Anesthetic Considerations

- Anesthetic implications of Trisomy 21: Cervical spine instability, large tongue, short trachea, difficult vascular access, early onset of PH
- Possible malnutrition, failure to thrive
- "Bubble" precautions
- If severe CHF: Intravenous induction preferred (see above, under "Management of Large VSD")
- Aiming for a stable PVR/SVR ratio and normoventilation
- Avoidance of hyperventilation and high $FiO_2$
- Avoidance of potent negative inotropic agents
- Risk of shunt reversal with severe hypotension, increase in PVR.

## Considerations for Patients With Repaired CAVC

- Residual mitral valve disease: Regurgitation, occasionally stenosis
- Pulmonary hypertension and right ventricle dysfunction
- Arrhythmias: Heart block, sinus node dysfunction

# Transposition of the Great Arteries

Transposition of the great arteries (TGA) is a complex mixing lesion that comprises 5–7 percent of all CHDs. It is the most common cyanotic CHD diagnosed in the newborn period. Abnormal rotation and septation of the arterial truncus results in transposition of the aorta and pulmonary artery.

## Pathophysiology

In the most common form, the d-TGA, the aorta arises anteriorly from the right ventricle and transports deoxygenated blood to the body, whereas the pulmonary artery originates posteriorly from the left ventricle and carries oxygenated blood back to the lungs. Thus, pulmonary and systemic circulations are in parallel. This is a fatal situation if not associated with an ASD, VSD, or PDA that will allow for some mixing of oxygenated and deoxygenated blood between the two circulations.

L-TGA is the so-called physiologically corrected form of transposition, where the aorta arises from a right ventricle that is connected to a left atrium, and the circulation is therefore in series but the right ventricle is supporting the systemic circulation.

## Associated Anomalies

TGA is rarely associated with extracardiac anomalies or syndromes. It is extremely unusual to see patients with unrepaired TGA presenting for noncardiac surgery.

## Considerations for Patients With Repaired TGA

- Arterial switch: Long-term problems are very rare
  - Supravalvular pulmonary stenosis or regurgitation into the neo-aorta are possible
  - Occasionally coronary artery stenosis
- Atrial switch: Mustard or Senning, nowadays only used as part of a "double switch" for L-TGA
  - Baffle leaks with shunting depending on location and pressure gradients
  - Increased risk of arrhythmias, sick sinus syndrome, etc. (scars around atrial sutures)
  - At risk for baffle obstruction, which leads to pulmonary edema and SVC syndrome.

# Single Ventricle Defects

Poor alignment, atresia of atrioventricular or semilunar valves, or incomplete septation of the ventricular chambers in utero can lead to complex cardiac defects with only one functional ventricle, most commonly tricuspid atresia, hypoplastic left heart syndrome, pulmonary atresia with intact ventricular septum, double outlet right ventricle, double inlet left ventricle or unbalanced CAVC. Palliative procedures in the neonatal period aim for balanced systemic and pulmonary blood flows, allowing the baby to grow for several months despite cyanosis and volume load on the ventricle (see Chapter 28 for a detailed description of the individual lesions and cardiac procedures).

## Pathophysiology

Systemic venous (deoxygenated) blood and pulmonary venous (oxygenated) blood is mixed in the one ventricle, depending on the lesion, at the atrial and/or ventricular level. The output of the single ventricle is divided into two parallel and competing circulations: the systemic and the pulmonary circulation. The relative proportion of the cardiac output for each vascular bed is determined by the ratio of PVR/SVR and various associated outflow obstructions (pulmonary stenosis/atresia, aortic stenosis, coarctation, hypoplastic arch, etc.). A patent ductus arteriosus is often essential for maintenance of adequate pulmonary or systemic blood flow (ductal-dependent lesions). A balanced circulation with Qp/Qs of 1:1 is characterized by good peripheral perfusion and oxygenation with systemic saturations of ~80–85 percent and $S_VO_2$ of ~60 percent. Unbalanced circulations, pulmonary over- or undercirculation, will result in tissue hypoxia either due to poor perfusion or severe cyanosis, and culminate in acidosis, rising lactate levels and cardiovascular collapse.

### Anesthetic Considerations for Unrepaired Cardiac Defects With Single Ventricle Physiology:

- Critically ill neonates: High-dose opioid technique for induction and maintenance
- For ductal-dependent lesions: Continue prostaglandin $E_1$ infusion to maintain ductal patency
- Careful balance of pulmonary and systemic circulations aiming for normotensive, well-perfused, non-acidotic patients with $SaO_2$ ~80–85 percent and $SvO_2$ around 60 percent
- Induction of anesthesia can cause unbalanced circulation due to decreased oxygen consumption, positive pressure ventilation, decreased PVR, etc.
- Pulmonary overcirculation with poor cardiac output should be treated by increasing the PVR (controlled hypoventilation with adequate tidal volumes, low respiratory rates, low $FiO_2$) and inotropic support
- Systemic overcirculation with profound cyanosis can be addressed by decreasing PVR (hyperventilation, higher $FiO_2$, alkalosis) and optimizing afterload
- Monitoring of ST-segments: Systemic hypotension can lead to poor coronary perfusion, cardiac ischemia, and sudden ventricular fibrillation
- Hematocrit levels should be maintained at ~40–45 percent to assure adequate oxygen delivery without compromising rheology
- Invasive monitoring is recommended: Capnography is often unreliable to assess adequacy of ventilation (often large $etCO_2$ to arterial $CO_2$ gradient)
- Consider perioperative inotropic support of volume-loaded ventricle
- Increased risk for postoperative complications and hemodynamic instability; recovery in cardiac ICU recommended.

### Anesthetic Considerations for Single Ventricle Defects After Stage 1 Palliation

- Preoperative review of most recent echo, postoperative course, and current respiratory status
- Management of the parallel circulation: see above
- Consider perioperative inotropic support of volume-loaded ventricle
- Consider invasive monitoring for prolonged procedures with fluid shifts and risk for hemodynamic or respiratory compromise (abdominal or thoracic surgery, laparoscopy etc.)
- Capnography is often unreliable to assess adequacy of ventilation; direct correlation with blood gas recommended
- Increased risk for postoperative complications and hemodynamic instability; recovery in highly monitored and specialized unit or cardiac ICU recommended
- Specifics for patients after a Norwood procedure for hypoplastic left heart syndrome (HLHS) (arch reconstruction, modified BT shunt):
  - Consider shunt thrombosis or kink if sudden onset of severe cyanosis, check shunt murmur
  - Pulmonary blood flow dependent on adequate pressure gradient across shunt: BP/PVR
  - Maintain adequate coronary perfusion (diastolic steal); at risk for arrhythmias
  - Decreased preload and acute afterload increases are poorly tolerated [11]
  - Good pain control and minimization of stress response important [12].
- Specifics for patients after a stage I Sano procedure for HLHS (right ventricle–pulmonary artery conduit, arch reconstruction)
  - Considered to be more stable, no diastolic steal
  - Potential for conduit stenosis or thrombosis

- Can "outgrow" conduit, resulting in progressive cyanosis.
    - S/p ventriculotomy: Ventricular dysfunction, risk for arrhythmias
- Specifics for patients after a stage I hybrid procedure for HLHS (ductal stenting, balloon septostomy and bilateral pulmonary artery banding)
    - Dislocation, obstruction or thrombosis of ductal stent possible
    - Ductus provides systemic blood flow: antegrade to body, retrograde to coronaries and brain
    - Careful management of parallel circulation: Bilateral pulmonary artery bands might be initially too loose, after several weeks too tight, resulting in progressive cyanosis
    - Will require extensive stage 2: Bidirectional Glenn plus arch reconstruction.

### Considerations for Patients After Bidirectional Glenn

Superior vena cava connected to right pulmonary artery, pulmonary blood flow dependent on pressure gradient, no pumping chamber, inferior vena cava blood continues to return directly to single ventricle.

- Pulmonary blood flow, and therefore oxygenation is dependent on transpulmonary pressure gradient (gradient between SVC and common atrium)
- Preload-dependent pulmonary blood flow: Prolonged dehydration and fasting periods should be avoided; preinduction fluid bolus of 10–15 ml kg$^{-1}$ is often beneficial
- Careful respiratory management with low intrathoracic pressures, low respiratory rates with prolonged expiration time (I:E ratio 1:3) and low PEEP to optimize PVR, higher $FiO_2$
- All factors that increase PVR (e.g., acidosis, atelectasis, hypoxia, severe hypercapnia, hypothermia) need to be corrected immediately
- Occasionally, oxygenation can be improved by mild hypoventilation: The ensuing cerebral vasodilation redirects a larger proportion of the cardiac output to the brain and then via the SVC to the pulmonary vascular bed
- Strict "bubble" precautions: All fluids entering the single ventricle via the IVC have direct access to the systemic circulation (paradoxical embolization, stroke)

- Considered to be the most stable stage of all single ventricle palliations: Blood flow via IVC can maintain cardiac output during periods of decreased pulmonary blood flow (bronchospasm, coughing, breath holding during emergence, etc.). "It's better to be blue and beating, then empty and dead."

## Pulmonary Hypertension

Pulmonary hypertension (PH) in neonates and infants can have many different etiologies: Cardiac defects with large left-to-right shunts (e.g., VSD, PDA, CAVC), alveolar hypoxia from chronic pulmonary disease, pulmonary venous hypertension (mitral stenosis, pulmonary vein stenosis), or primary disease of the pulmonary vasculature (idiopathic PH) [13,14].

### Pathophysiology

Triggers like longstanding increased pulmonary blood flow/pressure or hypoxia can lead to pulmonary vasoconstriction and endothelial dysfunction with imbalances of nitric oxide (NO) and endothelin release. The right ventricle responds to the afterload challenge with hypertension and hypertrophic changes. Patients with near systemic or suprasystemic right ventricle pressures and no "pop off" shunt (PFO, ASD, or VSD) are especially at risk for cardiac decompensation and cardiac arrest in the perioperative period. A pulmonary hypertensive crisis, due to a sudden rise in PVR (airway obstruction, hypoventilation, catecholamine surge, etc.), is characterized by a decrease in right ventricle stroke volume, resulting in poor left ventricle filling and loss of systemic output and coronary perfusion pressure. A leftward shift of the ventricular septum, caused by right ventricle dilation, further impairs left ventricle function. Hypotension and tachycardia dramatically reduce the coronary perfusion of the hypertrophied right ventricle. The subsequent ischemia of the conduction system can end in severe bradycardia and arrest.

### Anesthetic Considerations

- Careful risk–benefit analysis for all procedures: These are high-risk cases and should not be done without good indication, adequate preparation and preoperative discussion
- Avoidance of all triggers for sudden increases in PVR: hypoxia, hypercapnia, hypoventilation acidosis, hypothermia, sympathetic surges, light anesthesia, etc.

313

- Adequate levels of anesthesia during periods of intense stimulation (intubation, incision, etc.)
- Never discontinue a continuous prostacyclin infusion: Risk for severe rebound PH
- Continue specific therapy with sildenafil or bosentan in the perioperative period
- Higher levels of inspired $O_2$ and slight hyperventilation can be beneficial (except for unrepaired VSD, etc.)
- For severe cases: Consider NO for backup emergency therapy if positive vasodilator test; not effective for pulmonary venous hypertension or flow-related PH
- Maintenance of normal preload for hypertrophied right ventricle, positive pressure ventilation can decrease preload
- Early use of inotropic support for right ventricle
- Maintenance of adequate coronary perfusion pressure: Hypotension and tachycardia are especially dangerous for hypertrophied right ventricle at risk for ischemia
- Adequate postoperative monitoring and pain control: hypertensive pulmonary crisis can happen in the recovery room or on the floor; day surgery requires a specific individual risk–benefit assessment.

## Williams Syndrome

This syndrome is characterized by a combination of congenital heart defects (supravalvular aortic and pulmonary stenosis), developmental delay, as well as distinctive personality traits and facial features (elfin face). The incidence is about 1:20 000. A spontaneous deletion on chromosome 7q11.23 results in an elastin arteriopathy which leads primarily to supravalvular aortic stenosis with tubular narrowing of the ascending aorta, often including coronary ostia and coronaries. Other arteries (pulmonary, renal, or abdominal) can also be affected. Unfortunately, there is no correlation between the degree of supravalvular obstruction and the coronary involvement. In addition, echocardiography, the routine screening tool for ventricular function, hypertrophy and outflow obstruction, is very insensitive for assessment of coronary blood flow. Most other diagnostic studies (CT angiography, MRI or cardiac catheterization) often require some form of sedation or anesthesia and are therefore not helpful for the initial risk assessment [15].

### Pathophysiology

Bilateral ventricular hypertrophy from bilateral outflow obstructions with increased risk for myocardial ischemia and sudden death due to decreased coronary perfusion and/or increased myocardial oxygen consumption.

### Anesthetic Considerations

- Multiple case reports of sudden death and failed resuscitation attempts during sedation and general anesthesia
- Careful risk–benefit analysis for all elective procedures: These are high-risk cases and should not be done without good indication and preoperative discussion
- Careful choice of location, staffing, and potential support
- Meticulous attention to myocardial oxygen consumption and coronary perfusion pressures during the perioperative phase
- Avoid long NPO times; preload dependent stiff ventricles might benefit from preinduction fluid bolus
- Intravenous induction usually preferred, using agents which will maintain contractility and blood pressure
- Avoid hypotension and tachycardia; use α-adrenergic agents like phenylephrine to maintain adequate coronary perfusion pressure. Use β-adrenergic agents with caution: The resulting tachycardia and increased myocardial oxygen consumption may worsen the situation.
- Adequate postoperative pain control, fluid, and temperature management to prevent tachycardia and fever.

## Cardiomyopathies

Cardiomyopathies (CMs) can be classified as primary myocardial CMs or secondary CMs, associated with neuromuscular disorders, inborn errors of metabolism, iron overload, mitochondrial disease, or toxic/infectious agents (chemotherapy, Chagas). Cardiomyopathies fall into three types: dilated, hypertrophic, and restrictive, each with different risk factors, clinical courses, outcomes, and treatment options.

The published data on the anesthetic risk for neonates and infants with CM is very sparse, but data clearly highlight the importance of careful preoperative evaluation and preparation, as well as allocation of additional resources for high-risk patients (pre- and postoperative ICU, inotropic support, ECMO stand by, etc.) [16,17].

## Dilated Cardiomyopathy

Dilated cardiomyopathy (DCM) is the most common pediatric CM (>50 percent). It is often caused by genetic factors, but also by viral myocarditis, neuromuscular disorders, chemotherapeutic agents, and metabolic diseases. Treatment options include inotropic support, afterload reduction, diuretics, beta blockade and occasionally biventricular pacing or even ECMO support as a bridge to transplant. Survival rates are around 40–80 percent; the subgroup of viral myocarditis has the best chance of recovery.

### Pathophysiology

Progressive thinning of the left ventricle wall, ventricular dilation, and loss of systolic function result in severe CHF.

### Anesthetic Considerations

- Careful preoperative evaluation and assessment of ventricular function and end-organ disease
- For elective procedures in patients with severe ventricular dysfunction with fractional shortening (FS) <16 percent (normal 25–45 percent) or ejection fraction (EF) < 30 percent (normal 55–70 percent), a preoperative team discussion should address the need for preoperative admission and treatment optimization (sympathomimetics, milrinone) or ECMO stand by
- Meticulous fluid management: The volume-loaded, poorly contractile ventricle is unable to handle a rapid fluid bolus
- Avoid negative inotropic agents; may benefit from perioperative inotropic support and afterload reduction (dopamine, low-dose epinephrine or milrinone infusion)
- Ketamine has direct cardio-depressant effects in patients with CHF and depletion of catecholamine stores and can result in cardiovascular collapse.

## Hypertrophic Cardiomyopathy

Hypertrophic cardiomyopathy (HCM) constitutes about 25 percent of pediatric CMs, and is characterized by ventricular hypertrophy not caused by an underlying obstruction or stenosis. Seventy-five percent of cases are idiopathic (multiple genes, often autosomal dominant); the rest are associated with metabolic diseases (Pompe), malformation syndromes (Noonan), and neuromuscular disorders (Friedreich's ataxia). Children with inborn errors of metabolism and those with early presentation in infancy, lower shortening fraction and higher posterior wall thickness on echocardiography are at high risk for sudden death.

### Pathophysiology

The massive hypertrophy of the ventricle can be concentric, with symmetric thickening of the left ventricle wall or, more often, asymmetric with septal dominance. With contraction during systole the left ventricular outflow tract, and sometimes even the cavity itself, may become obstructed, a condition called hypertrophic obstructive CM (HOCM). Anterior motion of the mitral valve during systole (SAM) against the hypertrophied septum can be a contributing factor.

The hypertrophied ventricle has enhanced contractility, but impaired diastolic filling. Over time this will lead to dilation of the left atrium, pulmonary congestion and progressive heart failure.

The degree of outflow tract obstruction is highly dynamic and dependent on the intraventricular volume status and contractile state. Inotropic agents, low SVR, and poor preload will worsen the obstruction and result in poor cardiac output, coronary ischemia, arrhythmias, and sudden death.

### Anesthetic Considerations

- High-risk population: Careful risk–benefit evaluation
- Minimize NPO times, optimize preload; preinduction gentle fluid bolus recommended
- Do not discontinue beta blocker therapy due to risk of rebound tachycardia
- Increased preload, negative inotropic agents, and increased SVR will reduce outflow obstruction
- Consider esmolol to cover periods of significant stimulation and catecholamine surges
- Use pure α-agonists (phenylephrine) to treat hypotension. Avoid positive inotropic agents.

## Restrictive Cardiomyopathy

Restrictive cardiomyopathy (RCM) is a diastolic cardiac dysfunction defined as restrictive filling with normal ventricular size and wall thickness. It is relatively rare in children (2.5–3 percent) and responds poorly to medical or surgical treatment. Transplantation is usually considered early in the disease process.

### Pathophysiology

The stiff ventricles, often caused by infiltrative processes (e.g., sarcoidosis), impair diastolic filling which results in atrial enlargement (out of proportion to ventricular size) and PH.

### Anesthetic Consideration

- High-risk population: Careful risk–benefit evaluation
- Prone to thromboembolism, therefore often anticoagulated
- Meticulous fluid management: Poor tolerance for rapid fluid administration
- Management of PH and right ventricle dysfunction (see above).

## Transplant Recipients

Children account for about 12.5 percent of all cardiac transplantation; in infants ~60 percent occur for CHD and ~30 percent for cardiomyopathies. The average survival time for infants is currently 18 years [18].

### Physiology of the Transplanted Heart

After loss of sympathetic and parasympathetic innervation, the transplanted heart is dependent on an intact Frank Starling mechanism and circulating endogenous catecholamines to increase cardiac output. Additional characteristics are: elevated baseline heart rate and filling pressures, diastolic dysfunction, low normal left ventricle function, and altered responses to various medications.

### Anesthetic Considerations

- Thorough preoperative evaluation: Review of surveillance testing, cardiac function, current rejection status, infections, status of vascular access, organ dysfunction
- Review of current medications: Steroids and immunosuppressants, typical side-effects – hypertension, bone marrow suppression, liver and kidney dysfunction, osteoporosis, etc.
- Physiology of denervated heart:
  - Loss of cardiac reflexes, dependent on preload, circulating catecholamines

- Altered response to medications:
  - No heart rate response to atropine, glycopyrrolate, and digitalis
  - Possible severe bradycardia/cardiac arrest with neostigmine
  - Exaggerated response to Ca-channel blockers, beta blockers, adenosine
  - Exaggerated response to direct-acting sympathetic agents
  - Decreased response to indirect-acting agents like dopamine and ephedrine
- For hypotension: Careful fluid bolus and titration of a direct-acting sympathomimetic
- Increased risk of infection: Use aseptic techniques.

## Specific Situations

Recommendations for the perioperative management of children with complex CHD are largely based on small case series, retrospective chart reviews and institutional practice reports. Specific guidelines regarding the safety and optimal timing of elective procedures, prohibitive risk factors, suitability for laparoscopic or thoracoscopic surgery, the need for invasive monitoring, and postoperative ICU admission are clearly missing.

In one of the most recent retrospective reviews, Watkins et al. reported their institutional experience with complex cardiac patients who underwent noncardiac procedures from 2006 to 2011 [19]. The authors found that the majority of these procedures were gastrostomies and fundoplications (~50 percent), followed by peripherally inserted central catheter (PICC) and central venous line (CVL) placements (~20 percent), airway endoscopy (7.5 percent), and imaging studies like MRI or CT (5 percent). Over 60 percent of cases were done between stage 1 and 2 palliations for single ventricle physiology, and 70 percent of patients were younger than six months.

The following section will focus on these more frequently performed procedures and briefly review some of the available data and recommendations.

## Open Fundoplication and Gastrostomy After Stage 1 Palliation of HLHS [20]

A retrospective chart review of 39 patients with palliated HLHS who had these procedures between July 2006 and December 2009 found the following:

- Preoperative echo within one week of surgery: Review of ventricular function, outflow tract obstruction, neoaortic valve stenosis or insufficiency, residual arch gradient
- Average age of patients at time of surgery: 46 days (range 20–137 days)
- Average preoperative length of stay: 38 days (range 2–165 days)
- Hemodynamic instability during induction in 69.2 percent, during maintenance in 66.7 percent, in the emergence phase in 48.7 percent, and during recovery in 38.5 percent of patients
- 92 percent intravenous inductions, 50 percent regional anesthesia (mostly single-shot caudal, occasional epidural catheter)
- Regional anesthesia associated with increased instability during induction phase and increased need for intraoperative inotropic support; no correlation with extubation in operating room
- 79.5 percent extubated in operating room
- Within the first 24 h: 23.1 percent required escalation of respiratory management (increase of supplemental oxygen, noninvasive ventilation or reintubation); 15.4 percent required escalation of hemodynamic management (inotropic/vasoactive medications, afterload reduction, or antiarrhythmic drugs)
- 12.8 percent had unplanned ICU admissions
- Patients with neoaortic insufficiency had increased ventilator and ICU days
- Overall 30-day mortality: 2.7 percent.

The following conclusions can be drawn:

- Preoperative echo is important for risk assessment
- Perioperative instability is common, mainly during induction and the maintenance phase
- Many patients require perioperative inotropic support
- Regional anesthesia is associated with increased induction instability and need for inotropic support, has no significant benefit and is often contraindicated because of the need for anticoagulation
- Extubation in operating room is possible, but most postoperative complications were respiratory issues
- Adequate pain management is important; patients are often very opioid tolerant

- There is a strong recommendation to admit all patients directly from the operating room to the ICU for recovery.

# Laparoscopic Gastrostomy and Fundoplication After Stage 1 Palliation of HLHS

Abdominal $CO_2$ insufflation during laparoscopic surgery has significant implications for the anesthetic management of neonates and infants: changes in pulmonary mechanics ($\uparrow$ PIP, $\downarrow$ compliance, FRC, VC, TV and CV) as well as cardiovascular consequences of increased intra-abdominal pressure ($\downarrow$ venous return, preload and cardiac output, $\uparrow$ afterload, occurrence of left ventricle wall motion abnormalities) [21–23] are often poorly tolerated. $CO_2$ absorption increases with increasing inflation pressure, inflation time, and younger age [24]. In neonates, laparoscopic surgery times >100 min have been associated with an increased incidence of intraoperative events and need for postoperative ICU admission [25].

Patients with single ventricle physiology and limited cardiopulmonary reserves are even more susceptible to the deleterious effects of a pneumoperitoneum [11,12]:

- the volume-loaded ventricle is unable to handle increased afterload;
- loss of preload further decreases cardiac output;
- diastolic hypotension is poorly tolerated – risk for coronary ischemia;
- limited pulmonary blood flow decreases ability to eliminate additional $CO_2$;
- increases in PVR (hypercapnia, increased PIP, acidosis, hypothermia) can "unbalance" the circulation.

Nevertheless, several small studies and case series reported successful procedures with zero short-term mortality and no evidence of shunt thrombosis, using defined management protocols [7,26,27]:

- pre- and postoperative echocardiography;
- invasive blood pressure monitoring – end-tidal $CO_2$ is not a reliable reflection of $PaCO_2$ during laparoscopy;
- maintenance of anesthesia with low-dose isoflurane (0.5–1 percent) and fentanyl;
- low abdominal insufflation pressures (8–12 mmHg);

- transfusion to hematocrit of 40–45 percent;
- planned postoperative ICU admission.

## PICC or CVL Placement After Stage 1 Palliation

PICC or CVL placement is the second most frequent procedure for patients with single ventricle physiology:

- often performed off-site in interventional radiology suite or catheterization lab with poor access to patient;
- patients often have had a prolonged hospital stay, often have high opioid tolerance and poor vascular access;
- for stable patients with a clearly identified patent vessel and most likely short procedure, IV sedation with midazolam and ketamine is possible;
- for complex patients with borderline function, baseline oxygen requirements and high tolerance:
  - general anesthesia with endotracheal intubation and positive pressure ventilation is recommended; maintenance of body temperature is important;
  - for patients with extreme poor or borderline function, consider intubation and initial stabilization in the operating room or ICU with all available support systems;
  - preoperative discussion regarding the acceptable duration of access attempts and potential backup plan (short term CVL) to limit cardiovascular compromise;
  - careful management of parallel circulation, balancing systemic and pulmonary circulation;
  - many patients will require a fluid bolus prior to or shortly after induction;
  - close monitoring for possible hypoglycemia for patients on parenteral nutrition;
  - perioperative inotropic support often is beneficial;
  - risk for coronary ischemia during periods of hypotension with low diastolic pressures;
  - postoperative admission to ICU is recommended, especially after prolonged procedures.

## Direct Laryngoscopy and Bronchoscopy for Airway Evaluation in Patients After Stage 1 Palliation

- Requires individual preoperative assessment of ventricular function and pulmonary blood flow
- Careful management of parallel circulation, balancing systemic and pulmonary circulations
- Close communication with otolaryngologists is important
- Volume-loaded single ventricle with poor tolerance for deep inhalational or propofol anesthesia to maintain spontaneous ventilation. Alternative techniques or a multimodal approach is necessary (local anesthesia, ketamine, midazolam, low-dose inhalational agents, remifentanil, etc.)
- Consider perioperative inotropic support
- Prolonged periods of hypoxia and hypercapnia are often poorly tolerated
- Depending on airway status and extent of manipulations, consider postoperative admission to the ICU

## Imaging Studies (CT, MRI Brain, Cardiac MRI) After Stage 1 Palliation

- Off-site locations with limited support
- Single ventricle patients are often unable to tolerate deep sedation for prolonged immobility
- General anesthesia with controlled ventilation is usually preferred
- Requires careful management of parallel circulation (see above)
- Periods of breath holding for CT or cardiac MRI have to be limited or adequately spaced apart to avoid hypercapnia and atelectasis
- Consider recovery in main PACU or ICU; off-site recovery rooms are often inadequately staffed and equipped to handle complex cardiac patients.

## Duodenal Atresia, Trisomy 21 and CAVC [28]

- Neonatal urgent surgery, after initial stabilization, rehydration, and diagnostic evaluation
- Diagnostic tests are ultrasound, CT, CXR, labs
- Echo to evaluate CHD: patency of PDA, ventricular function, direction of shunts, AV

valve anatomy and function, degree of mitral regurgitation

- Anesthesia considerations for trisomy 21: large tongue, short trachea, possible cervical spine instability, difficult vascular access, small peripheral arteries, hypothyroidism
- "Bubble" precautions: possible bidirectional shunting at several levels
- Invasive monitoring: depending on extent and type of surgery (open versus laparoscopic), ventricular function and pulmonary status
- Fluid status: adequate rehydration if severe vomiting, correction of electrolyte deficits and metabolic status, alkalosis beneficial for elevated PVR
- Hemodynamic management:
  - high PVR and immature neonatal lungs – relative protection for pulmonary overcirculation
  - risk for significant right-to left shunting with increased PVR – avoid light anesthesia, suctioning, sudden PVR surges (hypercapnia, hypoxemia, hypothermia, acidosis, high peak pressures, etc.)
  - cardiac dysfunction: ↑ right ventricle afterload, AV regurgitation, etc.; consider low-dose inotropic support
- Postoperative recovery usually in the ICU.

## Tetralogy of Fallot and Tracheoesophageal Fistula [28]

- A neonatal urgent surgery, after diagnostic evaluation of CHD and other associated extracardiac anomalies (VACTERL)
- Echo to assess cardiac defect: type of ToF, pulmonary stenosis or atresia, source of pulmonary blood flow, PDA, extent of right ventricle outflow obstruction (valvular, supra- and subvalvular), evaluation of dynamic infundibular component, associated cardiac anomalies, especially right-sided aortic arch
- Right sided aortic arch usually requires a different surgical approach: left-sided thoracotomy
- Consider staged surgical repair for critically ill and unstable neonates: initial gastrostomy and ligation of fistula, full repair after cardiac surgery
- Maintenance of adequate pulmonary blood flow is important – avoidance of increases in right

ventricular outflow obstruction or decreases in preload and SVR

- Invasive monitoring recommended to assess adequacy of ventilation (right-to-left shunt)
- Hypotension should be treated with volume and pure α-agonist like phenylephrine
- All medications for treatment of hypercyanotic spells should be immediately available (see Table 29.4).

## References

1. Baum VC, Barton DM, Gutgesell HP. Influence of congenital heart disease on mortality after noncardiac surgery in hospitalized children. *Pediatrics.* 2000;105(2):332–5.

2. Flick RP, Sprung J, Harrison TE, et al. Perioperative cardiac arrests in children between 1988 and 2005 at a tertiary referral center: a study of 92,881 patients. *Anesthesiology.* 2007;106(2):226–37.

3. Ramamoorthy C, Haberkern CM, Bhananker SM, et al. Anesthesia-related cardiac arrest in children with heart disease: data from the Pediatric Perioperative Cardiac Arrest (POCA) registry. *Anesth Analg.* 2010;110(5):1376–82.

4. van der Griend BF, Lister NA, McKenzie IM, et al. Postoperative mortality in children after 101,885 anesthetics at a tertiary pediatric hospital. *Anesth Analg.* 2011;112(6):1440–7.

5. Chan DMSA. Congenital heart disease. In: Vacanti CASP, Urman RD, Derswitz M, Segal BS, editors. *Essential Clinical Anesthesia.* Cambridge: Cambridge University Press; 2011.

6. Wilson W, Taubert KA, Gewitz M, et al. Prevention of infective endocarditis: guidelines from the American Heart Association: a guideline from the American Heart Association Rheumatic Fever, Endocarditis, and Kawasaki Disease Committee, Council on Cardiovascular Disease in the Young, and the Council on Clinical Cardiology, Council on Cardiovascular Surgery and Anesthesia, and the Quality of Care and Outcomes Research Interdisciplinary Working Group. *Circulation* 2007;116:1736–54.

7. Wulkan ML, Vasudevan SA. Is end-tidal CO2 an accurate measure of arterial CO2 during laparoscopic procedures in children and neonates with cyanotic congenital heart disease? *J Pediatr Surg.* 2001;36(8):1234–6.

8. Sumpelmann R, Osthaus WA. The pediatric cardiac patient presenting for noncardiac surgery. *Curr Op Anaesth.* 2007;20(3):216–20.

9. White MC. Approach to managing children with heart disease for noncardiac surgery. *Paediatr Anaesth.* 2011;21(5):522–9.

10. Torres A, Jr., DiLiberti J, Pearl RH, et al. Noncardiac surgery in children with hypoplastic left heart syndrome. *J Pediatr Surg.* 2002;37(10):1399–403.

11. Wright GE, Crowley DC, Charpie JR, et al. High systemic vascular resistance and sudden cardiovascular collapse in recovering Norwood patients. *Ann Thorac Surg.* 2004;77(1):48–52.

12. Walker SG, Stuth EA. Single-ventricle physiology: perioperative implications. *Semin Pediatr Surg.* 2004;13(3):188–202.

13. Carmosino MJ, Friesen RH, Doran A, Ivy DD. Perioperative complications in children with pulmonary hypertension undergoing noncardiac surgery or cardiac catheterization. *Anesth Analg.* 2007;104(3):521–7.

14. Friesen RH, Williams GD. Anesthetic management of children with pulmonary arterial hypertension. *Paediatr Anaesth.* 2008;18(3):208–16.

15. Burch TM, McGowan FX, Jr., Kussman BD, Powell AJ, DiNardo JA. Congenital supravalvular aortic stenosis and sudden death associated with anesthesia: what's the mystery? *Anesth Analg.* 2008;107(6):1848–54.

16. Kipps AK, Ramamoorthy C, Rosenthal DN, Williams GD. Children with cardiomyopathy: complications after noncardiac procedures with general anesthesia. *Paediatr Anaesth.* 2007;17(8):775–81.

17. Lynch J, Pehora C, Holtby H, Schwarz SM, Taylor K. Cardiac arrest upon induction of anesthesia in children with cardiomyopathy: an analysis of incidence and risk factors. *Paediatr Anaesth.* 2011;21(9):951–7.

18. Schure AY, Kussman BD. Pediatric heart transplantation: demographics, outcomes, and anesthetic implications. *Paediatr Anaesth.* 2011;21(5):594–603.

19. Watkins SC, McNew BS, Donahue BS. Risks of noncardiac operations and other procedures in children with complex congenital heart disease. *Ann Thorac Surg.* 2013;95(1):204–11.

20. Watkins S, Morrow SE, McNew BS, Donahue BS. Perioperative management of infants undergoing fundoplication and gastrostomy after stage I palliation of hypoplastic left heart syndrome. *Pediatr Cardiol.* 2012;33(5):697–704.

21. Bannister CF, Brosius KK, Wulkan M. The effect of insufflation pressure on pulmonary mechanics in infants during laparoscopic surgical procedures. *Paediatr Anaesth.* 2003;13(9):785–9.

22. Huettemann E, Sakka SG, Petrat G, Schier F, Reinhart K. Left ventricular regional wall motion abnormalities during pneumoperitoneum in children. *Br J Anaesth.* 2003;90(6):733–6.

23. Gomez Dammeier BH, Karanik E, Gluer S, et al. Anuria during pneumoperitoneum in infants and children: a prospective study. *J Pediatr Surg.* 2005;40(9):1454–8.

24. McHoney M, Corizia L, Eaton S, et al. Carbon dioxide elimination during laparoscopy in children is age dependent. *J Pediatr Surg.* 2003;38(1):105–10.

25. Kalfa N, Allal H, Raux O, et al. Tolerance of laparoscopy and thoracoscopy in neonates. *Pediatrics.* 2005;116(6):e785–91.

26. Mariano ER, Boltz MG, Albanese CT, Abrajano CT, Ramamoorthy C. Anesthetic management of infants with palliated hypoplastic left heart syndrome undergoing laparoscopic nissen fundoplication. *Anesth Analg.* 2005;100(5):1631–3.

27. Slater B, Rangel S, Ramamoorthy C, Abrajano C, Albanese CT. Outcomes after laparoscopic surgery in neonates with hypoplastic heart left heart syndrome. *J Pediatr Surg.* 2007;42(6):1118–21.

28. Walker A, Stokes M, Moriarty A. Anesthesia for major general surgery in neonates with complex cardiac defects. *Paediatr Anaesth.* 2009;19(2):119–25.

**Chapter**

# 30

# Neonatal and Infant Tumors

Laura H. Leduc

Tumors in neonates and infants are rare but potentially life-threatening. According to the most recent data from 2007 through 2011, tracked by the National Cancer Institute through the Surveillance, Epidemiology, and End Results (SEER) Program, the rate of all cancers in children less than one year of age is 253.4 per 1 000 000 [1]. The rate of all childhood cancers is highest for infants as compared with all other pediatric age groups in the 1–19 years range, with infants having the lowest likelihood of survival at 77.7 percent [1]. This underscores the importance of accurate and prompt diagnosis, appropriate treatment, and quality-improvement measures.

Cancer in neonates often presents differently than cancer in older children, making diagnosis and management challenging in this age group. This review will focus on some of the more common tumors and their anesthetic implications. According to the International Classification of Childhood Cancer (ICCC) there are 12 categories of childhood cancer [2].

(1) leukemia
(2) lymphomas and reticuloendothelial neoplasms
(3) CNS and miscellaneous intracranial and intraspinal neoplasms
(4) neuroblastoma and other peripheral nervous cell tumors
(5) retinoblastoma
(6) renal tumors
(7) hepatic tumors
(8) malignant bone tumors
(9) soft tissue and other extra osseous sarcomas
(10) germ cell and trophoblastic tumors and neoplasms of gonads
(11) other malignant epithelial neoplasms and melanomas
(12) other and unspecified malignant neoplasms

Neonatal cancer is increasingly diagnosed by prenatal ultrasound, although this may lead to over-diagnosis due to the fact that many tumors regress spontaneously [3]. Ultrasound imaging combined with knowledge of location has been shown to correctly identify 94 percent of prenatal tumors [4]. Prenatal diagnosis can enable a pregnancy to be followed more closely for polyhydramnios or preterm labor, and delivery can occur under controlled circumstances.

Infants who are diagnosed with cancer in the perinatal period should be evaluated for a cancer predisposition syndrome [3]. Such risk would be higher in the setting of multifocal or bilateral disease, congenital malformations, or cancer in close relatives [5].

## Leukemia

The leukemias of infancy, including acute lymphoblastic leukemia (ALL), acute myelogenous leukemia (AML), and juvenile myelomonocytic leukemia (JMML) occur at a rate of 51.7 per 1 000 000 infants [1], and account for only 2 percent of childhood leukemias. They are a disease in which a stem cell gives rise to an unregulated proliferation of cells termed "blasts." The abnormal cells have an increased rate of proliferation and a decreased rate of spontaneous apoptosis which ultimately results in bone marrow failure.

Neonates with leukemia usually present with hyperleukocytosis and extensive tissue infiltration. Central nervous system (CNS) disease may be present, along with hepatosplenomegaly. Diffuse pulmonary infiltrates may cause tachypnea, and infants with AML may have subcutaneous nodules called leukemia cutis [6]. Older infants may present with nonspecific anorexia, fatigue, irritability, fevers, and bony pain. Bone marrow failure often results in bruising, bleeding, and pallor. Lymphadenopathy and hepatosplenomegaly may be noted. Compression of the airways by mediastinal lymph nodes can contribute to respiratory distress.

321

Genetic conditions that predispose to acute leukemia include Down syndrome, Bloom syndrome, ataxia-telangiectasia, Fanconi anemia, Li–Fraumeni syndrome, and neurofibromatosis type 1.

Neonatal leukemia has a guarded prognosis despite aggressive chemotherapy. Acute lymphoid leukemia and AML have a five-year relative survival of 56.5 percent and 65 percent respectively in this age group; however, patients can experience late-effects from treatment, including neurologic and cardiac sequelae.

Neonatal or infant ALL may respond well to oral steroids alone, but typically multiple chemotherapeutic agents including vincristine, L-asparaginase, and daunomycin are used for induction. Consolidation involves agents (e.g., cytarabine) more typically used in patients with AML with an intensive schedule.

Acute myeloid leukemia is as common as ALL in neonates [1]. The presentation is similar in terms of bone marrow failure, but can also include "blueberry muffin" lesions which are subcutaneous nodules, gingival infiltrates, disseminated intravascular coagulation, and chloromas or granulocytic sarcomas [3].

Up to 10 percent of patients with Down syndrome develop transient myeloproliferative disease (TMD), which is a transient clonal myeloproliferation [6]. It may be associated with hepatomegaly and liver fibrosis. Clinically symptomatic patients are treated with low-dose cytarabine. Patients will need careful follow-up as 20 percent will develop AML within the first four years of life [3].

Juvenile myelomonocytic leukemia is a rare leukemia that affects children less than two years of age. It consists of a clonal proliferation of hematopoietic stem cells. Patients may have rashes, lymphadenopathy, splenomegaly and hemorrhage [6]. While most cases resolve spontaneously, monocytosis and splenomegaly may persist for several years and approximately 10 percent of patients have a fatal progressive disease [1].

Patients with leukemia may present for anesthesia for diagnostic and treatment purposes. Newly diagnosed patients may receive general anesthesia for central line placement and associated procedures, and it is important to avoid administering dexamethasone to minimize the risk of tumor lysis syndrome or chemotherapy protocol violation. It is also important to avoid placing rectal thermometers in infants that are immunocompromised.

# CNS and Miscellaneous Intracranial and Intraspinal Neoplasms

Central nervous system, intracranial, and intraspinal neoplasms occur at a rate of 48.8 per 1 000 000 infants and have a five-year relative survival of 56.6 percent [1]. According to the World Health Organization (WHO), more than 100 categories and subtypes of primary CNS tumors occur in children [7]. Tumors of the CNS may be located in the supratentorial space, posterior fossa, parasellar region, or in the spinal cord. Infants are more likely than older children to present with tumors in the supratentorial space and the predominant tumor types are choroid plexus tumors and teratomas. There are several syndromes associated with pediatric brain tumors, including neurofibromatosis types 1 and 2 (NF-1/2), von Hippel–Lindau, tuberous sclerosis, Li–Fraumeni, Cowden, Turçot, and nevoid basal cell carcinoma [7].

The presenting symptoms for infants with CNS lesions vary depending on the location. Symptoms are usually due to increased intracranial pressure (ICP), are often nonspecific in infants, and may include vomiting, lethargy, irritability, and increasing head circumference. Infratentorial tumors may present with irritability due to headache pain, vomiting, papilledema, and nystagmus. Symptoms of brainstem tumors can include cranial nerve palsies and abnormal eye movements, weakness of an extremity, and upper motor neuron deficits. Supratentorial tumors present more commonly with focal neurologic deficits as well as a bulging fontanelle and the onset of seizures. Tumors of the parasellar may result in neuroendocrine abnormalities, failure to thrive, and visual abnormalities due to the proximity to the pituitary gland, optic pathways, and hypothalamus. Spinal cord tumors may present with crying and irritability due to pain and motor deficits as the tumor expands, causing compression within the spinal cord [7].

The evaluation of CNS tumors generally involves magnetic resonance imaging (MRI), which in most infants requires the administration of a general anesthetic to keep the child quiet during the imaging. In very young infants, swaddling and feeding the child just before the imaging has been successful. Tumors in the midline or suprasellar region should prompt an evaluation for neuroendocrine dysfunction. A lumbar puncture is indicated for tumors that are known to spread to the meninges, such as medulloblastoma/primitive neuroectodermal tumor (PNET), ependymoma, and germ cell tumors, but should be delayed until hydrocephalus and supratentorial midline shift is ruled out due to the potential for brain herniation and death [8].

Astrocytoma is the most common CNS malignancy of infancy and occurs at a rate of 15.5 per 1 000 000 infants and has a five-year relative survival of 76.5 percent [7]. It is most likely to occur in the cerebellum. Other locations include the hypothalamic/third ventricular region and the optic nerve and chiasmal region [7]. Astrocytoma tumors are graded I–IV according to their histological features as well as their clinicopathological characteristics. Pilocytic astrocytoma (PA) is a WHO grade I tumor because it has a low metastatic potential and rarely metastasizes [7]. There is a 15 percent incidence of PA of the optic nerve and chiasmal region in patients with NF-1. Fibrillary infiltrating astrocytoma is a WHO grade II tumor, which is still considered low grade. High-grade astrocytomas include anaplastic astrocytoma (WHO grade III) and glioblastoma multiforme (WHO grade IV), both of which have high malignant potential [7].

Treatment for astrocytomas in newborns and infants includes surgery and chemotherapy. Chemotherapeutic agents include carboplatin, vincristine, temozolomide, vinblastine, lomustine, and procarbazine [7]. Radiation is avoided for as long as possible because of potential long-term negative effects on brain development.

Ependymomas are tumors derived from the ependymal lining of the ventricular system. They are most likely to be in the posterior fossa. They are usually noninvasive, expanding in the ventricular system and eventually displacing normal structures, leading to obstructive hydrocephalus. Primary treatment is surgery, although chemotherapy and radiation are also indicated [7].

Choroid plexus tumors are rare, representing only 3 percent of all childhood brain tumors; however, most present within the first year of life. They are intraventricular epithelial neoplasms that arise from the choroid plexus. Tumors may be papillomas, which are considered low-grade tumors or carcinomas which are malignant tumors with the potential to metastasize to the CSF pathways [7]. The tumor is most likely to be supratentorial in the lateral ventricles. Choroid plexus papillomas have an excellent five-year survival rate of 95 percent, whereas choroid plexus carcinomas have a much poorer prognosis [7].

Primitive neuroectodermal tumors are malignant embryonal tumors. They can metastasize to the CNS and beyond and are classified as WHO grade IV tumors. Included in this group of tumors are medulloblastoma, supratentorial PNET, ependymoblastoma, medulloepithelioblastoma, and atypical teratoid/rhabdoid tumor (ATRT). Treatment can include surgery, chemotherapy, and radiation.

Craniopharyngioma is a rare pediatric tumor that is derived from ectodermal remnants, Rathke cleft, or other embryonal epithelium in the sellar or parasellar region [9]. The tumor usually arises in the region of the pituitary gland and endocrine abnormalities may be the presenting feature. Craniopharyngiomas are minimally invasive [7], but surgical resection can result in significant morbidity such as panhypopituitarism, growth failure, and visual loss due to the tumor location [7]. Life-threatening obesity in older children and adults can result from tumor resection due to damage to the hypothalamus [9]. Incomplete resection with less morbidity augmented by radiation to prevent local recurrence is one treatment approach.

There is significant morbidity associated with patients who survive neonatal brain tumors, including chronic neurologic deficits, seizure disorders, neurocognitive deficits, and neuroendocrine deficiencies [7]. Survivors are also at risk of secondary malignancies [7].

Infants with brain tumors undergo anesthesia for diagnostic neuroimaging, ventricular shunt placement, and surgical tumor resection. The preoperative assessment should include a thorough neurologic exam for signs of increased ICP. Typically premedication is not indicated. Anesthetic induction can be either intravenous or inhalational, depending on clinical symptoms. Intraoperative bleeding can be significant in tumor resections, and arterial line and large-bore intravenous catheters are essential. Blood should be immediately available. Positioning of the infant during tumor resection depends on the location of the tumor. In most cases, access to the airway will be limited; therefore careful attention should be made to securing the endotracheal tube (ETT) and to ETT positioning, especially if the infant is in the prone position with neck flexion. Intraoperative arterial blood gases, core temperature, urine output, and hemoglobin should be closely monitored. The operating room should be warmed and a forced-air warming blanket used to prevent hypothermia.

# Neuroblastoma

Neuroblastoma is a malignancy that arises from primordial neural crest cells which usually develop into sympathetic ganglia and the adrenal medulla. Pathologically, neuroblastoma is a small, round, blue cell tumor. Neuroblastoma and neuroganglioblastoma occur at a rate of 51 per 1 000 000 infants, with a five-year relative survival rate of 92 percent [1]. These tumors are by far the most common malignancy of infancy, followed by retinoblastoma and lymphoid leukemia [1].

Familial neuroblastoma accounts for approximately 1–2 percent of all cases and is associated with a younger age at diagnosis. The tumor is also associated with Hirschsprung disease, central hypoventilation syndrome, NF-1, Beckwith–Wiedemann syndrome, and hemihypertrophy [10].

Approximately half of neuroblastoma tumors arise in the adrenal glands [10]. Prenatal diagnosis is possible, but the tumor is difficult to distinguish from other adrenal pathology such as hemorrhage [11]. Metastatic spread is uncommon in infants and neonates, and likely contributes to the favorable prognosis for this age group.

Presentation of neuroblastoma is dependent on the location of the tumor. Localized disease may present as an asymptomatic abdominal mass. Larger masses may present with symptoms of respiratory distress, dysphagia, or vocal cord paralysis. There may be symptoms of spinal cord compression, bowel or bladder dysfunction, and superior vena cava syndrome. Alternatively, patients may be asymptomatic with an incidental finding on chest X-ray [12]. Spinal cord and nerve root compression result from invasion of the neural foramina by paraspinal neuroblastoma.

There are a number of clinical syndromes associated with neuroblastoma [10]. The opsoclonus myoclonus ataxia syndrome is a paraneoplastic syndrome of autoimmune origin and is characterized by myoclonic jerking, random eye movements, and cerebellar ataxia. While tumors that present this way tend to have a good outcome, the syndrome does not necessarily improve with tumor removal. Pepper syndrome refers to disease with massive liver metastases which may cause respiratory distress due to hepatomegaly. Horner syndrome occurs with a thoracic or cervical primary tumor but does not resolve with tumor resection. Kerner–Morrison syndrome is intractable secretory diarrhea due to secretion of vasoactive intestinal peptides. Neurocristopathy syndrome occurs when neuroblastoma is associated with other neural crest disorders [10].

Prenatal suspicion of neuroblastoma is followed by measurement of tumor markers, including catecholamine metabolites homovanillic acid and vanillylmandelic acid in urine. Tumor biopsy confirms the diagnosis. Workup for metastatic disease includes CAT scan (CT) or MRI of the chest and abdomen, bone scans, and bone marrow aspirates and biopsies. MIBG (iodine-123 meta-iodobenzylguanidine) scans may be used to define metastatic disease.

Treatment for neuroblastoma varies depending on the patient's age, tumor, and tumor biology. Patients who present with spinal cord compression may require urgent surgical intervention or chemotherapy. Low-risk tumors are treated with surgery. Intermediate-risk tumors are treated with surgery and chemotherapy. Patients with high-risk neuroblastoma undergo aggressive treatment with chemotherapy, autologous stem cell transplantation, surgery, radiation and immune modulation with 13-*cis*-retinoic acid, and monoclonal therapy. Chemotherapeutic agents used include cyclophosphamide, topotecan, doxorubicin, vincristine, cisplatin, and etoposide.

Infants and neonates with neuroblastoma will potentially undergo anesthesia for biopsies, port placement, and ultimately tumor resection. If neoadjuvant chemotherapy has been administered, the medications and potential effects on cardiovascular function must be noted. The preoperative evaluation should include a detailed history and physical examination for signs of respiratory distress, hypertension, and superior vena cava syndrome. Infants should be evaluated for associated syndromes such as congenital hypoventilation syndrome or Beckwith–Weideman syndrome. Preoperative imaging and laboratory values should be carefully reviewed. Large, abdominal operations can be accompanied by extensive blood loss due to the proximity of blood vessels to the tumor. Large-bore intravenous access and arterial monitoring are indicated. Infants undergoing abdominal procedures are at risk for hypothermia and increased evaporative losses. Careful attention should be paid to volume status and hemodynamic changes. Core temperature should be monitored and methods to prevent hypothermia should be used such as forced-air warming blankets, warmed irrigation fluids, and a warmed operating room. Patients may benefit from regional analgesia. Patients are typically cared for in the intensive care unit postoperatively.

# Retinoblastoma

The rate of retinoblastoma diagnosis in infants is 27.7 per 1 000 000, with a five-year relative survival rate of 98.1 percent [1]. It is the most common primary intraocular malignancy of childhood and there are approximately 300–350 new cases each year [13]. Children with hereditary retinoblastoma suffer from loss of the retinoblastoma gene (*RB1*) and generally present at a younger age with multifocal and bilateral disease [14]. The classical presentation is leukocoria, which is a white pupillary reflex as opposed to the normal red reflex. The diagnosis is confirmed by a dilated fundoscopic exam under anesthesia. An MRI may be required to evaluate the optic nerve and pineal region of the brain. Many neonates can undergo MRI scanning without anesthesia by using a feed-and-swaddle technique. However, it may be necessary to provide general anesthesia for extended scans or if other procedures are needed.

The treatment for retinoblastoma needs to be prompt, and early intervention is aimed at saving the globe if not vision. Treatment may be via laser, brachytherapy, local chemotherapy, systemic chemotherapy, and surgery [13]. Chemotherapeutic agents may include carboplatin and vincristine with or without etoposide. Each of 4–6 cycles of chemotherapy involves an exam under anesthesia [13]. External beam radiation is utilized only if absolutely necessary for infants due to the potential for significant orbital hypoplasia, cataract development, and increased incidence of secondary tumors later in life for patients with the retinoblastoma1 (*RB1*) gene [13].

The prognosis for children with retinoblastoma is excellent in this country, where most are diagnosed early, prior to metastatic spread of the tumor. However, children with the *RB1* germ line mutation are at significant risk for development of second malignancies, especially if radiation therapy was used during infancy [14].

# Renal Tumors

Renal tumors occur at a rate of 15.3 per 1 000 000 in the infant population [1]. Five-year survival rates are excellent at 90 percent [1]. Renal tumors in children include Wilms tumor, mesoblastic nephroma, clear cell sarcoma of the kidney, rhabdoid tumor of the kidney or renal cell carcinoma. Syndromes associated with renal tumors include Beckwith–Wiedemann, Denys–Drash, Simpson–Golabi–Behmel, and WAGR syndrome (Wilms, Aniridia, Genitourinary anomalies and mental Retardation) [15].

In the neonatal population, the most likely diagnosis for a renal tumor is congenital mesoblastic nephroma [16]. The vast majority of mesoblastic nephromas present prior to six months of age [15]. Prenatal ultrasound findings may include polyhydramnios, hydrops, and premature delivery [16]. Most patients not diagnosed prenatally will present with an abdominal mass. Patients may also present with hematuria and hypertension, as well as failure to thrive. The treatment for congenital mesoblastic nephroma is radical nephrectomy. Partial resections and positive margins are associated with recurrence of the tumor. Generally, chemotherapy is not indicated unless a patient is considered to be at high risk of recurrence [15].

Wilms tumor is an embryonal malignancy of the kidney and comprises about 20 percent of neonatal renal tumors [17,18]. Between 1 and 2 percent of patients have a familial case of Wilms tumor which has autosomal dominant inheritance with variable penetrance, and is more likely to present at a younger age and with bilateral disease [17]. Treatment for Wilms tumor is radical nephrectomy unless the tumor is bilateral. While some patients with early-stage tumors undergo surgery alone, most patients will also have treatment with chemotherapy and possibly radiation therapy. Lower-risk tumors are treated with vincristine and actinomycin. Higher-risk tumors may also be treated with doxorubicin, cyclophosphamide, and/or etoposide. As with mesoblastic nephroma, the most likely presentation is a palpable abdominal mass with increasing abdominal girth. However, imaging is more likely to demonstrate tumor invasion or thrombus in the renal vein or inferior vena cava (IVC) [15]. Patients may also present with hypertension (25 percent), hematuria (~20 percent), anemia, polycythemia, elevated platelet count, factor VII deficiency, and an acquired deficiency of von Willebrand factor [17]. Risk factors for local recurrence include advanced local stage, unfavorable histology, and spillage of tumor at the time of primary resection [12].

Other renal tumors in neonates are less common. Rhabdoid tumor of the kidney comprises approximately 11 percent of neonatal renal tumors [16]. The tumor is very aggressive and prognosis is poor, with an overall survival in neonates of <10 percent [15]. Metastases to lung, abdomen, lymph nodes, liver, bone, skin, and brain can be seen in nearly 10 percent of cases. Clear cell sarcoma of the kidney is also an aggressive tumor, with approximately 30 percent metastatic at diagnosis [15]. Early-stage tumors have an excellent prognosis. Treatment is radical nephrectomy, chemotherapy, and radiation.

Preoperative workup for infants with renal tumors is focused on cardiopulmonary and gastrointestinal function. Large tumors may impair gastric emptying and full stomach precautions may be indicated. While renal dysfunction is unusual, electrolytes may be abnormal if the patient has been vomiting and resuscitation may be warranted. Toxicity of chemotherapeutic agents should be considered. Intraoperative positioning requires additional consideration as the surgery may be prolonged. Intravenous lines should be placed above the diaphragm when possible in case of severe bleeding requiring cross-clamping of the IVC [12]. Access should be adequate for substantial blood loss in case of vascular involvement or injury. Ventilation may be quite challenging if a laparoscopic approach is planned, and discussion with the surgical team can be helpful in guiding the operative plan. Adjunctive regional anesthesia can be beneficial for postoperative pain control.

## Hepatic Tumors

Hepatic tumors that present in the first year of life can be malignant or benign. Malignant hepatic tumors occur at a rate of 10.1 per million children less than one year of age and the vast majority of these tumors are hepatoblastoma [1]. The five-year relative survival of infant hepatoblastoma is 83.7 percent [1]. Benign liver tumors include hamartomas and vascular lesions such as hemangiomas [15]. A final common pathway for liver tumors that are not treatable with medical management or surgical intervention can be liver transplantation.

Vascular lesions are the most common liver tumor in neonates. Many vascular liver lesions involute after about one year. They are frequently associated with hypothyroidism due to activity of type 3 iodothyronine deiodinase. Patients may present in high-output cardiac failure due to hemodynamic shunting. Symptomatic vascular lesions require surgical intervention only if medical intervention fails. Medical treatment includes propranolol, corticosteroids, and vincristine. For lesions not amenable to resection, hepatic artery ligation or arterial embolization are potential options. Ligation of the hepatic artery renders the lesion ischemic and controls the arteriovenous shunting. The liver maintains blood supply via the portal system [15].

Mesenchymal hamartoma is a benign liver tumor that generally presents as a palpable but asymptomatic abdominal mass. Prenatal diagnosis is possible; hydrops fetalis may occur and alpha-fetoprotein may be elevated. These tumors can be difficult to diagnose radiographically since they are composed of both solid and cystic components. The natural history of mesenchymal hamartomas ranges from possible spontaneous regression to malignant degeneration. Treatment is generally surgical resection for tumors that do not regress with efforts toward negative margins.

Hepatoblastoma also presents with an enlarging abdominal mass. It is the most common liver malignancy in children and most cases occur in infancy [15]. The risk of developing hepatoblastoma is increased in premature infants, especially those with birthweight <1500 g [15]. Development of hepatoblastoma has been associated with hemihypertophy, Beckwith–Wiedemann syndrome, polyposis coli, Wilms tumor, and fetal alcohol syndrome [12]. Patients may have anemia, jaundice, and ascites upon presentation, but liver function tests are likely to be normal [12]. The alpha-fetoprotein level is usually markedly elevated; however, normal alpha-fetoprotein levels do not rule-out the diagnosis. Radiologic features of hepatoblastoma include large tumors, multifocal tumors, calcifications, and vascular invasion. Metastatic spread may be present at diagnosis and is most likely to be in the lungs, brain, and bone [15]. Hepatoblastoma is derived from primitive epithelial parenchyma and there are four histological variants including fetal, embryonal, macrotrabecular, and anaplastic. The anaplastic, or small cell undifferentiated has a very poor prognosis. The highest survival rate is associated with fetal histology. Outcome is dependent upon complete resection. Eighty-five percent of the liver can be resected and there is hepatic regeneration postoperatively [18]. Chemotherapy includes cisplatin with vincristine and 5-fluorouracil or doxorubicin [18].

Anesthesia for liver surgery in neonates is a highly specialized endeavor. Patients may present with large tumors causing hemodynamic and respiratory compromise. Neoadjuvant chemotherapy can have significant repercussions for the cardiac and respiratory systems. Furthermore, massive blood volume replacement intraoperatively can result in coagulopathies, acid–base imbalance, electrolyte imbalance, hypothermia, and compromised oxygen delivery.

## Soft Tissue and Other Extra Osseous Sarcomas

Soft tissue sarcomas (STS) are the fifth most common malignancy in infants, with an overall rate of 19.6 per 1 000 000 infants [1]. Within the category of STS, rhabdomyosarcoma (RMS) is the most common in infants, followed by fibrosarcoma which occurs at a rate of 5.8 and 4.6 per 1 000 000 infants respectively. Five-year relative survival for STS is 63.1 percent [1]. There is a wide range of survival likelihood within the group, ranging from 94 percent for infants with fibrosarcoma to 24 percent for those with rhabdoid tumors [19].

Although rare, sarcomas should be considered in infants who present with soft tissue lesions. Ultrasound is the first-line imaging tool, followed by MRI. It may be difficult to distinguish the much more common vascular tumors from sarcomas by imaging alone, and biopsy may be indicated.

Vascular tumors result from active cell proliferation as opposed to vascular malformations which are a result of inborn defects in vascular morphogenesis [20]. Types of vascular tumors include infantile hemangioma, tufted angioma, kaposiform hemangioendothelioma, and epithelioid hemangioendothelioma.

Fibroblastic tumors of intermediate prognosis include lesions that may be locally aggressive but rarely metastasize. These tumors are juvenile fibromatosis, lipofibromatosis and desmoid-type fibromatosis. Infantile fibrosarcoma (IFS) occurs exclusively in the first two years of life, with 60 percent of cases presenting prior to three months of age. As many as 50 percent of the cases are present at birth [20]. Infantile fibrosarcoma presents as a large, non-inflammatory, enlarging mass most often located in the deep soft tissues of lower extremities, and less likely in the trunk or head and neck region [20]. While the tumor does not often metastasize, the greater concern is for local spread with infiltration of neuromuscular structures. Treatment is a combination of surgery and chemotherapy, including vincristine and actinomycin. Neoadjuvant chemotherapy can result in tumor shrinkage, enabling a more conservative surgery with less morbidity [20].

Malignant soft tissue tumors, including RMS and non-rhabdomyosarcoma soft tissue sarcomas (NRSTS) are characterized as high or low grade. The low-grade tumors are unlikely to metastasize but may still be aggressive locally, causing significant morbidity. The high-grade tumors are more likely to metastasize with a particular affinity for the lung [20].

Rhabdomyosarcoma, the most common pediatric soft tissue sarcoma, is an embryonal tumor of childhood. It is composed of cells resembling fetal skeletal muscle. It is typically a small, round, blue cell tumor. Generally, there is high-grade histology, local invasiveness, and high likelihood of metastasis. Congenital RMS is present at birth and accounts for 1–2 percent of cases. Between 5 and 10 percent of RMS is diagnosed in infancy. In order of frequency, RMS occurs in the head and neck, genitourinary tract, and extremities [20]. Presentation is highly variable and dependent upon tumor location. Symptoms may include nasal congestion, stridor, cranial nerve palsies, or enlarging masses [21]. Radiologic imaging does not easily distinguish between highly vascularized malignant soft tissue lesions such as RMS and benign vascular lesions, potentially leading to delayed diagnosis. Rhabdomyosarcoma metastasizes to the lung, bone marrow, bone, and brain in neonates. The diagnosis is confirmed by biopsy and the complete workup will include MRI or CT of the primary lesion, chest CT, bone scan, and bone marrow aspirate and biopsy. Prognostic factors are related to tumor histology, size, and location. Treatment is a combination of surgery, chemotherapy, and radiation therapy [20].

## Germ Cell and Trophoblastic Tumors and Neoplasms of Gonads

Germ cell tumors (GCTs) are the most common neoplasm in the newborn. They account for 35–40 percent of all tumors in the neonates. Most are teratomas and not considered to be malignant [22]. Germ cell tumors may arise in the gonad or in extragonadal sites. Newborns are most likely to have extragonadal GCTs (see Figure 30.1) [22]. These neoplasms are derived from primordial germ cells. The five histologic subtypes of GCTs are teratoma, yolk sac tumors (YSTs), germinoma, embryonal carcinoma, and choriocarcinoma [22].

Teratomas are the most common histology in neonates, followed by YSTs [22]. Teratomas may be mature or immature. Mature teratomas are cystic and

327

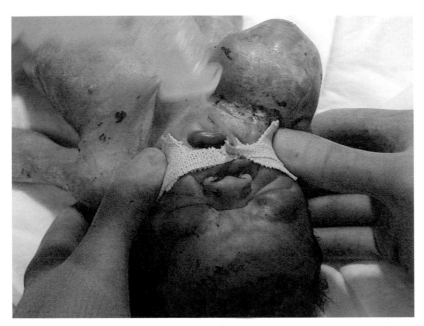

**Figure 30.1** Cervical teratoma in a newborn.
Photo courtesy of Dr. Jason Mouzakes, Albany Medical Center, Albany, New York.

contain differentiated tissue from at least one germ layer such as cartilage, bone, or hair. Immature teratomas have embryonal-appearing tissue that may be mixed with mature tissue.

Sacrococcygeal teratomas (SCTs) are germ cell tumors that occur most commonly in infants. Up to 25 percent of patients with SCT have other congenital abnormalities, including genitourinary malformations, congenital hip dislocation, esophageal atresia, and congenital heart disease [22]. Other perinatal GCTs may be located in the head and neck, oropharynx and nasopharynx, orbit, face, intracranial, cardiac, mediastinal, gastric, and fetus-in-fetu, as well as other sites [22]. Sacrococcygeal teratomas occur in 1 in 20 000–40 000 live births [22]. Prenatally, fetuses with SCT are at risk for developing hydrops fetalis due to high-output cardiac failure and anemia. Fetal interventions for tumor decompression are possible but carry a mortality rate of approximately 50 percent and are only recommended in a fetus at risk of hydrops. The treatment goal is complete resection after delivery, provided no metastatic disease is present. The entire tumor as well as the coccyx should be removed. Recurrence rates are >35 percent if the coccyx is not removed. However, highly morbid procedures involving removal of GI, GU, or neurologic structures are not indicated because even in the face of microscopically positive margins, recurrence rates and mortality are low [22]. Chemotherapy is indicated preoperatively

when complete resection is not considered possible. It is given postoperatively when complete resection was not successful. Even with metastatic disease present, cisplatin-based chemotherapy is very effective [23].

The resection of a sacrococcygeal teratoma is a high-risk procedure and requires much care and expertise in anesthetic management. Comorbid conditions include high-output cardiac failure from arteriovenous shunting in the tumor, prematurity, and coagulopathy. Tumors can be highly vascular and intraoperative blood loss can be rapid and massive. Patients are at risk for developing life-threatening hyperkalemia as the tumor is manipulated intraoperatively and hypocalcemia due to massive blood transfusion. Resuscitation drugs including calcium, sodium bicarbonate, and insulin should be readily available. Arterial monitoring and large-bore intravenous access is essential. Transfusions with fresh whole blood are preferable to packed red cells.

## Other and Unspecified Malignant Neoplasms: Pleuropulmonary Blastoma

Pleuropulmonary blastoma (PPB) is extremely rare but will be discussed briefly because of the potential anesthetic relevance. Pleuropulmonary blastoma is a malignant tumor arising from pleuropulmonary germ cells. Radiologically, this cystic or mixed solid and cystic tumor may be indistinguishable from congenital cystic adenomatoid malformation (CCAM). Diagnosis can be confirmed only by pathological analysis, but the implications of a diagnosis of PPB are significant as incomplete resection would require treatment with chemotherapy and close follow-up. Prenatal diagnosis is possible [24]. Neonatal presentation of PPB is most likely to be type I, which has an 85 percent long-term survival and is very unlikely to metastasize provided primary surgical resection margins are negative and chemotherapy is given [24].

## Diagnostic and Treatment Implications

Cancer treatment for infants is a highly specialized field of pediatric oncology. Treatment for childhood cancers is dependent on cancer type, subtype, location, and prognostic factors. Treatment may include chemotherapy alone or in combination with surgery, radiation therapy, and biologic agent therapy. Available treatments have a narrow therapeutic index and toxicity is a constant threat to all patients, especially neonates.

Chemotherapy generally involves combinations of drugs with different mechanisms of action [25]. Malignant cells have an increased metabolic cell cycle and are therefore more susceptible to toxicity than normal cells. Adverse effects are generally at sites of higher rates of cell turnover such as bone marrow, mucosa, epidermis, liver, and spermatogonia. Many patients experience thrombocytopenia and neutropenia due to bone marrow suppression. Other common side-effects are nausea and vomiting, mucositis, hepatic dysfunction, dermatitis, and alopecia. While these effects are often reversible, life-threatening complications are possible. Additionally, a few key complications are not reversible, such as cardiomyopathy due to anthracyclines, renal failure from platinum-based agents, and pulmonary fibrosis from bleomycin.

Corticosteroids are often used in the treatment of leukemias and lymphomas, although the latter is exceedingly rare in children under one year of age. Both prednisone and dexamethasone are used and the mechanism of action is lymphatic cell lysis. Steroids are also used in high doses to decrease swelling of the airway or in the CNS. Adverse effects are multiple and include Cushing syndrome, hyperglycemia, hypertension, cataract formation, myopathy, osteoporosis, avascular necrosis, infection, peptic ulcers, and

psychosis. Acute discontinuation from high doses can cause adverse effects. Chronic steroid use is of interest to anesthesiologists due to the inhibition of the adrenocortical axis and potential hypotension under general anesthesia.

Radiation therapy is avoided in neonates as much as possible due to their extreme susceptibility to adverse long-term events. Infants who will undergo radiation treatment generally require anesthesia. The treatments are usually five days per week for a variable number of weeks, and it is imperative that the patient maintains absolute stillness in an identical position for each treatment. Short-term complications from radiation treatment include nausea and vomiting, alopecia, somnolence after cranial irradiation, and swelling. Complications may have an impact on the anesthetic plan since the same patient positioning and set-up is required daily, and yet the patient's physiology may have changed. Long-term complications include growth impairment, endocrine dysfunction, cardiac or pulmonary insufficiency, abdominal strictures and adhesions, and infertility [25].

Tumor lysis syndrome is a metabolic disorder in which release of uric acid phosphates and potassium are released into the systemic circulation from the death of tumor cells. It can be induced by treatment initiation and in extreme cases can result in renal failure. It can occur prior to the initiation of treatment when there is a large tumor burden. Inadequate renal function can result in symptomatic hyperkalemia, hyperphosphatemia, and hypocalcemia [25].

Hematologic complications of cancer treatment result from bone marrow failure and include anemia, thrombocytopenia, disseminated intravascular coagulation, neutropenia, hyperleukocytosis, and graft-versus-host disease [25]. The presence of any of these situations would increase the risk of complications for patients presenting for anesthesia and only absolutely necessary procedures would be performed at this time.

There are a few oncologic emergencies that could require emergent intervention; these include spinal cord compression, increased intracranial pressure, superior vena cava syndrome, and tracheal compression. Anesthesia may be needed for diagnostic purposes such as imaging, for treatment with radiation, line placement for chemotherapy initiation, or urgent tumor resection or debulking. On rare occasions, a critical airway may need to be secured emergently. In this situation, a multidisciplinary team including pediatric anesthesiologists and pediatric otorhino-laryngologists should be assembled and a plan can be made for safe care of the patient.

Long-term effects of neonatal and infant tumors may not be apparent during the acute treatment phase. In addition to the medical complications previously covered, there are significant psychosocial and academic effects on survivors of childhood cancer and their entire families.

## Conclusion

Neonates with tumors may present with a variety of signs and symptoms including abdominal distention, respiratory or airway compromise, and increasing head circumference. Neonates can require anesthesia for diagnostic imaging as well as treatment-related procedures such as biopsies, tumor resections, and central venous access. The anesthetic management of neonates with tumors requires careful planning, a thorough understanding of neonatal physiology and pharmacology, and good communication between the surgical, anesthesia, and oncology teams.

## Acknowledgments

I would like to thank Dr. Vikramjit Kanwar for his contribution to the content of this chapter, Dr. Melissa Ehlers for her support throughout the project, and Pya Seidner for her editorial assistance.

## References

1. SEER. Age-adjusted and age-specific seer cancer incidence rates, 2007–2011 (Table 29.1). 2011. Available at: http://seer.cancer.gov/csr/1975_2011/results_merged/sect_29_childhood_cancer_iccc.pdf.

2. Steliarova-Foucer E, Stiller C, Lacour B, Kaatsch P. International classification of childhood cancer, third edition. *Cancer*. 2005;103:1457–67.

3. Orbach D, Sarnacki S, Brisse HJ, et al. Neonatal cancer. *Lancet Oncol*. 2013;14: e609–20.

4. Kamil D, Tepelmann J, Berg C, et al. Spectrum and outcome of prenatally diagnosed fetal tumors: ultrasound. *Obstet Gynecol*. 2008;31:296–302.

5. Merks JHM, Caron HN, Hennekam RCM. High incidence of malformation syndromes in a series of 1073 children with cancer. *Am J Med Genet*. 2005;134A: 132–43.

6. Tubergen DG, Bleyer A, Ritchey AK. The leukemias. In Kliegman RM, Stanton BMD, St Geme J, et al., editors. *Nelson Textbook of Pediatrics: Expert Consult Premium Edition*, 19th edn. Philadelphia, PA: Elsevier; 2011.

7. Kuttesch JF, Jr., Rush SZ, Ater JL. Brain tumors in childhood. In Kliegman RM, Stanton BMD, St Geme J, et al., editors. *Nelson Textbook of Pediatrics: Expert Consult Premium Edition*, 19th edn. Philadelphia, PA: Elsevier; 2011.

8. Lang S-S, Beslow LA, Gabel B, et al. Surgical treatment of brain tumors in infants younger than six months of age and review of the literature. *World Neurosurg*. 2012;78:137–44.

9. National Cancer Institute. Childhood craniopharyngioma treatment (PDQ®). 2017. Available at: www.cancer.gov/cancertopics/pdq/treatment/child-cranio/healthprofessional.

10. Zage PE, Ater JL. Neuroblastoma. In Kliegman RM, Stanton BMD, St Geme J, et al., editors *Nelson Textbook of Pediatrics: Expert Consult Premium Edition*, 19th edn. Philadelphia, PA: Elsevier; 2011.

11. Fisher JPH, Tweddle DA. Neonatal neuroblastoma. *Semi Fetal Neonatal Med*. 2012;17:207–15.

12. Hammer G, Hall S, Davis PJ. Anesthesia for general abdominal, thoracic, urologic, and bariatric surgery. In Davis PJ, Cladis FP, Motoyama EK, editors. *Smith's Anesthesia for Infants and Children*, 8th edn. Philadelphia, PA: Elsevier; 2011.

13. Gombos DS. Retinoblastomoa in the perinatal and neonatal child. *Semin Fetal Neonatal Med*. 2012;17:239–42.

14. Zage PE, Herzog CE. Retinoblastoma. In Kliegman RM, Stanton BMD, St Geme J, et al., editors *Nelson Textbook of Pediatrics: Expert Consult Premium Edition*, 19th edn. Philadelphia, PA: Elsevier; 2011.

15. Thompson PA, Chintagumpala M. Renal and hepatic tumors in the neonatal period. *Semin Fetal Neonatal Med*. 2012;17:216–21.

16. Anderson PM, Dhamne CA, Huff V. Neoplasmas of the kidney: other pediatric renal tumors. In Kliegman RM, Stanton BMD, St Geme J, et al., editors *Nelson Textbook of Pediatrics: Expert Consult Premium Edition*, 19th edn. Philadelphia, PA: Elsevier; 2011.

17. Anderson PM, Dhamne CA, Huff V. Neoplasmas of the kidney: Wilms tumor. In Kliegman RM, Stanton BMD, St Geme J, et al., editors *Nelson Textbook of Pediatrics: Expert Consult Premium Edition*, 19th edn. Philadelphia, PA: Elsevier; 2011.

18. Herzog C. Neoplasmas of liver. In Kliegman RM, Stanton BMD, St Geme J, et al., editors *Nelson Textbook of Pediatrics: Expert Consult Premium Edition*, 19th edn. Philadelphia, PA: Elsevier; 2011.

19. Sultan I, Casanova M, Al-Jumail U, et al. Soft tissue sarcomas in the first year of life. *Eur J Cancer*. 2010;46:2449–56.

20. Ferrari A, Orbach D, Sulton I, et al. Neonatal soft tissue sarcomas. *Semin Fetal Neonatal Med*. 2012;17:231–8.

21. Arndt CAS. Soft tissue sarcomas. In Kliegman RM, Stanton BMD, St Geme J, et al., editors *Nelson Textbook of Pediatrics: Expert Consult Premium Edition*, 19th edn. Philadelphia, PA: Elsevier; 2011.

22. Frazier AL, Wheldon C, Amatruda J. Fetal and neonatal germ cell tumors. *Semin Fetal Neonatal Med*. 2012;17:222–30.

23. Herzog CE, Huh WW. Gonadal and germ cell neoplasms. In Kliegman RM, Stanton BMD, St Geme J, et al., editors *Nelson Textbook of Pediatrics: Expert Consult Premium Edition*, 19th edn. Philadelphia, PA: Elsevier; 2011.

24. Miniati DN, Chintagumpala M, Langston C, et al. Prenatal presentation and outcome of children with pleuropulmonary blastoma. *J Ped Surg*. 2006;41:66–71.

25. Bleyer A, Ritchey AK. Principles of treatment. In Kliegman RM, Stanton BMD, St Geme J, et al., editors *Nelson Textbook of Pediatrics: Expert Consult Premium Edition*, 19th edn. Philadelphia, PA: Elsevier; 2011.

Chapter

31

# Anesthesia for Transplant Surgery

Evan Burke and Franklyn Cladis

## Introduction

Thomas E. Starzl performed the first successful orthotopic pediatric liver transplant in 1967 at the University of Colorado. The patient was an 18-month-old who survived for the next 400 days [1]. Between January 1988 and December 2013 there were 126 142 liver transplants performed in the United States. Just over one-tenth of these were performed in pediatric patients [2]. While the average number of pediatric transplants has stayed consistent over the past two decades, the pediatric percentage of total liver transplants has been halved. Due to the large number of those requiring transplants, several transplant options have been developed. Liver transplants can be either cadaveric or living donor. To make up for a lack of pediatric-size livers, smaller pediatric patients are able to receive reduced-size grafts or single segment grafts (segment III) or a reduced left lateral segment [3]. As the technique has developed, some studies are showing an improved outcome in living donor transplants over split liver transplants, possibly due to shorter cold and warm ischemia times [4].

## General Indications and Contraindications

There are several disease-specific indications for pediatric orthotopic liver transplant. The primary categories of disease include (1) extrahepatic cholestatic liver disease (biliary atresia accounts for half of transplanted patients); (2) metabolic disorders (maple syrup urine disease, $\alpha_1$-antitrypsin deficiency, urea cycle defects, primary oxaluria, Wilson's disease, and Criggler–Najjar syndrome); (3) intrahepatic cholestasis (TPN cholestasis, Alagille's syndrome, sclerosing cholangitis); and (4) acute liver failure. Hepatic neoplasms such as unresectable hepatoblastoma, hepatocellular carcinoma, and Budd–Chiari syndrome and cystic fibrosis are also indications for a transplant [1,5].

Absolute contraindications include active and untreated infections at the time of transplant, including actively replicating hepatitis B, acquired immune deficiency syndrome, and cancer outside the liver that is not curable. Relative contraindications include advanced cardiopulmonary disease, multi-organ failure, and human immunodeficiency virus. However, some contraindications may be specific to the individual transplant center.

## Pathophysiology and Systemic Manifestations of End-Stage Liver Disease

Some of the indications above, such as the inborn errors of metabolism or neoplasms, do not progress to end-stage liver disease (ESLD), and as such will not develop some of the associated pathophysiologic derangements. End-stage liver disease results from significant hepatic injury or insult and the liver's subsequent attempts at regeneration, which ultimately results in diffuse hepatic fibrosis and cirrhosis. As the liver becomes damaged, impaired glucose homeostasis and impaired drug clearance develop. Impaired protein synthesis may result in high free plasma levels of drugs that are normally protein-bound. Portal hypertension and liver dysfunction develop, affecting the cardiovascular, pulmonary, renal, neurologic, and hematologic systems [6].

Portal hypertension causes peripheral vasodilation and shunting, resulting in a lowered systemic vascular resistance (SVR) with a decreased sensitivity to vasopressors. This leads to a hyperdynamic state and a rise in cardiac output. The renin–angiotensin–aldosterone system (RAAS) is activated, and antidiuretic hormone is released, resulting in salt and water retention and a decrease in water excretion. This may lead to fluid overload, congestive heart failure, cirrhotic cardiomyopathy (over 70 percent of biliary atresia patients), and pulmonary hypertension [4].

From a respiratory standpoint, the patient develops a restrictive lung disease pattern, alveolar hypoventilation, and a decrease in functional residual capacity (FRC) secondary to abdominal ascites and pleural effusions. There is increased pulmonary blood flow from the fluid overload and increased cardiac output, but intrapulmonary shunting occurs and hypoxic pulmonary vasoconstriction is reduced, predisposing the patient to arterial hypoxemia. Hepatopulmonary syndrome is an abnormal pulmonary vasodilation that results in an increased V/Q mismatch severe enough to cause progressive hypoxemia on room air. Alternately, portopulmonary hypertension may develop as systemic endogenous vasoconstrictors bypass the liver where they are normally metabolized and directly enter the pulmonary circulation. This results in increased pulmonary vascular resistance and may cause acute right-sided heart failure and sudden death [7].

The kidneys are also prone to injury in ESLD from diuretics, acute tubular necrosis and hepatorenal syndrome. Diuretics are used to treat volume overload, as evidenced by ascites and peripheral edema, but patients remain intravascularly depleted due to the portal hypertension and hypoalbuminemia (secondary to decreased hepatic synthesis). Prerenal azotemia contributes to renal injury secondary to aggressive diuretic therapy and paracentesis without appropriate volume replacement. Acute tubular necrosis can develop from decreases in perfusion, secondary to relative hypovolemia and increased abdominal pressure from ascites. Hepatorenal syndrome may develop along with sodium retention and poor sodium excretion secondary to severe renal vasoconstriction. It does not respond to volume expansion as prerenal azotemia does. It has a very poor prognosis but is more common in adults than children. It also resolves with liver transplantation [8].

Neurologically, ESLD patients may develop hepatic encephalopathy. There are conflicting reports concerning its etiology, which is likely multifactorial. The liver metabolizes ammonia into urea, and thus ammonia toxicity is thought to be one of the contributing factors. With ESLD, more aromatic amino acids compared with branched chain amino acids develop. They cross the blood–brain barrier and may be neuroinhibitory in nature. Other neuroinhibitors, hypoglycemia, or decreased metabolism of various drugs may also play a role. Cerebral edema and increased intracranial pressure (ICP) may be present and may be exacerbated by the presence of hyponatremia [1].

The liver is responsible for the synthesis of all coagulation factors, except for von Willebrand's factor and factor VIII, which are made in the vascular endothelium (and are supranormal in liver disease states). Decreased synthetic liver function results in a coagulopathy. However, decreased levels of antithrombin III, protein C, and protein S may predispose to thrombosis. Anemia is common from variceal bleeding and a decrease in erythropoietin production from the underperfused kidney and bone marrow suppression. Thrombocytopenia is very common in these patients and is a result of decreased thrombopoietin and splenic sequestration.

# Surgical Technique

The following section highlights the surgical approach through four phases.

## Phase 1: The Pre-Anhepatic or Dissection Stage

Phase 1 occurs from the induction of anesthesia through the devascularization of the diseased liver. The main objective is the dissection of the liver from the surrounding tissues. In patients with previous abdominal surgery (Kasai, redo) this can take significant time and have considerable bleeding due to vascularized adhesions, collaterals, and portal hypertension. Careful attention is paid to the structures of the hilum. The hepatic artery and portal vein are assessed for adequacy of blood flow, which is imperative for the perfusion of the new liver. If needed, the surgical team will augment blood flow with vein or artery grafts, or bypass the native vessels. The next portion involves the dissection of the inferior vena cava (IVC). In the standard complete hepatectomy, this is accomplished with the complete excision of the IVC with the liver. This has significant consequence on preload. The piggyback hepatectomy is the alternative method of managing the IVC and is the one primarily used with pediatric liver transplants. It involves preserving the native IVC. The method may take additional dissection time, but by preserving the native IVC there is one less anastomosis to make later. Pediatric patients generally tolerate this better because complete IVC occlusion is avoided. The liver is then devascularized and the phase is concluded.

## Phase 2: The Anhepatic Stage

Phase 2 begins with the removal of the liver and concludes when the IVC and portal vein anastomoses are complete. In the standard hepatectomy, the suprahepatic IVC of the donor graft is clamped and anastomosed to the recipient's IVC. In the piggyback hepatectomy, a common cuff of the three ostia of hepatic veins is formed and anastomosed to the upper cava of the donor liver. Following this, a separate anastomosis is made between the lower cava of the donor liver and the infrahepatic IVC. Next, a vascular anastomosis is made between the donor portal vein and the recipient portal vein or a mesenteric vein graft. Resumption of flow through the portal vein signifies the end of this phase.

## Phase 3: The Reperfusion Stage

The third phase commences with reperfusion of the donor liver through the portal vein and ends when the hepatic artery is reconstructed. Immediately after reperfusion, initial hemostasis should be assessed and achieved. Once stability is maintained, attention can be turned to the hepatic artery anastomosis with the native hepatic artery or aortic graft. Due to the small and delicate nature of the artery, this portion can be time-intensive. Maintaining perfusion pressure and preventing thrombosis is imperative. During the hepatic artery reconstruction, the aorta may be cross-clamped. This typically results in hypertension but in pediatric patients is usually well tolerated.

## Phase 4: The Biliary Reconstruction Stage

The final phase of liver transplantation consists of biliary reconstruction. In larger children this is often done with a duct-to-duct anastomosis, as their native ducts are larger. In smaller children or those with diseased fragile ducts, the reconstruction requires a biliary-enteric anastomosis through a choledocho-jejunostomy to a Roux-en-Y limb. Integrity of this anastomosis is paramount for preventing biliary and enteric leaks, which can lead to significant morbidity and mortality. The final part of the surgery is the closure of the abdomen. Sometimes because of the different sizing ratios of the donor liver to the native body, as well as reperfusion associated inflammation and edema of the allograft, immediate abdominal closure (skin and fascia) is not possible secondary to intra-abdominal compartment syndrome. Even slight increases in intra-abdominal pressure with hemodynamic instability can result in vascular thrombosis (hepatic artery). Attention to ventilatory pressure changes or hemodynamic instability during abdominal closure is important. Delayed abdominal closure, temporary mesh closure, or skin closure alone without underlying fascia may be necessary until the edema subsides.

## Anesthesia Management

Preoperative evaluation of the pediatric transplant patient should focus on both the organ systems involved in the underlying disease as well as those affected by the diseased liver.

The cardiac preoperative evaluation should include a pulse oximetry, electrocardiogram, and a transthoracic echo to assess cardiac function, arrhythmias (heart block), valvular dysfunction, and oxygen saturation.

Lung disease in ESLD can be significant. Mild arterial hypoxemia is a common occurrence and results from the physiologic changes of ESLD, namely decreased FRC, total lung capacity, and V/Q mismatch. Hepatopulmonary syndrome, as described above with the classic triad of chronic liver disease, hypoxemia, and intrapulmonary shunting in absentia of primary pulmonary or cardiac disease, can be reversed with liver transplant. Portopulmonary hypertension can also occur secondary to liver disease. Pulmonary hypertension is not as common in pediatric patients, but if it is present it may predict intraoperative morbidity [7]. Underlying disorders such as $\alpha_1$-antitrypsin deficiency can have pulmonary involvement as well (emphysematous changes). Cystic fibrosis patients also have underlying pulmonary disease. Poor preoperative nutrition may result in delayed recovery and prolonged mechanical ventilation [5].

History and physical should elicit baseline hypoxemia, exertional dyspnea, ankle edema, chest pain, and syncope. Various studies to examine depend on history, and these include oxygen saturations, chest X-rays, arterial blood gas on room air and 100 percent oxygen, and transthoracic echocardiogram to assess ventricular performance and estimate pulmonary pressures.

Renal dysfunction may result from ESLD, and as described above the kidney may be susceptible to prerenal azotemia, acute tubular necrosis (ATN), and hepatorenal syndrome. Acute renal failure may result

**Table 31.1** Anesthesia for liver transplantation

| | |
|---|---|
| **Preop preparation** | Transthoracic echo, EKG |
| | Type and cross |
| | CBC, PLT, PT, PTT, metabolic profile |
| **IV access** | Two peripheral IVs |
| | In adolescents, consider a rapid infusion catheter (RIC line) |
| **Monitors** | One arterial line (avoid femoral artery because of arterial cross clamping) |
| | One central venous line |
| | Thromboelastography/ROTEM |
| | Standard ASA monitors |
| **Stage 1 Hepatectomy** | Goal: Resuscitate from dissection of native liver, may be > 1 blood volume |
| | Immunosuppression: if using Thymoglobulin, premedicate with diphenhydramine, solumedrol 2 mg kg$^{-1}$, acetaminophen 10 mg kg$^{-1}$ |
| | Antibiotics: piperacillin and tazobactam 75 mg kg$^{-1}$ |
| | Labs: Obtain baseline ABG, glucose and TEG, repeat as needed for resuscitation |
| **Stage 2 Anhepatic** | Goal: Continue resuscitation as needed and prepare for reperfusion, do not fluid overload, inotropic support may be required to maintain MAP without increasing CVP, correct acid–base status, lower K$^+$ to <4.5 meq l$^{-1}$, maintain hgb 8–9 g dl$^{-1}$ |
| | Immunosuppression: administer solumedrol 10 mg kg$^{-1}$ when graft is placed on surgical field |
| | Labs: Obtain as needed for resuscitation, and ABG just prior to reperfusion |
| **Stage 3 Reperfusion** | Goal: have epinephrine and calcium in line to treat hypotension after reperfusion |
| | Labs: recheck ABG and TEG 5 minutes after reperfusion and 30 minutes later, check lactate and continue to repeat lactate for trend |
| **Stage 4** | Goal: Continue resuscitation during hepatic artery, biliary and roux-en-Y reconstruction |
| | Labs: repeat CBC, PLT, PT, PTT, fibrinogen |
| | Antibiotics: redose piperacillin and tazobactam every 2 h x 2, and then every 6 h |
| **Emergence** | Intubation: Extubation may be performed in operating room if abd closed, hemodynamically stable, min. resp. acidosis, no hypoxia and no significant intraoperative events |

and require a combined renal/liver transplant. Studies may include electrolytes, BUN and creatinine, renal ultrasound, urinalysis, and calculating a fractional excretion of sodium (FENa). A metabolic panel will be important to evaluate for hyponatremia, hyperkalemia, and hypocarbia (metabolic acidosis). This information is essential for resuscitation and reperfusion. Low urine output from prerenal azotemia can be improved with a fluid challenge but not if it is secondary to hepatorenal syndrome. Both disorders have a FENa of less than 1 percent. Acute tubular necrosis has a FENa greater than 1 percent.

Anesthetic challenges will vary depending on the stage of the transplant. Induction of anesthesia depends on the current condition of the patient. Often a premedication such as midazolam is given prior to entry to the operating room, unless there is a contraindication (encephalopathy). Preoxygenation is important as the decrease in FRC can lead to rapid desaturation. If the patient doesn't have the stigmata of portal hypertension (variceal bleeding, ascites), full stomach, cardiac disease or multi-organ failure, then a standard inhalation or intravenous induction followed by endotracheal intubation is generally well tolerated. Otherwise a rapid sequence intravenous induction is more appropriate. A cuffed endotracheal tube (ETT) is used to allow positive pressure ventilation when the surgeons are retracting in the right upper abdomen, and guards against aspiration. If succinylcholine is used with induction, practitioners need to be aware that there may be decreased circulating pseudocholinesterase from decreased synthetic function of the liver and may result in longer duration of action. Also these patients may have impaired renal function and thus may have a preoperative hyperkalemia; succinylcholine may raise the potassium levels by 0.5 mmol L$^{-1}$.

Maintenance of anesthesia should include inhaled anesthetic agents, neuromuscular blockade, and intravenous pain medications. Nitrous oxide should be avoided in orthotopic liver transplantation (OLT) patients due to its tendency to cause bowel distention, which can obstruct the surgical field. General anesthesia and surgical compression have been shown to decrease hepatic perfusion, which is critical to maintain, especially during hepatic reperfusion. Sevoflurane and isoflurane have been shown to maintain the relationship of hepatic oxygen supply and demand better than halothane or enflurane at 1.2–1.4 MAC [9–13]. Neuromuscular blockade is ideally maintained with cisatracurium secondary to its consistent rate of metabolism by Hoffmann elimination and ester hydrolysis in patients with liver disease. Other nondepolarizing agents (some with active metabolites) are metabolized in the liver and excreted by the kidneys, and thus have variable metabolism. An opioid is an essential part of anesthetic maintenance. Fentanyl, morphine, or hydromorphone are commonly used.

Monitoring should include standard ASA monitors, urinary catheter, temperature, nerve stimulator, arterial blood pressure, and central venous pressure (CVP). Arterial monitoring is preferred in an upper extremity secondary to possible aortic cross-clamping during hepatic artery anastomosis. Two large-bore IVs should also be placed above the diaphragm to allow easy flow to the heart and circulation as blood loss can be massive and rapid during these cases, especially during retransplantation or previous abdominal surgeries [5]. Given the large abdominal incision, large surface area to volume ratio, and volume resuscitation, it is important to use warming blankets, fluid warmers, and heat the room as necessary.

The ventilation goal is to maintain a normal end-tidal $CO_2$ and to maintain peak airway pressures less than 20 $cmH_2O$ while maintaining adequate tidal volumes (6–8 ml $kg^{-1}$). This may be difficult depending on pulmonary compliance. PEEP is added to prevent progressive atelectasis.

During the pre-anhepatic stage hypotension is very common. Bleeding can be significant when the liver is dissected, collaterals are ligated, and adhesions are taken down. Preexisting coagulopathy can make the bleeding worse. The liver is lifted during the dissection of the major hepatic vessels on its posterior side, and this can temporarily obstruct the IVC, decreasing venous return. The goals during this phase are to maintain euvolemia, transfuse to maintain the hemoglobin at 8–9 g $dl^{-1}$, and correct coagulopathy

to minimize bleeding. It is important to not over-transfuse (hgb > 10 g $dl^{-1}$), or correct the coagulation to normal because this may increase the risk for hepatic artery thrombosis. Maintaining euvolemia is important for preparing the patient for vena cava cross-clamping in phase 2.

The second surgical phase is the anhepatic stage. The goals of anesthetic management for this phase are to maintain euvolemia, support the hemodynamics and prepare for reperfusion. Ideally the warm ischemia time for the donor liver is less than 60 minutes, so this phase may be shorter. In the standard complete hepatectomy, the portal vein and IVC is cross-clamped and the resulting decrease in cardiac preload or venous return decreases the cardiac output and CVP and increases the SVR and heart rate. Using the piggyback approach, these changes may be partly compensated since there is some flow through the IVC. The ability to tolerate vena cava cross-clamping depends on the development of collateral blood flow. A study comparing pediatric liver transplants for biliary atresia (BA) with those for glycogen storage diseases (GSDs) showed that the CVP and blood pressure were significantly lower and heart rate significantly higher for the GSD group, demonstrating that the cardiac output was more adversely affected during the vena cava cross-clamping. A possible explanation for this is that the BA group was more likely to have developed cirrhosis and significant collaterals than the GSD group (which did not progress to cirrhosis) and thus was better able to maintain venous return and tolerate caval cross-clamping [14]. Colloid or crystalloid should be used to maintain euvolemia but vasopressor support may be required to maintain the blood pressure. The donor liver is then flushed (retrograde direction) in order to eliminate hepatic air bubbles that can cause an embolus and preservatives that might lead to hyperkalemia or cardioplegic effects. Bleeding can be significant during this stage as well; the coagulation factors may be diluted and the platelets may be consumed.

The reperfusion stage is the third phase of the liver transplant. As the graft is reperfused, the preservation solution is flushed back into the recipient's circulation. This solution is cold, acidotic, heparin-containing, and high in potassium. A common preservative used for the liver graft is histidine-tryptophan-ketoglutarate (HTK). This solution has less potassium than University of Wisconsin solution (used for bowel transplantation) and results in less hyperkalemia immediately following reperfusion. The donor liver can also form endogenous heparinoids that are released upon reperfusion. Post-reperfusion syndrome is a phenomenon characterized by cardiovascular dysfunction, bradyarrhythmias, hypotension, and increased pulmonary artery pressure and CVP. Although the clinical severity may vary, all patients experience some form of reperfusion syndrome when the graft is reperfused [15,16]. Preparing for reperfusion is imperative to minimize the associated hemodynamic instability, arrhythmias, and possible left ventricular dysfunction. This includes increasing the inspired oxygen percentage, increasing minute ventilation, decreasing the inhaled anesthetic, correcting hyperkalemia prior to reperfusion, having calcium immediately available to treat hyperkalemia, and having vasopressors such as epinephrine and dopamine in-line for hemodynamic instability. Blood should be drawn immediately after reperfusion to evaluate for hyperkalemia. Lactate levels should also be measured after reperfusion and repeated during the reconstruction phase. A declining lactate level indicates graft function.

The management of coagulation is an essential part of anesthetic maintenance. In addition to major acute blood loss seen during surgery and the diseased liver's hypocoaguable state and thrombocytopenia, coagulation can change during the surgery because of consumption and dilution. Various coagulation tests such as prothrombin time (PT), partial thromboplastin time (PTT), D-dimer, hematocrit, and platelet count should be checked at certain time points during the case. Thromboelastography (TEG) is also used to help guide coagulation therapy. Fibrinolytic activity can increase during phase 2 and peak during phase 3, and can be observed on the TEG. This may necessitate the use of antifibrinolytics. These should only be started in consultation with the surgical team. Pediatric transplant patients are more prone to hepatic artery thrombosis (HAT) than their adult counterparts. Risk factors include age <2 years old, the hypercoagulability that develops secondary to a reduction in protein C and antithrombin III, high fibrinogen levels, and the increase in plasminogen activator inhibitor seen in children but not adults [17].

The type of graft may have an impact on the type of transfusions required during the intraoperative period. A study of 157 patients comparing deceased and live donor pediatric liver transplantations found that live donor transplants required more packed red blood cells (PRBCs), crystalloid, and colloid on a per kilogram basis, but required less fresh frozen plasma [18]. It should be noted that in this study the live donor transplants were significantly longer in duration.

Other metabolic changes that occur include derangement of plasma levels of sodium, potassium, glucose, calcium, magnesium, and temperature. Hyponatremia may be present at induction and care must be taken not to correct this deficiency too quickly because of the risk for central pontine myelinolysis. Sodium bicarbonate and 5 percent albumin have a higher sodium content and they may correct hyponatremia too quickly.

Hypokalemia may also be present at induction due to chronic diuretic use and metabolic alkalosis. It is not typically treated because a sudden acute rise in potassium levels following graft reperfusion will occur. Hypokalemia is the more common metabolic disturbance during the post-reperfusion period in pediatric liver transplants [19]. Hyperkalemia should always be treated. Packed red blood cells may be washed in a cell saver prior to being transfused, and acidosis should be treated to help prevent hyperkalemia.

Glucose metabolism is altered in chronic liver disease and glycogen stores may be depleted. In addition, insulin may not be degraded and thus persist longer in circulation. Hypoglycemia may occur and should be monitored throughout the intraoperative period. Conversely, hyperglycemia is common from intravenous steroids given to start immunosuppression. Hypocalcemia and hypomagnesemia can develop secondary to chelation from the citrate in PRBCs. This may result in coagulopathy, hemodynamic instability, and arrhythmias, and may require replacement.

Hypothermia is common from the large abdominal incision, cold donor, cold preservation solution, and cold intravenous fluids. Hypothermia may cause platelet dysfunction, fibrinolysis, and bleeding in an already coagulopathic patient. Measures to maintain euthermia include covering the head in plastic wrap, keeping the patient and operating room table dry, warming the operating room, using a humidifier in the anesthetic circuit, warming IV fluids, and using forced-air warmers. Finally, the head should be rotated every hour to minimize pressure sores on the scalp. This may result in permanent alopecia.

Following the end of the final phase of surgery, the abdomen may not be closed depending on the size differential between the donor liver and patient as well as edema of the bowels. Both of these can result in an abdominal compartment syndrome or may alter the perfusion of the new graft. The patients are often left intubated after the surgery. Some centers extubate these patients immediately after surgery. In general, fast-tracking extubation can occur if the patient is hemodynamically stable, the abdomen is closed (fascia may be open), and if there are no significant intraoperative complications. Patients that do not have portal hypertension (maple syrup urine disease) may bleed less and may be ideal candidates for fast-tracking. Risk factors for prolonged mechanical ventilation include intraoperative bleeding, mechanical ventilation prior to transplant, retransplantation, and acute liver failure. The data seem to indicate that impaired health prior to transplant is a major cause for prolonged ventilation [20].

## Postoperative Management

Early postoperative mortality is not common. In one study, various risk factors for early mortality (30 days) following OLT were examined and were found to include preoperative malnutrition, massive bleeding and transfusions, metabolic acidosis pre-perfusion, and post-reperfusion hyperglycemia and hyperlactatemia [21]. Patients often have ongoing blood and fluid requirements in the postoperative period. Urine output may decrease secondary to hypovolemia, poor graft function, or sepsis. Respiratory function can be impaired by the development of pleural effusions, fluid overload, or a large graft that compromises diaphragmatic function [1].

Postoperative pain control following pediatric liver transplant may be complicated. Adult studies suggest less morphine requirements for postoperative analgesia than controls undergoing liver resection [22,23] and open cholecystectomy [24]. Transplanted livers are surgically denervated and are therefore unlikely to feel capsular stretch or subcapsular hematoma. Increased levels of endogenous opioid peptides may explain the reduced analgesic requirements. The steroid bolus to start the immunosuppression may decrease pain levels as well. There are case reports of single injection caudal morphine, and thoracic epidural morphine, ropivacaine, and clonidine being used in pediatric liver transplants without coagulopathy. This may result in early extubation in the operating room and decreased analgesic requirements postoperatively [25,26].

## References

1. Bennett J, Bromley P. Perioperative issues in pediatric liver transplantation. *Int Anesthesiol Clin*. 2006;44(3):125–47.

2. United Network for Organ Sharing. www.unos.org/data/.

3. Guo CB, Li YC, Zhang MM, et al. Early postoperative care of liver transplantation for infants with biliary atresia during pediatric intensive care unit stay. *Transplant Proc*. 2010;42(5):1750–4.

4. Soler X, Myo Bui CC, Aronson LA, Saied AS. Current issues in pediatric liver transplantation. *Int Anesthesiol Clin*. 2012;50(4):54–65.

5. Uejima T. Anesthetic management of the pediatric patient undergoing solid organ transplantation. *Anesthesiol Clin N Am*. 2004;22(4):809–26.

6. Yudkowitz FS, Chietero M. Anesthetic issues in pediatric liver transplantation. *Pediatr Transplant*. 2005;9(5):666–72.

7. Condino AA, Ivy DD, O'Connor JA, et al. Portopulmonary hypertension in pediatric patients. *J Pediatr*. 2005;147(1):20–6.

8. Iwatsuki S, Popovtzer MM, Corman JL, et al. Recovery from "hepatorenal syndrome" after orthotopic liver transplantation. *New Eng J Med*. 1973;289(22):1155–9.

9. Matsumoto N, Rorie DK, Van Dyke RA. Hepatic oxygen supply and consumption in rats exposed to thiopental, halothane, enflurane, and isoflurane in the presence of hypoxia. *Anesthesiology*. 1987;66(3):337–43.

10. Merin RG, Bernard JM, Doursout MF, Cohen M, Chelly JE. Comparison of the effects of isoflurane and desflurane on cardiovascular dynamics and regional blood flow in the chronically instrumented dog. *Anesthesiology*. 1991;74(3):568–74.

11. Bernard JM, Doursout MF, Wouters P, et al. Effects of sevoflurane and isoflurane on hepatic circulation in the chronically instrumented dog. *Anesthesiology*. 1992;77(3):541–5.

12. Bernard JM, Doursout MF, Wouters P, et al. Effects of enflurane and isoflurane on hepatic and renal circulations in chronically instrumented dogs. *Anesthesiology*. 1991;74(2):298–302.

13. Frink EJ, Jr., Morgan SE, Coetzee A, Conzen PF, Brown BR, Jr. The effects of sevoflurane, halothane, enflurane, and isoflurane on hepatic blood flow and oxygenation in chronically instrumented greyhound dogs. *Anesthesiology*. 1992;76(1):85–90.

14. Huang HW, Lu HF, Chiang MH, et al. Hemodynamic changes during the anhepatic phase in pediatric patient with biliary atresia versus glycogen storage

disease undergoing living donor liver transplantation. *Transplant Proc.* 2012;44(2):473–5.

15. Aggarwal S, Kang Y, Freeman JA, Fortunato FL, Pinsky MR. Postreperfusion syndrome: cardiovascular collapse following hepatic reperfusion during liver transplantation. *Transplant Proc.* 1987;19(4 Suppl. 3):54–5.

16. Hilmi I, Horton CN, Planinsic RM, et al. The impact of postreperfusion syndrome on short-term patient and liver allograft outcome in patients undergoing orthotopic liver transplantation. *Liver Transplant.* 2008;14(4):504–8.

17. Ayala R, Martinez-Lopez J, Cedena T, et al. Recipient and donor thrombophilia and the risk of portal venous thrombosis and hepatic artery thrombosis in liver recipients. *BMC Gastroenterol.* 2011;11:130.

18. Alper I, Ulukaya S. Anesthetic management in pediatric liver transplantation: a comparison of deceased or live donor liver transplantations. *J Anesth.* 2010;24(3):399–406.

19. Xia VW, Du B, Tran A, et al. Intraoperative hypokalemia in pediatric liver transplantation: incidence and risk factors. *Anesth Analg.* 2006;103(3):587–93.

20. Glanemann M, Langrehr JM, Muller AR, et al. Incidence and risk factors of prolonged mechanical ventilation and causes of reintubation after liver transplantation. *Transplant Proc.* 1998;30(5):1874–5.

21. Castaneda-Martinez PD, Alcaide-Ortega RI, Fuentes-Garcia VE, et al. Anesthetic risk factors associated with early mortality in pediatric liver transplantation. *Transplant Proc.* 2010;42(6):2383–6.

22. Donovan KL, Janicki PK, Striepe VI, et al. Decreased patient analgesic requirements after liver transplantation and associated neuropeptide levels. *Transplantation.* 1997;63(10):1423–9.

23. Moretti EW, Robertson KM, Tuttle-Newhall JE, Clavien PA, Gan TJ. Orthotopic liver transplant patients require less postoperative morphine than do patients undergoing hepatic resection. *J Clin Anesth.* 2002;14(6):416–20.

24. Eisenach JC, Plevak DJ, Van Dyke RA, et al. Comparison of analgesic requirements after liver transplantation and cholecystectomy. *Mayo Clin Proc.* 1989;64(3):356–9.

25. Kim TW, Harbott M. The use of caudal morphine for pediatric liver transplantation. *Anesth Analg.* 2004;99(2):373–4.

26. Diaz R, Gouvea G, Auler L, Miecznikowski R. Thoracic epidural anesthesia in pediatric liver transplantation. *Anesth Analg.* 2005;101(6):1891–2.

**Chapter**

# 32

# Anesthesia for Interventional Radiology Procedures

Mary Landrigan-Ossar

## Introduction

Anesthesia for pediatric interventional radiology (IR) procedures is a rapidly increasing, highly challenging, very rewarding area of practice. Anesthesiologists are finding their services in greater demand than ever in radiology, both diagnostic and interventional [1,2]. Referring services increasingly recognize the expanding range of diagnostic questions that can be answered and the minimally invasive procedures which can be performed by radiologists. However, while an adult patient can tolerate these procedures with little or no anesthesia, a child may require at least sedation and often a general anesthetic for their safe completion. In our own institution, we have experienced a nearly two-fold increase in anesthesia cases in the IR suite over the past decade, such that there are now two or three dedicated anesthesia teams in IR each workday.

The purpose of this chapter is to describe the challenges inherent in IR and outfield anesthesia, the range of cases generally performed in the IR suite, and ways in which safe and successful anesthesia can be provided in this environment.

## Preoperative Workup and Safety

Any discussion of pre-anesthetic workup of patients for IR must perforce include the overall context of safe practice. The challenges inherent in administering anesthesia in IR and in any non-operating room location are myriad and well-described [3]. The physical obstacles are obvious: crowded, poorly lit procedure rooms with little leeway for anesthesia equipment, possibly unfamiliar or poorly maintained anesthesia equipment and monitors, physical separation of the patient from the anesthesiologist and remoteness from the main operating room anesthesia support. The nursing and support personnel in IR may be unfamiliar to the anesthesiologist. These personnel may also be less familiar with the fine points of anesthetic care and

how they can help the anesthesiologist, both with routine care and when a crisis develops [4].

Less overt but equally significant are the intrinsic challenges of the patients themselves [1]. There is a tendency among referring services to equate "less invasive" with "less risky." As a result, patients who are deemed to be poor surgical candidates for an open procedure will be sent to IR, where anesthesia or sedation will have to be administered nonetheless. The combination of a relatively minor interventional procedure with major patient comorbidities is a constant of life in IR anesthesia; an informal survey of cases in our institution found that up to 30 percent of cases in IR are emergent add-ons, with an ASA Physical Status of 3 or greater. Additionally, there may be greater variability in the workup of patients for radiology, increasing the risk that important information or the opportunity for timely pre-procedure medical corrections may be missed.

How, then, does one safely and successfully administer anesthesia in such a potentially daunting environment? A number of factors are crucial, and most involve standardizing practice in the outfield to that in the main operating room. Over the years, the practice of anesthesia in the operating room setting has achieved a high degree of safety and reliability, and rather than re-invent the wheel the goal of caregivers in the outfield should be to export these proven practices. It should be noted that standardization is not just good practice, it is a goal encouraged by both the Centers for Medicaid and Medicare and The Joint Commission [5].

Pre-anesthetic review of patients should be the same regardless of ultimate anesthetizing location. In our institution all pre-anesthesia patients have a chart review followed by a preoperative clinic visit or inpatient examination by an anesthesiologist when indicated. While emergent add-on patients – a significant percentage of cases in IR – may have an abbreviated review, this process allows a large number of patients to be reviewed and optimized well before they arrive for their procedure. Anesthesiologists need to act as the final arbiter of whether a child is able to undergo the physiologic stress of anesthesia for a procedure, regardless of the location in which that anesthetic will be delivered, and should be empowered by their institution to act in that role.

The presence of familiar equipment and monitors is essential. The IR suite should be equipped with the same anesthesia machines, monitors, and carts that are present in the main operating room, with the goal of reducing or eliminating errors due to unfamiliar or poorly maintained equipment. Stocking of anesthesia medications and supplies should likewise be standardized to that of the main operating room. Care of a complex patient should never be compromised by outdated equipment or inadequate supplies.

Post-anesthesia care should likewise be consistent with the main operating room. While in a busy radiology department it is often desirable to have a dedicated post-anesthesia recovery unit (PACU), standards for monitoring and discharge should be the same as those in the main PACU. Anesthesiologist coverage of these outfield PACUs should be explicitly delineated in case of emergency.

Emergency equipment such as defibrillators and "code carts" must be readily accessible and familiar to staff in the IR suite. While less-commonly used equipment such as difficult airway carts and malignant hyperthermia treatment carts may not be kept in the suite, protocols for their fast delivery must be well-understood. Protocols for summoning outside help, additional anesthesiologists, or the hospital "code team" must be well-delineated and easily activated in times of need. A very valuable exercise is regular simulation of emergency situations, so that everyone in the IR suite understands how they can contribute in the event of an emergency [6].

The most important element in the delivery of safe outfield care is communication within a committed, well-trained group of physicians, nurses, and radiology technologists. When the possibility of anesthesia backup is several minutes away, it is the personnel in IR who will be the anesthesiologist's first, best resource in an emergency. Having a team of people, all of whom know the case and are invested in the patient's safety, is crucial. One way to facilitate this is morning "board rounds" in which each patient is discussed in the presence of the radiologists, anesthesiologists, nurses, and technologists. At this time the procedure, expected complications, technology requirements, and anesthesia concerns are reviewed. This both clarifies the logistical issues of the day and helps foster a community approach to the care of the patient. It can be useful to have a core group of anesthesiologists who are familiar with both the procedures and the personnel in IR, who can work effectively in that setting and act as a resource for their colleagues who are less comfortable in that setting.

## Procedures

A day in a pediatric IR suite can include vascular procedures such as a cerebral angiogram or sclerotherapy of a peripheral vascular anomaly. Nonvascular procedures include abscess aspiration, ascites drainage, primary feeding tube placement, bone or soft tissue biopsy, and PICC line placement. These can be performed on patients ranging from a baby a few hours in age to an obese young adult – a range of cases and anesthetic requirements that can be dizzying.

Choice of anesthetic depends on a combination of patient-based and procedure-based factors. A mature older child may be able to tolerate a relatively minor procedure with light sedation and local anesthesia; however, in many cases the needs of the patient and procedure will necessitate a patient who is at minimum deeply sedated. Knowledge of the procedure to be performed, its length, the necessity for apneic episodes, likely complications, need for exams postoperatively, and pain medication requirements will all influence one's choice of technique.

## Biopsies and Drain Placements

Drainage of fluid collections and biopsies are some of the most common procedures performed in any IR suite. The patient population can run the gamut from the otherwise healthy child with a suspicious lump to a child after liver transplant with a bile collection and septic physiology. These can often be performed with ultrasound guidance, although deeper targets or those near vital structures can require CT guidance.

The location of the tissue to be biopsied or drained and the imaging mode to be used help determine the type of anesthesia required, although the patient's overall health will always be the final determinant. For patients who cannot be placed supine, such as those with large pleural effusions or an anterior mediastinal mass, the radiologist can perform the procedure under ultrasound guidance with the patient in a semi-recumbent or even frank upright position. This is a situation where good pre-procedure communication will ensure safe and speedy completion.

Ultrasound-guided procedures generally can be done with moderate to deep sedation even in young infants, since the radiologist will be able to watch the needle continuously during the procedure. Soft tissue biopsies are not very painful postoperatively, particularly if local anesthetic has been utilized, and moderate intraoperative narcotic may be sufficient. Placement of a drainage catheter does involve more discomfort, although infiltration of local anesthesia can mitigate this.

CT-guided procedures, e.g., biopsy of bony lesions, require an immobile patient under general anesthesia since any motion necessitates another round of scanning and more patient irradiation. Bone biopsies tend to be more painful than soft tissue biopsies, and should be treated accordingly. Ketorolac is quite helpful, if the child is old enough for it to be safely administered.

Complications from these procedures are quite rare. They include bleeding and puncture of non-target structures [7]. Biopsies of solid organs should all have blood bank specimens sent, although the chance of needing transfusion is quite low [8]. Drainage of an abscess will occasionally result in changes in hemodynamics reminiscent of sepsis. These are generally short-lived and responsive to supportive therapy [7].

## PICC Placement

This procedure is often done on some of the sickest patients in the hospital. Everything else being equal, which it rarely is, patients for percutaneously inserted central catheter (PICC) insertions only require sedation to lie still. If a patient is very small (5 kg or less) or has had multiple lines placed previously, it is very possible for this procedure to require multiple attempts and take well over an hour, in which case it may be desirable to place a laryngeal mask airways (LMA) or endotracheal tube (ETT). Pain medication is rarely necessary, as local anesthetic can be given at the insertion site. As above, if a patient's status is such that little sedation can be safely given, i.e., a patient with poorly palliated congenital heart disease, it is essential to communicate this to the radiologist before the procedure so that they can decide if they will be able to perform the procedure on a patient who may not be completely still.

## Sclerotherapy of Vascular and Lymphatic Malformations

Vascular malformations (VMs) and lymphatic malformations (LMs) are slow-flow congenital vascular lesions which can be treated by a variety of IR methods [9,10]. The most common is chemical sclerotherapy to scar a lesion's endothelium. The various agents are discussed below. Additionally, endovenous and cutaneous laser therapy may be employed, glue may be injected or coils deployed. Patients may have isolated lesions of a few centimeters' diameter or syndromes such as Klippel–Trenaunay or CLOVES, whose lesions encompass an entire extremity or more (see Figure 32.1) [11,12]. In the past, common practice was to not treat asymptomatic VMs and LMs until the patient was old enough to complain about cosmesis. However, recent evidence suggests these lesions will inevitably continue to grow and become more difficult to treat [13,14], making it increasingly common for younger patients to present for treatment.

These cases and embolizations of intracranial vascular anomalies (see below) tend to be the longest procedures in IR, lasting 8–10 hours for extensive

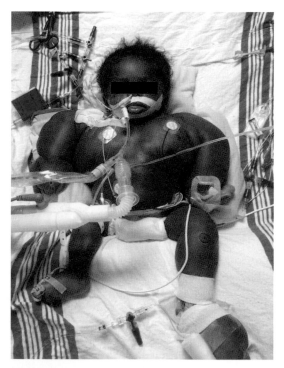

**Figure 32.1** Infant with CLOVES syndrome. Note deformity of extremities and lipomatous overgrowth of trunk.

lesions. Depending on positioning and length of procedure, these cases can be done with an ETT, LMA, or even sedation. Blood loss is not significant as a general rule, but good access to ensure adequate hydration is a must, and arterial lines are rarely necessary.

These procedures may begin with significant contrast loads from venography. Euvolemia to slightly hypervolemia is recommended to offset the osmotic diuretic effect of IV contrast [15]. Sclerosants such as alcohol and sodium tetradecyl sulfate (STS) cause hemolysis in a dose-dependent fashion. If hematuria is noted or expected, our practice is to infuse saline with bicarbonate at the maintenance rate and use crystalloid for any other needed hydration, which should be generous [16].

Large ectatic veins with slow flow are at high risk of intralesional thrombosis. This can act both as a source of potentially fatal thromboembolism, and as a nidus of consumptive coagulopathy [17,18]. Treatment for this is anticoagulation, which slows clot formation in the lesion and makes clotting factors available for the rest of the body. A similar coagulopathy can develop in a patient with a large macrocystic LM if there is hemorrhage into the cyst. Periprocedure anticoagulation should be discussed with a hematologist familiar with this pathophysiology.

Cervicofacial VMs or LMs can be particularly challenging (see Figure 32.2). Intubation may be difficult due to involvement of the tongue or floor of the mouth, and in some severe cases a tracheostomy tube may be placed before a course of treatment starting in early infancy. Even if intubation is accomplished, it is important to recognize that post-procedure swelling

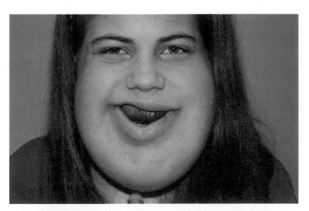

**Figure 32.2** Twelve-year-old female with cervicofacial lymphatic malformation. This patient required tracheostomy as an infant due to severe airway obstruction.

from all chemical sclerosants will increase for several hours after instillation, and extubation should be carefully considered if a lesion is treated near the airway. Our practice is to slightly undersize endotracheal tubes for a low initial air leak. If the leak has increased at the end of the case, maintaining intubation for a few hours to determine if extubation is safe after swelling peaks may be advisable. Postoperative intubation can be necessary for several days.

### Sclerotherapy Agents

**STS.** Sodium tetradecyl sulfate is moderately painful on injection, and causes tissue swelling that adds to postoperative pain. STS's potential for causing hematuria is mentioned above. Post-procedure pain responds well to moderate doses of narcotics with ketorolac when appropriate. Skin ulceration is possible if STS is injected into vessels immediately under the skin, but more systemic adverse effects are rare [19].

**Alcohol.** Alcohol is quite painful at the time of injection, and the patient will often respond with transient increases in heart rate and blood pressure. It is important not to over-treat this acute response; it is possible to over-narcotize a patient with a potentially significant blood alcohol level [20]. Possible hematuria is mentioned above. There can also be local swelling and postoperative skin ulceration. Serious systemic effects up to cardiovascular collapse have been described with larger doses [21]. Alcohol can be quite nauseating in the postoperative period, and aggressive PONV prophylaxis is required. Postoperative pain usually requires moderate narcotics and ketorolac.

**Doxycycline.** Doxycycline is less painful on injection, but due to its acidity (pH 1–2) it is very painful postoperatively. Patients report the worst pain for the first few hours post-procedure. These patients need generous doses of narcotic, with ketorolac if indicated. Clonidine can be helpful as an analgesic and slight sedative in the postoperative period. Deep extubation is often helpful as patients can then sleep through the most painful postoperative period. Of all the sclerosants, doxycycline causes the most significant postoperative swelling [22,23].

**Bleomycin.** Bleomycin is the newest agent being used for treatment primarily of head and neck lesions. It causes less swelling than doxycycline, and may be less painful, with pain medicine requirements similar to those for STS. While pulmonary fibrosis and interstitial pneumonia have been reported with chemotherapy doses, bleomycin doses for sclerotherapy are much lower and such complications have not been described [24,25].

## Lymphangiography

This procedure is performed by accessing lymph nodes in the groin with a tiny needle, through which a lipid-contrast mixture is slowly infused to define the central conducting lymphatics [26]. Patients may present with thoracic effusions or chylous ascites from congenital defects in lymphatics or after cardiac or thoracic surgery. Appropriate management of these patients' comorbidities is the most challenging aspect of their anesthetic. It is essential that the patient be absolutely still since once access to a lymph node is lost it cannot be reestablished. While this can be achieved with very deep sedation, the need for apnea should be discussed with the radiologist. This is not a painful procedure, but can take anywhere from one hour to several hours for cases of disordered lymphatic flow. Embolization of the conducting lymphatics can take many hours and similarly requires an absolutely still patient.

## Diagnostic Cerebral Angiography

Diagnostic cerebral angiograms are generally quick procedures, taking less than one hour. They are the gold standard for delineating vascular pathology, such as arteriovenous malformations (AVM) and vasculitis [3,27]. As an infant or young child cannot cooperate either with being still or the required intermittent apnea, these cases are performed with endotracheal intubation. Arterial catheters are rarely necessary. Contrast loads can be significant, so generous hydration is recommended. The most common complication is bleeding at the femoral puncture site [28,29]. Thus, for both diagnostic angiograms and for AVM embolizations, deep extubation possibly supplemented by α2 agonists prior to extubation should be considered, as patients need to lie flat for several hours after arterial decannulation [30,31]. Pain is not usually significant after these procedures.

## Embolization of Cerebral Arteriovenous Malformations

Intracranial AVMs requiring treatment are uncommon in the very young patient, but are particularly challenging to manage when they do manifest. In utero or in young infants these lesions, which are often Vein of Galen malformations, tend to present with heart failure [6,32]. Depending on the severity of heart failure, the prognosis even after treatment for Vein of Galen malformations is poor. Older children with either Vein of Galen malformations or other AVMs more commonly present with hydrocephalus or intracranial hemorrhage, which can be devastating [33].

Cerebral AVMs can be treated in a variety of ways. Coils or balloons can be deployed, particulate matter can be injected, and sclerosing agents or various forms of glue can be injected. Cerebral embolization procedures tend to be quite prolonged. They are almost universally performed with endotracheal intubation and consistent muscle relaxation, as motion could be catastrophic. Blood loss from these cases is usually minimal, but good access for hydration is necessary to offset the diuretic effect of intravenous contrast [15]. The radiologist instills heparinized saline via the femoral catheter to reduce the chance of microemboli [34]; this can result in a significant amount of fluid over a long case. Close blood pressure control is generally required for treatment of intracranial AVMs, requiring an arterial catheter. Vasoactive medications are rarely necessary to keep blood pressure below a predetermined maximum, but must be readily available. Pain is not usually significant after these procedures. As mentioned above, deep extubation possibly supplemented by α2 agonists should be considered, as patients need to remain flat postoperatively.

Hemodynamic changes may occur during AVM embolization. In some patients with heart failure due to high cardiac output, treatment of the AVM can result in almost immediate improvement in the patient's physical status [35]. Embolization with ethylene vinyl alcohol copolymer glue (Onyx, Covidien, Plymouth, MN) has been reported to induce bradycardia [36]. Due to alterations in flow dynamics in a treated AVM, there may be a period of increased risk of hemorrhage [37,38]. This is particularly true if embolization has not been complete, as in the case of embolizations done presurgical resection [39].

Post-embolization care emphasizes control of blood pressure to avoid sudden increases [39], although there are few descriptions of how to achieve this in pediatric patients. Our group has had success with a continuous low-dose infusion of dexmedetomidine, but we have not attempted this on young infants, who we tend to keep intubated and sedated.

The most common complication is again bleeding at the femoral artery puncture site. With injection of embolic agents, there is always the possibility of inadvertent closure of arteries supplying nearby normal brain tissue, either through glue migration or because the target vessel supplies both normal and abnormal tissue. This latter risk is fortunately extremely low [35].

## Intra-Arterial Chemotherapy Injection

Injection of chemotherapy into a tumor's feeding artery is a therapy described for retinoblastoma, and thus may be performed in quite young children [40]. Access is obtained via the femoral artery, and chemotherapeutic agents are injected specifically into the affected ophthalmic artery. Anesthesiologists can assist by giving oxymetazoline nasal spray to the ipsilateral nostril just prior to chemotherapy injection to shrink the nasal branch of the ophthalmic artery and drive flow to the ophthalmic portion [41]. Albuterol is given at the same time since this protocol is associated with a not insignificant incidence of bronchospasm. Prophylaxis for PONV should be given even in young patients.

## Conclusion

In many institutions, including my own, the not-quite-joking question to any anesthesiologist who is often assigned to IR is "Who's mad at *you*?" It can certainly seem like a less-desirable assignment to be sent outside the familiar surroundings of the main operating rooms if one is unprepared for it. I recommend fluency with the proposed procedures, proper equipment selection and setup, adequate preoperative workup of patients, and an IR staff with the training and motivation to provide effective backup in an emergency. Once this is ensured, the anesthesiologist can focus on providing exceptional care to some of the most challenging patients in the hospital

## References

1. Schenker MP, Martin R, Shyn PB, Baum RA. Interventional radiology and anesthesia. *Anesthesiol Clin.* 2009;27:87–94.

2. Wachtel RE, Dexter F, Dow AJ. Growth rates in pediatric imaging and sedation. *Anesth Analg.* 2009;108:1616–21.

3. Kaufman T, Kallmes D. Diagnostic cerebral angiography: archaic and complication-prone or here to stay for another 80 years? *Am J Roentgenol.* 2008;190:1435–7.

4. Frankel A. Patient safety: anesthesia in remote locations. *Anesthesiol Clin.* 2009;27(1):127–39.

5. The Joint Commission. *The Joint Commission Comprehensive Accreditation and Certification Manual.* Oak Brook, IL: Joint Commission Resources; 2014.

6. Li AH, Armstrong D, terBrugge KG. Endovascular treatment of vein of Galen aneurysmal malformation: management strategy and 21-year experience in Toronto. *J Neurosurg Pediatr.* 2011;7(1):3–10.

7. Lorenz J, Thomas JL. Complications of percutaneous fluid drainage. *Semin Intervent Radiol.* 2006;23(2):194–204.

8. Govender P, Jonas MM, Alomari AI, et al. Sonography-guided percutaneous liver biopsies in children. *AJR Am J Roentgenol.* 2013;201(3):645–50.

9. Cahill AM, Nijs ELF. Pediatric vascular malformations: pathophysiology, diagnosis, and the role of interventional radiology. *Cardiovasc Intervent Radiol.* 2011;34:691–704.

10. Greene AK, Alomari AI. Management of venous malformations. *Clin Plast Surg.* 2011;38(1):83–93.

11. Schook CC, Mulliken JB, Fishman SJ, et al. Differential diagnosis of lower extremity enlargement in pediatric patients referred with a diagnosis of lymphedema. *Plast Reconstr Surg.* 2011;127(4):1571–81.

12. Alomari AI. Characterization of a distinct syndrome that associates complex truncal overgrowth, vascular, and acral anomalies: a descriptive study of 18 cases of CLOVES syndrome. *Clin Dysmorphol.* 2009;18(1):1–7.

13. Hassanein AH, Mulliken JB, Fishman SJ, et al. Venous malformation: risk of progression during childhood and adolescence. *Ann Plast Surg.* 2012;68(2):198–201.

14. Greene AK, Perlyn CA, Alomari AI. Management of lymphatic malformations. *Clin Plast Surg.* 2011;38(1):75–82.

15. Lenhard DC, Pietsch H, Sieber MA, et al. The osmolality of nonionic, iodinated contrast agents as an important factor for renal safety. *Invest Radiol.* 2012;47(9):503–10.

16. Barranco-Pons R, Burrows PE, Landrigan-Ossar M, Trenor CC,III, Alomari AI. Gross hemoglobinuria and oliguria are common transient complications of sclerotherapy for venous malformations: review of 475 procedures. *AJR Am J Roentgenol.* 2012;199(3):691–4.

17. Adams DM. Special considerations in vascular anomalies: hematologic management. *Clin Plast Surg.* 2011;38(1):153–60.

18. Kelly M. Kasabach–Merritt phenomenon. *Pediatr Clin N Am.* 2010;57:1085–9.

19. Duffy DM. Sclerosants: a comparative review. *Dermatol Surg.* 2010;36(Suppl 2):1010–25.

20. Mason K. Pediatric procedures in interventional radiology. *Int Anesth Clin.* 2009;47(3):35–43.

21. Bisdorff A, Mazighi M, Saint-Maurice JP, et al. Ethanol threshold doses for systemic complications during sclerotherapy of superficial venous malformations: a retrospective study. *Neuroradiology.* 2011;53(11):891–4.

22. Burrows PE, Mitri RK, Alomari A, et al. Percutaneous sclerotherapy of lymphatic malformations with doxycycline. *Lymphat Res Biol.* 2008;6(3–4):209–16.

23. Nehra D, Jacobson L, Barnes P, et al. Doxycycline sclerotherapy as primary treatment of head and neck lymphatic malformations in children. *J Pediatr Surg.* 2008;43(3):451–60.

24. Bajpai H, Bajpai S. Comparative analysis of intralesional sclerotherapy with sodium tetradecyl sulfate versus bleomycin in the management of low flow craniofacial soft tissue vascular lesions. *J Maxillofac Oral Surg.* 2012;11(1):13–20.

25. Muir T, Kirsten M, Fourie P, Dippenaar N, Ionescu GO. Intralesional bleomycin injection (IBI) treatment for haemangiomas and congenital vascular malformations. *Pediatr Surg Int.* 2004;19(12):766–73.

26. Rajebi MR, Chaudry G, Padua HM, et al. Intranodal lymphangiography: feasibility and preliminary experience in children. *J Vasc Interv Radiol.* 2011;22(9):1300–5.

27. Wolfe TJ, Hussain SI, Lynch JR, Fitzsimmons B, Zaidat OO. Pediatric cerebral angiography: analysis of utilization and findings. *Pediatr Neurol.* 2009;40:98–101.

28. Burger I, Murphy K, Jordan L, Tamargo R, Gailloud P. Safety of digital subtraction angiography in children: complication rate analysis in 241 consecutive diagnostic angiograms. *Stroke.* 2006;37:2535–9.

29. Hoffman CE, Santillan A, Rotman L, Gobin Y, Souweidane MM. Complications of cerebral angiography in children younger than 3 years of age. *J Neurosurg Pediatr.* 2014;13(4):414–19.

30. Logemann T, Luetmer P, Kaliebe J, Olson K, Murdock DK. Two versus six hours of bed rest following left-sided cardiac catheterization and a meta-analysis of early ambulation trials. *Am J Cardiol.* 1999;84:486–8.

31. Landrigan-Ossar M, McClain CD. Anesthesia for interventional radiology. *Paediatr Anaesth.* 2014;24(7):698–702.

32. Deloison B, Chalouhi GE, Sonigo P, et al. Hidden mortality of prenatally diagnosed vein of Galen aneurysmal malformation: retrospective study and review of the literature. *Ultrasound Obstet Gynecol.* 2012;40(6):652–8.

33. Krings T, Geibprasert S, Terbrugge K. Classification and endovascular management of pediatric cerebral vascular malformations. *Neurosurg Clin N Am.* 2010;21(3):463–82.

34. Blanc R, Deschamps F, Orozco-Vasquez J, Thomas P, Gaston A. A 6F guide sheath for endovascular treatment of intracranial aneurysms. *Neuroradiology.* 2007;49:563–6.

35. Theix R, Williams A, Smith E, Scott R, Orbach D. The use of Onyx for embolization of central nervous system arteriovenous lesions in pediatric patients. *Am J Neuroradiol.* 2010;31:112–20.

36. Lv X, Li C, Jiang Z, Wu Z. The incidence of trigeminocardiac reflex in endovascular treatment of dural arteriovenous fistula with Onyx. *Intervent Neuroradiol.* 2010;16:59–63.

37. Lv X, Wu Z, Li Y, Yang X, Jiang C. Hemorrhage risk after partial endovascular NBCA and ONYX embolization for brain arteriovenous malformation. *Neurol Res.* 2012;34:552–6.

38. Henkes H, Gotwald T, Brew S, et al. Pressure measurements in arterial feeders of brain arteriovenous malformations before and after endovascular embolization. *Neuroradiology.* 2004;46:673–7.

39. Natarajan S, Ghodke B, Britz G, Born D, Sekhar L. Multimodality treatment of brain arteriovenous malformations with microsurgery after embolization with Onyx: single-center experience and technical nuances. *Neurosurgery.* 2008;62:1213–26.

40. Gobin YP, Dunkel IJ, Marr BP, Brodie SE, Abramson DH. Intra-arterial chemotherapy for the management of retinoblastoma. *Arch Opthalmol.* 2011;129:732–7.

41. Abruzzo T, Patino M, Leach J, Rahme R, Geller J. Cerebral vasoconstriction triggered by sympathomimetic drugs during intra-arterial chemotherapy. *Pediatr Neurol.* 2013;48:139–42.

# Anesthesia for Conjoined Twins

## Chapter 33

Philip D. Bailey and Lynne G. Maxwell

Conjoined twins are identical twins whose bodies are joined in utero. The prevalence is estimated to range from 1 in 50 000 to 1 in 100 000 births, with a somewhat higher occurrence in Southwest Asia and Africa [1]. The condition is more frequently found among females, with a ratio of 3:1 [2]. Many are born with abnormalities incompatible with life. The overall survival rate for conjoined twins is approximately 20 percent [3].

The term conjoined twinning refers to an incomplete splitting of monozygotic twins after day 12 of embryogenesis. The fetuses are physically joined at some anatomical location as a result. The point of union is used to classify twins; the suffix used is the Greek word *pagos*, which means "that which is fixed" [4].

- Thoraco-omphalopagus: Fusion from the upper chest to the lower abdomen. These twins usually share a heart, and may also share the liver or part of the digestive system.
- Thoracopagus: Fusion of the upper thorax of variable extent. The heart is always involved.
- Omphalopagus: Fusion at the abdomen. Unlike thoracopagus, the heart is never involved; however, the twins often share a liver, digestive system, diaphragm, and other organs.
- Ischiopagus and pyopagus: Fusion at the pelvis or sacrum. Usually genitourinary and intestinal tract are involved. May have limb abnormalities.
- Craniopagus: Fused skulls, but separate bodies. These twins can be conjoined at the back of the head, the front of the head, or the side of the head, but not on the face or the base of the skull. The brains may be separate or fused with variable amounts of shared brain tissue, CSF spaces, and blood vessels.
- Parasitic twins: Twins that are asymmetrically conjoined, resulting in one twin that is small, less formed, and dependent on the larger twin for survival. This is known as heteropagus twinning.

Thoracopagus, thoraco-omphalopagus, and omphalopagus twins comprise approximately 70 percent of all conjoined twins. Other classification terms are symmetrical or equal conjoined twins (i.e., two well-developed babies) and asymmetrical or unequal conjoined twins (i.e., a small part of the body is duplicated, or an incomplete twin is attached to a fully developed twin). The later the incomplete embryologic separation occurs, the higher the likelihood of a complicated fusion [5].

Two opposing theories exist to explain the origin of conjoined twins. The older theory is *fission*, in which the fertilized egg splits incompletely. More recently, fusion has been proposed, which is now more generally accepted. In the process of fusion, the fertilized egg completely separates, but stem cells find like-stem cells on the other twin and fuse the twins together. Conjoined twins share a single common chorion, placenta, and amniotic sac, although these characteristics are not exclusive to conjoined twins as there are some rarely occurring monozygotic, monoamniotic twins which are non-conjoined [4].

Treating conjoined twins can be a formidable challenge for the multidisciplinary team. Furthermore, these cases often have religious, moral, ethical, and legal implications.

## Preoperative Planning

Conjoined twinning can usually be diagnosed in the first trimester by ultrasound and MRI. It is important to make the diagnosis as early as possible to identify associated anomalies, predict prognosis, plan obstetrical management as well as allow appropriate counseling for the family. Cardiac and neurologic anomalies are key factors in determining prognosis and outcomes. Perinatal care should be directed to centers that have experience managing conjoined twins. Cesarean delivery is almost always the delivery method of choice.

The moral and ethical aspects of separation must be considered once the diagnosis is confirmed, especially in the following circumstances [6]:

- A choice must be made concerning single organ systems. The twin who receives the organ system will live and thrive, whereas the other twin will suffer or die. A similar problem arises when unequal limbs are present.
- The twins have conjoined hearts. Surgical separation of the cardiac complex has been mostly unsuccessful. In some cases, one twin is allowed to live with the entire cardiac complex.
- The twins are craniopagus and have complete brain junction. These twins are usually inseparable.

Additionally, the following will need to be addressed prior to separation [7].

- Consent for surgery: Informed consent is the recommended practice. The decision to separate should involve detailed discussions of the procedure and associated risks with the parents.
- One person or two? Should be considered two individuals except in the case of parasitic twins, one heart, or one head.
- Acceptable operative risks: Operative mortality should not exceed 50 percent and potential for major permanent disability should be considered.

Almost every organ system will need to be investigated thoroughly, taking into consideration shared organs and body parts. Basic laboratory studies (CBC, metabolic panel, liver function, and coagulation studies) are obtained. The most widely used diagnostic tests are X-rays, ultrasound, CT, MRI/MRA/MRV and echocardiography. Catheterization may be necessary to determine complex cardiac anomalies. An accurate assessment of all major inflow and outflow tracts needs to be determined.

A systematic approach to the workup is necessary in conjoined twins. The type of conjoining determines the specific studies needed; the possible areas of fusion are predictable in each type. Three-dimensional models should be built to depict the shared anatomy [8]. The shared structures must be divided, if possible, in order to maintain maximum functional integrity for each twin. Some shared organs (e.g., a single rectum) may not be divisible.

Shared organs need to be evaluated. Mixing of blood is an issue in shared organs as well as direct intervascular communications between twins. The anesthesia team must evaluate the condition of the twins several times before surgery (posture, preferred position, experimenting with different positions, assessing intubation difficulties). Cardiac evaluation and direct communication with a cardiologist is essential to determine potential issues perioperatively. Problems with intravenous access issues should be anticipated and addressed prior to the day of separation. Large-bore central venous access such as Broviac catheters may need to be placed in each twin by a surgeon or interventional radiologist prior to the day of surgery.

The timing of surgery is determined by several factors. Associated anomalies, which may preclude survival or lead to major handicap interfering with acceptable life, need to be determined prior to proceeding with separation. Cardiac anomalies are the most common cause preventing separation followed by brain involvement. The decision has to be made with caution after thorough investigation and several meetings with the multidisciplinary team. Preoperative team conferences should be held specifically aimed at reviewing all the information available. Additionally, moral, ethical, and legal issues will need to be fully addressed prior to separation. Separation is best performed on an elective basis at 9–12 months of age, with a preferred combined weight of at least 8 kg. Such a weight will provide greater skin surface area for coverage and blood volume to tolerate and allow for successful surgery. Experience with separation of large numbers of conjoined twins is limited to only a few centers in the world [9–12].

## Staging and Planning Procedures

Most conjoined twins will require anesthesia for medical imaging studies prior to separation. The general principles of anesthesia for conjoined twins discussed below must be adhered to, with some modification. It may be safer to intubate in the operating room and transfer to the radiology suite. In addition, most will require one or more surgical operations: most of these procedures are relatively minor, short in duration, and not associated with blood loss.

Tissue expanders are usually placed several months prior to the planned separation. They are placed with the aim of recruiting skin to facilitate coverage, but may also contribute to complications such as organ compression, sepsis and breakdown, as well as possible compromise of respiration and ventilatory mechanics [13].

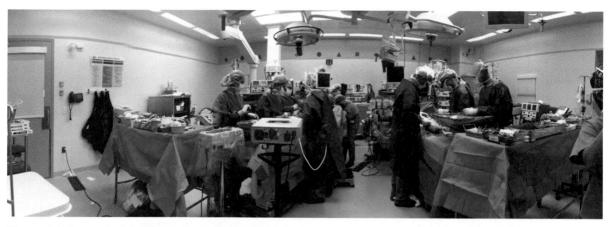

**Figure 33.1** Panoramic photo of operating room after separation of twins and transfer to two separate operating tables.

The multidisciplinary team is made up of different specialties that are involved in the management of the twins before, during, and after separation. The parents are part of the team since they must be informed of procedures and risks to which their children will be exposed in detail, the likelihood of separation and quality of life after separation. The multidisciplinary team leader is responsible for the overall management of the case. The anesthesia team leader is usually someone who has prior experience in the separation of conjoined twins. In addition, two different anesthesiologists should be assigned to manage each of the twins. Each anesthesiologist, with an assistant and technician, is assigned to manage one twin throughout surgery (Figure 33.1).

## Surgical Separation

Separation is usually planned at 6–12 months of age and around 8 kg. Surgical separation is a complex surgery involving different phases with several steps in each phase. Positioning of a large amount of equipment, movement, and location must be determined before surgery. Personnel and equipment assigned to each twin should be identified by different color labels and readily recognizable clothing, such as hats. Live rehearsal with the multidisciplinary team addresses these issues as well as positioning of the patients for induction, line placement, and then surgery, draping, and moving the twins after separation. The parents should be asked if they would like to attend the rehearsal/simulation to help them understand what their children will undergo.

Blood loss may be sudden and massive during the separation, necessitating that blood and component products are available in the room. Blood for each twin must also be color coded. Circulatory collapse at separation secondary to unappreciated volume and blood loss must be planned for and anticipated. Frequent laboratory testing during the procedure is necessary.

Routine noninvasive monitors, as well as adequate vascular access and arterial access are absolutely essential. If neurological function is at stake, SSEP (somatosensory evoked potentials) and MEP (motor evoked potentials) monitoring is indicated. An attempt to synchronize ventilation to some degree may be beneficial. Maintaining normothermia may be challenging secondary to the surface area exposed throughout the procedure: forced warmed air, plastic drapes, warmed fluids, etc. are useful in achieving this goal.

The longest part of the operation is the reconstruction phase after separation. Fluid requirements are substantial and blood loss, which may be concealed, can be massive. Normothermia may be especially hard to achieve during this stage of the operation. A primary closure that is too tight may compromise cardiac and pulmonary, as well as, gastrointestinal and renal function.

Prepping and draping and planning for the point of separation have several issues, mainly transferring the just-separated twins onto separate operating room tables while maintaining a sterile field. Once the babies have been separated and transferred to separate operating tables, continued sterility needs to be ensured. Moving from one to two operating tables should be done slowly and in a coordinated fashion. During the transfer gentle handling is essential since it will be necessary to protect the airway, support and protect the limbs, and reestablish lines; many hands are necessary to accomplish this. It is one of the biggest logistical challenges of the entire procedure.

Lap pad, instrument, and needle counts need to be verified, and it is not unreasonable to obtain plain films on both twins to ensure nothing has been inadvertently left inside the infants.

Of all types of conjoined twins, omphalo-ischiopagus twins are the most favorable candidates for elective surgery because of good survival rates [12]. Historically, conjoined twins in general have been placed into three groups [10] :

- Group 1: Those who do not survive delivery and those who die shortly after birth.
- Group 2: Those who survive to undergo an elective procedure.
- Group 3: Those in whom an emergent procedure is required.

Emergent conditions may arise at any time and include intestinal obstruction, rupture of an omphalocele, congestive cardiac failure, severe degree of respiratory compromise, and life-threatening illness in one of the twins. The following are indications for emergent separation [14]:

- one or both twins are in a life-threatening situation;
- a correctable, life-threatening associated congenital anomaly (e.g., intestinal atresia, malrotation with midgut volvulus, ruptured exomphalos, anorectal agenesis) is present.

## Anesthetic Considerations and Challenges

The anesthesia team usually consists of a team leader, two lead anesthesiologists (one to care for each twin), trainees, and technicians. Executing the anesthetic plan involves careful planning and several rehearsals prior to separation; experience helps with these cases.

Premedication is generally not required since most surgical procedures are performed on young infants who have been hospitalized since birth, who are familiar with the hospital environment and personnel. If needed, oral midazolam 0.5 mg kg$^{-1}$ (or an equipotent dose of intravenous midazolam) may be administered to each twin. If the twins appear equal in size the combined weight can be divided in half; however, if the twins differ in size then the weight may be estimated according to their ratio of size difference.

One should not give a double dose to one twin assuming it will be distributed equally, due to incomplete cross-circulation. Ideally, intravenous access should be obtained prior to arrival in the operating room.

Cross-circulation is always present to varying degrees. The extent of the shared organs and vasculature and the effect on the pharmacokinetics and pharmacodynamics of a drug, as well as fluid and blood administration, needs to be appreciated and ideally determined before separation [15]. Communication between the anesthetic teams is critical.

Induction of anesthesia should commence in sequential fashion, not simultaneously; the induction and intubation of one twin followed by the other. Inhalation or intravenous induction of anesthesia in one twin does not usually produce significant sedation in the other twin; however, when a drug is administered intravenously to one twin in the usual individual dose, it will distribute to the whole body and shared organs. Some of the drug that reaches the shared organs may cross over to the other twin; this dose is usually too small to produce a significant clinical effect; muscle relaxants may be an exception, because of the possibility of the premature onset of weakness in the unintubated twin. Inhalational or intravenous induction with ketamine and atropine is appropriate. The first twin is induced and usually intubated nasally without the administration of muscle relaxant. The second twin is then induced and intubated nasally after administration of a muscle relaxant if needed. The advantage of intubating the first twin without the use of muscle relaxant is to avoid the possibility of subclinical paralysis with hypoventilation and desaturation in the second twin. Elevating one twin to optimize induction/intubation of the other twin should be avoided if possible since it may lead to hypotension in the elevated twin.

Airway management in thoraco-omphalopagus twins is predictably more difficult: these twins have difficult airways until proven otherwise. Opisthotonus, hyperextension of the neck, and inability to position each twin supine may make visualizing the cords difficult. Also, since their faces are close to one another access to the mouth and larynx is often difficult, making instrumentation of the mouth challenging. Placing the tracheal tube is often difficult since it tends to get hung-up in the subglottic space due to angulation of the trachea (Figure 33.2).

When the diaphragm is involved, and/or the chest wall is involved, lung compliance is usually affected.

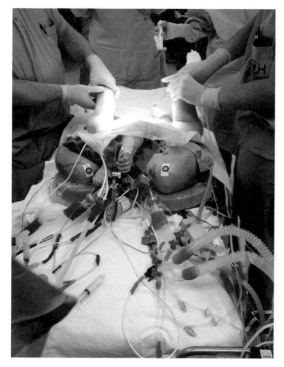

**Figure 33.2** Positioning of twins after intubation. Note color-coding of all equipment and IV lines for each twin. Note face-to-face position in thoraco-omphalopagus twins, which may cause difficulty in positioning for intubation.

As one of the twins develops cardiorespiratory embarrassment the other twin is almost always affected. Separating thoracopagus twins creates flail chests requiring both twins to have sternal and chest wall reconstruction [15].

Color-coding is used from the time the twins are born until they are separated, even if they look different. Colored stickers are attached to each patient's file, wristband, etc. The color-coding scheme continues through the perioperative period – use of colored elastic wrap attached to the anesthesia machine, lines, monitors, syringes, etc. Color-coding prevents administering the wrong drug to the wrong twin and allows lines and circuits to be identified during surgery when the twins are completely covered as well as at the time of separation. The color-coding extends to the anesthesia and surgical team members assigned to each twin.

The layout and traffic system must be discussed and determined during the meetings and rehearsals of the multidisciplinary team, including placement of the team members and equipment. Rehearsals should include color-coding of all team members and

equipment, and incorporate a life-like replica of the twins' physical orientation (Figure 33.3). The twins will start on one operating table and a second table will be brought in at the time of separation.

When positioned on the operating room table, most types of conjoined twins will have one or more body parts lying beneath them. Pressure injury is a risk, so meticulous attention to detail is necessary to ensure adequate protection and padding.

Monitoring during the surgery is similar to any major surgery in infants. Each twin needs its own set of monitors. EKG sites need to be carefully planned for both pre- and post-separation. Pulse oximeter probes on lower extremities should be avoided if possible. An arterial line, central vascular access, urinary catheter, and esophageal or rectal temperature probe for each twin should be standard. The presence of an arterial/ventricular septal defect is high, making embolization a possibility.

Maintenance of anesthesia throughout surgical separation usually consists of sevoflurane 1–2 percent with low-flow oxygen/air plus fentanyl. Combined general and epidural anesthesia has been used successfully without complications, but most avoid it since the risk of possible damage to the spinal cord due to unfavorable positioning outweighs the benefits, especially since the patients will be intubated and ventilated for several days postoperatively [16].

Extensive surgical incisions and long operative times lead to massive third-space fluid losses. Often crystalloid solutions must be administered to each baby at 15 ml kg$^{-1}$ h$^{-1}$ or greater for maintenance. Central venous pressure (CVP), arterial blood pressure and tracing, as well as urine output should guide fluid replacement. When large amounts of crystalloid have been given, 5 percent albumin should be considered. Glucose should be monitored hourly and dextrose-containing solution administered when required. Arterial blood gases and electrolytes should be monitored as indicated, with ionized calcium tracked if large blood loss and replacement is occurring.

It may be difficult to determine which twin is losing blood and to what extent. Only laboratory tests can confirm which twin is losing blood. Blood should be given when the hematocrit reaches 30 percent. It should not be assumed that blood transfused to one twin will be equally distributed to the other twin. Blood loss is variable, depending on the extent of surgery and type of joining. Preparation, cross-matching,

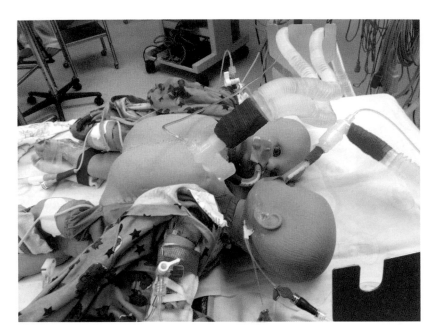

**Figure 33.3** Doll models used for simulation of separation prior to procedure. Note stents around endotracheal tubes to prevent kinking, and color-coding of IVs and airway equipment.

and transfusion practice should be done as for any two different patients.

Vasopressor infusion (e.g., dopamine, epinephrine) may be used to support circulation and improve perfusion in spite of adequate fluid replacement. Vasodilation of one infant may lead to a steal scenario where blood is diverted to this infant, thereby causing hypotension in the other twin.

The goal of intraoperative management is to provide ideal surgical conditions: analgesia, amnesia, and muscle relaxation. Control of the airway, ventilation, hemodynamic stability, and temperature regulation are critical. Challenges with cardiovascular depression, difficult ventilation, and unpredictable drug absorption and responses with uncertain degrees of cross-circulation all necessitate regular adjustments in anesthetic agents and muscle relaxants [4]. Drugs may need to be dosed more frequently secondary to ongoing blood losses. Communication between anesthesia teams and surgical teams is critical.

Additionally, extensive interest can result in a potentially unacceptable number of people in the operating room at one time; therefore, someone needs to be tasked with controlling traffic during the procedure. Real-time video streaming to multiple locations allows the event to be telecast outside the operating room in order to minimize the presence of extraneous personnel.

Sudden unexpected deterioration may occur in thoracopagus twins, and death in this group may occur secondary to respiratory and cardiovascular failure; cardiac failure in the neonatal period is common. Anatomically the twins may have a single heart, separate hearts, or compound hearts. Any maneuver that alters intrathoracic pressures and moves the hearts and lungs of each infant back and forth between them may result in cardiovascular and respiratory instability. Airway management is often difficult, as previously mentioned, and becomes more difficult the higher the point of fixation, and may cause hypoxemia of one or both twins during induction. Central intravenous access may be difficult because the usual anatomic landmarks are frequently unreliable.

In omphalopagus twins, extreme variability from a small fibrous connecting band to a complex hepatobiliary and vascular fusion may be present. Gastrointestinal sharing of organs is common. Difficulty with airway management (both intubation and ventilation) are similar to thoracopagus twins.

In ischiopagus and pyopagus twins, blood loss may be extensive during pelvic osteotomies. Neuraxial abnormalities may be present and neuromonitoring may be needed. Airway management is usually not an issue in these anatomic variants.

In craniopagus twins, airway management is usually a challenge, as is securing the endotracheal tube (ETT). Air embolism is a potential issue because of opening of large intracranial veins and dural venous sinuses during exposure. Venous sinus fusion with the potential for massive and terminal blood loss is often what makes them inseparable. Central venous access may be limited to femoral vessels.

## Physical Impact of Separation

Once the surgical procedure is complete the twins will need careful monitoring in the ICU. Postoperative issues usually relate to blood loss/massive transfusion, tight closure, prolonged surgery, as well as alterations in postoperative anatomy. Monitoring for continued blood loss, hypoxia, acidosis, hypothermia, electrolyte imbalance, and organ dysfunction (especially renal and hepatic) is mandatory. One of the most challenging issues is fluid management. Massive fluid shifts require hour-by-hour monitoring and replacement. Cardiovascular and respiratory complications remain the most common cause of death [4]. Altered ventilatory mechanics from diaphragmatic dysfunction and sternal/chest wall insufficiency need to be appreciated. Post-surgical infection and sepsis may be a problem. Good pain relief is obligatory. Attempts should be made to manage the newly separated twins in the same room when feasible to avoid separation anxiety. Physiotherapy and rehabilitation are essential. The importance of the team approach cannot be overemphasized and must be continued in the postoperative period and during follow-up. Immediate and long-term survival is variable, although the twins tend to do better if they do not share vital organs. Extensive rehabilitation and future reconstructive surgeries will frequently be necessary.

## References

1. Spitz L, Kiely EM. Conjoined twins. *JAMA*. 2003;289(10):1307–10.

2. Spitz L. Conjoined twins. *Prenat Diagn*. 2005;25(9):814–19.

3. Mackenzie TC, Crombleholme TM, Johnson MP, et al. The natural history of prenatally diagnosed conjoined twins. *J Pediatr Surg*. 2002;7(3):303–9.

4. Thomas J. Anesthesia for conjoined twins. In Davis PJ, Cladis FP, Motoyama EK, editors. *Smith's Anesthesia for Infants and Children*, 8th edn. St. Louis, MO: Mosby; 2011; 950–70.

5. El-Gammal M. Conjoined twins: anesthetic considerations. In: Bissonnette B, Anderson BJ, Bosenberg A, et al, editors. *Pediatric Anesthesia: Basic Principles-State of the Art-Future*. Shelton, CT: People's Medical Publishing House; 2001; 1877–90.

6. Cowley C. The conjoined twins and the limits of rationality in applied ethics. *Bioethics*. 2003;17(1):69–88.

7. Lee M, Gosain AK, Becker D. The bioethics of separating conjoined twins in plastic surgery. *Plast Reconstr Surg*. 2011;128(4):328e–334e.

8. Rhodes JL, Yacoe M. Preoperative planning for the separation of omphalopagus conjoined twins: the role of a multicomponent medical model. *J Craniofac Surg*. 2013;24(1):175–7.

9. O'Neill JA Jr., Holcomb GW III, Schnaufer L, et al. Surgical experience with thirteen conjoined twins. *Ann Surg*. 1988;208(3):299–312.

10. Spitz L, Kiely EM. Experience in the management of conjoined twins. *Br J Surg*. 2002;89(9):1188–92.

11. Leelanukrom R, Somboonviboon W, Bunburaphong P, Kiatkungwanklai P. Anaesthetic experiences in three sets of conjoined twins in King Chulalongkorn Memorial Hospital. *Paediatr Anaesth*. 2004;14(2):176–83.

12. Brizot ML, Liao AW, Lopes LM, et al. Conjoined twins pregnancies: experience with 36 cases from a single center. *Prenat Diagn*. 2011;31(12):1120–5.

13. Clifton MS, Heiss KF, Keating JJ, et al. Use of tissue expanders in the repair of complex abdominal wall defects. *J Pediatr Surg*. 2011;46(2):372–7.

14. Walton JM, Gillis DA, Giacomantonio JM, et al. Emergency separation of conjoined twins. *J Pediatr Surg*. 1991;26(11):1337–40.

15. Szmuk P, Rabb MF, Curry B, Smith KJ, et al. Anaesthetic management of thoracopagus twins with complex cyanotic heart disease for cardiac assessment: special considerations related to ventilation and cross-circulation. *Br J Anaesth*. 2006;96(3):341–5.

16. Greenberg M, Frankville DD, Hilfiker M. Separation of omphalopagus conjoined twins using combined caudal epidural-general anesthesia. *Can J Anaesth*. 2001;48:478–82.

**Chapter**

# 34

# Anesthesia for Fetal Surgery

Linda A. Bulich, Arielle Y. Mizrahi-Arnaud, and Kha M. Tran

## Introduction

Fetal intervention is a fascinating, unique, and rapidly developing field of medicine that involves the expertise and teamwork of many subspecialties including surgery, anesthesia, obstetrics, radiology, and neonatology. It is unique in that one is asked to provide care to two patients – the maternal patient who can communicate her needs and discomforts, is easily monitored, and can readily have medications administered, and the frequently "hidden" fetal patient, whom one can only get intermittent glimpses of through advanced imaging techniques. In the fetus, one can only assume or infer nociceptive capabilities, and monitoring is intermittent and often unreliable. Drug administration is usually difficult and many times indirect.

The first successful fetal intervention was performed by Sir William Liley in 1963, and involved blind, intraperitoneal blood transfusion to a fetus affected with erythroblastosis fetalis. It was not until almost 20 years later that Harrison and his group at the University of California at San Francisco reported the first open fetal surgical intervention in a 21-week-old fetus with severe obstructive hydronephrosis. Through bilateral ureterostomies, the urinary tract of the fetus was decompressed and the fetus was able to continue to grow and develop for three months prior to delivery. Unfortunately, because of extensive renal and pulmonary damage, the infant died within a day of delivery [1]. Despite this initial disappointment, a group of pioneers in the field of fetal surgery joined with other subspecialists to study the pathophysiology and natural course of many fetal anomalies and diseases. The goal was to both arrest the progression of the disease and allow definitive postnatal repair, or to correct the disease outright. A consensus document was drafted in 1982 by the newly created International Fetal Medicine and Surgery Society that is still referenced today (Table 34.1) [2]. A period of enormous research followed with randomized multicenter trials

involving human patients, which established the role of in utero surgery as a clinical reality designed to help once-doomed fetuses. It is estimated that approximately 1000 fetal surgeries were performed in 2012 in the United States alone, and this number is predicted to rise substantially in the near future [3]. Another evolution in fetal medicine is underway, with many current areas of research focusing on stem cell and gene therapy [4]. Promising candidates for human application include those fetuses affected with hemophilia, muscular dystrophy, and central nervous system disorders. Although great progress has been made over the last 40 years, much remains to be discovered and accomplished.

## The Maternal Patient

Implicit in the criteria for fetal surgery is the understanding that one must "Do No Harm." The mother has been referred to as an "innocent bystander" who, although exposed to significant surgical and postpartum risk, receives no direct health benefits. It is essential that the anesthesiologist taking care of the fetus has an awareness that whatever hemodynamic changes affect the mother also affect the fetus. Although virtually every organ system in the mother undergoes physiological changes during pregnancy, it is most important for the fetal anesthesiologist to focus on the maternal cardiovascular, respiratory, and nervous system changes of pregnancy and the anesthetic implications in the perioperative period.

### Cardiovascular

Cardiac output will increase by as much as 35–40 percent by the end of the first trimester [5]. It will continue to rise throughout the second trimester until it reaches a level that is 50 percent greater than nonpregnant women. The majority of the increase in cardiac output in early pregnancy is due to increases in heart rate of 15–25 percent above prepregnancy

**Table 34.1** Criteria for Fetal Surgery

| | |
|---|---|
| 1. | Accurate diagnosis and staging of the disease with noted exclusion of other associated anomalies. |
| 2. | The natural history of the disease is documented and the prognosis is established. |
| 3. | In utero surgery proven feasible in animal models, reversing deleterious effects of the conditions. |
| 4. | There is no current effective postnatal treatment. |
| 5. | Intervention can only be ethically justified if there is a reasonable probability of benefit. |
| 6. | The family is counseled about risks and benefits and should agree to treatment including long-term follow-up to determine efficacy. |
| 7. | Interventions should be performed at specialized multidisciplinary fetal treatment centers after approval by an institutional review board. |
| 8. | All case material should be reported, regardless of outcome, to a fetal-treatment registry and/or in the medical literature , so that the benefits and liabilities of fetal therapy can continue to be established |

levels that then remain stable after the second trimester [6]. Stroke volume will progressively increase by 25–30 percent by the end of the second trimester and remain this way until term [7].

The gravid uterus may decrease preload, cardiac output, and maternal blood pressure by compressing the aorta and/or vena cava of supine women. This becomes most pronounced at term. Although the majority of women will experience minimal if any hypotension when supine due to increased systemic vascular resistance, any anesthetic that decreases sympathetic tone (such as neuraxial blockade or some general anesthetics) will worsen the effects of aortocaval compression, resulting in significant hypotension. Maternal hypotension will decrease uteroplacental perfusion and impair fetal oxygenation. For these reasons, the more traditional left uterine displacement or in some cases right uterine displacement must be provided.

For many open fetal interventions, high concentrations of volatile anesthetics may be necessary for adequate uterine relaxation to prevent preterm labor and inadvertent placental separation. These agents are potent vasodilators and at higher doses are cardiac depressants. Therefore prompt treatment of hypotension is very important. Because uteroplacental blood flow is not autoregulated, falls in maternal blood pressure will result in decreased blood flow to the fetus with resultant hypoxia and acidosis. Intravenous ephedrine and/or phenylephrine are drugs of choice used in most cases to treat maternal hypotension. Although fluid boluses may also help in improving preload and maternal blood pressure, careful attention must be paid to the fluid status of the mother. Aggressive fluid resuscitation combined with the abundant use of prophylactic tocolytics has been implicated in occurrences of pulmonary edema in some fetal surgery patients [8].

## Pulmonary

Pregnancy results in progressive increases in oxygen consumption and minute ventilation along with a reduced functional residual capacity and residual volume [9]. These increases in metabolic demand make the pregnant patient more prone to hypoxia during periods of apnea or hypoventilation. Prior to anesthetic induction, it is imperative to adequately preoxygenate the mother and immediately intubate following a rapid sequence induction. Maternal hypoxia will obviously result in fetal hypoxia.

Resting maternal $PaCO_2$ decreases from 40 mmHg to approximately 30 mmHg by 12 weeks' gestation and remains at this level until term [9]. Ventilating the pregnant patient demands meticulous attention. Excessive hyperventilation below a $PaCO_2$ of 20 mmHg will likely lead to uterine vessel vasoconstriction and decreased placental perfusion, jeopardizing the fetus [10].

## Nervous System

Pregnancy will decrease the minimal alveolar concentration (MAC) of volatile anesthetics by approximately 30 percent [11]. While the concentration of inhaled agent required to achieve a desired anesthetic effect is decreased, one must remember that high concentrations are often required for many open fetal procedures. Local anesthetic dose requirements for spinal and epidural anesthesia are also lower than for the nonpregnant patient and hence adequate doses are usually about one-third less than those of nonpregnant women.

## The Fetal Patient

The combination of immature organ systems and the stress of a surgical intervention place the fetus at a considerable anesthetic risk. The well-being of the fetus is dependent on both maternal oxygenation as well as the adequacy of fetoplacental perfusion.

## Fetal Oxygenation

The supply of oxygen to the fetus depends on a number of factors. First, the mother must be adequately oxygenated. Second, there must be sufficient flow of well-oxygenated blood to the uteroplacental circulation. As discussed in the previous section, maternal hypotension can result from aortocaval compression as well as the direct cardiac depressant effects of the inhaled anesthetics or the vasodilatory effects of local anesthetics. Significant maternal hemorrhage reduces maternal blood flow and thus uterine blood flow. It is also known that the surgical incision of hysterotomy that is required for open fetal procedures reduces uteroplacental blood flow by as much as 73 percent in the sheep model, whereas fetoscopic procedures have no effect [12]. Furthermore, anything that increases maternal catecholamine production (i.e., light anesthesia) will increase uteroplacental vascular resistance and decrease flow.

Tocolytic agents are often required to prevent preterm labor in fetal surgery patients. Uterine contractions are particularly dangerous during a fetal intervention, not only because uterine blood flow is reduced, but also because inadvertent placental separation can occur, leading to disastrous outcomes.

Even if the uterine circulation is adequate, the fetus will still rely on blood flow to the placenta and the umbilical vein for tissue oxygenation. Increased amniotic fluid volume will increase intra-amniotic pressure and will impair uteroplacental perfusion [13,14]. Studies in animals suggest that uteroplacental perfusion has to be reduced by >50 percent before there are adverse effects on fetal gas exchange [15]. In the setting of increased fetal catecholamine production (i.e., fetal stress), fetoplacental vascular resistance will rise, which will in turn increase fetal cardiac afterload [16]. Other factors that can impair umbilical blood flow and hence fetal oxygenation include umbilical cord kinking, umbilical vessel spasm, or significant fetal hemorrhage. Rapid, uncontrolled loss of amniotic fluid may result in kinking of the umbilical vessels, or even direct compression of the umbilical vessels by a fetus that is no longer suspended in the amniotic fluid.

## Fetal Cardiovascular Response

Unlike adults and older children, fetal cardiac output depends more on heart rate than on stroke volume [17]. Because fetal myocardial contractility is likely maximally stimulated, the fetus has a limited ability to increase stroke volume. In animal studies, increases in preload had a limited effect on cardiac output – volume loading increased cardiac output by only 15–20 percent [18].

The choice of a maternal anesthetic will impact the fetus. All inhaled anesthetics rapidly cross the placental barrier [19], yet the uptake occurs more slowly in the fetus than in the mother. The partial pressures of volatile anesthetics are also lower in the fetal umbilical vessels than in maternal arterial blood [20]. However, MAC in the fetus is below that of the mother [21]. During moderately deep (1.5 MAC) isoflurane or halothane anesthesia, maternal arterial pressure and cardiac output were decreased. Uterine vasodilation occurred and uteroplacental perfusion was maintained [22]. Fetal oxygenation and base excess were also maintained. However, at higher concentrations of inhaled anesthetic (2.0 MAC), maternal hypotension resulted in reduced uteroplacental perfusion despite uterine vasodilation leading to fetal hypoxia and acidosis [22,23]. The administration of 1.5–2.0 MAC of anesthesia should result in fetal anesthesia as long as uteroplacental gas exchange is maintained.

## Fetal Pain

Because pain is a subjective experience, some may argue whether the fetus even feel pain and, if it does, when does it feel pain? It has been suggested that to feel pain one needs to be aware, or conscious, and consciousness cannot be demonstrated in the fetus. The fetus cannot tell us what it is feeling, and there is no objective method available to measure pain. Given current knowledge, one must rely on anatomic evidence and the fetal stress response to help guide the anesthetic management of the fetus during surgery.

It is known that cutaneous receptors are present in the human fetus by the 20th week of gestation. However, the fetal awareness of noxious stimuli requires functional thalamocortical connections which appear at 23–30 weeks' gestation [24]. Electroencephalogram patterns are discontinuous before 25 weeks. From 25 to 29 weeks, periods of activity increase, such that by 30 weeks, electroencephalogram patterns show a distinction between wakefulness and sleep [25]. At this point in development, it seems certain that the fetus has the necessary neuroanatomic connections to feel pain. In fact, the descending inhibitory pathways are not complete until after birth so conceivably the fetus may be even more sensitive to painful stimuli than the older child.

Activation of the hypothalamic–pituitary–adrenal axis (i.e., stress response) may also be an indicator of pain. Human fetal endocrine responses to stress have been demonstrated as early as 20 weeks' gestation. Giannakoulopoulos and colleagues demonstrated a fetal endocrine stress response after obtaining blood samples from fetuses at 20–34 weeks' gestation with intrauterine needling [26]. Needling of the innervated intrahepatic vein (IHV) resulted in increases in fetal plasma concentrations of cortisol and beta-endorphin (known stress hormones), whereas needling of the denervated placental cord failed to showed these pronounced hormonal responses. Fetal plasma levels of noradrenaline were also significantly elevated in those fetuses (18–37 weeks' gestation) who had IHV sampling when compared with those fetuses who had umbilical venous blood sampling from the placental cord [27]. Convincing evidence for the importance of providing analgesia to the fetus came from the landmark study by Fisk and colleagues in which intravenous fentanyl (10 μg kg$^{-1}$ estimated fetal weight × 1.25 placental correction) ablated the beta-endorphin response in fetuses having IHV cannulation [28]. Further support for providing analgesia to fetuses undergoing invasive procedures comes from primate studies indicating that periods of perinatal stress during critical times of development can have permanent detrimental effects on hippocampal development and stress behavior [29–31]. A final reason for providing anesthesia and analgesia to the fetal patient is a humanitarian and ethical one. As Glover and Fisk so eloquently stated in a 1996 editorial, "We don't know better; better to err on the safe side from mid-gestation" [32].

# Diseases and Interventions

## Cardiac

Pharmacological fetal cardiac interventions have been attempted when the fetus is at risk for demise or severe morbidity due to arrhythmia or fetal heart block. Maternal oral administration of digoxin, propranolol, and more specific antiarrhythmics are part of the treatment for fetal arrhythmias and high-grade AV block. When transplacental passage is compromised as in the setting of hydrops, a more direct administration can be achieved with intramuscular or intravenous injection to the fetus, under ultrasound guidance [33].

Anatomic cardiac defects are the most common congenital newborn malformation and they can be diagnosed prenatally as early as 14 weeks' gestation. The advances in fetal imaging techniques allow for a better understanding of the natural history and progression of these lesions. Clinicians struggle to improve outcome in instances when the survival of the fetus is at stake or when significant neonatal morbidity is anticipated. Fetal interventions for congenital cardiac malformations have seen a tremendous growth and are now therapeutic options for specific conditions. By and large, minimally invasive, percutaneous, and image-guided fetal cardiac interventions are typically performed at mid or late gestation. A team that includes an experienced ultrasonographer, obstetrician, interventional cardiologist, maternal anesthesiologist, and fetal anesthesiologist work together in the operating room. The immediate risks to the fetus are mitigated by the goals of improving survival and morbidity. Appropriate follow-up will help define long-term risks and benefits of these techniques. Before attempting difficult and high-risk procedures, it is imperative to define their anticipated goals (Table 34.2). Currently three cardiac conditions fit criteria for prenatal intervention and each has specific objectives (Table 34.3).

Obstructive cardiac valve lesions progress during pregnancy and according to the flow theory, normal blood flow through the heart contributes to normal growth of the ventricles. Ultimately the decision to intervene is guided by the objective of avoiding single ventricle physiology in the postnatal period. Despite an increased survival in specialized centers

**Table 34.2** Fetal cardiac interventions

| Goals |
|---|
| Prevent fetal death |
| Prevent arrhythmias |
| Normalize hemodynamics |
| Normalize pulmonary development |
| **Lesions** |
| Aortic stenosis |
| Pulmonary stenosis or atresia with intact ventricular septum |
| Hypoplastic left heart syndrome with intact or restrictive atrial septum |

**Table 34.3** Goals of specific fetal cardiac interventions

| Aortic valvuloplasty | Pulmonary valvuloplasty | Atrial septostomy |
|---|---|---|
| Decrease LV afterload | Increase RV growth | Decompress LA |
| Promote flow through left heart | Improve pulmonary vasculature | Prevent pulmonary venous hypertension |
| Prevent HLHS | Reverse hydrops | Prevent postnatal hypoxia |

with expertise managing single ventricle patients, the long-term complications after palliative surgery remain quite debilitating. Two-ventricle circulation is preferred as it is a superior predictor of improved life expectancy and quality of life [34].

## Fetal Aortic Valvuloplasty

### Rationale for Intervention

Echocardiographic predictors of the evolution of critical aortic stenosis (AS) to hypoplastic left heart syndrome include (1) valvar aortic stenosis with dilated or normal size left ventricle; (2) reversed flow in the transverse aortic arch and foramen ovale; and (3) monophasic mitral inflow [35]. With critical AS and impaired left ventricular growth the left ventricle becomes hypoplastic. Endocardial fibroelastosis (EFE) contributes to impaired filling and redirection of flow across the foramen ovale to the right ventricle, now in charge of the whole cardiac output. A different picture evolves when the increase in left ventricle pressure results in rapid left ventricle dilation and mitral regurgitation. The absence of synchronous left ventricle contractions combined with EFE and impaired coronary perfusion cause progressive and irreversible myocardial damage. Extreme left ventricle dysfunction and dilation with severe mitral regurgitation and increased left atrial pressure can cause closure of the foramen ovale, thus rendering the left atrium unable to decompress into the right atrium. The pulmonary veins are dilated and ultimately congestive heart failure (CHF) or hydrops occur when the right ventricle is unable to maintain cardiac output.

The technical steps involve the advancement of a needle through the maternal abdomen into the amniotic sac under continuous ultrasound guidance. The left ventricle is reached through the fetal chest. After alignment of the insertion needle with the left ventricle outflow tract, a coronary balloon catheter is introduced through the needle and inflated across the obstructed valve. A technically successful procedure results in flow across the valve accompanied with moderate to severe aortic regurgitation and decrease in left ventricular size.

### Results

The group at Boston Children's Hospital performed their first fetal aortic valvuloplasty in 2000. After the obligatory learning curve, the Boston group now reports an 80 percent technical success rate [36]. In their most recent review they report that 30 percent of fetuses after a technically successful procedure are born with biventricular circulation, while 8 percent are converted to two-ventricle physiology after initial univentricular palliation. Half of the fetuses experienced hemodynamic instability during the procedure, namely bradycardia requiring treatment with intramuscular or intracardiac injections of epinephrine and bicarbonate and drainage of pericardial effusions. There were no maternal complications, but there was a 10 percent rate of fetal death or premature delivery.

The Austrian group published the second largest series with 24 procedures and a 67 percent technical success rate [37]. Of these, 63 percent achieved biventricular physiology after birth. It seems reasonable to eliminate candidates for fetal valvuloplasty when there is high velocity forward flow in the aortic arch and good ventricular function, as these patients can wait for postnatal treatment. Fetuses with ventricles that are too small to avoid univentricular circulations should not be candidates for the procedure.

## Fetal Pulmonary Valvuloplasty

### Rationale for Intervention

In contrast to the left ventricle, after interruption or limitation of blood flow from pulmonary valve obstruction, the right ventricle does not dilate but develops excessive muscular hypertrophy. Impaired filling and growth can result in CHF or univentricular circulation at birth. Ten percent of pulmonary valve stenosis cases progress to pulmonary atresia. Patient selection is critical since the postnatal outcome for the majority of cases of pulmonary atresia with intact atrial septum is favorable with postnatal balloon valvuloplasty. Fetal tricuspid valve size has emerged as a possible predictor of postnatal outcome. Fetuses with hypoplasia of the tricuspid valve annulus and a significant transvalvular pressure gradient are the best candidates. The optimal timing to intervene would be before right ventricular hypoplasia and coronary fistula develop. The fetal right ventricular outflow tract is accessed percutaneously with a balloon catheter through a subcostal or intercostal approach.

### Results

With their series of 30 fetuses undergoing midgestation pulmonary valvuloplasty, Tworetzky et al. report technical success for 75 percent of cases but no decisive evidence that the intervention changed the natural course of the disease [38].The risks for the fetus remain the same as for aortic valvuloplasty, but hemopericardium is more likely due to a larger needle and bigger balloon.

### Fetal Atrial Septostomy

#### Rationale for Intervention

In fetuses with left-sided obstructions, an open foramen ovale is crucial for drainage of the pulmonary venous return. Increased left atrial pressure resulting in premature closing of the foramen ovale will generate high pressure in the pulmonary vascular bed resulting in increased morbidity and mortality at birth despite urgent atrial septostomy. Chronic pulmonary venous hypertension in utero has been shown to reduce the survival rate of Norwood stage 1 from 90 percent to 52 percent [39].

### Results

The largest series to date, from the Boston experience, contains 21 procedures performed between 24 and 34 weeks' gestation [40]. The creation of a defect of at least 3 mm in diameter is associated with better oxygenation and less frequent need for emergent postnatal intervention, but the impact on survival has not been demonstrated. Two fetal deaths were directly attributed to the intervention. To prevent the risk of re-stenosis after a single dilation, the authors have questioned the benefit of stenting rather than catheter and balloon inflation. In the future, short bursts of

YAG laser directed at the atrial septum could achieve longer lasting results.

## Airway

### Extrinsic Obstruction

Lymphangiomas and teratomas around the airway do not often cause fetal demise, but this extrinsic airway obstruction will very likely result in mortality in the perinatal period. These fetuses must be delivered via ex utero intrapartum therapy (EXIT) so the airway can be secured in a controlled fashion. The EXIT procedure will give the team time to work on the fetus while the placenta still serves as the organ of fetal respiration. Direct laryngoscopy, rigid bronchoscopy, tracheostomy, neck dissection with retrograde intubation, or even tumor resection may be accomplished during an EXIT procedure. After the fetal procedure is complete, the umbilical cord is clamped and the child is delivered to a neonatal team for further resuscitation. Ideally, the EXIT will occur at or near term, but this may not always be feasible for a variety of reasons, such as preterm labor, a shortening cervix, or very rarely, worsening hydrops and impending fetal demise.

In a series of patients with a broad range of pathology cared for between 1996 to 2002, long-term survival was 89 percent [41]. Specific pathology and pathophysiology will influence survival. Giant cervical teratoma was the diagnosis in a series of 17 EXIT procedures performed from 1995 to 2010. While all patients survived the procedure, prematurity and mass effect from the giant teratomas led to pulmonary hypoplasia which resulted in a neonatal mortality rate of 23 percent [42]. Fetuses with oropharyngeal tumors seem to fare better. All four patients with oropharyngeal tumors delivered between 2006 and 2012 survived [43].

### Intrinsic Obstruction

Atresia, webs, cysts, or agenesis at the laryngeal or tracheal level may cause intrinsic obstruction of the fetal airways. This condition is commonly called CHAOS (congenital high airway obstruction syndrome) and is associated with a set of findings on prenatal imaging which includes the following: large dilated lungs, flattened or everted diaphragms, distal airway dilation, and hydrops fetalis [44]. Mortality in cases of CHAOS occurs for two reasons, and the fetus must make it past these two hurdles to survive. The first hurdle occurs during gestation. Death is due to massively enlarged lungs compressing the fetal heart. This compression of the heart by the lungs will result in a physiology similar to cardiac tamponade. Fetal hydrops and death may result. The second hurdle occurs at birth. Simple airway obstruction is the cause of demise.

In the fetal period, decompression of the fetal airway and lungs is necessary to relieve pressure on the fetal heart, and this may allow resolution of the hydrops. Decompression may occur spontaneously [45]. Fetoscopic laser decompression of the airways has been performed in selected cases [46]. A fetus with CHAOS palliated by airway decompression has made it past the first hurdle, and may survive longer in utero, hopefully delivering closer to term. At this time the fetus must clear the second hurdle and be delivered via EXIT procedure to secure the airway. Long-term survival is possible [45,47].

## Myelomeningocele

### Rationale

Myelomeningocele does not threaten the life of the fetus, and it is not a direct cause of neonatal mortality, but it is a cause of serious morbidity, such as paralysis, bowel and bladder dysfunction, Arnold–Chiari II malformation, and hydrocephalus. Repair of the myelomeningocele in utero would hopefully improve neurologic function by decreasing the exposure of the developing spinal cord to the amniotic fluid and by helping improve the hindbrain herniation that occurs with the Chiari II malformation.

### Results

A randomized trial of prenatal versus postnatal repair of myelomeningocele was conducted between 2003 and 2010 [48]. The trial was stopped after an interim analysis as it demonstrated efficacy of prenatal surgery. The trial found a difference between the groups for the composite primary outcome of neonatal death or need for placement of a ventriculoperitoneal shunt (68 percent in the prenatal surgery group vs. 98 percent in the postnatal repair group). Another outcome was a composite score of mental development and motor function. This composite score was improved in the prenatal repair group. The procedure is not without risk to the fetus. In the prenatal surgical group, bradycardia occurred in 10 percent,

death occurred in 3 percent, and mean gestational age at delivery was 34 weeks. While maternal morbidity was not a primary outcome studied in this trial, this large series of mothers undergoing open fetal surgery allowed some quantification of the risk to the mothers undergoing mid-gestation surgery and subsequent Cesarean delivery. Chorioamniotic membrane separation occurred in 26 percent of mothers undergoing the prenatal repair, while 21 percent developed oligohydramnios. Only 64 percent of the mothers were found to have a well-healed, intact uterus at the time of delivery, and 9 percent had to be transfused at the time of delivery. The Cesarean section that must be performed after open fetal surgery is more complex, as the omental flap must be taken down, and the prior hysterotomy must also be inspected and repaired if needed.

## Thoracic Tumors

Two common thoracic tumors encountered in the fetal period are congenital cystic adenomatoid malformation (CCAM) and bronchopulmonary sequestration (BPS). The CCAM results from overgrowth of terminal bronchioles, so there is a connection between the tumor and the tracheobronchial tree. The CCAM may be primarily cystic, solid, or mixed. A BPS does not originate from lung tissue, and there is no connection to the fetal airways, but the BPS does have a connection to the systemic vascular supply, typically via one or several arterial feeding vessels. Occasionally a "hybrid lesion" develops, which has characteristics of both CCAM and BPS in that connections to both the airways and the systemic vasculature exist. In utero, tumors may cause cardiac compression, and may also grow enough to impede cardiac filling and function. This will result in hydrops [49]. Postnatally, neonates are at risk for respiratory compromise as these tumors do not participate in gas exchange. Additionally, mass effect from the tumor causes hypoplasia of the normal lung tissue.

The size, growth rate, pathology, and gestational age at which symptoms appear will dictate the therapy for the fetus. In most cases small tumors do not perturb the development of the fetus, and the child may be delivered normally and go home with the family after a period of observation. The child may then return at several weeks to months of age for elective resection of the tumor. Larger, growing tumors may cause symptoms of hydrops, and frequent prenatal observation is warranted. If steroids are given to the mother, the growth may slow or tumors may shrink [50]. If symptoms persist and occur before lung maturity, fetal surgical intervention is warranted. Intervention may be as minimally invasive as aspirating and decompressing a cystic lesion, or may be as complex as performing a mid-gestation hysterotomy and fetal thoracotomy with pulmonary lobectomy for solid lesions not amenable to decompression.

In some cases, if the symptoms of hydrops do not develop until later in gestation, or if the size and mass effect of the tumor are deemed too great, delivery may be via an EXIT procedure with neonatal pulmonary lobectomy before the umbilical cord is clamped [51,52]. Survival in a series of nine patients undergoing EXIT for lung resection was 89 percent [52]. The neurodevelopmental outcome of the majority of children undergoing these procedures is age-appropriate, with 77 percent scoring in the normal range for neuromotor outcome and 23 percent in the mildly delayed range [53].

### Congenital Diaphragmatic Hernia

As pulmonary hypoplasia and pulmonary hypertension are major factors in the mortality of children with congenital diaphragmatic hernia (CDH), the rationale for fetal therapy is clear. If the herniated bowel could be returned to the abdominal cavity during fetal life, the lungs would have more time to grow. Open fetal procedures involving fetal laparotomy were not successful, so less invasive strategies involving fetal tracheal occlusion were developed [54]. The goal of tracheal occlusion was to stimulate lung growth, as in cases of CHAOS. Unfortunately, after much work in this field, trials of minimally invasive fetal surgical intervention with tracheal occlusion have not been shown to be better than optimal postnatal care [55]. The approach consists of tracheal fetal occlusion and subsequent delivery via EXIT procedure. This approach is still a major undertaking in terms of risk and potential morbidity for the mother. European centers are studying an even less invasive approach that involves percutaneous, fetoscopically guided placement of a balloon to occlude the fetal trachea. This balloon is removed several weeks later, also minimally invasively. This approach limits maternal risk and morbidity [56,57]. Some centers in the United States may be participating in trials in the future utilizing this less invasive strategy.

## Sacrococcygeal Teratoma

### Rationale

A prenatal diagnosis of sacrococcygeal teratoma (SCT) carries a high mortality rate. Death can be due to high-output heart failure from the large, rapidly growing SCT or simply from tumor rupture and fetal anemia. Symptomatic tumors will result in fetal hydrops, and a variety of ultrasound findings can be used to assess the gravity of the situation. Serial fetal echocardiography will allow for trending of fetal heart function and measurement of the combined cardiac output. Evidence of an enlarging placenta, increasing diameter of the fetal inferior vena cava, and increased blood flow to the descending aorta are all signs that the fetal status is worsening [58,59]. Palliative fetal treatment is aimed at decreasing the tumor size, whether by open surgical debulking, or minimally invasive ablation of the tumor. If the tumor burden can be decreased, the high-output failure will hopefully resolve, allowing the fetus to survive to delivery and definitive surgical resection in the postnatal period.

### Results

Fetal treatment for these tumors is risky and the path is not as clear as that for lung tumors. Minimally invasive therapy has been attempted, but this is not yet an optimal technique. Approaches have included laser ablation, radiofrequency ablation, sclerotherapy, electrocautery, and vascular coiling. Survival rate after minimally invasive therapy is 30 percent. Radiofrequency ablation has caused iatrogenic trauma to the surrounding area, including the ischium, gluteal region, the femoral head, and sciatic nerve. Open fetal surgery has a survival rate of 50 percent, but is a significant undertaking, with all the attendant risks to both the mother and the fetus [60]. Open surgery involves a hysterotomy, fetal vascular access, and debulking of the tumor. The anatomy of the tumor must be considered when planning open fetal surgery. The tumors should be primarily external with a small stalk. Broad-based tumors would pose technical challenges given the time constraints of open fetal surgery. Early Cesarean delivery with early or immediate postnatal surgery in an adjacent operating room has also been proposed as a management approach [61,62].

## Complicated Multiple Gestations

### Rationale

Twin and higher order multiple gestations are at risk for complications. Monozygotic twins are at higher risk than dizygotic pregnancies, as a monozygotic twin pair may develop into a monochorionic–diamniotic or monochorionic–monoamniotic pregnancy. The monochorionic twins may share blood flow from the placenta to varying degrees, and in some cases this blood flow is uneven, with one twin getting more net blood flow than the other. The recipient twin can develop hypervolemia, polyuria, and polyhydramnios. The donor twin develops hypovolemia, oliguria, and oligohydramnios. Both twins are at risk for neurologic and cardiac complications, and death [63]. The goal is to save both twins, and treatment has ranged from aspiration of amniotic fluid from the twin with poly-hydramnios, to creation of a microseptostomy between the twins' amniotic membranes, to laser ablation of the vessels that are allowing unequal blood flow. In some cases, selective feticide via ablation of the umbilical cord to one of the twins is performed to try to optimize the chances for survival of one of the twins. Aspiration of excess amniotic fluid (amnioreduction) was intended as a symptomatic treatment to prevent preterm labor, but the fetuses may be helped by a reduction of uterine wall tension, and improved uteroplacental blood flow, as evidenced by improved Doppler waveforms. Microseptostomy, similarly, may equalize pressures between the two amniotic sacs to allow better utero-placental blood flow. Laser ablation of the vessels on the placenta allowing the unequal blood flow is more directly targeted to the pathophysiology, but also carries more risk than either amnioreduction or micro-septostomy. Selective feticide may decrease risk of neurologic injury or death to the surviving twin [64].

### Results

A 2014 update of a Cochrane review remains supportive of the use of endoscopic laser ablation of the placental anastomoses to improve neurodevelopmental outcomes. This review included three studies and synthesized data for 253 women. When septostomy was compared with amnioreduction, no significant differences were found [65]. When taken together, the two trials comparing amnioreduction and endoscopic laser surgery showed no difference in overall death, but did show improved neurologic outcome [66,67]. The techniques continue

to be adjusted, and a recent trial supports ablation of all vessels at the vascular "equator" between both twins as compared to selective ablation [68].

## Anesthetic Management

To provide adequate maternal and fetal surgical conditions, optimal positioning, and stable hemodynamics, we work with a dedicated team knowledgeable of the challenges and differences of each procedure.

## Anesthesia for Fetal Cardiac Interventions

### Maternal Anesthesia

Regardless of the indications, all fetal cardiac interventions (FCIs) are currently performed percutaneously under ultrasound guidance, thus resulting in minimal maternal discomfort. General anesthesia with endotracheal intubation was standard practice when procedures lasted a few hours and a mini-laparotomy was occasionally required. The Boston group has accomplished steady technical progress and since 2012 has performed all FCIs under neuraxial anesthesia with a T4 sensory level. After placement of an epidural or combined spinal epidural dosed with bupivacaine and fentanyl the mother is positioned with left uterine displacement. She receives high-flow oxygen, is fitted with headphones, and encouraged to listen to music for distraction. Small doses of benzodiazepines, opioids, or inducing agents can be beneficial to decrease anxiety and agitation. Maternal blood pressure is maintained at 20 percent of baseline with a combination of crystalloids, phenylephrine, and ephedrine. As with any regional technique for obstetric patients, the maternal risks include failed block, intravascular injection, high spinal or aspiration from excessive sedation. In the immediate postoperative period mothers are monitored for preterm labor, and fetal cardiac ultrasound is performed prior to discharge.

### Fetal Anesthesia

With the advent of regional anesthesia, the fetus is no longer exposed to anesthetic medications via transplacental passage. All cardiac procedures involve insertion of a needle through the fetus chest wall and heart. Complete fetal immobility is paramount at a time when wires, catheters, and balloons are inflated in the tiny cardiac cavity. The existence of a fetal stress response and its impact on outcome and preterm labor is well established, as is the need to blunt or attenuate this response. Once in optimal position, the fetus receives an intramuscular injection of vecuronium 0.2 mg kg$^{-1}$ or 1–2 mg kg$^{-1}$ rocuronium, fentanyl 50 μg kg$^{-1}$, and atropine 20 μg kg$^{-1}$. This anesthetic provides suitable conditions for these procedures, which rarely exceed two hours. Monitoring of the fetus is currently limited to Doppler ultrasonography. Continuous observation of the fetal heart rate and function while still in the operating room are required for up to ten minutes after the procedure ends. Fetal hemodynamic instability, specifically profound bradycardia and hemopericardium, have been reported irrespective of the indications for fetal cardiac interventions [69]. Given the limited access to the fetus, a plan for fetal resuscitation must always be put in place [70]. Based on the estimated fetal weight, syringes of epinephrine, 10–20 μg kg$^{-1}$ and bicarbonate1–2 mEq kg$^{-1}$ are prepared under sterile conditions for intramuscular or intracardiac administration should fetal resuscitation be necessary. Special attention must be paid to the total volume injected into the fetal cardiac cavity. An improvement of cardiac function frequently follows the administration of resuscitative medications and/or drainage of large pericardial effusion. In extreme circumstances maternal transabdominal compressions can be attempted, although with limited success. The contingencies for emergent delivery of a viable albeit severely compromised fetus must be discussed with the parents during the pre-procedure meeting, with input from the neonatologist, cardiologist, and obstetrician.

## Anesthesia for Mid-Gestation Open Fetal Surgery

### Maternal Anesthesia

The preoperative evaluation of the mother should include the standard anesthetic history and physical with particular attention paid to symptoms of reflux and supine hypotension, and the exam of the airway and spine. Mothers should be quite healthy overall to minimize the risks of other anesthetic complications. A complete blood count, serum electrolytes, blood urea nitrogen, and creatinine should be measured, with other laboratory and diagnostic studies as indicated by the history, physical, and procedure. An electrocardiogram is helpful to diagnose previously asymptomatic conduction abnormalities that may come to the surface under the deep general anesthesia.

Blood should be cross-matched for the mother, and type O, Rh-negative blood for the fetus can be cross-matched against the mother's sample, as maternal antibodies can cross the placenta. Fetal blood should be available as indicated by the surgical procedure.

A high lumbar or low thoracic epidural catheter may be placed for maternal postoperative analgesia. Indomethacin is also given to the mother. Aspiration prophylaxis, and left uterine displacement precede rapid sequence induction of general anesthesia. After intubation, an arterial catheter and large-bore intravenous catheter are placed. Administration of intravenous crystalloid is often kept to a minimum as fetal surgical patients are at increased risk for pulmonary edema [8]. While other options are possible, the central feature of many anesthetics for open fetal surgery is deep maternal general anesthesia with high-dose volatile anesthetics [71]. Profound uterine relaxation is required by the surgical team to allow easy access to the fetus, to decrease resistance to uterine blood flow, and to minimize the potential risks of abruption. Desflurane is often chosen because its low solubility allows for rapid titration. Approximately twice the minimum alveolar concentration of volatile anesthetic is used. This strategy is obviously not without risks, which include maternal hypotension and fetal cardiac depression [72]. Some centers are advocating a lower dose of volatile anesthetic supplemented by intravenous anesthetics [73,74]. Open mid-gestation surgery should be technically feasible with a pure neuraxial technique and intravenous nitroglycerin for uterine relaxation, but the length of the procedure, stress for the mother, hemodynamic shifts, and need for the operating room team to be able to concentrate fully on the needs at hand while possibly being distracted by an awake patient would make this a challenging proposition.

After the laparotomy, the uterus is exposed, uterine tone is assessed and adjusted as needed, the placental edges are mapped using ultrasound, and the hysterotomy is made with special uterine staplers which keep the edges of the chorionic and amniotic membranes together with the uterine edges. Warmed crystalloid is infused into the amniotic space to maintain fetal warmth and adequate amniotic fluid volume. Fetal incision is made, usually after an intramuscular injection of opioid and muscle relaxant. When the procedure is completed, the uterine edges are closed, and a flap of omentum is also sewn over the hysterotomy site to encourage blood flow and healing. As the uterus is being closed, an intravenous bolus of magnesium sulfate is started, the epidural catheter is activated, and the volatile anesthetic is decreased. The mother is extubated awake.

### Fetal Anesthesia

Fetal pain is a controversial topic, but there is clear hormonal and hemodynamic evidence of a fetal stress response to noxious stimuli [24,28]. The fetal stress response can be attenuated by opioids, which are often administered as an intramuscular injection (20 $\mu$g kg$^{-1}$ fentanyl), along with a nondepolarizing muscle relaxant (0.2 mg kg$^{-1}$ vecuronium). Atropine (20 $\mu$g kg$^{-1}$) may be added in cases where the fetus is felt to be at higher risk for bradycardia. As previously mentioned, volatile anesthetics cross the placenta.

Vascular access to the fetus depends on the needs of the procedure. In cases of myelomeningocele repair, tubing is prepared and primed, but an intravenous catheter would only be placed in emergent situations. In cases where blood loss is likely, peripheral venous access is obtained in the fetus. Monitoring of the fetus is accomplished by direct observation, intermittent assessment of fetal heart rates by ultrasound, or continuous fetal echocardiography, depending on the case. Continuous fetal pulse oximetry can also be used if a hand or foot is accessible. Normal fetal saturations should be between 40 and 70 percent, and the heart rate should be between 110 and 160 bpm. If the fetus becomes bradycardic, the anesthesia team must quickly assess the well-being of the mother, and ensure adequate uteroplacental flow. The patency of the umbilical cord must also be assessed, amniotic fluid volume must be assured, and pressure on the placenta or the fetus itself should be relieved. Echocardiography can guide fluid resuscitation, medication administration, and chest compressions on the fetus.

## Anesthesia for the EXIT Procedure

### Maternal Anesthesia

The basics of maternal anesthesia for an EXIT procedure are largely the same as for in an open mid-gestation procedure, with a few differences. Since the child will be delivered at the end of the procedure, and no magnesium bolus is needed, maternal fluid administration can be liberalized; 3–5 liters of crystalloid is usually well tolerated. After delivery of the child,

reversal of the uterine atony is often accomplished simply by decreasing the volatile anesthetic along with administration of oxytocin, but it is prudent to have additional uterotonics available.

### Fetal Anesthesia

The basic principles of anesthesia, in terms of vascular access, medications, and monitoring for the fetus during an EXIT procedure are also the same as for an open mid-gestation procedure, with some exceptions. Some specifics to the EXIT follow. As the fetus will be delivered in a deeply anesthetized state and will likely still be paralyzed from the intramuscular injection, intubation should occur on the field. The fetus is not ventilated, however, until the umbilical cord is about to be clamped, as ventilation and oxygenation of the fetus may start a cascade of events leading to placental separation. Surfactant is often given to the fetus before ventilation. Once the fetal chest has been observed to rise, and the oxygen saturations have begun to increase, the umbilical cord can be clamped and the baby is delivered to a team of neonatologists for further resuscitation or to another operating room for further surgery.

Another difference between an EXIT and midgestation open fetal surgery is the need for a second operating room. This room is staffed with another team of nurses and anesthesiologists, and is prepared and ready to go in case the fetus does not tolerate the EXIT procedure, or in case a further procedure is planned.

## Anesthesia for Minimally Invasive Noncardiac Procedures

### Maternal/ Fetal Anesthesia

The vast majority of minimally invasive noncardiac procedures can be performed with maternal sedation or neuraxial anesthesia. Advances in technology have resulted in smaller instruments [75], and advances in the skills of the operators has allowed a decrease in anesthetic requirement. Anesthetic techniques have ranged from general anesthesia with an endotracheal tube to sedation alone. As for any anesthetic, the needs of the patient and the procedure are taken into consideration in the formulation of an anesthetic plan. A thorough discussion with all team members and with the patient is essential. In many cases, light sedation with local anesthetic infiltration is all that is required. The preoperative evaluation should consider the patient's expectations of level of awareness, feelings of anxiety, history of panic attacks, symptoms of supine hypotension, and severity of gastroesophageal reflux. The ability of the mother to lie still in a particular position for an hour or more should be explored, as patient position is quite variable for these cases, depending on the location of the placenta. Mild airway obstruction with paradoxical abdominal movement will make the procedure technically more difficult. The gestational age of the fetus should also be considered. If the fetus is considered viable, contingency plans should be made for the emergent delivery and resuscitation of a very premature infant.

Sedation regimens can be quite variable. Various combinations of diazepam and morphine have been used, as have propofol and fentanyl. Midazolam and remifentanil allow rapid titration of analgesia, while the mothers are typically lucid enough to participate in their own positioning for these cases. Local anesthetic infiltration is important if a neuraxial technique is not being used. Regardless of the particular agents used, the goal is to minimize motion and stress in the fetus, while achieving a slightly decreased but safe level of consciousness in the mother.

The fetus is rarely given any medication directly in these procedures, as transplacental passage of the maternal anesthetics is often adequate to decrease fetal motion. If fetal motion persists, intramuscular injection of medications such as opioids or nondepolarizing muscle relaxants can be considered.

# The Future

Multidisciplinary teams involved in fetal interventions face numerous challenges. The anesthesiologist plays a major role in the selection of suitable maternal candidates and safe anesthetic techniques for both mother and fetus. Enhanced imaging techniques and improved instrumentation will facilitate the procedures and the field promises to grow steadily. Long-term follow-up is essential to justify and evaluate the interventions.

# References

1. Harrison MR, Golbus MS, Filly RA, et al. Fetal surgery for congenital hydronephrosis. *N Engl J Med*. 1982;306(10):591–3.

2. Harrison MR, Filly RA, Golbus MS, et al. Fetal treatment 1982. *N Engl J Med*. 1982;307(26):1651–2.

3. Zoler ML. Myelomeningocele repair drives changes in fetal surgery. *Pediatic News Digital Network*. October 17, 2012.

4. Roybal JL, Santore MT, Flake AW. Stem cell and genetic therapies for the fetus. *Semin Fetal Neonatal Med*. 2010;15(1):46–51.

5. Thornburg KL, Jacobson S-L, Giraud GD, Morton MJ. Hemodynamic changes in pregnancy. *Semin Perinatol*. 2000;24(1):11–14.

6. Robson SC, Hunter S, Boys RJ, Dunlop W. Serial study of factors influencing changes in cardiac output during human pregnancy. *Am J Physiol*. 1989;256(4):H1060–5.

7. Hunter S, Robson SC. Adaptation of the maternal heart in pregnancy. *Br Heart J*. 1992;68(6):540–3.

8. DiFederico EM, Burlingame JM, Kilpatrick SJ, Harrison M, Matthay MA. Pulmonary edema in obstetric patients is rapidly resolved except in the presence of infection or of nitroglycerin tocolysis after open fetal surgery. *Am J Obstet Gynecol*. 1998;179(4):925–33.

9. Rosen MA. Management of anesthesia for the pregnant surgical patient. *Anesthesiology*. 1999;91(4):1159–63.

10. Motoyama EK, Rivard G, Acheson F, Cook CD. The effect of changes in maternal pH and P-CO2 on the P-O2 of fetal lambs. *Anesthesiology*. 1967;28(5):891–903.

11. Chan MT, Mainland P, Gin T. Minimum alveolar concentration of halothane and enflurane are decreased in early pregnancy. *Anesthesiology*. 1996;85(4):782–6.

12. Luks FI, Johnson BD, Papadakis K, Traore M, Piasecki GJ. Predictive value of monitoring parameters in fetal surgery. *J Pediatr Surg*. 1998;33(8):1297–301.

13. Bower SJ, Flack NJ, Sepulveda W, Talbert DG, Fisk NM. Uterine artery blood flow response to correction of amniotic fluid volume. *Am J Obstet Gynecol*. 1995;173(2):502–7.

14. Fisk NM, Tannirandorn Y, Nicolini U, Talbert DG, Rodeck CH. Amniotic pressure in disorders of amniotic fluid volume. *Obstet Gynecol*. 1990;76(2):210–14.

15. Skillman CA, Plessinger MA, Woods JR, Clark KE. Effect of graded reductions in uteroplacental blood flow on the fetal lamb. *Am J Physiol*. 1985;249(6 Pt 2):H1098–105. Available at: http://proxy.library.upenn.edu:2205/content/249/6/H1098.long.

16. Fenton KN, Heinemann MK, Hickey PR, et al. Inhibition of the fetal stress response improves cardiac output and gas exchange after fetal cardiac bypass. *J Thorac Cardiovasc Surg*. 1994;107(6):1416–22.

17. Rudolph AM, Heymann MA. Cardiac output in the fetal lamb: the effects of spontaneous and induced

changes of heart rate on right and left ventricular output. *Am J Obstet Gynecol.* 1976;124(2):183–92.

18. Gilbert RD. Control of fetal cardiac output during changes in blood volume. *Am J Physiol.* 1980;238(1):H80–6.

19. Warren TM, Datta S, Ostheimer GW, et al. Comparison of the maternal and neonatal effects of halothane, enflurane, and isoflurane for cesarean delivery. *Anesth Analg.* 1983;62(5):516–20.

20. Dwyer R, Fee JP, Moore J. Uptake of halothane and isoflurane by mother and baby during caesarean section. *Br J Anaesth.* 1995;74(4):379–83.

21. Myers LB, Cohen D, Galinkin J, Gaiser R, Kurth CD. Anaesthesia for fetal surgery. *Paediatr Anaesth.* 2002;12(7):569–78.

22. Biehl DR, Yarnell R, Wade JG, Sitar D. The uptake of isoflurane by the foetal lamb in utero: effect on regional blood flow. *Can J Anaesth.* 1983;30(6):581–6.

23. Palahniuk RJ, Shnider SM. Maternal and fetal cardiovascular and acid–base changes during halothane and isoflurane anesthesia in the pregnant ewe. *Anesthesiology.* 1974;41(5):462–72.

24. Lee SJ, Ralston HJP, Drey EA, Partridge JC, Rosen MA. Fetal pain: a systematic multidisciplinary review of the evidence. *JAMA.* 2005;294(8):947–54.

25. Torres F, Anderson C. The normal EEG of the human newborn. *J Clin Neurophysiol.* 1985;2(2):89–103.

26. Giannakoulopoulos X, Glover V, Sepulveda W, Kourtis P, Fisk NM. Fetal plasma cortisol and β-endorphin response to intrauterine needling. *The Lancet.* 1994;344(8915):77–81.

27. Giannakoulopoulos X, Teixeira JM, Fisk NM, Glover V. Human fetal and maternal noradrenaline responses to invasive procedures. *Pediatr Res.* 1999;45(4):494–9.

28. Fisk NM, Gitau R, Teixeira JM, et al. Effect of direct fetal opioid analgesia on fetal hormonal and hemodynamic stress response to intrauterine needling. *Anesthesiology.* 2001;95(4):828–35.

29. Meaney MJ, Aitken DH. The effects of early postnatal handling on hippocampal glucocorticoid receptor concentrations: temporal parameters. *Brain Res.* 1985;354(2):301–4.

30. Clarke AS, Wittwer DJ, Abbott DH, Schneider ML. Long-term effects of prenatal stress on HPA axis activity in juvenile rhesus monkeys. *Dev Psychobiol.* 1994;27(5):257–69.

31. Schneider ML, Coe CL, Lubach GR. Endocrine activation mimics the adverse effects of prenatal stress on the neuromotor development of the infant primate. *Dev Psychobiol.* 1992;25(6):427–39.

32. Glover V, Fisk N. Do fetuses feel pain? We don't know; better to err on the safe side from mid-gestation. *BMJ.* 1996;313(7060):796.

33. McElhinney DB, Tworetzky W, Lock JE. Current status of fetal cardiac intervention: circulation. *Am Heart Assoc.* 2010;121(10):1256–63.

34. van den Bosch AE, Roos-Hesselink JW, van Domburg R, et al. Long-term outcome and quality of life in adult patients after the Fontan operation. *Am J Cardiol.* 2004;93(9):1141–5. Available at: http://proxy.library.upenn.edu:2080/science/article/pii/S0002914904001328.

35. Makikallio K. Fetal aortic valve stenosis and the evolution of hypoplastic left heart syndrome: patient selection for fetal intervention. *Circulation.* 2006;113(11):1401–5.

36. McElhinney DB, Marshall AC, Wilkins-Haug LE, et al. Predictors of technical success and postnatal biventricular outcome after in utero aortic valvuloplasty for aortic stenosis with evolving hypoplastic left heart syndrome. *Circulation.* 2009;120(15):1482–90. Available at: http://circ.ahajournals.org/cgi/doi/10.1161/CIRCULATIONAHA.109.192655.

37. Arzt W, Wertaschnigg D, Veit I, et al. Intrauterine aortic valvuloplasty in fetuses with critical aortic stenosis: experience and results of 24 procedures. *Ultrasound Obstet Gynecol.* 2011;37(6):689–95.

38. Tworetzky W, McElhinney DB, Marx GR, et al. In utero valvuloplasty for pulmonary atresia with hypoplastic right ventricle: techniques and outcomes. *Pediatrics.* 2009;124(3):e510–18.

39. Vlahos AP. Hypoplastic left heart syndrome with intact or highly restrictive atrial septum: outcome after neonatal transcatheter atrial septostomy. *Circulation.* 2004;109(19):2326–30.

40. Marshall AC, Levine J, Morash D, et al. Results of in utero atrial septoplasty in fetuses with hypoplastic left heart syndrome. *Prenat Diagn.* 2008;28(11):1023–8.

41. Hedrick HL. Ex utero intrapartum therapy. *Semin Pediatr Surg.* 2003;12(3):190–5.

42. Laje P, Johnson MP, Howell LJ, et al. Ex utero intrapartum treatment in the management of giant cervical teratomas. *J Pediatr Surg.* 2012;47(6):1208–16.

43. Laje P, Howell LJ, Johnson MP, et al. Perinatal management of congenital oropharyngeal tumors: the ex utero intrapartum treatment (EXIT) approach. *J Pediatr Surg.* 2013;48(10):2005–10.

44. Hedrick MH, Ferro MM, Filly RA, et al. Congenital high airway obstruction syndrome (CHAOS): a potential for perinatal intervention. *J Pediatr Surg.* 1994;29(2):271–4.

45. Roybal JL, Liechty KW, Hedrick HL, et al. Predicting the severity of congenital high airway obstruction syndrome. *J Pediatr Surg.* 2010;45(8):1633–9.

46. Kohl T, Van de Vondel P, Stressig R, et al. Percutaneous fetoscopic laser decompression of congenital high airway obstruction syndrome (CHAOS) from laryngeal atresia via a single trocar: current technical constraints and potential solutions for future interventions. *Fetal Diagn Ther.* 2009;25(1):67–71.

47. Saadai P, Jelin EB, Nijagal A, et al. Long-term outcomes after fetal therapy for congenital high airway obstructive syndrome. *J Pediatr Surg.* 2012;47(6):1095–100.

48. Adzick NS, Thom EA, Spong CY, et al. A randomized trial of prenatal versus postnatal repair of myelomeningocele. *N Engl J Med.* 2011;364(11):993–1004.

49. Adzick NS. Management of fetal lung lesions. *Clin Perinatol.* 2003;30(3):481–92.

50. Peranteau WH, Wilson RD, Liechty KW, et al. Effect of maternal betamethasone administration on prenatal congenital cystic adenomatoid malformation growth and fetal survival. *Fetal Diagn Ther.* 2007;22(5):365–71.

51. Tran KM, Johnson MP, Almeida-Chen GM, Schwartz AJ. The fetus as patient. *Anesthesiology.* 2010;113(2):462.

52. Hedrick HL, Flake AW, Crombleholme TM, et al. The ex utero intrapartum therapy procedure for high-risk fetal lung lesions. *J Pediatr Surg.* 2005;40(6):1038–43.

53. Danzer E, Siegle J, D'Agostino JA, et al. Early neurodevelopmental outcome of infants with high-risk fetal lung lesions. *Fetal Diagn Ther.* 2012;31(4):210–15.

54. Harrison MR, Mychaliska GB, Albanese CT, et al. Correction of congenital diaphragmatic hernia in utero IX: fetuses with poor prognosis (liver herniation and low lung-to-head ratio) can be saved by fetoscopic temporary tracheal occlusion. *J Pediatr Surg.* 1998;33(7):1017–22.

55. Harrison MR, Keller RL, Hawgood SB, et al. A randomized trial of fetal endoscopic tracheal occlusion for severe fetal congenital diaphragmatic hernia. *N Engl J Med.* 2003;349(20):1916–24.

56. Deprest J, Jani J, Gratacos E, et al. Fetal intervention for congenital diaphragmatic hernia: the European experience. *Semin Perinatol.* 2005;29(2):94–103.

57. Doné E, Gratacos E, Nicolaides KH, et al. Predictors of neonatal morbidity in fetuses with severe isolated congenital diaphragmatic hernia undergoing fetoscopic tracheal occlusion. *Ultrasound Obstet Gynecol.* 2013;42(1):77–83.

58. Flake AW. Fetal sacrococcygeal teratoma. *Semin Pediatr Surg.* 1993;2(2):113–20.

59. Hedrick HL, Flake AW, Crombleholme TM, et al. Sacrococcygeal teratoma: prenatal assessment, fetal intervention, and outcome. *J Pediatr Surg.* 2004;39(3):430–8.

60. Mieghem TV, Al-Ibrahim A, Deprest J, et al. Minimally invasive therapy for fetal sacrococcygeal teratomas: case series and systematic review of the literature. *Ultrasound Obstet Gynecol.* 2014;43(6):611–19.

61. Roybal JL, Moldenhauer JS, Khalek N, et al. Early delivery as an alternative management strategy for selected high-risk fetal sacrococcygeal teratomas. *J Pediatr Surg.* 2011;46(7):1325–32.

62. Tran KM, Flake AW, Kalawadia NV, Maxwell LG, Rehman MA. Emergent excision of a prenatally diagnosed sacrococcygeal teratoma. *Paediatr Anaesth.* 2008;18(5):431–4.

63. Lewi L, Van Schoubroeck D, Gratacós E, et al. Monochorionic diamniotic twins: complications and management options. *Curr Opin Obstet Gynecol.* 2003;15(2):177–94.

64. Roberts D, Neilson JP, Kilby MD, Gates S. Interventions for the treatment of twin-twin transfusion syndrome. *Cochrane Database Syst Rev.* 2014;1(1):1–35.

65. Moise KJ Jr., Dorman K, Lamvu G, et al. A randomized trial of amnioreduction versus septostomy in the treatment of twin–twin transfusion syndrome. *Am J Obstet Gynecol.* 2005;193(3):701–7.

66. Crombleholme TM, Shera D, Lee H, et al. A prospective, randomized, multicenter trial of amnioreduction vs selective fetoscopic laser photocoagulation for the treatment of severe twin–twin transfusion syndrome. *Am J Obstet Gynecol.* 2007;197(4):396.e1–9.

67. Senat M-V, Deprest J, Boulvain M, et al. Endoscopic laser surgery versus serial amnioreduction for severe twin-to-twin transfusion syndrome. *N Engl J Med.* 2004;351(2):136–44.

68. Slaghekke F, Lopriore E, Lewi L, et al. Fetoscopic laser coagulation of the vascular equator versus selective coagulation for twin-to-twin transfusion syndrome: an open-label randomised controlled trial. *The Lancet.* 2014;383(9935):2144–51.

69. Mizrahi-Arnaud A, Tworetzky W, Bulich LA, et al. Pathophysiology, management, and outcomes of fetal hemodynamic instability during prenatal cardiac intervention. *Pediatr Res.* 2007;62(3):325–30.

70. Brusseau R, Mizrahi-Arnaud A. Fetal anesthesia and pain management for intrauterine therapy. *Clin Perinatol.* 2013;40(3):429–42.

71. Lin EE, Tran KM. Anesthesia for fetal surgery. *Semin Pediatr Surg*. 2013;22(1):50–5.

72. Rychik J. Acute cardiovascular effects of fetal surgery in the human. *Circulation*. 2004;110(12):1549–56.

73. Boat A, Mahmoud M, Michelfelder EC, et al. Supplementing desflurane with intravenous anesthesia reduces fetal cardiac dysfunction during open fetal surgery. *Pediatr Anesth*. 2010;20(8):748–56.

74. Ngamprasertwong P, Michelfelder EC, Arbabi S, et al. Anesthetic techniques for fetal surgery: effects of maternal anesthesia on intraoperative fetal outcomes in a sheep model. *Anesthesiology*. 2013;118(4):796–808.

75. Klaritsch P, Albert K, Van Mieghem T, et al. Instrumental requirements for minimal invasive fetal surgery. *BJOG*. 2008;116(2):188–97.

# Pain Management in Neonates and Infants

Christine Greco and Charles Berde

## Introduction

The treatment of pain is a fundamental aspect in caring for neonates. Optimal pain management should be individualized and requires an understanding of the neurobiology of pain, developmental analgesic pharmacology, pain assessment, and techniques for providing pain relief.

## Developmental Neurophysiology of Pain

There is substantial maturation of peripheral, spinal, and supraspinal neurologic pathways necessary for nociception by late in the second trimester of human gestation [1]. Cutaneous sensory terminals are present in the perioral region at 7 weeks' gestation and spread to all body areas by 20 weeks' gestation. Peripheral nociceptive fibers extend into the dorsal spinal cord at 8–10 weeks' gestation [2]. At birth, A- and C-fiber territories are overlapping in the substantia gelatinosa while cortical descending inhibitory pathways such as the dorsolateral funiculus develops postnatally [3–5]. Neurobiological studies in infant rats and humans show hyper-responsiveness to noxious stimulation compared to older infants [6]. Migration of cortical neurons and establishment of cortico-thalamic connections progresses from 20 weeks' gestation to term. Myelination extends to the spinal cord and brain stem by 22–30 weeks' gestation and extends up to the cortex by 37 weeks or term. Research using near-infrared spectroscopy (NIRS) shows activation of the contralateral somatosensory cortex after noxious stimulation in premature infants as young as 25–28 weeks post-menstrual age (PMA) [6,7], though in the youngest of preterm infants the patterns of activation differ little between noxious and non-noxious stimulation. Studies have suggested that infants have the ability to form memory of pain and that there are potentially short- and long-term consequences of untreated pain.

Neonatal males circumcised without analgesia had an enhanced pain response to immunizations at two, four, and six months [8]. Infants undergoing major surgery who received deeper anesthetic techniques had improved suppression of stress response compared to infants who received lighter anesthesia [9]. Conversely, in a prospective randomized trial, the routine administration of morphine infusions to critically ill infants receiving mechanical ventilation had no clear benefits compared to intermittent morphine boluses for painful procedures [10,11]. Infant rats exposed to repeated noxious stimuli showed increased responses to painful stimuli and had loss of nociceptive primary afferents compared to control infant and adult rats [12]. Studies of pain-conditioned behaviors in adult rats who had persistent noxious stimuli as neonates showed a decrease in pain threshold and re-organization in the dorsal horn structure [13]. A study of extremely low birth-weight-infants who experienced painful stimuli in the neonatal intensive care unit (NICU) had increased somatic complaints as toddlers compared to a control group of children who had been full-term healthy neonates [14]. In general, patterns of opioid dosing for neonates undergoing intensive care have changed considerably over the past 20 years, and it remains difficult to recommend a particular dosing regimen as better than others, both for the immediate aim of reducing pain and distress and the longer term aim of minimizing adverse effects on neurodevelopment.

## Pain Assessment in Neonates

Pain assessment in neonates and other vulnerable populations is particularly challenging. Infants show predictable response pain patterns to pain with respect to stress hormone levels, behavior patterns and changes in physiologic parameters. Nevertheless, physiologic and behavioral parameters can be nonspecific indicators and may not necessarily reflect measures of pain. Studies using NIRS have attempted to evaluate whether pain assessment tools reflect cortical pain responses. A study by Slater et al. showed an overall fair correlation between the Premature Infant Pain Profile (PIPP) and cortical activity for infants undergoing heel lances; however, cortical pain responses were recorded in some infants who did not display facial expression of pain, concluding that infants with low pain scores may not necessarily be pain-free [15]. Physiologic measures of pain can be confounded by autonomic activation unrelated to pain, particularly in infants who are critically ill and receiving vasopressors. Behavioral responses are unavailable as measures during neuromuscular blockade. There are several pain assessment tools that have been studied in neonates [16–19]. Most tools are easily used at the bedside and combine behavioral parameters such as crying, facial expression, and posture with physiologic parameters such as blood pressure and heart rate. Pain assessment tools most commonly used for neonates include the PIPP [16], the Neonatal Infant Pain Scale (NIPS) [17] and Neonatal Pain Agitation and Sedation Scale (N-PASS) [18], and the CRIES scale (**C**rying, **R**equires oxygen, **I**ncreased vital signs, **E**xpression, and **S**leeplessness) [19] (see Tables 35.1–35.4). Currently used neonatal pain assessment tools may not be reliable for neonates experiencing persistent, untreated pain since neonates will often have an attenuation of their hemodynamic response and behavior in response to persistent pain [20,21].

# Principles of Developmental Analgesic and Local Anesthetic Pharmacology

There are several pharmacokinetic and pharmacodynamic factors that produce age-related differences in responses to analgesics [22]. Neonates and young infants have immature hepatic enzyme systems involved in conjugation, glucuronidation, and sulfation of opioids and amide local anesthetics, which results in prolongation of elimination half-life and increased risk of drug toxicity. Most neonates and young infants will have maturation of hepatic enzyme systems involved in biotransformation and conjugation by the age of six months; however, enzyme maturation rates can vary. Pharmacogenomic differences can further introduce variability in hepatic metabolism of opioids. This effect is especially prominent for codeine, which acts as a pro-drug and provides analgesia only with conversion to morphine [23].

Glomerular filtration and renal tubular secretion are reduced in the first several weeks of life, resulting in slower elimination of many renally eliminated drugs and active metabolites of drugs that have undergone hepatic metabolism. Delayed elimination of glucuronides of morphine and hydromorphone can lead to sedation, analgesia, and respiratory depression. Delayed renal clearance of MEGX, a primary metabolite of lidocaine, can have neuro-excitatory effects. Neonates and young infants have decreased levels of $\alpha_1$-acid glycoprotein and albumin, which results in decreased plasma protein binding for many drugs including amide local anesthetics and opioids. Reduced plasma protein binding can result in increased concentrations of pharmacologically active, unbound drug, and increased risk of drug toxicity. Infants have immature ventilatory reflexes in response to hypoxia [24,25] and hypercarbia [26], increasing the risk of apnea associated with opioids. Abnormal ventilatory reflexes may persist through the first year of life in some infants with chronic lung disease and in some with abnormal brainstem development, including some infants with myelomeningocele and Arnold–Chiari malformation [27].

# Management of Pain

## Nonpharmacologic Approaches

Infants experience a number of routine and often daily painful procedures such as endotracheal suctioning and heel lances. In general, attempts should be made to reduce the number of painful events, but in many cases painful interventions such as endotracheal suctioning are necessary for optimal care [28]. Several studies have shown benefit of nonpharmacologic therapies such as sucrose, facilitated tucking and kangaroo care with respect to reduction of pain scores during mildly painful routine procedures in neonates [29–31]. Current American Academy of Pediatrics (AAP) guidelines recommend the use of nonpharmacologic methods to reduce pain from minor routine procedures in neonates [28]. A study of facilitated tucking during endotracheal tube (ETT) suctioning showed that the facilitated tucking group had significantly lower PIPP scores compared to a control group [32]. There is some controversy over whether sucrose's action should be regarded as a "calming" action or an analgesic action *per se* [33]. A randomized controlled trial showed that sucrose, especially when combined

**Table 35.1** Neonatal Pain Agitation And Sedation Scale

| Assessment Criteria | Sedation | | Normal | Pain/agitation | |
|---|---|---|---|---|---|
| | **−2** | **−1** | **0** | **1** | **2** |
| Crying/irritability | No cry with painful stimuli | Moans or cries minimally with painful stimuli | Appropriate crying<br>Not irritable | Irritable or crying at intervals<br>Consolable | High-pitched or silent-continuous cry<br>Inconsolable |
| Behavior state | No arousal to any stimuli<br>No spontaneous movement | Arouses minimally to stimuli<br>Little spontaneous movement | Appropriate for gestational age | Restless, squirming<br>Awakens frequently | Arching, kicking<br>Constantly awake OR<br>Arouses minimally/no movement (not sedated) |
| Facial expression | Mouth is lax<br>No expression | Minimal expression with stimuli | Relaxed<br>Appropriate | Any pain expression is intermittent | Any pain expression is continual |
| Extremities tone | No grasp reflex<br>Flaccid tone | Weak grasp reflex<br>Reduced muscle tone | Relaxed hands and feet<br>Normal tone | Intermittent clenched toes, fists or finger splay<br>Body is not tense | Continual clenched toes, fists or finger splay<br>Body is tense |
| Vital sign: HR < RR, BP, $SaO_2$ | No variability with stimuli<br>Hypoventilation or apnea | <10 percent variability from baseline with stimuli | With baseline or normal for gestational age | Increased 10–20 percent from baseline<br>$SaO_2$ increases quickly with stimulation | Increased >20 percent from baseline<br>$SaO_2$ < 75 percent and increases slowly with stimulation<br>Out of sync with ventilation |

Adjustment:
- +3 if less than 28 weeks' gestational age
- +2 if 28–31 weeks' gestational age
- +1 if 32–35 weeks' gestation age

with non-nutritive sucking, was effective in providing analgesia for heel-sticks in newborns [34]. However, a controlled trial using electroencephalography in neonates to measure pain-specific brain activity evoked by a heel lance showed that sucrose did not significantly affect activity in the neonatal brain, concluding that reductions in observational pain scores with sucrose should not necessarily be interpreted as pain relief [33]. In addition, there is controversy about the long-term effect of frequent dosing of oral sucrose in preterm infants and the developing brain [35,36].

## Pharmacologic Approaches

### Acetaminophen

Acetaminophen is one of the most widely used analgesics, although its actual mechanism of analgesic and antipyretic action remains uncertain. Putative targets of acetaminophen have included a range of peripheral, spinal, and supraspinal sites, including cox-isoenzymes, TRPV1, and TRPA1 receptors and cannabinoid receptors. Acetaminophen exerts little anti-inflammatory effect and is associated with significantly less gastropathy, platelet dysfunction, and renal dysfunction than NSAIDs. The majority of acetaminophen undergoes sulfation and glucuronidation to renally eliminated water-soluble products. There are limited data on hepatic enzyme profiles of acetaminophen in neonates, but preliminary studies show good hepatic tolerance [37]. A small portion of acetaminophen is metabolized by the CYP450 system to a toxic metabolite that binds to glutathione to form a nontoxic conjugate. Inadvertent overdosing errors have led to fulminant hepatic necrosis. Some initial analgesic trials with either oral or rectal acetaminophen in newborns were negative. More recently, a randomized

**Table 35.2** Premature Infant Pain Profile

| Indicators | Score | | | |
|---|---|---|---|---|
| | **0** | **1** | **2** | **3** |
| Gestational age | 36 weeks or more | 32–35weeks + 6 days | 28–31 weeks + 6 days | Less than 28 weeks |
| Behavioral state | Active, awake, eyes open, facial movements | Quiet, awake, eyes open, no facial movements | Active, awake, eyes closed, facial movements | Quiet, asleep, eyes closed, no facial movements |
| Heart rate maximum | 0 bpm increase | 5–15 bpm increase | 15–24 bpm increase | 24 bpm increase |
| $O_2$ sats | 92–100 percent | 89–91 percent | 85–88 percent | 84 percent or less |
| Brow bulge | None | Minimum | Moderate | Maximum |
| Eye squeeze | None | Minimum | Moderate | Maximum |
| Naso-labial furrow | None | Minimum | Moderate | Maximum |

**Table 35.3** Neonatal Infant Pain Scale

| Indicator | Score | | |
|---|---|---|---|
| | **0** | **1** | **2** |
| Facial expression | Relaxed – restful face, neutral expression | Grimace – tight facial muscles, furrowed brow, chin, jaw | – |
| Cry (if infant is intubated, score silent cry based on facial movement) | No cry | Whimper – mild moaning, intermittent | Vigorous crying – loud screaming, shrill, continuous |
| Breathing pattern | Relaxed – usual pattern for this infant | Change in breathing – irregular, faster than usual, gagging, breath holding | – |
| Arms | Relaxed – no muscular rigidity, occasional random movements | Flexed/extended – tense, straight arms, rigid and/or rapid extension, flexion | – |
| Legs | Relaxed – no muscular rigidity, occasional random movements | Flexed/extended – tense, straight arms, rigid and/or rapid extension, flexion | – |
| State of arousal | Quiet, peaceful sleeping or awake, alert and settled | Fussy – alert, restless, and thrashing | – |

**Table 35.4** CRIES scale

| Indicator | Score | | |
|---|---|---|---|
| | **0** | **1** | **2** |
| Crying | No | High pitched | Inconsolable |
| Requires oxygen | No | <30 percent | >30 percent |
| Increased vital signs | Heart rate and blood pressure less than or equal to baseline | Heart rate and blood pressure increase of less than 20 percent from baseline | Heart rate and blood pressure increase more than 20 percent from baseline |
| Expression | None | Grimace | Grimace/grunt |
| Sleeplessness | No | Wakes at frequent intervals | Constantly awake |

controlled trial by Ceelie et al., showed that postoperative use of intermittent IV acetaminophen resulted in lower cumulative morphine dose in the first 48 hours in neonates and infants undergoing thoracic and abdominal surgery with no difference in pain scores or adverse effects between groups [38]. Conversely, a recent systematic review of the use of acetaminophen for the treatment of pain in neonates concluded there was lack of data for efficacy and that additional trials are needed to determine efficacy [39]. Despite the negative conclusion of this Cochrane review, we continue to prescribe acetaminophen for neonates undergoing major surgery. In our view several factors may have contributed to false-negative conclusions in some of the trials pooled in the Ohlsson systematic review: (1) overly generous rescue opioid dosing washing out between-group differences; (2) slow and inefficient absorption following rectal dosing; and (3) insensitivity of measures and the heterogeneity of behavioral and physiologic pain ratings in studies of postoperative neonates where some are receiving mechanical ventilation and others are not. There remains a possibility the target(s) of acetaminophen are not yet developed or connected in neonates, analogous to the studies by Ririe et al. [40] for NSAIDs described in the next section. Nevertheless, we believe that acetaminophen has a favorable safety profile in comparison to several other analgesics in neonates, and this factor supports its use for post-surgical pain.

Pharmacokinetic studies of intravenous acetaminophen show reduced clearance with younger gestational age infants, with clearance at 27 weeks' PMA

less than half that of a full-term newborn [41,42]. Recommended doses are found in Table 35.5. There is inadequate pharmacokinetic data for infants younger than 28 weeks' PMA to allow for safe dosage recommendations.

## Nonsteroidal Anti-Inflammatory Agents

Nonsteroidal anti-inflammatory agents reversibly inhibit the actions of COX enzymes, which are responsible for the conversion of arachidonic acid to prostaglandins that have diverse roles contributing to pain, inflammation, gastric mucosal integrity, vasodilation, and hypersensitivity. There are very few safety or efficacy data on the use of NSAIDs in newborns and premature infants. A clinical trial of 70 preterm infants less than 37 weeks received either high- or low-dose ibuprofen for patent ductus arteriosus (PDA) closure; there were no gastrointestinal, hematologic, or renal adverse effects reported [43]. A recent systematic review concluded that compared to indomethacin, ibuprofen was associated with reduced risk of necrotizing enterocolitis and transient renal insufficiency [44]. There are animal data showing that intraspinal and systemic administration of a COX-1 inhibitor in infant rats produced no reduction in response to incisional pain; infant rats, unlike more mature rats, had no increase in COX-1 protein in the spinal cord [40]. This raises the question of whether COX-inhibitors are effective in infants due to developmental differences in COX-enzyme expression in the spinal cord microglia [40].

**Table 35.5** Acetaminophen dosing

| | |
|---|---|
| Intravenous dosing | |
| PMA 28–32 weeks | 10 mg kg$^{-1}$ dose$^{-1}$ every 12 hours (max. 22.5 mg kg$^{-1}$ day$^{-1}$) |
| PMA 33–36 weeks | 10 mg kg$^{-1}$ dose$^{-1}$ every 8 hours (max. 40 mg kg$^{-1}$ day$^{-1}$) |
| PMA ≥ 37 weeks | 10 mg kg$^{-1}$ dose$^{-1}$ every 6 hours (max. 40 mg kg$^{-1}$ day$^{-1}$) |
| Oral dosing | |
| PMA 28–32 weeks | 10–12 mg kg$^{-1}$ dose$^{-1}$ every 6–8 hours; max. daily dose: 40 mg kg$^{-1}$ day$^{-1}$ |
| PMA 32–37 weeks and term neonates <10 days | 10–15 mg kg$^{-1}$ dose$^{-1}$ every 6 hours; max. daily dose: 60 mg kg$^{-1}$ day$^{-1}$ |
| Term neonates ≥10 days | 10–15 mg kg$^{-1}$ dose$^{-1}$ every 4–6 hours; max. daily dose: 75 mg kg$^{-1}$ day$^{-1}$ |
| Rectal dosing | |
| PMA 28–32 weeks | 20 mg kg$^{-1}$ dose$^{-1}$ every 12 hours; max. daily dose: 40 mg kg$^{-1}$ day$^{-1}$ |
| PMA 32–37 weeks and term neonates <10 days | Loading dose: 30 mg kg$^{-1}$; then 15 mg kg$^{-1}$ dose$^{-1}$ every 8 hours; max. daily dose: 60 mg kg$^{-1}$ day$^{-1}$ |
| Term neonates ≥10 days | Loading dose: 30 mg kg$^{-1}$; then 20 mg kg$^{-1}$ dose$^{-1}$ every 6–8 hours; max. daily dose: 75 mg kg$^{-1}$ day$^{-1}$ |

**Table 35.6** Doses of non-steroidal anti-inflammatory drugs

| | Dose |
|---|---|
| Ibuprofen | 5–10 mg kg$^{-1}$ dose$^{-1}$ every 6–8 hours; maximum dose 40 mg kg$^{-1}$ day$^{-1}$ |
| Ketorolac | 0.5 mg kg$^{-1}$ dose$^{-1}$ every 6 hours for a maximum of 12 doses |

Dosing guidelines refer to infants under six months of age. Ibuprofen and ketorolac at Q8–12 hour dosing intervals have been used in neonates and young infants but there are limited safety and efficacy data in infants under six months.

Ketorolac is a commonly prescribed parenteral NSAID often used for postoperative pain in older infants and children. There are minimal efficacy data, pharmacokinetic data, and conflicting safety data on the use of ketorolac in neonates and preterm infants. In a randomized controlled trial of infants and children undergoing cardiac surgery, ketorolac did not increase the risk of surgical bleeding or gastrointestinal bleeding [45]. However, other studies have found increased risk for bleeding events in infants younger than 21 days and less than 37 weeks' PMA who received ketorolac after surgery [46]. Small case series have not reported harm with use after surgeries in neonates and young infants [47,48], though larger prospective studies and pharmacokinetic studies are needed to better define the risks of NSAIDs in neonates and premature infants. Recommended doses are found in Table 35.6.

## Opioid Therapy

### Morphine

Opioids such as morphine are commonly used in the treatment of pain in neonates. Opioid receptors are widely distributed in the forebrain, brainstem, and spinal cord by mid-gestation; functional maturation of opioid receptors occurs prenatally and continues postnatally. Several studies have shown beneficial as well as adverse short-term effects with morphine. Long-term outcome studies among former preterm neonates have also shown mixed results [49,50]. Results from the Neurologic Outcomes and Pre-emptive Analgesia in Neonates (NEOPAIN) trial showed no differences in mortality, intraventricular hemorrhage (IVH), or periventricular leukomalacia in ventilated preterm neonates randomly assigned to receive either morphine infusions or placebo, and there was no evidence of benefit on distress measures [51]. A randomized trial by Simons et al. showed

no differences in analgesia between ventilated preterm infants receiving morphine infusion vs. placebo; although the morphine group had a decreased incidence of IVH, there were no differences in poor neurologic outcomes, leading to the conclusion that routine morphine infusions are not warranted in ventilated preterm neonates [52]. Morphine appears to be effective for acute postoperative pain in preterm neonates, but there is evidence suggesting it does not provide adequate analgesia for procedural pain such as endotracheal tube suctioning or heel lances [53,54]. There is evidence that morphine may improve respiratory synchrony in ventilated neonates; however, a randomized trial showed that morphine infusions in preterm infants with respiratory distress syndrome did not improve short-term pulmonary outcomes among ventilated preterms [10,55].

In a long-term follow-up study of former ventilated preterm infants aged 5–7, those who received preemptive morphine had smaller head circumference, more social problems, and performed more poorly in memory tasks than those who had received placebo; however, there were no differences in overall IQ or academic performance [56]. A study by Valkenburg et al. found continuous morphine infusions in former preterm neonates at ages 8 or 9 years had no long-term adverse effects on quantitative sensory testing, the development of chronic pain, or overall neurologic functioning [57].

Morphine metabolism occurs in the liver through glucuronidation to morphine-3-glucuronide, which has excitatory action, and morphine-6-glucuronide, which has analgesics, sedative, and respiratory depressant actions. Both are renally eliminated and can accumulate in renal insufficiency. A randomized trial of 68 neonates receiving either intermittent doses or continuous infusions of morphine showed that younger neonates had significantly reduced postoperative morphine requirements and seemed to preferentially metabolize morphine to morphine-3-glucuronide [58]. The clearance of morphine is reduced in preterm neonates compared to term neonates [54], and is less than half that measured in adults. Dosing should be adjusted based on age, weight, and side-effects since there is considerable individual variation in pharmacokinetics. For nonventilated neonates, doses should be titrated with careful monitoring of respiratory status since neonates can develop apnea in response to hypoxia and hypercarbia. Typical starting doses for intermittent morphine bolus dosing is 0.02 mg kg$^{-1}$

**Table 35.7** Typical opioid starting doses

|  | Typical starting opioid intravenous bolus doses and intervals | Typical starting opioid intravenous infusion doses | Typical starting opioid oral doses and intervals |
|---|---|---|---|
| Morphine | 0.025–0.1 mg kg$^{-1}$ every 2–4 h | 0.01–0.03 mg kg$^{-1}$ h$^{-1}$ | 0.15–0.3 mg kg$^{-1}$ every 3–4 h |
| Hydromorphone | 0.005–0.02 mg kg$^{-1}$ every 2–4 h | 0.002–0.006 mg kg$^{-1}$ h$^{-1}$ | 0.02–0.04 mg kg$^{-1}$ every 3–4 h |
| Fentanyl | 0.25–1.0 µg kg$^{-1}$ every 1–2 h | 0.5–2.0 µg kg$^{-1}$ h$^{-1}$ | N/A |

Effective starting doses vary considerably.
All doses are approximate and should be adjusted according to clinical circumstances with careful titration and close monitoring for side effects.
Dose reductions are recommended for premature infants and non-ventilated infants.

and 0.015 mg kg$^{-1}$ h$^{-1}$ for continuous infusions (see Table 35.7).

### Fentanyl

Fentanyl undergoes metabolism in the liver primarily by CYP3A4 to inactive metabolites, and can be useful for patients with renal failure. The effect of a single dose of fentanyl is terminated by redistribution rather than metabolism, whereas the effect of continuous infusion is terminated more by metabolism and can have a prolonged duration of action. The context-sensitive half-life of fentanyl in neonates is particularly prolonged [59]. Fentanyl can induce glottic and chest wall rigidity, particularly in neonates; treatment can consist of neuromuscular blockade and controlled ventilation; naloxone is variably effective. A randomized controlled trial showed that ventilated newborns who received fentanyl infusions had lower pain scores but longer controlled ventilation time compared to a placebo group who received intermittent fentanyl doses [60]. Other opioids such as remifentanil are sometimes used for brief painful procedures, but there are few data on efficacy or safety [61].

### Hydromorphone

Hydromorphone has a similar duration of action to morphine and can be used in nurse-controlled analgesia and epidural analgesia. Because of its greater potency compared to morphine, dose titration of hydromorphone is more difficult in young infants and smaller weight patients. Hydromorphone is frequently used in patients with renal insufficiency; however, there is little supportive evidence and active metabolites for both morphine and hydromorphone can be

associated with neurotoxic effects. Because hydromorphone is more hydrophilic than fentanyl, we generally avoid using hydromorphone-based epidural solutions in young infants due to the risk of respiratory depression. See Table 35.7 for typical opioid starting doses.

## Tolerance and Withdrawal

A consequence of prolonged opioid therapy in critically ill infants is the development of opioid tolerance and subsequent risk of withdrawal as opioids are withdrawn. Primary factors that affect the development of opioid tolerance include age and duration of opioid therapy. The function of opioid and NMDA receptors, regulation of G-protein signaling and other components of opioid signaling systems undergo age-related changes [62]. Evidence suggests that infants are more vulnerable to developing opioid tolerance than children and adults [63]. Evidence from a recent multicenter trial evaluating the efficacy of protocolized sedation for critically ill infants and children showed that adherence to a goal-directed comfort algorithm resulted in fewer days of opioid administration and exposure to fewer drug classes, and may help in preventing tolerance by allowing for proactive weaning of opioids when clinical condition permits [64]. Elements of the sedation protocol included daily team discussion of the patient's illness trajectory and adjustment of pain and sedation medications at least every eight hours. Patients who received opioids for less than five days were able to have their opioids discontinued without weaning or signs of withdrawal. Every eight hours adjustments in pain and sedation medications were well tolerated and there were no differences in occurrence of iatrogenic withdrawal between the protocolized group and the group who received usual ICU care. Clonidine is an alpha-2-agonist that attenuates the noradrenergic effects of withdrawal, and can be useful in preventing withdrawal symptoms as opioids are weaned. A controlled trial of clonidine in ventilated newborns showed that clonidine reduced fentanyl requirements with no difference in frequency of side-effects [65].

## Methods of Opioid Administration

Intermittent parenteral dosing of opioids can be useful for episodic pain or as a loading dose to achieve a rapid rise in plasma opioid concentration. However, intermittent dosing results in wide variations in plasma opioid concentrations and subsequent pain intensity and side effects. Continuous infusions are often used in neonates and infants who are mechanically ventilated with additional boluses of opioids given for endotracheal tube suctioning and painful procedures. A continuous infusion provides a steady plasma opioid concentration with near-constant level of analgesia; however, this does not take into account fluctuations in pain intensity as with chest physiotherapy or coughing. Patient-controlled and nurse-controlled analgesia takes into account both individual variations in opioid pharmacokinetics and pain intensity as well as provides ease of opioid administration. Morphine is more commonly used in NCA in young infants. Cardiorespiratory monitoring should be used for all patients receiving continuous infusions and for patients at risk for opioid-induced respiratory depression. See Table 35.8 for typical NCA starting doses.

**Table 35.8** Typical starting doses for nurse-controlled analgesia

| | Bolus dose | Continuous rate | 1-hour limit |
|---|---|---|---|
| Morphine | 0.02 mg kg$^{-1}$ | 0.005–0.015 mg kg$^{-1}$ h$^{-1}$ | 0.1 mg kg$^{-1}$ |
| Hydromorphone | 0.005 mg kg$^{-1}$ | 0.001–0.003 mg kg$^{-1}$ h$^{-1}$ | 0.02 mg kg$^{-1}$ |
| Fentanyl | 0.25 µg kg$^{-1}$ | 0.15 µg kg$^{-1}$ h$^{-1}$ | 1 µg kg$^{-1}$ |

Effective starting doses vary considerably.
All doses are approximate and should be adjusted according to clinical circumstances with careful titration and close monitoring for side effects.
Dose reductions are recommended for premature infants and non-ventilated infants.

## Regional Analgesia

Epidural analgesia and continuous peripheral nerve blockade can provide excellent postoperative analgesia for infants undergoing a variety of surgical procedures, including thoracic, lower extremity, and abdominal procedures. Regional analgesia can reduce overall opioid use, thereby reducing opioid side-effects and the development of tolerance. A detailed discussion of regional blocks can be found in Chapter 36. To avoid direct needle placement in the thoracic region and associated risk of neurologic complications, an alternative method of epidural catheter placement is to advance catheters from the caudal and lumbar regions cephalad to thoracic dermatomes. This may be performed blindly, with guidance by fluoroscopy, ultrasound [66], and nerve stimulation [67]. Blind placement without confirmation is generally not recommended when advancing catheters cephalad since there is a 30 percent failure associated with blind placement. The clearance of amide local anesthetics is much slower in infants and lower local anesthetic infusion rates are necessary to avoid systemic toxicity. Because of the limitations of using safe local anesthetic infusion rates, it is crucial in infants to place epidural catheter tips in the correct surgical dermatome. A radio-opaque catheter can be used and visualized while advancing cephalad using fluoroscopy. Another method of radiographic confirmation is to inject a small volume of radiocontrast dye (0.5–1 ml) through the epidural catheter and observe proper tip location on a plain radiograph (epidurogram).

It is sometimes necessary to confirm proper position of an epidural catheter postoperatively for patients who have pain despite adequate dosing of epidural infusions. Due to concerns of toxicity with amide local anesthetics, one method is to confirm epidural position by administering a test dose of 2 percent chloroprocaine in incremental doses and observing for behavioral signs of pain relief such as relaxed posture and ceasing of crying as well as more objective signs such as return of blood pressure and heart rate to baseline. Alternatively, an epidurogram using radiocontrast dye can also be used to confirm epidural catheter position postoperatively.

Epidural drug selection should be individualized and varies with surgical and patient-specific factors. In most cases, we recommend infusions of local anesthetics in combination with opioids and/or clonidine due to the synergistic effect of combining local anesthetics with adjuvants. Pharmacokinetic studies measuring unbound, pharmacologically active bupivacaine in infants receiving continuous epidural bupivacaine infusions showed plasma bupivacaine levels rise and can accumulate to reach toxic levels after the first 48 hours, despite increases in serum α-1-acid glycoprotein levels [68,69]. Based on these pharmacokinetic studies, epidural bupivacaine infusion rates in neonates and infants younger than four months should be limited to 0.2 mg kg$^{-1}$ h$^{-1}$. In a study by Olsson, however, a substantial number of neonates had a continued rise in serum bupivacaine levels at 48 hours even with limiting the dose to 0.2 mg kg$^{-1}$ h$^{-1}$ [70]. Epidural bupivacaine infusion rates of 0.4 mg kg$^{-1}$ h$^{-1}$ appear to be safe for children over the age of six months. Pharmacokinetic data of ropivacaine in infants show that clearance is reduced in neonates and young infants compared to older children [71–73]. Ropivacaine infusion rates up to 0.2 mg kg$^{-1}$ h$^{-1}$ appear to be safe in neonates, although pharmacokinetic data are limited [74].

Because of the risks and limitations in dosing of amide local anesthetics in neonates and young infants, the amino ester local anesthetic chloroprocaine can be used as an alternative local anesthetic for epidural and peripheral nerve catheter infusions. Studies of continuous epidural infusions of chloroprocaine showed good surgical anesthesia [74–76].

The addition of opioids to epidural solutions can potentiate analgesia but may increase the likelihood of respiratory depression. Because of the increased risk of cephalad spread and potential for respiratory depressant effects, we rarely use hydromorphone neuraxially in nonventilated infants less than four months of age. Fentanyl is used selectively in epidural infusions in infants less than four months of age, although there remains some risk of respiratory depression. Clonidine can prolong and enhance the analgesic effect of local anesthetics. Although continuous epidural infusions containing dilute solutions of clonidine tend to be well tolerated without respiratory depression or hypotension in neonates, there have been reports of apnea associated with bolus dosing of clonidine in caudal blocks in preterm infants [77]. Due to the increased risk of toxicity in neonates and potential accumulation of amide local anesthetics during continuous infusions, our practice is to use chloroprocaine-based solutions for peripheral nerve catheter and epidural catheter infusions in neonates (see Tables 35.9 and 35.10).

**Table 35.9** Recommended neonatal and infant peripheral nerve catheter infusion rates

| Solution | <2 months | 2–6 months | >6 months |
|---|---|---|---|
| Ropivacaine 0.1% | 0.2 ml kg$^{-1}$ h$^{-1}$ | 0.3 ml kg$^{-1}$ h$^{-1}$ | 0.3–0.4 ml kg$^{-1}$ h$^{-1}$ |
| Chloroprocaine 1.5% | 0.5–0.8 ml kg$^{-1}$ h$^{-1}$ | | |

Consider chloroprocaine-based infusions due to risk of accumulation and toxicity of amide local anesthetics in neonates.
Little information is available on how best to adjust these rates based on degrees of prematurity.
Infusion rates and solutions should be modified according to clinical circumstances.
Monitoring and close observation are recommended.

# References

1. Fitzgerald M, Walker SM. Infant pain management: a developmental neurobiological approach. *Nat Clin Pract Neurol.* 2009;5(1):35–50.

2. Flaris NA, Shindler KS, Kotzbauer PT, et al. Development of the primary afferent projection in human spinal cord. *J Comp Neurol.* 1995;354(1):11–12.

3. Kostovic I. Structural and histochemical reorganization of the human prefrontal cortex during perinatal and postnatal life. *Prog Brain Res.* 1990;85:223–39.

4. Cornelissen L, Fabrizi L, Patten D, et al. Postnatal temporal spatial and modality tuning of nociceptive cutaneous flexion reflexes in human infants. *PLoS One.* 2013;8(10). doi: https://doi.org/10.1371/journal.pone.0076470.

5. Fitzgerald M. Alterations in the ipsi- and contralateral afferent inputs of dorsal horn cells produced by capsaicin treatment of one sciatic nerve in the rat. *Brain Res.* 1982;248(1):97–107.

6. Slater R, Cantarella A, Gallella S, et al. Cortical pain responses in human infants. *J Neurosci.* 2006;26(14):3662–6.

7. Bartocci M, Bergqvist LL, Lagercrantz H, Anand K. Pain activates cortical areas in the preterm newborn brain. *Pain.* 2006;122(1–2):109–17.

8. Taddio A, Katz J, Ilersich AL, Koren G. Effect of neonatal circumcision on pain response during subsequent routine vaccination [comment]. *The Lancet.* 1997;349(9052):599–603.

9. Anand KJS, Hansen DD, Hickey PR. Hormonal-metabolic stress responses in neonates undergoing cardiac surgery. *Anesthesiology.* 1990;73(4):661–70.

10. Bhandari V, Bergqvist L, Kronsberg S, Barton B, Anand K; NEOPAIN Trial Investigators Group.

**Table 35.10** Recommended neonatal and infant epidural infusion rates

| Epidural solution | <2 months | 2–6 months | >6 months |
|---|---|---|---|
| Bupivacaine 0.1%<br>± fentanyl 0.3 µg ml⁻¹<br>± clonidine 0.05 µg ml⁻¹ | 0.2 ml kg⁻¹ h⁻¹ | 0.2 ml kg⁻¹ h⁻¹ | |
| Ropivacaine 0.1%<br>± fentanyl 0.3 µg ml⁻¹<br>± clonidine 0.05 µg ml⁻¹ | 0.2 ml kg⁻¹ h⁻¹ | 0.3 ml kg⁻¹ h⁻¹ | |
| Chloroprocaine 1.5%<br>± fentanyl 0.3 µg ml⁻¹<br>± clonidine 0.05 µg ml⁻¹ | 0.2–0.5 ml kg⁻¹ h⁻¹ thoracic<br>0.5–0.8 ml kg⁻¹ h⁻¹ lumbar | 0.2–0.5 ml kg⁻¹ h⁻¹ thoracic<br>0.5–0.8 ml kg⁻¹ h⁻¹ lumbar | |
| Bupivacaine 0.1%<br>± fentanyl 2 µg ml⁻¹<br>± clonidine 0.4 µg ml⁻¹ | | 0.2 ml kg⁻¹ h⁻¹ | 0.3–0.4 ml kg⁻¹ h⁻¹ |
| Ropivacaine 0.1%<br>± fentanyl 2 µg ml⁻¹<br>± clonidine 0.4 µg ml⁻¹ | | 0.3 ml kg⁻¹ h⁻¹ | 0.3–0.4 ml kg⁻¹ h⁻¹ |
| Ropivacaine 0.1%<br>± hydromorphone 10 µg ml⁻¹<br>± clonidine 0.4 µg ml⁻¹ | | | 0.3–0.4 ml kg⁻¹ h⁻¹ |

Consider chloroprocaine-based infusions due to risk of accumulation and toxicity of amide local anesthetics in neonates; little information is available on how best to adjust these rates based on degrees of prematurity.

Rates shown reflect upper end of usual infusion rates.

Infusion rates and solutions should be modified according to clinical circumstances; solutions containing hydrophilic opioids may increase the risk of respiratory depression.

Cardiorespiratory monitoring and close observation are recommended for all patients receiving epidural infusions.

Morphine admininstration and short-term pulmonary outcomes among ventilated preterm infants. *Pediatrics.* 2005;116(2):352–9.

11. Carbajal R, Lenclen R, Jugie M, et al. Morphine does not provide adequate analagesia for acute procedural pain among preterm neonates. *Pediatrics.* 2005;115(6):1494–500.

12. Knaepen L, Patijn J, van Kleef M, et al. Neonatal repetitive needle pricking: plasticity of the spinal nociceptive circuit and extended postoperative pain in later life. *Dec Neurobiol.* 2013;73(1):85–97.

13. Anand KJ, Coskun V, Thrivikraman KV, Nemeroff CB, Plotsky PM. Long-term behavioral effects of repetitive pain in neonatal rat pups. *Physiol Behav.* 1999;66(4):627–37.

14. Grunau R, Whitfield M, Petrie H. Pain sensitivity and temperament in extremely low-birth-weight premature toddlers and preterm and full-term controls. *Pain* 1994;58:341–6.

15. Slater R, Cantarella A, Franck L, Meek J, Fitzgerald M. How well do clinical pain assessment tools reflect pain in infants? *PLoS Med.* 2008;5(6).

16. Stevens B, Johnston C, Petryshen P, Taddio A. Premature Infant Pain Profile: development and intial validation. *Clin J Pain.* 1996;12(1):13–22.

17. Lawrence J, Alcock D, McGrath P, et al. The development of a tool to assess neonatal pain. *Neonatal Netw.* 1993;12(6):59–66.

18. Hummel P, Puchalski M, Creech S, Weiss M. Clinical reliability and validity of the N-PASS: neonatal pain, agitation and sedation scale with prolonged pain. *J Perinatol.* 2008;28(1):55–60.

19. Krechel S, Bildner J. CRIES: a new neonatal postoperative pain measurement score. Initial testing of validity and reliability. *Paediatr Anaesth.* 1995;5(1):53–61.

20. van Ganzewinkel C, Anand K, Kramer B, Andriessen P. Chronic pain in the newborn: toward a definition. *Clin J Pain.* 2014;30(11):970–7.

21. Pillai Riddell R, Stevens B, McKeever P, et al. Chornic pain in hopsitalized infants: health professionals' perspectives. *J Pain.* 2009;10(12):1217–25.

22. Kearns G, Abdel-Rahman S, Alander S, et al. Developmental pharmacology-drug disposition,

action, and therapy in infants and children. *N Engl J Med.* 2003;349(12):1157–67.

23. Lam J, Woodall K, Solbeck P, et al. Codeine-related deaths: the role of pharmacogenetics and drug interactions. *Forensic Sci Int.* 2014;239:50–6.

24. Cohen G, Malcolm G, Henderson-Smart D. Ventilatory response of the newborn infant to mild hypoxia. *Pediatr Pulmonol.* 1997;24(3):163–72.

25. Bissonnette JM. Mechanisms regulating hypoxic respiratory depression during fetal and postnatal life. *Am J Physiol.* 2000;278(6):R1391–400.

26. Anwar M, Marotta F, Fort MD, et al. The ventilatory response to carbon dioxide in high risk infants. *Early Hum Dev.* 1993;35(3):183–92.

27. Calder N, Williams B, Smyth J, et al. Absence of ventilatory responses to alternating breaths of mild hypoxia and air in infants who have had bronchopulmonary dysplsia: implications for the risk of sudden infant death. *Pediatr Res.* 1994;35(6):677–81.

28. American Academy of Pediatrics Committee on Fetus and Newborn; American Academy of Pediatrics Section on Surgery; Canadian Paediatric Society Fetus and Newborn Committee, et al. Prevention and management of pain in the neonate: an update. *Pediatrics.* 2006;118(5):2231–41.

29. Stevens B, Yamada J, Lee GY, Ohlsson A. Sucrose for analgesia in newborn infants undergoing painful procedures. *Cochrane Database Syst Rev.* 2013;1:CD001069.

30. Johnston C, Campbell-Yeo M, Fernandes A, et al. Skin-to-skin care for procedural pain in neonates. *Cochrane Database Syst Rev.* 2014;1:CD008435.

31. Lopez O, Subramanian P, Rahmat N, et al. The effect of facilitated tucking on procedural pain control among premature babies. *J Clin Nurs.* 2015;24(1–2):183–91.

32. Alinejad-Naeini M, Mohagheghi P, Peyrovi H, Mehran A. The effect of facilitated tucking during endotracheal suctioning on procedural pain in preterm neonates: a randomized controlled crossover study. *Glob J Health Sci.* 2014;6(4):278–84.

33. Slater R, Cornelissen L, Fabrizi L, et al. Oral sucrose as an analgesic drug for procedural pain in newborn infants: a randomized controlled trial. *The Lancet.* 2010;376(9748):1225–32.

34. Thakkar P, Arora K, Goyal K, et al. To evaluate and compare the efficacy of combined sucrose and non-nutritive sucking for analgesia in newborns undergoing minor painful procedure: a randomized controlled trial. *J Perinatol.* 2016;36(1):67–70.

35. Holsti L, Grunau RE. Considerations for using sucrose to reduce procedural pain in preterm infants. *Pediatrics.* 2010;125(5):1042–7.

36. Johnston CC, Filion F, Snider L, et al. Routine sucrose analgesia during the first week of life in neonates younger than 31 weeks' postconceptional age. *Pediatrics.* 2002;110(3):523–8.

37. Allegaert K, Rayyan M, Vanhaesebrouck S, Naulaers G. Developmental pharmacokinetics in neonates. *Expert Rev Clin Pharmacol.* 2008;1(3):415–28.

38. Ceelie I, de Wildt SN, van Dijk M, et al. Effect of intravenous paracetamol on postoperative morphine requirements in neonates and infants undergoing major noncardiac surgery: a randomized controlled trial. *JAMA.* 2013;309(2):149–54.

39. Ohlsson A, Shah PS. Paracetamol (acetaminophen) for prevention or treatment of pain in newborns. *Cochrane Database Syst Rev.* 2015;6:CD011219.

40. Ririe DG, Prout HD, Barclay D, et al. Developmental differences in spinal cyclooxygenase 1 expression after surgical incision. *Anesthesiology.* 2006;104(3):426–31

41. Allegaert K, Anderson BJ, Naulaers G, et al. Intravenous paracetamol (propacetamol) pharmacokinetics in term and preterm neonates. *Eur J Clin Pharmacol.* 2004;60(3):191–7.

42. Allegaert K, Palmer GM, Anderson BJ. The pharmacokinetics of intravenous paracetamol in neonates: size matters most. *Arch Dis Child.* 2011;96:575–80.

43. Dani C, Vangi V, Bertini G, et al. High-dose ibuprofen for patent ductus arteriosus in extremely preterm infants: a randomized controlled study. *Clin Pharmacol Ther.* 2012;91(4):590–6.

44. Ohlsson A, Walia R, Shah SS. Ibuprofen for the treatment of patent ductus arteriosus in preterm or low birth weight (or both) infants. *Cochrane Database Syst Rev.* 2015;2:CD003481.

45. Gupta A, Daggett C, Drant S, Rivero N, Lewis A. Prospective randomized trial of ketorolac after congenital heart surgery. *J Cardiothorac Vasc Anesth.* 2004;18(4):454–7.

46. Aldrink JH, Ma M, Wang W, et al. Safety of ketorolac in surgical neonates and infants 0 to 3 months old. *J Pediatr Surg.* 2011;46(6):1081–5.

47. Burd RS, Tobias JD. Ketorolac for pain management after abdominal surgical procedures in infants. *South Med J.* 2002;95(3):331–3.

48. Moffett BS, Wann TI, Carberry KE, Mott AR. Safety of ketorolac in neonates and infants after cardiac surgery. *Paediatr Anaesth.* 2006;16(4):424–8.

49. de Graaf J, van Lingen RA, Valkenburg AJ, et al. Does neonatal morphine use affect neuropsychological outcomes at 8 to 9 years of age? *Pain*. 2013;154(3):449–58.

50. de Graaf J, van Lingen RA, Simons SH, et al. Long-term effects of routine morphine infusion in mechanically ventilated neonates on children's functioning: five-year follow-up of a randomized controlled trial. *PAIN*. 2011;152:1391–7.

51. Anand KJ, Hall RW, Desai N, et al. Effects of morphine analgesia in ventilated preterm neonates: primary outcomes from the NEOPAIN randomised trial. *The Lancet*. 2004;363(9422):1673–82.

52. Simons SH, van Dijk M, van Lingen RA, et al. Routine morphine infusion in preterm newborns who received ventilatory support: a randomized controlled trial. *JAMA*. 2003;290(18):2419–27.

53. Carbajal R, Lenclen R, Jugie M, et al. Morphine does not provide adequate analgesia for acuteprocedural pain among preterm neonates. *Pediatrics*. 2005;115(6):1494–500.

54. Anand KJ, Anderson BJ, Holford NH, et al. Morphine pharmacokinetics and pharmacodynamics in preterm and term neonates: secondary results from the NEOPAIN trial. *Br J Anaesth*. 2008;101(5):680–9.

55. Boyle EM, Freer Y, Wong CM, McIntosh N, Anand KJ. Assessment of persistent pain or distress and adequacy of analgesia in preterm ventilated infants. *Pain*. 2006;124(1–2):87–91.

56. Ferguson SA, Ward WL, Paule MG, Hall RW, Anand KJ. A pilot study of preemptive morphine analgesia in preterm neonates: effects on head circumference, social behavior, and response latencies in early childhood. *Neurotoxicol Teratol*. 2012;34(1):47–55.

57. Valkenburg AJ, van den Bosch GE, de Graaf J, et al. Long-term effects of neonatal morphine infusion on pain sensitivity: follow-up of a randomized controlled trial. *J Pain*. 2015;16(9):926–33.

58. Bouwmeester NJ, Hop WC, van Dijk M, et al. Postoperative pain in the neonate: age-related differences in morphine requirements and metabolism. *Intensive Care Med*. 2009;29(11):2009–15.

59. Santeiro ML, Christie J, Stromquist C, Torres BA, Markowsky SJ. Pharmacokinetics of continuous infusion fentanyl in newborns. *J Perinatol*. 1997;17(2):135–9.

60. Ancora G, Lago P, Garetti E, et al. Efficacy and safety of continuous infusion of fentanyl for pain control in preterm newborns on mechanical ventilation. *J Pediatr*. 2013;163(3):645–51.

61. Lago P, Tiozzo C, Boccuzzo G, Allegro A, Zacchello F. Remifentanil for percutaneous intravenous central catheter placement in preterm infant: a randomized controlled trial. *Paediatr Anaesth*. 2008;18(8):736–44.

62. Zhao J, Xin X, Xie GX, Palmer PP, Huang YG. Molecular and cellular mechanisms of the age-dependency of opioid analgesia and tolerance. *Mol Pain*. 2012;8:38.

63. Wang Y, Mitchell J, Moriyama K, et al. Age-dependent morphine tolerance development in the rat. *Anesth Analg*. 2005;100(6):1733–9.

64. Curley MA, Wypij D, Watson RS, et al. Protocolized sedation vs usual care in pediatric patients mechanically ventilated for acute respiratory failure: a randomized clinical trial. *JAMA*. 2015;313(4):379–89.

65. Hünseler C, Balling G, Röhlig C, et al. Continuous infusion of clonidine in ventilated newborns and infants: a randomized controlled trial. *Pediatr Crit Care Med*. 2014;15(6):511–12.

66. Willschke H, Bosenberg A, Marhofer P, et al. Epidural catheter placement in neonates: sonoanatomy and feasibility of ultrasonographic guidance in term and preterm neonates. *Reg Anesth Pain Med*. 2007;32(1):34–40.

67. Tsui BC, Wagner A, Cave D, Kearney R. Thoracic and lumbar epidural analgesia via the caudal approach using electrical stimulation guidance in pediatric patients: a review of 289 patients. *Anesthesiology*. 2004;100(3):683–9.

68. Meunier JF, Goujard E, Dubousset AM, Samii K, Mazoit JX. Pharmacokinetics of bupivacaine after continuous epidural infusion in infants with and without biliary atresia. *Anesthesiology*. 2001;95(1):87–95.

69. Mazoit JX, Dalens BJ. Pharmacokinetics of local anaesthetics in infants and children. *Clin Pharmacokinet*. 2004;43(1):17–32.

70. Larsson BA, Lonnqvist PA, Olsson GL. Plasma concentrations of bupivacaine in neonates after continuous epidural infusion. *Anesth Analg*. 1997;84(3):501–5.

71. Rapp HJ, Molnar V, Austin S, et al. Ropivacaine in neonates and infants: a population pharmacokinetic evaluation following single caudal block. *Paediatr Anaesth*. 2004;14(9):724–32.

72. McCann ME, Sethna NF, Mazoit JX, et al. The pharmacokinetics of epidural ropivacaine in infants and young children. *Anesth Analg*. 2001;93(4):893–7.

73. Lonnqvist PA, Westrin P, Larsson BA, et al. Ropivacaine pharmacokinetics after caudal block in 1–8 year old children. *Br J Anaesth*. 2000;85(4):506–11.

74. Bosenberg A, Thomas J, Cronie L, et al. Pharmacokinetics and efficacy of ropivacaine for

continuous epidural infusion in neonates and infants. *Paediatr Anaesth*. 2005;15(9):739–49.

75. Veneziano G, Iliev P, Tripi J, et al. Continuous chloroprocaine infusion for thoracic and caudal epidurals as a postoperative analgesia modality in neonates, infants, and children. *Paediatr Anaesth*. 2016;26(1):84–91.

76. Henderson K, Sethna NF, Berde CB. Continuous caudal anesthesia for inguinal hernia repair in former preterm infants. *J Clin Anesth*. 1993;5(2):129–33.

77. Bouchut JC, Dubois R, Godard J. Clonidine in preterm-infant caudal anesthesia may be responsible for postoperative apnea. *Reg Anesth Pain Med*. 2001;26(1):83–5.

## Chapter 36

# Regional Anesthesia in Neonates and Infants

Karen Boretsky

Pain management is especially challenging in neonates and, increasingly, regional anesthesia is being employed as a major pain management technique for neonates and young infants. The implementation of multimodal analgesia with the inclusion of regional anesthesia may be especially important in neonates, where the side-effects of opioids are common and frequently severe. The majority of regional anesthetic techniques provided to neonates are blocks of the neuraxis; although most of these are single-shot caudals, the use of peripheral nerve blocks is increasing in neonatal anesthesia practice [1–3]. Safety must always be a primary consideration and existing safety data are overall reassuring, with the incidence of serious complications reported in neonates at 1 percent [3,4]. While all of the complications occurred in patients having neuraxial blocks, and consisted mostly of dural punctures and total spinals with transient apnea, there were no reports of permanent sequellae. No complications occurred in neonates receiving peripheral nerve blocks, suggesting an added safety advantage of peripheral nerve blocks compared to neuraxial. These data mirror the results found in studies of older children [3].

Regional anesthesia can be performed in neonates for operative anesthesia, postoperative analgesia, or the treatment of painful nonoperative traumatic or medical conditions. Contraindications to peripheral nerve blocks in neonates are similar to those identified in older children and consist of absolute allergy to local anesthetic agents, guardian refusal, or infection at the insertion site. Although coagulopathy and treated bacteremia are not necessarily absolute contraindications, when present, the risk and benefits of the peripheral nerve block need to be carefully considered.

Most neonates need to be unconscious when the peripheral nerve block is inserted, and there is a good record of safety for performing regional anesthesia on infants while heavily sedated or under general anesthesia. Regardless of the type of sedation, all infants must have standard monitoring in place and resuscitation equipment must be immediately available when regional anesthesia is being administered. If the block is performed with the infant awake, topical or local anesthesia should be applied to the injection site(s) and a sucrose pacifier, although providing no analgesia, may give the infant comfort.

## Anatomic and Developmental Differences

Myelination of peripheral nerve axons begins in utero but is not complete until 1–2 years of age. This relative lack of myelination allows the nerves to be more easily blocked with local anesthetics. Lower volumes – for example 0.1–0.2 ml kg$^{-1}$– of bupivacaine and ropivacaine solutions are usually sufficient to block most peripheral nerves.

Ultrasound has become an important adjunct in regional anesthesia and the use of ultrasound for visualization of nerves and adjacent anatomy is especially advantageous in neonates due to the miniscule size of the target structures and the close proximity of adjacent structures. The ultrasound pictures of soft tissue structures are similar to those in adults and older children when corrected for size. Neonatal bone, however, is largely cartilaginous and the relative lack of ossification in neonates produces different ultrasound images of the bones. During performance of a sciatic block, the femoral head lacks the characteristic echogenicity of the bone and may be difficult to visualize. The lack of bone density of the vertebrae also creates some acoustic windows that are not normally present in older infants and children, providing unique opportunities for access to the neuraxis. During real-time imaging for a paravertebral block, the structures of the entire neuraxis may be visible due to lack of ossification in the overlying vertebra. These differences in imaging must be considered when searching for appropriate landmarks.

The integrity of the coagulation system is important when performing perineural procedures [5]. Differences exist in the neonatal coagulation system for both premature and term infants when compared to adults and older children, and result in different "normal" values when considering laboratory studies of coagulation function. Fortunately, any maturational differences are considered to be functionally balanced and do not affect overall hemostasis and thrombosis. It is, therefore, important to use normal values for gestation and age when making decisions about the performance of regional anesthesia.

The risk of local anesthetic systemic toxicity in neonates is higher compared to older children and adults for a variety of reasons. Local anesthetics are highly bound to plasma proteins, the most important of which is alpha1-acid glycoprotein. Infants have lower blood levels of alpha 1-acid glycoprotein (AAG), about 50 percent of the adult value, which results in less protein binding of local anesthetics and greater free fraction of unbound drug. Fortunately, AAG is an acute phase reactant protein and levels can rise in response to stress, providing some protection to the stressed neonate [6]. In addition, amide local anesthetic drugs are metabolized in the liver and neonates have reduced metabolism and clearance due to immaturity of the cytochrome P450 enzymes. Consequently, bolus dosing of amide local anesthetic should be reduced in neonates and young infants by at least 30 percent [7]. Pharmacokinetic data suggest that serum levels of amide local anesthetics can continue to rise with continuous infusions in neonates, even at low dosing [8]. Local anesthetic dosing recommendations are provisional and based on extrapolation of data in older children, infant animal studies, and limited pharmacokinetic data. All bolus doses should be administered incrementally with careful monitoring for toxic effects.

Ester local anesthetics are metabolized by plasma pseudocholinesterase, and although neonates have reduced levels of pseudocholinesterase, elimination of the most commonly used esters is very rapid and complete. Due to concerns about increased risk of amide local anesthetic accumulation and toxicity in neonates and young infants, infusions of 2-chloroprocaine have been advocated for use in neonates and young infants, and appear to be safe [9].

# Peripheral Nerve Blocks

## Indications

Almost all of the blocks performed in older pediatric populations have been used in neonates (Table 36.1).

**Table 36.1** Surgical sites and their peripheral nerve blocks

| | |
|---|---|
| Supraorbital | Frontal craniotomy, VP shunt, forehead surgery |
| Infraorbital | Upper lip surgery |
| Mandibular division of trigeminal | Lower lip surgery, mandibular distraction |
| Greater occipital | Posterior fossa craniotomy |
| Infraclavicular | Peripherally inserted central catheter (PICC), upper extremity amputation, syndactyly, polydactyly |
| Digital | Finger surgery |
| Axillary | Syndactyly, polydactyly, upper extremity amputation, upper extremity ischemia |
| Paravertebral, intercostal | Rib fx, TEF, esophageal atresia, abdominal surgery |
| Transversus abdominis plane | Ileostomy/colostomy creation and takedown, laparotomy, closure gastroschesis or omphalocele, pyloromyotomy |
| Ilioinguinal | Herniorrhaphy |
| Rectus sheath | Laparoscopy, periumbilical incision |
| Sciatic | Lower extremity amputation, syndactyly, polydactyly |
| Femoral | Lower limb amputation, muscle biopsy |
| Fascia iliaca | Muscle biopsy |
| Penile/pudendal | Circumcision |

# Techniques

Many sources describe the technical aspects of regional anesthesia for use in infants and children. A comprehensive review of all blocks is beyond the scope of this chapter, but descriptions of the most common peripheral blocks with clinical pearls specific to neonates are included.

## Transversus abdominis plane (TAP)

The abdomen is innervated by the thoracoabdominal nerves that are the continuation of the corresponding thoracic spinal nerves. These nerves travel between the deep investing fascia of internal oblique (IO) and the transversus abdominis (TA) muscles. The TAP block in neonates is used for surgery of the abdominal wall and is usually performed with ultrasound guidance. The muscle layers of the abdominal wall assume a characteristic pattern of three parallel hyperechoic muscles separated by hyperechoic fascia. In adult studies, injection at the midaxillary line results in dermatomal spread inferior to the umbilicus and is suitable for surgeries below the umbilicus, while injection more posterior, at the termination of the TA muscle, results in more extensive cephalad spread, reported as high as T7 [10]. This block has been used successfully for major and minor operations of the abdominal wall with both single injections and placement of unilateral indwelling catheters. Bilateral TAP catheters in this age group are impractical due to limitations in safe local anesthetic dosing. The TAP block is feasible in patients for whom thoracic epidurals may be contraindicated or undesirable, but no direct comparative studies are available.

### Equipment

(1) Needle/catheter:
  (a) Single injection: 22–24G × 40–50 mm needle
  (b) Catheter: 18G × 50 mm Tuohy with 20G catheter; alternatively, a 20G needle with an 18G catheter over the needle system.
(2) Portable ultrasound with a high-frequency (6–13/18 MHz) linear transducer with a limited footprint (25–38 mm).

### Dosing

(1) Single bolus: 0.2–0.50 ml kg$^{-1}$ of 0.2 percent ropivacaine, 0.25 percent bupivacaine (optimal dose/dermatomal spread is not yet determined).

### Technique

The ultrasound transducer is placed in a transverse orientation at the midaxillary line between the iliac crest and the 12th rib. The characteristic landmarks are identified to include the external oblique, IO, TA muscles, and the transversalis fascia and parietal peritoneum.

(1) Lateral TAP: Injection at the level of midaxillary line between the iliac crest and the 12th rib will result in reliable coverage of T11–L1. The needle is advanced in-plane with continuous visualization until the tip penetrates the fascia below the IO muscle. A small amount of saline is injected to confirm placement. After careful aspiration, the local anesthetic is injected and viewed for appropriate spread with real-time ultrasound.
(2) Posterior TAP: If more cephalad dermatomal coverage is desired, after identification of landmarks in the midaxillary line, the transducer is moved posterior until the termination of the TA muscle is identified and injection placed in the fascia at the termination of the TA muscle. If desired, a catheter can be advanced into the space and secured.

### Tips

(1) Saline should be used to identify the fascial plane to limit dose of local anesthetic.
(2) For bilateral single-shot injections, local anesthetic can be diluted to 0.1 percent.
(3) Fascial planes are difficult to distinguish in lower weight infants.
(4) Echogenic needles facilitate needle visibility.
(5) Complications are rare but the close proximity to the abdominal cavity may predispose to injury of the bowel or liver if the needle is advanced into the peritoneum.

## Ilioinguinal/Iliohypogastric

The ilioinguinal/iliohypogastric nerves arise from L1 (and sometime T12) and provide the sensory innervation to the skin of the lower abdominal wall, upper thigh, and lateral hip, making this an excellent block for analgesia following inguinal hernia repair, a frequent operation in former preterm infants. The terminal portions of the ilioinguinal/iliohypogastric nerves travel between the TA and IO just medial to the anterior superior iliac spine (ASIS) and can be identified with both ultrasound and landmarks [11,12]. The use of portable ultrasound to identify the landmarks and nerves has resulted in more reliable analgesia with fewer reported complications, but if resources are limited a landmark technique is a good option [13]. Bowel perforation and hepatic laceration have been reported with the landmark technique, while intraperitoneal trespass of the needle has been reported in the ultrasound group without negative consequences.

### Equipment

(1) Needle: 22–24G × 40–50 mm needle
(2) Portable ultrasound with a high-frequency (6–13/18 MHz) linear transducer with a limited footprint (25–38 mm).

### Dosing

0.2–0.40 ml kg$^{-1}$ of 0.2 percent ropivacaine or 0.25 percent bupivacaine

### Technique

(1) Ultrasound-guided technique: The transducer is placed at the edge of the ASIS and oriented toward the umbilicus. The three characteristic muscular layers of the abdominal wall, external oblique (EO), IO, and TA are identified. At this level the EO may be an aponeurotic sheath leaving just the IO and TA identifiable. In the fascial plane between the IO and the TA, the ilioinguinal nerve, when visible, will be located approximately 2 mm and the iliohypogastric will be about 4 mm away from the ASIS. The nerves appear as ellipsoid in shape with a hyperechoic sheath and hypoechoic center. Advance the needle slowly in-plane to a point midway between the two nerves and, after careful aspiration, inject immediately below the fascia beneath the IO.

(2) Landmark technique: Palpate and identify the ipsilateral ASIS and mark a point 3–4 mm away from the ASIS in a line connecting the ASIS to the umbilicus [14]. Following aseptic technique, the block needle is inserted perpendicular to the skin and advanced slowly to allow the operator to appreciate two "pops" associated with fascial planes between the EO and the IO and the IO and the TA. The needle must be advanced carefully as the fascial "pops" are subtle in the neonate.

### Tips

Same considerations as the TAP block

## Paravertebral

The thoracic spinal nerves exit the intervertebral foramen into the paravertebral space en-route to becoming the intercostal nerves. A nerve block at this level provides excellent analgesia for unilateral surgery on the thorax or abdomen. The paravertebral space is a triangular-shaped space bounded by the parietal pleura, the costotransverse ligament, and the posterolateral aspect of the vertebral bodies. This space containing the nerves is continuous between thoracic levels and injection at one level provides coverage of adjacent nerves in a dose-dependent fashion. Studies indicate that 0.2 ml kg$^{-1}$ covers 5–6 dermatomes and 0.4 ml kg$^{-1}$ covers 6–8 dermatomes [15]. Single injections and unilateral catheters are both used. Bilateral catheters are used in larger patients, but the small size of neonates and the limits on safe dosing of local anesthetic makes bilateral catheters impractical. Pediatric studies indicate a high success rate and no major complications, although pneumothorax, subarachnoid block, and hypotension have been reported in adults. This block was first described in neonates using a landmark technique in 1992 and has since been described using an ultrasound-guided technique.

### Equipment

(1) Needle/catheter:
    (a) Single injection: 22–24G × 40–50 mm needle
    (b) Catheter: 18G × 50 mm Tuohy with 20G catheter; alternatively, a 20G needle with an 18G catheter over the needle system.
(2) Portable ultrasound with a high-frequency (6–13/18 MHz) linear transducer with a limited footprint (25–38 mm)

### Dosing

0.2–0.40 ml kg$^{-1}$ of 0.2 percent ropivicaine or 0.25 percent bupivacaine; dermatomal spread is dose-dependent. See Chapter 35 for peripheral nerve catheter infusions.

### Ultrasound-guided Technique

The appropriate thoracic level is identified and marked. Following aseptic technique, the transducer is placed in a transverse orientation over the spinous process of the desired thoracic level. The probe is then moved lateral until the transverse process is visualized as a thumb-like hyperechoic structure above a hyperechoic sliding shimmering line representing the parietal pleura. When visible, the internal intercostal membrane (IICM) will be seen as a hyperechoic structure connecting the bottom of the transverse process to the internal intercostal muscle. The needle is advanced in-plane in a lateral to medial direction until the tip of the needle penetrates the IICM and rests in the space between the pleura and the transverse process. Proper location is confirmed by downward displacement of the pleura with injection of 1 ml of sterile saline. If desired, a catheter can be advanced into the space and secured.

## Tips

(1) Saline should be used to identify proper needle tip placement to limit dose of local anesthetic.
(2) The acoustic shadow characteristically seen below the transverse process on older patients will be absent due to the lack of ossification.
(3) For bilateral single-shot injections, local anesthetic can be diluted to 0.1 percent.
(4) Echogenic needles facilitate needle visibility.

## Rectus Sheath

The terminal branches of the T8–T11 thoracoabdominal nerves exit the TAP plane (from between the IO and the TA), pierce the posterolateral border of the rectus sheath (RS) and course through the rectus abdominus (RA) muscle. These branches innervate the center of the abdominal wall between the lateral edges of the RA muscle, including the umbilicus. This block provides excellent analgesia for midline surgeries including laparoscopies, pyloromyotomies, and midline laparotomy incisions.

## Equipment

(1) Needle: 22–24G × 40–50 mm needle
(2) Portable ultrasound with a high-frequency (6–13/18 MHz) linear transducer with a limited footprint (25–38 mm)

## Dose

0.1 ml kg$^{-1}$ of 0.2 percent ropivacaine or 0.25 percent bupivacaine.

## Technique

The dermatomal level to be blocked is identified and marked. (The umbilicus is the most common level

to block.) Using aseptic technique, the transducer is placed in a transverse orientation with the lateral edge of the transducer lined up with the lateral edge of the RA muscle (the linea semilunaris). The RA muscle is identified and the probe is moved slightly lateral until the medial edges of the muscles of the lateral abdominal wall are just visible. Two hyperechoic lines beneath the RA muscle represent the transversalis fascia and the parietal peritoneum.

Using an in-plane technique, the needle is inserted slowly to reach a target at the lateral-most edge of the posterior RA at a point just above the transversalis fascia. Injection into this space will cause the RA muscle to "roll up" away from the transversalis fascia.

## Tips

(1) The epigastric vessels run within the RA muscle and Doppler can be used for identification.
(2) Saline should be used to identify proper needle tip placement to limit dose of local anesthetic.
(3) For multiple single-shot injections, local anesthetic can be diluted to 0.1 percent.
(4) Echogenic needles facilitate needle visibility.

## Dorsal Penile

Male circumcision is commonly performed in the neonatal period, and penile nerve block has been shown to decrease the associated pain and stress response [16,17]. The penis is innervated by the pudendal nerve (S2–3), which divides into the right and left dorsal nerves of the penis and travels in the subpubic space just below the scarpas fascia. The nerves are lateral to the dorsal veins and arteries. The traditional landmark technique is described.

## Equipment

(1) 25–30G × ¾–1¼ needle.

## Medication

Bupivacaine 0.25 percent; 1 ml with total dose not to exceed 1.5 mg kg$^{-1}$. Since the penile block is a fixed-needle procedure, the risk of inadvertent intravascular injection is higher.

## Technique

Following aseptic preparation of the base of the penis, the penis is retracted gently in a caudal direction. At a point just below the inferior ramus of the pubic bone, two separate injections are made at the 10 o'clock and 2 o'clock positions as measured from the midline [18].

The needle is advanced slowly until first a gentle "give" (superficial fascia) is felt followed by a more definitive "pop" of the deep fascia. After aspiration, 0.5 ml of local anesthetic is injected. Injection is repeated on the contralateral side.

### Tips

(1) Always aspirate due to the proximity of several arteries and veins.
(2) Solutions containing epinephrine should never be used.
(3) Local anesthetic systemic toxicity should be suspected with the occurrence of cardiac irregularities.

### Femoral Nerve Block

The femoral nerve is composed of branches of the L2–L4 spinal nerves and innervates the femur, the skin of the anterior aspect of the upper leg, and the knee joint. The nerve travels with the femoral artery and can be best accessed just caudal to the inguinal ligament. The fascia surrounding the iliopsoas muscle, the fascia iliaca, runs on top of the nerve and separates the nerve from the artery. This block can be used for lower limb salvage surgery and muscle biopsies. To avoid entering the hip joint, this block is best performed using ultrasound guidance.

### Equipment

(1) Needle/catheter:
  (a) Single injection: 22–24G × 40–50 mm needle
  (b) Catheter: 18G × 50 mm Tuohy with 20G catheter; alternatively, a 20G needle with an 18G catheter over the needle system.
(2) Portable ultrasound with a high-frequency (6–13/18 MHz) linear transducer with a limited footprint (25–38 mm)

### Dosing

0.1 ml $kg^{-1}$ of 0.2 percent ropivacaine or 0.25 percent bupivacaine.

### Technique

Using aseptic technique, the transducer is placed at the level of and parallel to the inguinal crease. The landmarks of this block include the femoral artery, the iliopsoas muscle, and the fascia iliaca. The nerve lies lateral to the artery and under the fascia iliaca, and it assumes a triangular or compressed oval shape. Using an in-plane approach, the needle is advanced slowly to a target position under the fascia iliaca and lateral to the nerve. Once the needle is through the fascia iliaca, an injection of saline can be used to confirm placement beneath the fascia iliaca. After careful aspiration, local anesthetic can be injected. If desired, a catheter can be inserted and secured.

### Tips

(1) Manual compression of the vein with the ultrasound transducer confirms lateral to medial orientation.
(2) Saline should be used to identify needle tip placement to limit dose of local anesthetic.
(3) The needle tip must be under the fascia iliaca.

### Infraclavicular Brachial Plexus

The brachial plexus is composed of the ventral rami of the fifth cervical through the first thoracic spinal nerves, and supplies all of the innervation to the upper extremity. The brachial plexus can be blocked at multiple locations along its course, but the most accessible site in small infants is the infraclavicular approach that accesses the nerves as cords of the brachial plexus after they pass under the clavicle. This block can be used to facilitate peripheral insertion of central catheters (PICC lines) without the need for general anesthesia, and can facilitate limb salvage [19].

### Equipment

(1) Needle/catheter:
  (a) Single injection: 22–24G × 40–50 mm needle
  (b) Catheter: 18G × 50 mm Tuohy with 20G catheter; alternatively, a 20G needle with an 18G catheter over the needle system.
(2) Portable ultrasound with a high-frequency (6–13/18 MHz) linear transducer with a limited footprint (25–38 mm).

### Dosing

0.1 ml $kg^{-1}$ of 0.2 percent ropivicaine or 0.25 percent bupivacaine.

### Technique

Using aseptic technique, the ultrasound transducer is placed in a cephalad to caudad orientation adjacent

387

to the medial aspect of the corocoid process with the edge of the transducer at the inferior edge of the clavicle. Slide the probe as needed to visualize the axillary artery in short axis. The two muscles overlying the artery are the pectoralis major and minor. The brachial plexus at this level consists of three cords, with the medial cord located at 9 o'clock, the posterior cord at 6 o'clock, and the lateral cord at 3 o'clock relative to the artery. If individual cords cannot be identified it will suffice to surround the artery with local anesthetic. The block needle is advanced in-plane to the bottom of the artery, initially targeting the posterior cord. Additional passes of the needle are performed to surround all of the cords and the artery with local anesthetic. If desired, a catheter can be passed through the needle and secured.

### Tips

(1) Use a cephalad to caudad needle approach and position the transducer and needle as lateral as possible to minimize the possibility of pneumothorax.

## Epidural Anesthesia

Epidural anesthesia continues to occupy a major role in pediatric regional anesthesia and represents almost half of the regional anesthetics in children less than three years of age [20]. In parallel with the use of ultrasound in all regional anesthesia, the use of ultrasound for guidance of epidural anesthesia has evolved quickly. When imaging and accessing the neuraxial structures in infants and children it is important to be aware of the developmental changes in the spine and the spinal canal that affect the ultrasound images.

The location of the spinal cord and dural sac within the spinal canal changes over time. During the development of the fetus in utero, the spinal cord extends the entire length of the spinal canal. This position ascends as the fetus develops and in a newborn the spinal cord extends as low as the L3 level, with termination of the dura sac at the S4 level [21]. As the child grows, the vertebral column grows faster than the spinal cord and the termination of the spinal cord moves to a progressively higher level; L1/L2 for spinal cord and S2 for dura at one year of age [22,23]. These may be important details to keep in mind in order to avoid complications such as inadvertent dural puncture and/or spinal cord trauma [23].

The limited ossification of the pediatric vertebral column allows better visualization of the neuraxis in pediatric patients. The newborn skeleton is predominantly cartilaginous at birth and proceeds to deposit calcium and ossify progressively until puberty. This relative lack of ossification allows the easy penetration of ultrasound waves and a clear view of the neuraxial structures up until three months of age, after which ultrasound imaging becomes progressively more difficult [24]. Around nine months of age the bony mass of the vertebral arches start to impose ultrasound shadows over the underlying structures, but anatomic information remains available in the ultrasound windows between adjacent vertebrae.

Ultrasound can be used in multiple ways to help with accessing the pediatric epidural space at different levels. Pre-puncture scanning gives information about the location and depth of the epidural space and adjacent structures. Alternatively, ultrasound imaging is used for real-time scanning to guide and direct the needle and catheter insertion into the epidural space. The ultrasound imaging is also used after the catheter or needle is inserted to confirm position.

## Single-Shot Caudal Approach to the Epidural Space

**Background and Indications.** The relative popularity of epidural analgesia can be attributed to the relative ease with which the epidural space can be accessed via the sacral hiatus in infants and young children. A single injection of local anesthetic into the caudal epidural space, the "kiddie caudal," is appropriate for most surgeries below the umbilicus and results in low complication rates and high success rates. Inadvertent spinal anesthesia, with an incidence of dural puncture of 0.19 percent [25], and perforation of adjacent viscera from improper position of the needle, have, however, been reported. Ultrasound guidance offers a way to identify sacrum anatomy and perform caudal blocks in the patients at risk for dural puncture (neonates and very small infants), and patients with difficult anatomy (older patients and patients with lumbosacral spinal dysraphism), potentially increasing the success rate and reducing the rate of complications [26–28].

**Anatomy.** The sacrum is composed of five fused sacral vertebrae (Figure 36.1). Its dorsal surface is convex and has a raised interrupted median crest with four (sometimes three) spinous tubercles representing fused sacral spines. The posterior surface is formed

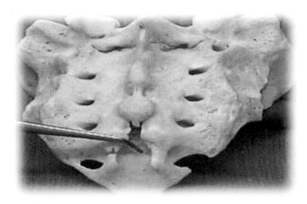

**Figure 36.1** The sacrum structures are visualized in both the short axis (transverse) and the midline long axis (longitudinal).

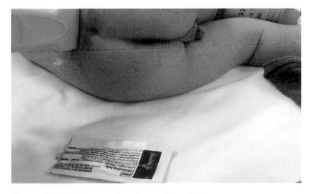

**Figure 36.2** Ultrasound probe position for transverse scan over sacrum.

by fused laminae. Below the fourth (or third) spinous tubercle an arched sacral hiatus is identified due to failure of the fifth pair of laminae to meet, exposing the sacral canal, a continuation of the lumbar spinal canal. This caudal opening of the canal, or sacral hiatus, is covered by the sacrococcygeal ligament, which is an extension of the ligamentum flavum. The fifth inferior articulate processes project caudally and flank the sacral hiatus as prominent boney sacral cornua. The sacral canal contains the cauda equina (including the filum terminale) and the spinal meninges, epidural venous plexus, and adipose tissue. The lowest margin of the filum terminale emerges at the sacral hiatus and transverses the dorsal surface of the fifth sacral vertebra.

**Short axis.** (See Figure 36.2.) The two bony prominences of the sacral cornua appear as hyperechoic reversed U-shaped structures (Figure 36.3). Two hyperechoic band-like structures lie between the two cornua. The band-like structure on top of the sacral cornua is the sacrococcygeal ligament and the band-like structure at the bottom is the bone of the dorsal surface of the anterior sacrum. The sacral hiatus is the hypoechoic region between the two band-like structures.

**Long axis.** (See Figure 36.4.) With the caudad edge of the transducer resting between the two cornua, the most prominent rounded hyperechoic structure observed is the bony prominence of the S4 spinous tubercle of the sacrum (Figure 36.5). The

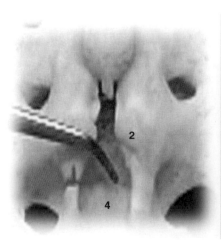

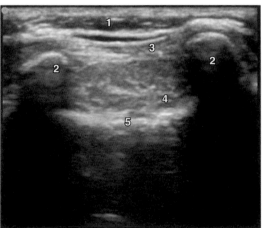

**Figure 36.3** Sacrum and ultrasound transverse view over sacrum.(1) is subcutaneous tissue, (2) is sacrum cornua, (3) is sacrococcygeal ligament, (4) is sacral hiatus, (5) is sacrum bone.

sacrococcygeal ligament presents as a thick band beyond the end of the S4 spinous process and the sacral hiatus is the hypoechoic region under the sacrococcygeal ligament.

**Patient position.** Prone or lateral position with hips, knees, and neck flexed.

**Transducer.** 25–35 mm linear array oscillating at 6–13 MHz.

**Transducer orientation.** Initially transverse over the two bony prominences of sacral cornua to identify sacrum structure. Then the transducer is rotated 90° for real-time and/or confirmatory needle placement.

**Needle.** 22-gauge, 4–5 cm blunt needle.

**Local anesthetic.** Since the single-shot caudal block involves a fixed needle position, the risk of inadvertent intravascular injection is increased. If larger volumes of local anesthetic are used, the concentration should be reduced so that the dose does not exceed 1.5 mg kg$^{-1}$ of bupivacaine or 1.8 mg kg$^{-1}$ of ropivacaine.

### Technique

After proper disinfection of the skin, the sterile covered transducer is placed with a transverse orientation over the sacrum at the level where the sacral cornua can be palpated, the S4–S5 level. The sacral hiatus is identified as the hypoechoic space between the hyperechoic upside-down U-shaped structures of the sacral cornua deep to the sacrococcygeal ligament. The probe is rotated to the longitudinal position while still visualizing the sacral hiatus and the lower edge of the probe is placed at the level of the cornua. Under ultrasound longitudinal view the needle is inserted through the sacrococcygeal ligament from a caudad to cephalad direction using an in-plane approach. The needle appears as a hyperechoic structure positioned in the sacral hiatus. The local anesthetic administration is observed in real time as a turbulence moving cephalad in the sacral hiatus. A final transition back to a transverse view may permit visualization of the local anesthetic between the sacrococcygeal ligament and the sacrum.

### Tips

A prone position with rolls placed transversely under the hips achieves a flatter skin surface at the sacral hiatus area for the placement of the ultrasound transducer.

In the lateral position with hips, knees, and neck flexed, the dural sac shifts significantly cephalad, providing some safety margin to avoid dural puncture [27].

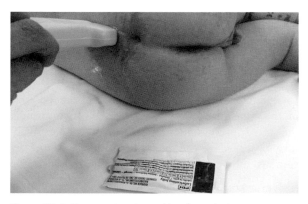

**Figure 36.4** Ultrasound probe position for sagittal scan over sacrum.

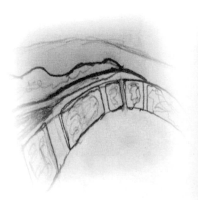
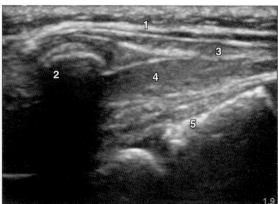

**Figure 36.5** Ultrasound longitudinal view over sacrum. (1) is subcutaneous tissue, (2) is spinous tubercle of S4, (3) is sacrococcygeal ligament, (4) is epidural space, (5) is floor of sacral canal.

The technique can be done under the ultrasound transverse view, using an out-of-plane technique.

The optimal angle for needle insertion is between 10° and 38° [29].

The characteristic "give "or "pop" can be detected when the sacrococcygeal ligament is penetrated.

## Lumbar and Thoracic Epidural Catheters via the Caudal Approach

**Background and indications.** In the smallest patients, accessing the epidural space via a direct approach at the desired lumbar or thoracic level is technically challenging because of the diminutive size and the close proximity of vulnerable anatomic structures and the fear of complications such as spinal cord trauma. Since 1988 a technique of accessing the epidural space via the sacral hiatus and threading a catheter cephalad to the desired dermatomal level is frequently used in infants and young children [30]. Ultrasound imaging can be used to confirm placement of the needle and catheter through the sacral hiatus into the epidural space and to confirm passage of the catheter to the appropriate lumbar or thoracic level. Ensuring that the tip of the epidural catheter is placed at the appropriate surgical dermatome allows for effective and safe local anesthetic infusion rate.

**Anatomy.** (See Figure 36.7) The vertebral column contains 12 thoracic and five lumbar vertebrae bones. Each vertebra is composed of a body anteriorly and an arch posteriorly which enclose a canal housing the spinal cord. Protruding from the posterior midline of each arch is the spinous process and extending laterally are the paired transverse processes. The spinal cord lies within the vertebral canal and is covered by three membranes. The two outermost layers, the dura mater and the arachnoid mater, are closely adherent. The space between the arachnoid mater and the third layer, the pia mater, is the subarachnoid space, which contains the cerebrospinal fluid (CSF). The spinal cord is thickest at the thoracic level and decreases in size as it sheds nerve roots and tapers to its termination in a bundle of loose nerve roots called the cauda equina. The ligamentum flavum is a tough ligament that extends from C1 to S1 and connects the vertebrae to each other. The potential space created between the ligamentum flavum and the dura is the epidural space. The anatomy and sonoanatomy of the sacral hiatus and caudal canal are described above.

The lumbar and thoracic spine structures can be visualized in both the short axis/transverse view (Figure 36.6) and the long axis/longitudinal view (see Figure 36.9).

**Short axis.** (See Figures 36.6 and 36.7.) The spinous process is represented as a hyperechoic upside-down V-shaped structure with an acoustic shadow below. The spinal cord and dura are seen as two hyperechoic concentric circles deep to the spinous process; the hypoechoic spinal cord cased by the hyperechoic pia is represented by the innermost circle; the CSF is the hypoechoic concentric rim; and the dura is the outermost hyperechoic circle. The ligamentum flavum is difficult to visualize and usually appears indistinguishable from the dura. The ligamentum flavum can best be seen when separated from the dura by hydrodissection into the epidural space (Figure 36.8).

**Long Axis.** (See Figure 36.9 and 36.10.) The long axis can be best visualized from a longitudinal paramedian view. The spinous processes are now visualized as thick, slanted hyperechoic lines creating acoustic windows occurring at regular intervals. Between these acoustic windows the elements of the spinal canal can be identified by layer. The dura mater is represented by the topmost (anatomically posterior) hyperechoic line between the acoustic windows. The hypoechoic layer beneath this represents the CSF below which the hyperechoic pia mater is seen. The appearance of the neural element layer is dependent on the vertebral level being viewed. It appears as either a homogeneous

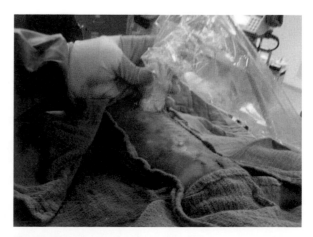

**Figure 36.6** Ultrasound probe position for transverse scan over thoracic spine for caudal catheter insertion in an infant.

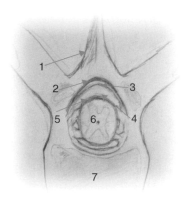
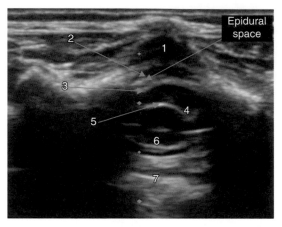

**Figure 36.7** Ultrasound transverse view over thoracic spine for an infant.(1) is spinous process, (2) is ligamentum flavum, (3) is dura mater, (4) is cerebrospinal fluid, (5) is pia mater, (6) is spinal cord, (7) is vertebral body.

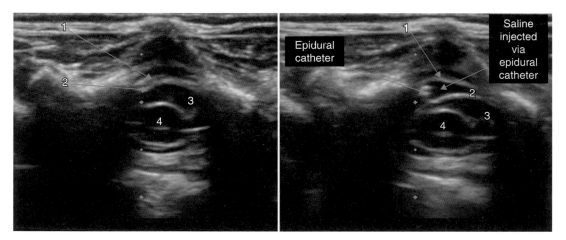

**Figure 36.8** Epidural space before (left) and after (right) hydro expansion with normal saline.(1) is ligamentum flavum, (2) is dura mater, (3) is cerebrospinal fluid, (4) is spinal cord.

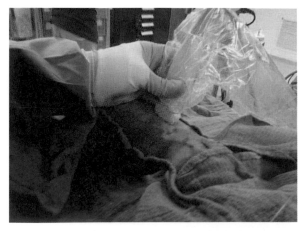

**Figure 36.9** Long axis; (longitudinal) probe position for epidural in infant.

hyperechoic area representing the solid spinal cord or a bundle of hyperechoic linear structures representing the cauda equina. The vertebral bodies can be identified ventrally. The degree of acoustic shadowing cast by the spinous processes is dependent upon the amount of ossification.

**Patient Position.** (See Figure 36.11.) Prone, with rolls placed transversely under the hips and shoulders to allow free excursion of the abdomen and flatten the lumbar curve. Alternatively, a lateral position with the patient flexed forward and curled inward can be used.

**Transducer.** 25–50 mm linear array oscillating at 6–17 MHz.

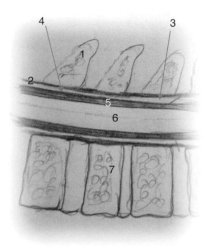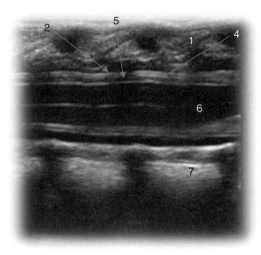

**Figure 36.10** Ultrasound longitudinal view over thoracic spine for an infant.(1) is spinous process, (2) is ligamentum flavum, (3) is epidural space, (4) is dura mater, (5) is subarachnoid space, (6) is spinal cord, (7) is vertebral body.

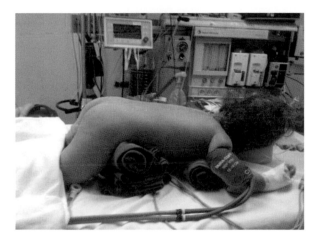

**Figure 36.11** Prone position for caudal catheter placement.

**Transducer Orientation**.

- Transverse: visualize/locate sacral cornua
- Longitudinal: visualize needle and catheter insertion
- Transverse: confirm catheter tip location

**Needle**. 18-gauge 5 cm Tuohy needle
**Local Anesthetic**.

- Initial bolus
- 0.4–0.5 ml kg$^{-1}$ of 0.2 percent ropivacaine, 0.25 percent bupivacaine, or 3 percent chloroprocaine for lumbar approach
- 0.3–0.4 ml kg$^{-1}$ of 0.2 percent ropivacaine, 0.25 percent bupivacaine, or 3 percent chloroprocaine for thoracic approach

- Maximum of 1.7 mg kg$^{-1}$ for ropivacaine and 1.5 mg kg$^{-1}$ for bupivacaine

See Chapter 35 for recommended epidural infusion rates.

## Technique

Palpate and mark: (1) presumed position of the sacral cornua; and (2) desired lumbar or thoracic level for final catheter tip location. Using sterile technique, prep and drape a field to include the top of the intergluteal crease to the desired dermatomal level for the tip. Using an ultrasound probe with a sterile sheath, locate the cornua (two upside-down Us) and sacral hiatus via the short-axis view and rotate the probe 90° to a long-axis view while keeping the sacral hiatus in sight. Position the lower end of the probe at the level of the sacral cornua. Position and insert the needle as described above for the single-shot technique and carefully advance under ultrasound guidance. The needle will appear as a hyperechoic structure. Between 2 and 5 ml of pre-servative free normal saline is injected and used to confirm placement and open up the epidural space. With the probe still in a longitudinal orientation, the catheter is inserted through the needle and visualized entering the epidural space. The hyperechoic catheter can sometimes be continually visualized during inser-tion by sliding the transducer cephalad in the longi-tudinal orientation along the vertebral column as the catheter is inserted. The ability to follow the catheter insertion in real time continually to the desired der-matome is poor and becomes increasingly less reliable

393

as the vertebrae ossify. Once the catheter is inserted to the desired dermatomal distance the tip location can be confirmed by: (1) direct visualization of the tip if it contains sonoreflective material such as metal; or (2) administration of small amounts of preservative free saline under ultrasound visualization in the short-axis view and viewing the expansion of the epidural space and displacement of tissue. With increasing age, visualization will rely more on information contained in ultrasound windows between vertebra. Caudal catheters should be tunneled subcutaneously to reduce the risk of bacterial colonization to equal that of lumbar epidural catheters [31].

### Tips

- View both the long axis and short axis to provide two points of reference.
- The epidural space is a potential space that is visualized best when the space is hydrodissected.
- The lumbar spine offers better ultrasound visualization than the thoracic spine [32].
- Before insertion of the catheter, measure the distance to the desired dermatome and insert the catheter initially the measured distance. If the catheter doesn't coil, it can then be found near the desired dermatome and small adjustments more easily made.

## Lumbar and Thoracic Continuous Epidural Analgesia via the Direct, Intervertebral Approach

**Background and Indications.** For pediatric patients, the loss-of-resistance (LOR) technique using saline solution is the classic technique for the placement of the epidural catheters directly at lumbar or thoracic levels. Ultrasonography with a linear high-frequency ultrasound probe can be used to identify neuroaxial structures, to measure skin-to-epidural space and dura depth, may permit visualization of the local anesthetic spread in epidural space, and can be used to confirm the catheter position [32–34].

**Anatomy.** Anatomy and sonoanatomy of the spine were described above.

**Needle.** 18 gauge 5–10 cm Tuohy needle.

### Technique

After proper disinfection of the skin, the sterile covered transducer is placed with a paramedian/

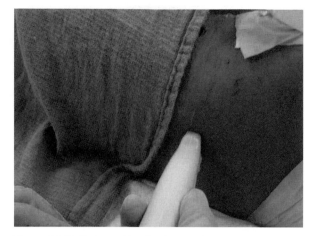

**Figure 36.12** Probe position for short-axis/transverse view over the thoracic spine.

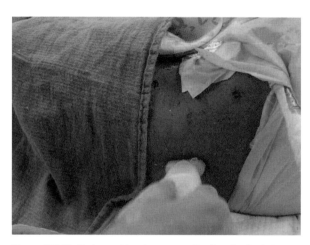

**Figure 36.13** Probe position for paramedian/longitudinal view over the thoracic spine.

longitudinal orientation (Figure 36.12) to identify the longitudinal view of spinous process, dura, and epidural space (Figure 36.13). The distance from the skin to the ligamentum flavum/epidural space and from the skin to dura mater should be measured. These distances should be considered when the Tuohy needle is inserted for LOR technique. After the placement of the epidural catheter, the ultrasound transducer is placed with a transverse orientation at the level where the tip of the catheter is expected to be found. A short/transverse ultrasound view of the spine was presented above. The spine is better visualized in infants than in older children (Figure 36.14). Injection of normal saline/local anesthetic through the epidural catheter will visualize the downward displacement of the dura.

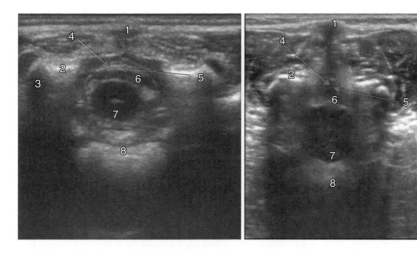

**Figure 36.14** Ultrasound transverse view over the thoracic spine for an infant (left) and a seven-year-old child (right). (1) is spinous process, (2) is lamina, (3) is transverse process, (4) is epidural space, (5) is dura mater, (6) is subarachnoid space, (7) is spinal cord, (8) is vertebral body.

If the transducer is moved longitudinally above and below the injection sites, the local anesthetic in the epidural space is confirmed by the displacement of the dura as the epidural space is expanded by the injected local anesthetic.

Ultrasound imaging can be used to place an epidural catheter under direct visualization [24]. With the transducer placed with a paramedian/longitudinal orientation, the needle is inserted using a midline approach and can be visualized penetrating the ligamentum flavum (if visible) and lying on the top of the dura. The injection of local anesthetic through the Touhy needle in the epidural space can be visualized during continuous technique for LOR. A final transition back to a transverse view may permit visualization of the local anesthetic as described above. A second person is needed to manipulate the ultrasound probe.

**Local anesthetic.** The same as epidural catheter placement via the caudal approach.

### Tips

- The dura mater is more easily visualized than the ligamentum flavum.
- Ultrasound provides better visualization for catheter placement in children younger than six months of age rather than older children [35].
- Ultrasound visualization of the neuroaxial structures at the thoracic spine is more difficult than ultrasonography at the lumbar spine secondary to narrower acoustic windows at the thoracic level.

- A correlation of 0.88 could be estimated between ultrasound depth of the epidural space and measured LOR [34].

## References

1. Polaner DM, Taenzer AH, Walker BJ, et al. Pediatric Regional Anesthesia Network (PRAN): a multi-institutional study of the use and incidence of complications of pediatric regional anesthesia *Anesth Analg.* 2012;115(6):1353–64. doi: 10.1213/ANE.0b013e31825d9f4b.

2. Walker BJ, Long JB, De Oliveira GS, et al. Peripheral nerve catheters in children: an analysis of safety and practice patterns from the pediatric regional anesthesia network (PRAN). *Br J Anaesth.* 2015;115(3):457–62. doi: 10.1093/bja/aev220.

3. Ecoffey C, Lacroix F, Giaufré E, Orliaguet G, Courrèges P; Association des Anesthésistes Réanimateurs Pédiatriques d'Expression Française (ADARPEF). Epidemiology and morbidity of regional anesthesia in children: a follow-up one-year prospective survey of the French-Language Society of Paediatric Anaesthesiologists (ADARPEF). *Paediatr Anaesth.* 2010;20(12):1061–9. doi: 10.1111/j.1460-9592.2010.03448.

4. Giaufre E, Dalens B, Gombert A. Epidemiology and morbidity of regional anesthesia in children: a one-year prospective survey of the French-Language Society of Pediatric Anesthesiologist. *Anesth Analg.* 1996;83(5):904–12.

5. Horlocker TT, Wedel DJ, Rowlingson JC, et al. Regional anesthesia in the patient receiving antithrombotic or thrombolytic therapy: American Society of Regional Anesthesia and Pain Medicine

Evidence-Based Guidelines (Third Edition). *Reg Anesth Pain Med*. 2010:35(1):64–101.

6. Booker PD, Taylor C, Saba G. Perioperative changes in alpha-1-acid glycoprotein concentrations in infants undergoing major surgery. *BJA*. 1996;76:365–8.

7. Suresh A, Polaner D, Cote C. Regional anesthesia. In: Cote C, Lerman J, Anderson B, editors. *A Practice of Anesthesia for Infants and Children*, 5th edn. Philadelphia, PA: Elsevier Saunders; 2013.

8. Meunier JF, Goujard E, Dubousset AM, et al. Pharmacokinetics of bupivacaine after continuous epidural infusion in infants with and without biliary atresia. *Anesthesiology*. 2001;95(1):87–95.

9. Henderson K, Sethna N, Berde CB. Continuous caudal anesthesia for inguinal hernia repair in former preterm infants. *J Clin Anesth*. 1993;5(2):129–33.

10. Sondekoppam RV, Brookes J, Morris L, Johnson M, Ganapathy S. Injectate spread following ultrasound-guided lateral to medial approach for dual transversus abdominis plane blocks. *Acta Anaesthesiol Scand*. 2015;59(3):369–76.

11. Weintrad M, Marhofer P, Bosenberg A, et al. Ultrasound-guided ilioinguinal/iliohypogastric blocks in children: where do we administer the local anesthetic without direct visualization? *Anesth Analg*. 2008:106:89–93.

12. Willschke H, Marhofer P, Bosenberg A, et al. Ultrasonography for ilioinguinal/iliohypogastric nerve blocks in children. *Br J Anaesth*. 2005;95(2):226–30.

13. Shuying L, Tan SWK. Ultrasonography-guided ilioinguinal-iliohypogastric nerve block for inguinal herniotomies in ex-premature neonates. *Singapore Med J*. 2013;54(11):e218–e220.

14. van Schoor AN, Bosman MC, Bosenberg AT. Revisiting the anatomy of the ilioinguinal/iliohypogastric nerve block. *Paediatr Anaesth*. 2013;23(5):390–4.

15. Albokrinov AA, Fesenko UA. Spread of dye after single thoracolumbar paravertebral injection in infants: a cadaveric study. *Eur J Anaesthesiol*. 2014;31:305–9.

16. Stang HJ, Gunnar MR, Snellman L, Condon LM, Kestenbaum R. Local anesthesia for neonatal circumcision: effects on distress and cortisol response. *JAMA*. 1988;259(10):1507–11.

17. Williamson PS, Williamson ML. Physiologic stress reduction by a local anesthetic during newborn circumcision. *Pediatrics*. 1983;71(1):36–40.

18. Dalens B, Vanneuville G, Dechelotte P. Penile block via the subpubic space in 100 children. *Anesth Analg*. 1989;69:41–5.

19. Mislovic, V. Multimodal analgesia including infraclavicular block in perioperative management of upper extremity amputation in neonate. *Pediatr Anesth*. 2011;21(12):1272–3.

20. Ecoffey C, Lacroix F, Giaufre E, Orliaguet G, Courreges P, Association des Anesthesistes Reanimateurs Pediatriques d'Expression F. Epidemiology and morbidity of regional anesthesia in children: a follow-up one-year prospective survey of the French-Language Society of Paediatric Anaesthesiologists (ADARPEF). *Paediatr Anaesth*. 2010;20(12):1061–9. doi: 10.1111/j.1460-9592.2010.03448.x.

21. Johr M, Berger TM. Caudal blocks. *Paediatr Anaesth*. 2012;22(1):44–50. doi: 10.1111/j.1460-9592.2011.03669.x.

22. Malas MA, Seker M, Salbacak A, et al. The relationship between the lumbosacral enlargement and the conus medullaris during the period of fetal development and adulthood: surgical and radiologic anatomy: *SRA*. 2000;22(3–4):163–8.

23. Willschke H, Marhofer P, Bosenberg A, et al. Epidural catheter placement in children: comparing a novel approach using ultrasound guidance and a standard loss-of-resistance technique. *Br J Anaesth*. 2006;97(2):200–7. doi: 10.1093/bja/ael121.

24. Beyaz SG, Tokgoz O, Tufek A. Caudal epidural block in children and infants: retrospective analysis of 2088 cases. *Ann Saudi Med*. 2011;31(5):494–7. doi: 10.4103/0256-4947.84627.

25. Chen CP, Tang SF, Hsu TC, et al. Ultrasound guidance in caudal epidural needle placement. *Anesthesiology*. 2004;101(1):181–4.

26. Koo BN, Hong JY, Kim JE, Kil HK. The effect of flexion on the level of termination of the dural sac in paediatric patients. *Anaesthesia*. 2009;64(10):1072–6. doi: 10.1111/j.1365-2044.2009.06031.x.

27. Visoiu M, Lichtenstein S. 25 years of experience, thousands of caudal blocks, and no dural puncture: what happened today? *Paediatr Anaesth*. 2012;22(3):304–5. doi: 10.1111/j.1460-9592.2011.03785.x.

28. Park JH, Koo BN, Kim JY, et al. Determination of the optimal angle for needle insertion during caudal block in children using ultrasound imaging. *Anaesthesia*. 2006;61(10):946–9. doi: 10.1111/j.1365-2044.2006.04795.x.

29. Bösenberg AT, Bland BA, Schulte-Steinberg O, Downing JW. Thoracic epidural anesthesia via caudal route in infants. *Anesthesiology*.1988;69(2):265–9.

30. Marhofer P, Bosenberg A, Sitzwohl C, et al. Pilot study of neuraxial imaging by ultrasound in infants and children. *Paediatr Anaesth*. 2005;15(8):671–6. doi: 10.1111/j.1460-9592.2004.01521.x.

31. Bubeck J, Boos K, Krause H, Thies KC. Subcutaneous tunneling of caudal catheters reduces the rate of bacterial colonization to that of lumbar epidural catheters. *Anesth Analg*. 2004;99(3):689–93. doi: 10.1213/01.ANE.0000130023.48259.FB.

32. Vallejo MC, Phelps AL, Singh S, Orebaugh SL, Sah N. Ultrasound decreases the failed labor epidural rate in resident trainees. *Int J Obstet Anesth*. 2010;19(4):373–8. doi: 10.1016/j.ijoa.2010.04.002.

33. Kil HK, Cho JE, Kim WO, et al. Prepuncture ultrasound-measured distance: an accurate reflection of epidural depth in infants and small children. *Region Anesth Pain Med*. 2007;32(2):102–6. doi: 10.1016/j.rapm.2006.10.005.

34. Rapp HJ, Folger A, Grau T. Ultrasound-guided epidural catheter insertion in children. *Anesth Analg*. 2005;101(2):333–9. doi: 10.1213/01.ANE.0000156579.11254.D1.

35. Chawathe MS, Jones RM, Gildersleve CD, et al. Detection of epidural catheters with ultrasound in children. *Paediatr Anaesth*. 2003;13(8):681–4.

## Chapter 37

# Procedural Sedation

Mary Ellen McCann and Christine Greco

The safe sedation of infants for procedures and imaging can be very difficult. It requires a careful presedation evaluation to determine whether there are underlying medical issues that would put the infant at higher risk. Infants with congenital cardiac defects may be poor candidates for sedation, in part because they may not tolerate adverse events such as even short episodes of hypoxia or hypercarbia. The hepatic and renal function of the infant will have an impact on the dosing of the sedatives as well as plans for discharge. Other medications that the child takes are important to note because they may alter the pharmacokinetics and dynamics of sedatives, which could lead to sedation failures or oversedation. Practitioners must be ready with both a sedation plan as well as a rescue plan for an infant that develops a deeper plane of sedation than planned for. Although it is not necessary for all practitioners who perform sedations to be anesthesiologists, it is necessary that they have the appropriate training and skills in airway management to allow rescue of the patient. Correct age- and size-appropriate equipment for airway management and venous access, appropriate medications, and reversal agents must be immediately available. Careful monitoring by a dedicated person not doing the procedure as well as a properly staffed and equipped recovery area is essential for safe pediatric sedation.

For infants, sometimes pharmacologic sedation for imaging procedures is not necessary. Protocols to maximize the chance that an infant will naturally sleep through an MRI examination have been utilized in several centers. A typical protocol would involve fasting and avoiding a nap for the infant for a four-hour period, bringing the caregiver into the MRI suite where the infant is either breast- or bottle-fed, placed on a warmed mattress, either swaddled in blankets or gently restrained with straps. Earplugs or specially designed ear-muffs for infants, or a sound attenuation helmet, can be placed on the infant after they are

asleep. Pacifiers should be avoided because they can introduce motion artifact for cranial scans. A retrospective study of infants with aortic arch abnormalities less than six months of age scheduled for cardiac MRIs found that 23 out of 24 infants were successfully imaged without sedation, giving a success rate of 96 percent [1]. The scanning time, however, was very short at less than ten minutes. A prospective series using similar "feed and sleep" technique for neonates and infants less than six months of age for cardiac MRIs found a 100 percent success rate in 20 infants imaged [2]. The mean length of the scans in this series was 46 minutes. These techniques avoid sedation but do put a burden on the imaging staff. The scanners must be available when it is the correct time to feed the fasting infant. These techniques obviously will not work for procedures in infants that are painful.

## Planes of Sedation [3]

Minimal sedation is a drug-induced state during which patients respond normally to verbal commands. Although cognitive function and coordination may be impaired, ventilatory and cardiovascular functions are unaffected. Although older children who have received minimal sedation generally do not require more than observation and intermittent assessment of their level of sedation, infants should be assessed continuously.

Moderate sedation is a drug-induced depression of consciousness during which patients respond purposefully to verbal commands. For very young infants, crying or opening their eyes to a verbal stimulus or light tactile stimulation constitutes a moderate plane of sedation. Generally patients receiving moderate sedation are able to maintain a patent airway, and have adequate spontaneous ventilation and normal cardiovascular function. However, patients can obstruct and may need some support in maintaining an open airway.

Deep sedation is a state of consciousness in which infants are not easily arousable but will respond purposefully to a painful stimulus. Infants in particular may have difficulty in maintaining a patent airway and may hypoventilate or become apneic. Partial or complete loss of airway reflexes is common. Cardiovascular function is usually intact. The boundary between deep sedation and general anesthesia is very easy to cross and all practitioners planning on deeply sedating infants should be prepared and qualified to perform general anesthesia on young infants. They should have expertise with placing airway devices (endotracheal intubation, mask airways, laryngeal mask airways, oral airways) and with methods to support cardiovascular function (fluid and pressors).

Measuring the depth of sedation in young infants can be very difficult. Many of the available scales involve verbally or tactilely stimulating the patient to test their ability to respond, which of course is the opposite goal of a successful procedural sedation, in which the goal is to keep the patient still throughout the procedure. Scales such as the Observer's Assessment of Alertness/Sedation (OAAS) and the University of Michigan Sedation Scale (UMSS) have been validated in infants and found to correlate closely with each other [4]. They are most reliable during minimal to moderate sedation and less reliable during deep sedation. The Neonatal Pain, Agitation and Sedation Scale (N-PASS) was found to reliably measure oversedation, but did not differentiate between adequate and undersedation in neonates requiring sedation in the NICU [5]. Processed EEG monitors such as the bispectral index can be used to reliably measure anesthetic and sedation depth in children aged two and older. The algorithms used in the monitors were based on the adult EEG patterns found during general anesthesia. Research is currently being done to better determine the expected EEG changes found in young infants undergoing anesthesia, and it is hoped that in the future there may be a processed EEG anesthetic depth monitor that can be used in infants.

## Presedation Evaluation

All infants need a health evaluation prior to undergoing sedation for a procedure. This evaluation can be done by a licensed practitioner and reviewed by the sedation team or be done by the sedation team. This evaluation can be used to screen for patients in whom a simple sedation is unsafe or unlikely to succeed

secondary to premorbid conditions that could affect the patient's ability to maintain airway patency or cardiovascular stability.

A history of the medications the infant is taking is very important. Both prescribed and over-the-counter medications need to be evaluated. Many herbal medications can alter sedation drug pharmacokinetics by inhibiting or enhancing liver metabolism, leading to increased or decreased serum concentrations of sedatives. Prescribed medications such as erythromycin and cimetidine can inhibit the cytochrome P450 system, leading to prolonged sedation. Anticonvulsant medications can also lead to tolerance for some sedatives. A careful medical history including drug and environmental allergies, a family history, and a thorough review of systems is essential. Physical examination should include the infant's age and weight, baseline vital signs, and evaluation of the airway and pulmonary, cardiac system, neurologic system, and ASA status.

This evaluation should focus on the infant's airway, looking for anatomic airway abnormalities as well as enlarged tonsils which may predispose the infant to airway obstruction while sedated. The pulmonary status of the infant should be evaluated to determine whether the infant will be able to maintain effective spontaneous ventilation while sedated. A careful evaluation of the child's neurocognitive development is important – children with delays have more adverse events during sedation compared with normally developing children [6].

## Fasting

Almost all sedatives can, in a dose-related manner, impair protective airway reflexes. Since most airways are not "protected" by endotracheal intubation, pulmonary aspiration of gastric contents is a risk in sedated infants. Although the risk of aspiration is likely to be less than that found in general anesthesia, the absolute risk is unknown so it is prudent for elective sedation cases to follow the same fasting rules as for elective general anesthesia in infants. The recommendations from the ASA guidelines on pediatric sedation are the same as for general anesthesia. For infants, the suggested fasting times are two hours for clear liquids, four hours for breast milk, and six hours for solids or infant formulas. However, there is very little evidence that shows an effect on preoperative fasting in infants and later adverse events during procedures requiring sedation. For emergency procedures of short duration, the risks and benefits of doing sedation versus a general anesthetic need to be evaluated on a case-by-case basis.

## Monitoring

Monitoring of infants during procedures requiring sedation should include continuous heart rate and pulse oximetry and blood pressure and respiratory rates every five minutes. One of the factors associated with adverse events in children undergoing procedural sedation is failure to monitor patients appropriately [6]. Capnography is not essential but is very helpful during procedural sedation. There is a time lag of seconds to minutes between the onset of apnea and oxygen desaturation. When this is coupled with the fact that infants are often sedated in locations where the sedation provider is in the next room observing the infant, and not immediately at the patient's bedside, the need for a more sensitive monitor for apnea is apparent. Surveillance for apnea is enhanced by a factor of 17 when capnography is used compared to monitoring without capnography [7]. Capnography of infants can be accomplished by placing a small cannula either in a face mask or in the nares. These are sometimes not well tolerated by infants, especially those that are minimally or moderately sedated. Newer respiratory monitors such as acoustic impedance monitoring, which measures acoustically the infant's respiratory rate by an adhesive sensor placed on the neck, may be better tolerated. In the postsedation care unit, standard monitoring should be used until the infant is fully conscious.

## Sedation Record

Infants undergoing sedation should have continuous monitoring of their oxygen saturation, heart rate, and ventilation by capnography and intermittent noninvasive blood pressure monitoring. A sedation record should be kept that notes values for the heart rate, respiratory rate, blood pressure, oxygen saturation, and expired carbon dioxide values every five minutes. This record should also note the medications and fluid the infant has received as well as any events, adverse or otherwise, that occur during the sedation or recovery period after the procedure is complete. The fasting time should also be recorded. For elective sedations, fasting times should mirror fasting times for elective procedures. For emergencies, the risks of aspiration

or other adverse event from a full stomach should be balanced against the benefits of sedation to perform needed procedures.

## Post-Procedure

Infants that have received moderate sedation should recover in a setting where they are closely observed and where there is the capacity to deliver positive pressure ventilation, to suction secretions and to oxygenate with greater than 90 percent oxygen. Vital signs should be monitored every ten minutes. Infants that have received longer-acting sedatives may be observed in a stepdown unit until they have returned completely to baseline in terms of sedation. The observation period for those patients who have received reversal agents such as naloxone or flumazenil needs to be prolonged because resedation can occur after the antagonist action has subsided.

## Medications

### Midazolam

Midazolam is a short-acting benzodiazepine with sedative, amnestic, anxiolytic, anticonvulsant, and muscle relaxant properties. It binds to the gamma amino butyric acid receptor (GABA), one of the brain's major inhibitory neurotransmitters. It has a very fast onset of action when administered intravenously, but can be given orally, mucosally (rectal, nasal, or sublingual), and intramuscularly. Adverse reactions include hypoventilation, oxygen desaturation, apnea, hypotension, and paradoxical excitement. It is a relatively weak sedative when given in standard doses (0.05–0.1 mg $kg^{-1}$ IV initial dose) for infants >6 months and thus is inadequate for procedural sedation when given alone. Adequate sedation can occur when it is combined with other sedative/hypnotic drugs such as fentanyl, ketamine, dexmedetomidine, or propofol, although the risk of respiratory depression and hemodynamic changes may be increased. It has been used as an infusion for neonatal intensive care sedation, but in preterm infants it has been associated with lower blood pressures, adverse neurologic events, and an increased stay in a NICU [8]. Despite concerns about its safety in the NICU setting, a retrospective review of a large database consisting of information on infants admitted to the NICU from 2005 through 2010 in the United States found that midazolam was one of the most commonly prescribed drugs [9].

## Propofol

Propofol is a sedative hypnotic that is believed to act through potentiation of the $GABA_A$ receptor and act as a sodium channel blocker. It is metabolized by conjugation in the liver with a half-life in older children and adults of 2–24 hours, although its clinical effect is much shorter. The median clearance and volume of distribution at steady state is decreased in preterm and term neonates compared with older infants [10,11]. However, infants ages 2–6 months have a higher volume of distribution and clearance than older infants and children [12]. Although one trial found propofol to be superior to morphine, atropine, and suxamethonium for intubation for surfactant administration in preterm infants, another trial in premature infants found that even a low dose of 1 mg kg$^{-1}$ of proprofol led to moderate hypotension for longer than ten minutes after administration [13,14].

In older infants and children, propofol is the most commonly used sedation agent for procedural sedation directed by a pediatric anesthesiologist. It has a higher incidence of hemodynamic and respiratory adverse events compared with dexmedetomidine, which is the reason that most institutions only permit anesthesiologists or critical care specialists to administer it. Its benefit over other agents is its rapid onset and rapid recovery times. A review of over 90 000 pediatric procedural sedations found an incidence of 5 percent for adverse events. The most commonly reported event was airway obstruction (1.6 percent), desaturation (1.5 percent), coughing (1 percent), and emergent airway intervention (0.7 percent) [15]. Risk factors included low weight, prematurity, ASA status, upper and lower respiratory diagnoses, and sedation for painful procedures. Propofol has very little analgesic property, so for some painful procedures some centers combine it with a low-dose narcotic infusion such as remifentanil or low doses of ketamine.

## Ketamine

Ketamine is a noncompetitive antagonist of the N-methyl-D-aspartate receptor (NMDAR) which is responsible for its anesthetic, amnesic, dissociative, and hallucinogenic effects. It is also an inhibitor of the reuptake of serotonin, dopamine, and norepinephrine, which contributes to increased sympathetic tone including bronchodilation, although ketamine is also a myocardial depressant. It has analgesic properties because it blocks NMDA receptors in the dorsal horn of the spinal cord, preventing transmission of nociceptive impulses to the brain. Ketamine is biotransformed in the liver to norketamine, which has one-third the potency as an anesthetic of ketamine. There is a paucity of pharmacokinetic and pharmacodynamic data about the actions of ketamine in neonates and preterm infants. One study found that an intravenous dose of 2 mg kg$^{-1}$ was effective in decreasing pain during endotracheal suctioning in ventilated neonates [16]. It is associated with anesthetic-induced neurotoxicity in immature animals and thus is not recommended for routine sedation of very young infants. In an evidence-based practice guideline published in the *Annals of Emergency Medicine*, it was suggested that ketamine never be administered to infants less than three months of age because of laryngospasm and other airway concerns [17]. Although many emergency rooms do not permit the use of ketamine in infants less than 12 months of age, there is little evidence to suggest that older infants are at an enhanced risk from airway adverse events compared with very young children. The incidence of laryngospasm following ketamine sedation is low at 0.4 percent and is usually easily treated with assisted ventilation and oxygen [18]. It can be administered by almost any route imaginable, but is most commonly administered intravenously, intramuscularly, or orally.

## Triclofos and Chloral Hydrate

Triclofos and chloral hydrate are prodrugs that are metabolized in the liver to the active drug trichlorethanol (TCE). Triclofos is slightly less potent than chloral hydrate (600 mg of chloral hydrate =1 g of triclofos). TCE binds to the $GABA_A$ receptors to induce sedation. In neonates given a single dose, the peak concentration of serum TCE occurred 1–12 hours later. The average elimination half-life was 37 hours, which was more than three times longer than the elimination half-life for adults [19].

A significant relationship exists between TCE half-life and age, with preterm infants averaging 39 hours, term infants averaging 27 hours, and older infants and children averaging 10 hours. There is also a relationship between peak concentrations and age, with peak concentrations declining with increasing age [20]. A retrospective cohort study of over 1000 infants who received chloral hydrate for sedation for MRIs found that 20 percent of all patients required supplemental oxygen to maintain an oxygen saturation

>90 percent during the procedure [21]. Young infants receiving chloral hydrate should be monitored during and after the procedure to prevent apnea and airway obstruction. A review of over 405 infants and children who received chloral hydrate for sedation for cardiac echography found that the average dose used was 77 mg kg$^{-1}$, with a range of 25–125 mg kg$^{-1}$ [22]. Adequate sedation was achieved in 98 percent of the children, with 82 percent achieving it within 30 minutes. Children younger than age three were more likely to be successfully sedated, and 6 percent of patients required supplemental oxygen to maintain adequate oxygen saturation. Drawbacks of chloral hydration as a sedative in children include a prolonged onset of action, a prolonged duration of action, and lack of reversibility.

In a large pediatric review of 95 adverse events associated with pediatric sedation, it was found that chloral hydrate was the medication most associated with adverse events in the nonhospital setting [6]. Almost half of the 15 cases of adverse events associated with chloral hydrate resulted in death or permanent neurologic injury. In ten of the cases, chloral hydrate was administered with another sedative and in five of the cases it was the sole medication administered.

## Dexmedetomidine

Dexmedetomidine is an anxiolytic, sedative agent with some analgesic properties. It is an alpha-adrenergic agonist similar to clonidine. It is associated with less respiratory depression than GABA$_A$ agonists. However, it is associated with effects on blood pressure, with low doses causing decreased blood pressure and higher doses associated with elevated blood pressures from baseline [23]. It has not been studied extensively in neonates, but a small safety, efficacy, and pharmacokinetic study of preterm and term infants found that there were very few adverse reactions [24]. In preterm infants less than 36 weeks' postconceptual age, the plasma clearance at 0.3 L h$^{-1}$ was only one-third that of term neonates from 36 weeks to 44 weeks at 0.9 L h$^{-1}$. The elimination half-life for the preterm infant was more than double that of the term infant at 7.6 and 3.2 hours, respectively. The dosing regimen in this study was much less than the doses given to older infants and children. The three escalating dosing regimens were a loading dose of 0.1 mg kg$^{-1}$ followed by an infusion of 0.1 mg kg$^{-1}$ h$^{-1}$, a loading dose of 0.2 mg kg$^{-1}$ followed by an infusion of 0.2 mg kg$^{-1}$ h$^{-1}$, and a loading dose of 0.3 mg kg$^{-1}$ followed by an infusion of 0.3 mg kg$^{-1}$ h$^{-1}$.

The dosing of dexmedetomidine in older infants for procedural sedation can be high. Failure rates are up to 10–15 percent of infants and children receiving 1–1.5 µg kg$^{-1}$ bolus followed by an infusion of 1–1.5 µg kg$^{-1}$ min$^{-1}$ [25]. In a large cohort study, increasing the loading dose and infusion to a loading dose of 2–3 µg kg$^{-1}$ and 2–3 µg kg$^{-1}$ min$^{-1}$ increased the success rate for sedation to 97.6 percent [26]. However, this was accompanied by a 16 percent incidence of bradycardia, with several toddlers developing heart rates less than 50 bpm. When dexmedetomidine was paired with midazolam, it provided superior sedation with stable hemodynamics with tachycardia prevention when used postoperatively for sedation following pediatric cardiac surgery [27].

**Table 37.1** Key components of the presedation evaluation

| | |
|---|---|
| 1 | Demographic data: patient's name, age, weight, and sex |
| 2 | Past medical history |
| | Comorbid medical conditions including history of snoring suggestive of obstructive sleep apnea |
| | Acute medical conditions |
| | Previous sedation and anesthetic history |
| 3 | Allergies |
| 4 | Current medications |
| 5 | Family history of anesthetic complications |
| 6. | Nil per os status |
| 7 | Social history |
| | Tobacco or illicit drug use |
| | Exposure to second-hand tobacco smoke |
| 8 | Perceived urgency for the procedure |
| 9 | Pregnancy history |
| | Mandatory screening may be indicated based on institutional guidelines |
| 10 | Physical examination |
| | Baseline vital signs including room air oxygen saturation |
| | Airway examination |
| | Cardiac and pulmonary examination |
| 11 | Laboratory evaluation (if appropriate) |
| 12. | Summary statement including ASA status |
| 13 | Plan |
| 14 | Risks discussed and informed consent obtained |

ASA, American Society of Anesthesiologists.

Recovery times, especially when large doses of dexmedetomidine are used, are prolonged, especially compared with propofol. But even with high doses of dexmedetomidine, airway reflexes and patency and normal ventilation are maintained.

## Conclusion

The role of procedural sedation in the care of young infants is extremely important. Many procedures formerly done in the operating room are now being done less invasively in the radiologic suites, gastrointestinal suites, and procedure rooms. It is necessary for all practitioners performing sedations on infants to provide the safest possible environment for these patients. Understanding the unique challenges that infants undergoing sedation present with will minimize the chance that these vulnerable patients suffer an adverse event.

## References

1. Fogel MA, Pawlowski TW, Harris MA, et al. Comparison and usefulness of cardiac magnetic resonance versus computed tomography in infants six months of age or younger with aortic arch anomalies without deep sedation or anesthesia. *Am J Cardiol.* 2011;108:120–5.

2. Windram J, Grosse-Wortmann L, Shariat M, et al. Cardiovascular MRI without sedation or general anesthesia using a feed-and-sleep technique in neonates and infants. *Pediatr Radiol.* 2012;42:183–7.

3. Cote CJ, Wilson S. Guidelines for monitoring and management of pediatric patients during and after sedation for diagnostic and therapeutic procedures: an update. *Pediatrics.* 2006;118:2587–602.

4. Malviya S, Voepel-Lewis T, Tait AR, et al. Depth of sedation in children undergoing computed tomography: validity and reliability of the University of Michigan Sedation Scale (UMSS). *Br J Anaesth.* 2002;88:241–5.

5. Hummel P, Puchalski M, Creech SD, Weiss MG. Clinical reliability and validity of the N-PASS: neonatal pain, agitation and sedation scale with prolonged pain. *J Perinatol.* 2008;28:55–60.

6. Cote CJ, Karl HW, Notterman DA, Weinberg JA, McCloskey C. Adverse sedation events in pediatrics: analysis of medications used for sedation. *Pediatrics.* 2000;106:633–44.

7. Waugh JB, Epps CA, Khodneva YA. Capnography enhances surveillance of respiratory events during procedural sedation: a meta-analysis. *J Clin Anesth.* 2011;23:189–96.

8. Anand KJ, Barton BA, McIntosh N, et al. Analgesia and sedation in preterm neonates who require ventilatory support: results from the NOPAIN trial. Neonatal Outcome and Prolonged Analgesia in Neonates. *Arch Pediatr Adolesc Med.* 1999;153:331–8.

9. Hsieh EM, Hornik CP, Clark RH, et al. Medication use in the neonatal intensive care unit. *Am J Perinatol.* 2014;31:811–21.

10. Allegaert K, Peeters MY, Knibbe C. Propofol in (pre) term neonates: consider the extensive interindividual variability in clearance within the neonatal population. *Paediatr Anaesth.* 2011;21:174–5.

11. Allegaert K, Peeters MY, Verbesselt R, et al. Inter-individual variability in propofol pharmacokinetics in preterm and term neonates. *Br J Anaesth.* 2007;99:864–70.

12. Sarhan TS, El-attar, A. Propofol pharmacokinetics in infants: BAPCAP1–1. *Eur J Anaesthesiol.* 2010;27:1.

13. Ghanta S, Abdel-Latif ME, Lui K, et al. Propofol compared with the morphine, atropine, and suxamethonium regimen as induction agents for neonatal endotracheal intubation: a randomized, controlled trial. *Pediatrics.* 2007;119: e1248–55.

14. Welzing L, Kribs A, Eifinger F, et al. Propofol as an induction agent for endotracheal intubation can cause significant arterial hypotension in preterm neonates. *Paediatr Anaesth.* 2010;20:605–11.

15. Kamat PP, McCracken CE, Gillespie SE, et al. Pediatric critical care physician-administered procedural sedation using propofol: a report from the Pediatric Sedation Research Consortium Database. *Pediatr Crit Care Med.* 2015;16:11–20.

16. Saarenmaa E, Neuvonen PJ, Huttunen P, Fellman V. Ketamine for procedural pain relief in newborn infants. *Arch Dis Child Fetal Neonatal Ed.* 2001;85: F53–6.

17. Green SM, Krauss B. Clinical practice guideline for emergency department ketamine dissociative sedation in children. *Ann Emerg Med.* 2004;44:460–71.

18. Green SM, Rothrock SG, Lynch EL, et al. Intramuscular ketamine for pediatric sedation in the emergency department: safety profile in 1,022 cases. *Ann Emerg Med.* 1998;31:688–97.

19. Ghershanik JJ Boecler B, Lertora JJL, et al. Monitoring levels of trichloroethanol during chloral hydrate administration to sick neonates [abstract]. *Clin Res.* 1981;29:895.

20. Mayers DJ, Hindmarsh KW, Sankaran K, Gorecki DK, Kasian GF. Chloral hydrate disposition following single-dose administration to critically ill neonates and children. *Dev Pharmacol Ther.* 1991;16:71–7.

21. Litman RS, Soin K, Salam A. Chloral hydrate sedation in term and preterm infants: an analysis of efficacy and complications. *Anesth Analg.* 2010;110:739–46.

22. Napoli KL, Ingall CG, Martin GR. Safety and efficacy of chloral hydrate sedation in children undergoing echocardiography. *J Pediatr.* 1996;129(2):287–91.

23. Ebert TJ, Hall JE, Barney JA, Uhrich TD, Colinco MD. The effects of increasing plasma concentrations of dexmedetomidine in humans. *Anesthesiology.* 2000;93:382–94.

24. Chrysostomou C, Schulman SR, Herrera Castellanos M, et al. A phase II/III, multicenter, safety, efficacy, and pharmacokinetic study of dexmedetomidine in preterm and term neonates. *J Pediatr.* 2014;164:276–82 e1–3.

25. Tobias JD. Sedation of infants and children outside of the operating room. *Curr Opin Anaesthesiol.* 2015;28:478–85.

26. Mason KP, Zurakowski D, Zgleszewski SE, et al. High dose dexmedetomidine as the sole sedative for pediatric MRI. *Paediatr Anaesth.* 2008;18:403–11.

27. Hasegawa T, Oshima Y, Maruo A, et al. Dexmedetomidine in combination with midazolam after pediatric cardiac surgery. *Asian Cardiovasc Thorac Ann.* 2015;23:802–8.

Chapter

# 38

# Ambulatory Anesthesia in Infants

Sharon Redd and Ethan Sanford

Perioperative risk assessment and management is increasingly an important role for pediatric anesthesiologists. Balancing operating room schedules, hospital costs, and patient care needs is challenging. Evidence addressing perioperative risk for elective procedures in pediatric patients has accumulated over the past 20 years in an effort to guide decision-making.

There are many considerations to be weighed before doing ambulatory surgery on an infant. First and foremost, it is important to educate family members about the postoperative care of infants. Infants whose family structure is unstable or whose family members are uncomfortable caring for an infant who has had recent surgery are not good candidates for ambulatory surgery. It is also important to manage parental expectations during and after the surgical procedure. It is generally not recommended to allow parents into the operating room for a parent-present induction until the child has demonstrated some stranger anxiety. This is a normal developmental stage of infants and generally occurs around nine months of age.

Ambulatory facility requirements in free-standing surgical centers or as part of a larger hospital are identical [1]. An anesthesiologist who is trained in pediatric anesthesia and has regular or special clinical privileges to take care of infants and children should administer the pediatric anesthesia service in an ambulatory surgical center. There should be dedicated preoperative evaluation areas that offer privacy and a comforting environment suited to pediatric patients. The operating rooms should be equipped with age-appropriate equipment and medications and equipment to maintain normothermia in infants. There should be a resuscitation cart also equipped with age-appropriate equipment, including pediatric defibrillator paddles. In the PACU there should be a dedicated area for infants and children manned by nurses who are comfortable and competent in taking

care of young patients. Finally, there should be an agreement with an inpatient pediatric facility to admit infants that require further care after an ambulatory procedure.

## Age Considerations

The minimum age for ambulatory surgery has been decreasing as general anesthesia has become safer for very young infants. In the past, many institutions used a rule of four – the infants had to be born full term and be at least 44 weeks postconceptual age, be at least four weeks old, and be at least 4 kg in weight. A survey published in 2007 querying 44 ACGME-accredited pediatric anesthesiology programs in the United States found that 23 percent had no policy with regards to age for full-term infants and 58 percent allowed ambulatory surgery in full-term infants who had reached a postconceptual age between 41 and 44 weeks [2].

Infants born preterm are at higher risk for postoperative apnea after receiving general anesthesia. In a large meta-analysis, the risk of postoperative apnea diminished to less than 1 percent when preterm infants reached a postconceptual age of 56 weeks [3]. Other studies have shown the risk of postoperative apnea is inversely related to the postconceptual age of the infant and positively related to the gestational age at birth of the infant [4]. A recent prospective study known as the GAS trial examined risk factors for postoperative apnea of 359 infants undergoing sevoflurane general anesthesia and found that the risk factors for postoperative apnea included prematurity, decreasing gestational age at birth, decreasing weight, decreasing postmenstrual age, a history of recent apnea, methylxanthine receipt, endotracheal intubation, and ventilation or oxygen support [5].

This study found that there was a higher risk of postoperative apnea in infants who received general anesthesia compared to those who received regional anesthesia, but only in the first half-hour postoperatively. A possible limitation of this study is that the apnea was diagnosed clinically rather than by pneumograph or other monitoring methods. This study did not find an association between postoperative apnea and anemia (hematocrit <30 percent), but other studies have [5,6]. The GAS trial would suggest that young infants should be monitored for at least 12 hours postoperatively.

There is no consensus in the pediatric anesthesia community about the minimum age for ambulatory surgery in infants born prematurely. A recent survey of pediatric anesthesia programs found that 13 percent allowed ambulatory surgery once preterm infants reached a postconceptual age of 45–49 weeks, 58 percent at 50–55 weeks, 10 percent at 55–59 weeks, and 26 percent after 60 weeks, respectively [2].

## Concurrent Upper Respiratory Infections

A frequently encountered dilemma in pediatric anesthesia is the infant or child with an upper respiratory tract infection presenting for an elective procedure

(Figure 38.1). An association between infections of the respiratory tract and perioperative adverse events has long been known from clinical experience; this section reviews the literature with respect to pediatric respiratory tract infections (URIs) and anesthesia. In a community-based study, pediatric patients were found to have 3–8 respiratory illnesses each year. Importantly, children <1 year of age had the highest mean incidence per year at 6.1 [7].

Early studies focusing on risk factors for perioperative respiratory events, such as laryngospasm and bronchospasm, found a strong link to concurrent URI. This is clearly important to pediatric clinicians as ~30 percent of perioperative cardiac arrests in children are due to respiratory events [8]. Overall incidence of respiratory events in pediatric anesthesia is 5–15 percent. In children with URI, this risk increases to 15–27 percent [9–13]. More recently, clinicians have focused on which clinical symptoms and history better predict those at risk and anesthetic techniques that might mitigate those risks.

An effective model used in other reviews categorizes patient risk factors for respiratory events into three groups as follows.

**Figure 38.1** Decision-making guide.

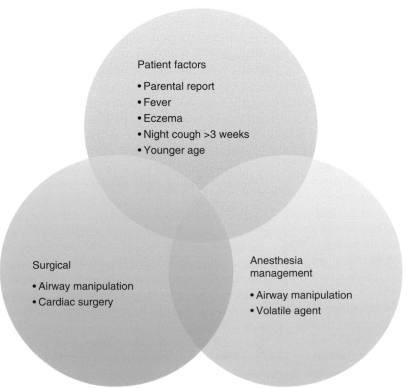

Patient factors

• Parental report
• Fever
• Eczema
• Night cough >3 weeks
• Younger age

Surgical

• Airway manipulation
• Cardiac surgery

Anesthesia management

• Airway manipulation
• Volatile agent

## Patient-Related Risk Factors

The preponderance of clinical studies demonstrates that concurrent URI as defined by clinical symptoms or parental history has been linked to respiratory events [9–11]. Studies proposing to discern what clinical factors carry the greater risk have found varied results. In the largest prospective study to date, certain historical factors were significant predictors of risk: parental report of fever, nocturnal dry cough, wheezing more than three times in the preceding month, and a history of eczema [9].

If concurrent URI increases risk, when is it safe to proceed with a general anesthetic after a patient has an infection? Scheduling elective procedures, especially in young patients, can be burdensome for parents and multiple procedural delays can impede quality of care and the infant's development. Many centers advise that four weeks pass after a URI prior to planned anesthetic. This is based on persistence of cough for this time interval and some inconclusive data. More recently, two weeks appears to be a safe interval of time to proceed [9,10].

Two other factors consistently appear as significant factors in risk stratification. Younger patients have had more respiratory events in nearly every study. There is an approximately 11 percent decrease in relative risk for each yearly increase in age [9]. Passive exposure to smoking has also been significantly linked in a majority of studies [14]. Comorbid conditions, especially involving the respiratory tract, increase risk and exacerbate morbid effects of respiratory events. Respiratory syncytial virus (RSV) infection, active asthma exacerbation, prematurity, bronchopulmonary disease, cystic fibrosis, pneumonia, anatomic airway anomalies, and pulmonary hypertension should be investigated prior to anesthetic administration in order to plan for a safe anesthetic and to adequately inform parents about the risks of general anesthesia.

## Anesthesia-Related Risk Factors

When anesthesia must be induced in a patient with concurrent URI, some techniques may be better than others. Several studies in children have shown that inhalational general anesthesia with facemask is associated with fewer complications than endotracheal intubation [9,12]. This is consistent with the theory that inflamed airways are more sensitive to physical manipulation, thus instrumentation of the airway should be avoided when possible. Further, only experienced providers should manipulate the infant's airway in order to avoid many attempts to secure the airway.

The use of laryngeal mask airways (LMAs) as opposed to endotracheal tube (ETT) in the setting of URI is less clear, with several reports offering different conclusions [9,11,15,16]. However, LMA use may pose greater risk for laryngospasm when removed in conscious infants rather than done when the infants are deeply unconscious (deep extubation). Caution should be exercised in LMA removal in awake infants with URI as the LMA continues to stimulate the airway without preventing obstruction at the level of the larynx.

Anesthetic agents also offer differing safety profiles. Intravenous induction and maintenance with propofol should be considered in infants with active URIs. Care should be taken to avoid hypotension in very young infants who are given propofol because they are more prone to this compared to older children and adults. Volatile agents are known to increase airway sensitivity. Despite sevoflurane's improved safety profile over agents such as desflurane and halothane, the instance of laryngospasm with volatile agents is increased compared than the intravenous agents [9]. Although it is sometimes difficult to place an intravenous line preoperatively in an infant, it should be considered if the infant has an active URI.

Several other techniques have been used to mitigate respiratory events in pediatric anesthesia, with varying reports of success. Topical lidocaine spray of larynx/vocal cords may attenuate airway reactivity, though administration of the spray itself can cause laryngospasm [17]. Preoperative use of bronchodilator therapy is also a relatively benign intervention, with some limited reports of efficacy [18]. These interventions may be helpful especially in specific patient populations (history of wheeze/asthma/passive smoke exposure) or surgical procedures (airway surgery).

## Surgery-Related Risk Factors

Similar to anesthetic technique, the surgical procedures that involve manipulation of the airway carry higher risk of respiratory events both in the operating room and in the postoperative care unit (PACU). Some infants with chronic upper airway infections require surgical procedures to alleviate their conditions. Thus, resolution of symptoms such as cough or congestion may not be feasible. Providers should take this under consideration when delaying cases, especially in patients who have already undergone prior delays. Cardiac surgery patients have also been shown to have worse outcomes when concurrent URI is present [18]. Tonsillectomies are rarely done in infants less than one year and almost always done in this age group because of moderate to severe obstructive sleep apnea. These infants are not candidates for ambulatory procedures and need to be cared for in a monitored bed situation postoperatively.

There are also procedures in infants that need to be performed in a time-sensitive manner. Conditions such as cranial synostosis, cleft palate, and strabismus, if not repaired during a particular developmental window, can lead to long-term deficits in infants. Some of the procedures are usually done on an ambulatory basis, such as dental appliance insertion for cleft palate and strabismus. In the setting of an active URI, if the surgical determination is that the procedure cannot be delayed, then planning for a postoperative observation admission should be considered.

Newborns undergoing invasive procedures present many unique challenges for clinicians. The presence of URI in this population has been clearly linked with respiratory events. This risk must be balanced with benefits of the procedure. The younger the infant, the greater the risk and, therefore, more caution is advised. Querying family about symptoms, especially fever, cough, and wheeze, is critical. Also considering the surgical procedure and how it might influence complications is important. In circumstances in which anesthesia is needed, techniques minimizing airway manipulation and exposure to volatile anesthetics have been found to mitigate risk. Neonates with a comorbid disease including a URI are not candidates for ambulatory surgery.

The decision to permit ambulatory surgery in young infants is dependent on the postoperative pain requirements of the infants. There is no consensus within the pediatric anesthesia community on what the minimum age for ambulatory surgery should be to permit infants to be treated postoperatively with narcotics. Many centers will admit infants less than six months of age if it is felt that their postoperative pain is great enough to warrant narcotic therapy. Regional and peripheral nerve blocks administered while the infants are anesthetized can effectively control postoperative pain in many cases. In general, postoperative pain in infants can be treated with acetaminophen in ambulatory cases.

# Infants With Chronic Disease

Although the vast majority of infants having ambulatory surgery will be healthy and classified as having an ASA I or II status, there are an increasing number of children with chronic illnesses also being seen in ambulatory surgery. Some of the chronic illnesses seen include infants with epilepsy, bronchospastic disorders, cystic fibrosis, repaired or unrepaired congenital heart disease, and those that have undergone organ transplantation. Careful preoperative screening should be done to determine whether these patients are suitable candidates for day surgery. Preoperative consultation and planning with pediatric specialists and surgeons can allow many of these complex and chronically ill infants to have their procedures done on an outpatient basis. Very often these patients will need preoperative blood work to determine that their medication levels such as digoxin and anticonvulsant levels are within the normal range. Since some of these medications can affect liver, renal function, and hematopoietic function, preoperative laboratory studies may be warranted. Most patients should receive their chronic medications on the day of the procedure. It is wise to consult with the cardiologist for all patients with cardiac disease prior to an ambulatory general anesthetic. For these patients, very often diuretics and antihypertensives are held in anticipation of the vasodilatory effects of general anesthesia. Venous air embolism precautions may be necessary for those patients with an intra- or extracardiac shunt.

# References

1.  American Society of Anesthesiologists. Statement on practice recommendations for pediatric anesthesia, 2011

2.  Castro PE. At what age is ambulatory surgery safe in infants? A survey of practices of pediatric anesthesiology programs in the United States. Society for Pediatric Anesthesia Winter Meeting, 2007

3.  Cote CJ, Zaslavsky A, Downes JJ, et al. Postoperative apnea in former preterm infants after inguinal herniorrhaphy: a combined analysis. *Anesthesiology*. 1995;82:809–22.

4.  Kurth CD, Spitzer AR, Broennle AM, Downes JJ. Postoperative apnea in preterm infants. *Anesthesiology*. 1987;66:483–8.

5.  Davidson AJ, Morton NS, Arnup SJ, et al. Apnea after awake regional and general anesthesia in infants: the general anesthesia compared to spinal anesthesia study – comparing apnea and neurodevelopmental

outcomes, a randomized controlled trial. *Anesthesiology*. 2015;123(1):38–54.

6. Welborn LG, Hannallah RS, Luban NL, Fink R, Ruttimann UE. Anemia and postoperative apnea in former preterm infants. *Anesthesiology*. 1991;74:1003–6.

7. Monto AS, Ullman BM. Acute respiratory illness in an American community: the Tecumseh study. *JAMA*. 1974;227:164–9.

8. Bhananker SM, Ramamoorthy C, Geiduschek JM, et al. Anesthesia-related cardiac arrest in children: update from the Pediatric Perioperative Cardiac Arrest Registry. *Anesth Analg*. 2007;105:344–50.

9. von Ungern-Sternberg BS, Boda K, Chambers NA, et al. Risk assessment for respiratory complications in paediatric anaesthesia: a prospective cohort study. *Lancet*. 2010;376:773–83.

10. Flick RP, Wilder RT, Pieper SF, et al. Risk factors for laryngospasm in children during general anesthesia. *Paediatr Anaesth*. 2008;18:289–96.

11. Rachel Homer J, Elwood T, Peterson D, Rampersad S. Risk factors for adverse events in children with colds emerging from anesthesia: a logistic regression. *Paediatr Anaesth*. 2007;17:154–61.

12. Mamie C, Habre W, Delhumeau C, Argiroffo CB, Morabia A. Incidence and risk factors of perioperative respiratory adverse events in children undergoing elective surgery. *Paediatr Anaesth*. 2004;14:218–24.

13. Tait AR, Malviya S, Voepel-Lewis T, et al. Risk factors for perioperative adverse respiratory events in children with upper respiratory tract infections. *Anesthesiology*. 2001;95:299–306.

14. Seyidov TH, Elemen L, Solak M, Tugay M, Toker K. Passive smoke exposure is associated with perioperative adverse effects in children. *J Clin Anesth*. 2011;23:47–52.

15. Tait AR, Pandit UA, Voepel-Lewis T, Munro HM, Malviya S. Use of the laryngeal mask airway in children with upper respiratory tract infections: a comparison with endotracheal intubation. *Anesth Analg*. 1998;86:706–11.

16. von Ungern-Sternberg BS, Boda K, Schwab C, et al. Laryngeal mask airway is associated with an increased incidence of adverse respiratory events in children with recent upper respiratory tract infections. *Anesthesiology*. 2007;107:714–19.

17. Hamilton ND, Hegarty M, Calder A, Erb TO, von Ungern-Sternberg BS. Does topical lidocaine before tracheal intubation attenuate airway responses in children? An observational audit. *Paediatr Anaesth*. 2012;22:345–50.

18. Scalfaro P, Sly PD, Sims C, Habre W. Salbutamol prevents the increase of respiratory resistance caused by tracheal intubation during sevoflurane anesthesia in asthmatic children. *Anesth Analg*. 2001;93:898–902.

**Chapter**

**39**

# Apnea and Bradycardia

Puneet Sayal and Samuel Rodriguez

## Introduction

The risk of apnea and bradycardia in infants and neonates, both premature and full-term, has been described in the literature as early as the 1980s [1,2]. Many premature neonates have apneic episodes periodically, and this is exacerbated in the postoperative period [3]. The most commonly used definition of apnea of prematurity (AOP) specifies a pause of breathing for more than 15–20 s, or accompanied by oxygen desaturation ($SpO_2 \leq 80$ percent for $\geq 4$ s) and bradycardia (heart rate less than two-thirds of baseline for $\geq 4$ s) in infants born less than 37 weeks' gestation [4,5]. Apnea can be further subdivided into either central or obstructive apnea. Central apnea is secondary to absent diaphragmatic activity, and alone accounts for approximately 40 percent of apnea in infancy. Obstructive apnea (OA) is defined as the inability to ventilate, despite continued respiratory effort secondary to physical obstruction at some point in the airway, and alone accounts for only 10 percent of apneas. Mixed apnea, defined as a combination of central and OA, accounts for 50 percent of apneas. Some infants with obstructive sleep apnea also have disordered, immature reflexes to hypercapnia and hypoxia, predisposing them to apneic episodes [6]. The most common form of mixed apnea starts with central apnea and progresses to include an obstructive component. Bradycardia in an infant is defined as a heart rate less than 80 bpm for any period of time, and is frequently associated with an apneic episode [7].

As apnea and bradycardia of infancy has been further studied, the pathophysiology, risk factors, and treatment/prevention strategies are being better understood. The differential diagnosis includes periodic breathing, subtle seizures, and primary cardiac conditions [8]. Periodic breathing, defined as hypoventilation with two breathing pauses in 20 seconds, is not a precursor to apnea [9]. The natural progression of an apneic episode was described by Daily et al. as an episode in which for the initial 20–30 seconds the infant appeared well-perfused and did not show signs of distress and subsequently became cyanotic, lost muscle tone, and proceeded to unresponsiveness rapidly [5].

## Incidence

The incidence of postoperative apnea and bradycardia has been estimated to be as high as 49 percent, although recent meta-analyses place the incidence closer to 5 percent, occurring in 20–30 percent of preterm infants in the first month of life [2,8,10,11]. The onset of AOP generally occurs after 1–2 days of life and peaks in frequency at 5–7 days of life [5,8]. The risk of apnea increases with the degree of prematurity and the risk decreases with birth weight. As premature infants approach a postconceptual age (gestational age at birth + age since birth) of 60 weeks the risk of postoperative apnea diminishes and approaches zero (see Figure 39.1) [5,12]. Most studies have focused on premature infants, although there are case reports of full-term infants with comorbidities and congenital defects having apneic episodes in the postoperative period [13–15].

## Pathophysiology

The pathophysiology of AOP has been postulated to be multifactorial, stemming from immature chemoreceptor function, lung muscle mechanics, airway anatomy, and contributions from specific comorbidities.

Central chemoreceptor function and immature brainstem respiratory control has been postulated as the basis for central apnea. A number of studies demonstrating a higher resting $PaCO_2$, flattened/right-shifted $CO_2$ response curve, upregulated peripheral chemoreceptor activity, and an increased ventilatory response to hypoxia relative to hypercapnia in premature infants exhibiting apneic episodes support

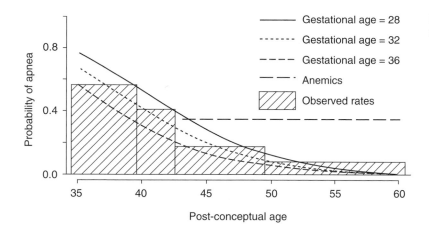

**Figure 39.1** Incidence of apnea at each postconceptual age. Source: [12].

this theory [8,11]. Rigatto et al. further demonstrated mature activity of peripheral chemoreceptors by 28 weeks' gestation, suggesting they are unlikely to be involved in periodic breathing or apnea [16,17]. Knill et al. also demonstrated that peripheral chemoreceptor responses were abolished under halothane anesthesia, furthering the idea that the peripheral chemoreceptors are unlikely to be involved in the increased risk postoperatively [18].

The lungs of premature infants are prone to early fatigue and being overworked, coupled with an increased incidence of pulmonary comorbidities in this age group [2,11]. Increased compliance of the rib cage demands increased diaphragmatic work, and this distorts the chest wall, creating a decreased distending force on the lungs. This combined with tachypnea can lead to early respiratory muscle fatigue [11]. Keens demonstrated that with chronically increased respiratory work, diaphragmatic changes included increased oxidative capacity (where previously it was relatively low) and additional slow-twitch fiber acquisition [19]. Tachypnea, causing an increased respiratory load, results from a variety of stimuli, such as halothane anesthesia and discomfort from the operation itself [2]. Anesthetics can also cause increased respiratory work, depending relatively more on diaphragmatic than intercostal muscle work as the intercostals are recruited much less under the influence of anesthesia [19]. Increased chest wall compliance results in failure to maintain functional residual capacity (FRC), necessitating tachypnea to maintain FRC and greatly decreasing FRC during apnea [11].

Premature infants are susceptible to OA through a variety of mechanisms and therefore there is often an obstructive component following central apneic

episodes leading to hypoxemia [8]. Immature airway reflexes and a propensity for glottic closure lead to airway obstruction, both of which are exacerbated by general anesthesia [20]. Specific attention should be paid to infants with Treacher Collins, Pierre Robin, and Nager syndrome, as they are at increased risk of obstructive sleep apnea [21].

A number of comorbidities predispose premature infants to apnea, as described in Table 39.1. Joshi et al. postulated that anemia resulted in an irregular and unstable respiratory pattern by hypoxic respiratory center depression, secondary to increased susceptibility to tissue hypoxia by the decreased $O_2$ carrying capacity of the blood [22]. Infants with obstructive sleep apnea and night-time hypoxemia have been demonstrated to have lower opioid requirements postoperatively, and this sensitivity predisposes them to respiratory complications with increased opioid doses. Steward also proposed a degree of nutritional deprivation in premature infants, influencing the energy requirements of respiratory muscles [2]. Further research is required to elucidate the mechanisms relating apnea to many of the comorbidities that increase its risk.

The pathophysiology of bradycardia in prematurity has been postulated to be multifactorial, with most emphasis placed on vagal reflexes, but also its relationship with concomitant apneic episodes (Table 39.2). Henderson-Smart et al. propose that the mechanism of bradycardia of prematurity is immature vagal reflexes/increased vagal tone. They propose that during upper airway obstruction during apneic episodes, the vagus nerve is stimulated which activates muscarinic acetylcholine receptor $M_2$ receptors on the sinoatrial node [23].

**Table 39.1** Risk factors for apnea

Prematurity (gestational age at birth), presence and degree

Postconceptual age less than 46 weeks without comorbidities, and less than 60 weeks with comorbidities

Low birth weight*

Previous apneic episodes and hypoventilation, at home and postoperative period

Anemia

Sepsis

Necrotizing enterocolitis

Pneumonia

Use of postoperative opioids

Bronchopulmonary dysplasia

Temperature instability, specifically hypothermia

Obstructive sleep apnea, presence and severity

General anesthesia

Neuraxial anesthetic with ketamine sedation

Epidural clonidine

Caudal epidural anesthetic, controversial

Gastroesophageal reflux

Codeine

Central nervous system lesions

Infections

Cardiac abnormalities

Metabolic arrangements

Upper respiratory structural abnormalities

Drug administration (e.g., narcotics)

* Some studies have demonstrated that small for gestational age infants are somewhat protected from apnea relative to large for gestational age [13].
Source: [7,8,10–12,16–25].

**Table 39.2 Risk factors for bradycardia**

Prematurity

Low ASA physical status

Prolonged apnea, hypoxia

Severe hypotension

Anesthetic overdose

Down syndrome

Congenital heart disease

Source: [27–29].

# Prevention and Treatment

The mainstay of prevention of apnea and bradycardia is avoiding elective surgery during high-risk periods and decreasing morbidity through overnight observation and monitoring devices following surgery. Recent meta-analyses support previous suggestions of overnight admission postoperatively for premature infants at a postconceptual age of 46 weeks or less, and a plan made on a case-by-case basis for premature infants at a postconceptual age of 46–60 weeks with comorbidities [2,10–12]. However, many hospital guidelines suggest that premature and former premature infants be admitted for observation after general anesthesia until they reach 60 weeks postconceptual age.

Other methods of prevention focus on modification of risk factors. To address anemia, Welborn et al. recommend delaying elective surgery and iron supplementation to achieve a hematocrit greater than 30 percent [24]. Tailoring the anesthetic plan to decrease risk has also been demonstrated to possibly reduce the risk of postoperative apnea, such as utilizing desflurane for a shorter recovery time, using spinal/regional anesthesia without sedation, and decreasing opioid use in infants with obstructive sleep apnea [25]. A recent Cochrane review demonstrated the benefits of spinal anesthesia to include decreased postoperative apnea with the use of spinal anesthesia without sedation, but noted significant anesthetic placement failure [26]. Welborn et al. demonstrated that in comparing spinal anesthesia with and without ketamine, the ketamine group had an increased risk of apnea in the postoperative period [27]. Opiate management in the perioperative period can be difficult, especially in patients with obstructive sleep apnea, and the recommendation is to reduce doses of opioids secondary to their increased sensitivity.

The mainstay of postoperative monitoring includes pulse oximetry and movement sensors – thoracic impedance monitors, respiratory inductive plethysmography, and magnetometers. Murphy et al. suggest that selecting infants at high risk of apnea to be monitored in the neonatal or intensive care unit postoperatively may have savings in terms of resources and costs [28].

The immediate management of an apneic episode with or without hypoxemia focuses on maintaining airway, breathing, and circulation. The ultimate goal is treatment of the underlying cause, with the appropriate intervention, such as medications, CPAP, or mechanical ventilation [8]. Although hyperox-emia is a concern in premature infants less than 44 weeks PCA, treatment of acute episodes of apnea may require administration of 100 percent oxygen during the immediate resuscitation period.

Pharmacologic treatment of apnea consists of methylxanthines, namely caffeine, theophylline, and aminophylline. When pharmacologic therapy is being considered, caffeine's efficacy is the best studied but its prophylactic use in at-risk infants is debatable. Benefits include once-daily dosing and decreased risk of toxicity relative to theophylline [29]. A stable, therapeutic blood concentration has also been dem-onstrated, despite both a prolonged half-life in neo-nates and infants with hepatic/renal comorbidities. Theophylline is another methylxanthine that has dem-onstrated efficacy in preventing serious apneas, but its use is limited by a narrow therapeutic index and risk of serious toxicity (tachyarrhythmias and CNS excita-tion/seizures). Aminophylline is also another methyl-xanthine that has been demonstrated to stimulate the respiratory centers and myocardium directly, but has a side-effect profile similar to theophylline. If patients fail pharmacologic therapy with methylxanthines, continuous positive airway pressure (CPAP) and ulti-mately intubation may be necessary to prevent serious apneic episodes.

Most bradycardic episodes in the neonatal intensive care unit (NICU) are accompanied by either an episode of apnea or oxygen desaturation, lending plausibility to the belief that the initial event is a disturbance in respiration. However, infants can develop episodes of bradycardia that are not related to prematurity or anes-thetic exposure. New onset of bradycardic or apneic episodes in an infant, especially a term infant, could be due to underlying cardiac or neurologic disease, infec-tion, hypoglycemia, hypoxia, hypo- or hyperthermia, or excessive stress. The mainstay of therapy is to treat the underlying cause of the bradycardia.

Certain medications administered during gen-eral anesthesia can predispose infants to bradycar-dia. Pretreatment with anticholinergics has been demonstrated to be effective in preventing bradycar-dia and increasing heart rates. The most commonly used anticholinergic medication during infancy is atropine, which has been associated with unpleas-ant side-effects such as dry mouth, urinary retention, and agitation even in infancy. Young children can also develop "atropine fever in early infancy," first described in the *New England Journal of Medicine* in 1935 [30].

Succinylcholine is the preferred muscle relaxant for multiple anesthetic situations due to its rapid onset and limited duration of action, but may carry the risk of bradycardia. Previously it was recommended to rou-tinely premedicate with atropine before succinylcholine administration in children, but this practice has been questioned. Data does suggest that the risk of bradycar-dia increases with repeated doses of succinylcholine and decreases with increasing age after the first few months of life [31]. Bradycardia in the setting of a rescue situ-ation should be treated with epinephrine as a first-line medication, with anticholinergics reserved for infants and children whose bradycardia is known to be due to increased vagal tone or primary atrioventricular block. If pharmacologic treatment is unsuccessful or the heart rate drops below 60, chest compressions should be ini-tiated according to the PALS algorithm [32].

# References

1. Liu LM, Coté CJ, Goudsouzian NG, et al. Life-threatening apnea in infants recovering from anesthesia. *Anesthesiology*. 1983;50(5):506–10.

2. Steward D. Preterm infants are more prone to complications following minor surgery then the term infants. *Anesthesiology*. 1982;55:304–6.

3. Sims C, Johnson CM. Postoperative apnoea in infants. *Anaesth Intensive Care*. 1994;22(1):40–5.

4. Moriette G, Lescure S, El Ayoubi M, Lopez E. Apnea of prematurity: what's new? *Arch Pediatr*.2010;17(2):186–90. doi: 10.1016/j.arcped.2009.09.016.

5. Daily WJ, Klaus M, Meyer HB. Apnea in premature infants: monitoring, incidence, heart rate changes, and an effect of environmental temperature. *Pediatrics*. 1969;43(4):510–18.

6. Kerbl R, Zotter H, Schenkeli R, et al. Persistent hypercapnia in children after treatment of obstructive sleep apnea syndrome by adenotonsillectomy. *Wiener klinische Wochenschrift*. 2001;113(7–8):229–34.

7. Krane EJ, Haberkern CM, Jacobson LE. Postoperative apnea, bradycardia, and oxygen desaturation in formerly premature infants: prospective comparison of spinal and general anesthesia. *Anesth Analg*. 1995;80(1):7–13.

8. Mishra S, Agrwal R, Jeevasankar M, et al. Apnea in the newborn. *Indian J Pediatr*. 2008;75(1):57–61.

9. Barrington K, Finer N. The natural history of the appearance of apnea of prematurity. *Pediatr Res*. 1991;29:372–5.

10. Lee SL, Gleason JM, Sydorak RM. A critical review of premature infants with inguinal hernias: optimal

timing of repair, incarceration risk, and postoperative apnea. *J Pediatr Surg.* 2011;46(1):217–20.

11. Gregory GA, Steward DJ. Life-threatening perioperative apnea in the ex-"premie". *Anesthesiology.* 1983;59(6):495–8.

12. Coté CJ, Zaslavsky A, Downes JJ, et al. Postoperative apnea in former preterm infants after inguinal herniorrhaphy: a combined analysis. *Anesthesiology.* 1995;82(4):809–22.

13. Coté CJ, Kelly DH. Postoperative apnea in a full-term infant with a demonstrable respiratory pattern abnormality. *Anesthesiology.* 1990;72(3):559–61.

14. Tetzlaff JE, Annand DW, Pudimat MA, Nicodemus HF. Postoperative apnea in a full-term infant. *Anesthesiology.* 1988;69(3):426–8.

15. Noseworthy J, Duran C, Khine HH. Postoperative apnea in a full-term infant. *Anesthesiology.* 1989;70(5):879–80.

16. Rigatto H, Brady JP, de la Torre Verduzco, R. Chemoreceptor reflexes in preterm infants: I. The effect of gestational and postnatal age on the ventilatory response to inhalation of 100% and 15% oxygen. *Pediatrics.* 1975;55(5):604–13.

17. Rigatto H, Brady JP, de la Torre Verduzco, R. Chemoreceptor reflexes in preterm infants: II. The effect of gestational and postnatal age on the ventilatory response to inhaled carbon dioxide. *Pediatrics.* 1975;55(5):614–20.

18. Knill RL, Gelb AW. Ventilatory responses to hypoxia and hypercapnia during halothane sedation and anesthesia in man. *Anesthesiology.* 1978;49(4):244–51.

19. Keens TG, Chen V, Patel P, et al. Cellular adaptations of the ventilatory muscles to a chronic increased respiratory load. *J App Physiol.* 1978;44(6):905–8.

20. Kurth CD, LeBard SE. Association of postoperative apnea, airway obstruction, and hypoxemia in former premature infants. *Anesthesiology.* 1991;75(1):22–6.

21. James D, Ma L. Mandibular reconstruction in children with obstructive sleep apnea due to micrognathia. *Plast Reconst Surg.* 1997;100(5):1131–7.

22. Joshi A, Gerhardt T, Shandloff P, Bancalari E. Blood transfusion effect on the respiratory pattern of preterm infants. *Pediatrics.* 1987(80):79.

23. Henderson-Smart DJ, Butcher-Puech MC, Edwards DA. Incidence and mechanism of bradycardia during apnoea in preterm infants. *Arch Dis Child.* 1986;61:227–32.

24. Welborn LG, Greenspun JC. Anesthesia and apnea: perioperative considerations in the former preterm infant. *Pediatr Clin North Am.* 1994;41(1):181–98.

25. Davidson AJ, Morton NS, Arnup SJ. Apnea after awake regional and general anesthesia in infants: the general anesthesia compared to spinal anesthesia study – comparing apnea and neurodevelopmental outcomes, a randomized controlled trial. *Anesthesiology.* 2015;123(1):38–54.

26. Craven PD, Badawi N, Henderson-Smart DJ, O'Brien M. Regional (spinal, epidural, caudal) versus general anaesthesia in preterm infants undergoing inguinal herniorrhaphy in early infancy. *Cochrane Database Syst Rev.* 2003;3:CD00366.

27. Welborn LG, Rice LJ, Hannallah RS, et al. Postoperative apnea in former preterm infants: prospective comparison of spinal and general anesthesia. *Anesthesiology.* 1990;72(5):838–42.

28. Murphy JJ, Swanson T, Ansermino M, Milner R. The frequency of apneas in premature infants after inguinal hernia repair: do they need overnight monitoring in the intensive care unit? *J Pediatr Surg.* 2008;43(5):865–8.

29. Henderson-Smart DJ, De Paoli AG. Prophylactic methylxanthine for prevention of apnoea in preterm infants. *Cochrane Database Syst Rev.* 2010;12:CD000432.

30. . Johnson CK. Atropine fever in early infancy. *N Engl J Med.* 1935;213:620–2.

31. McAuliffe G, Bissonnette B, Boutin C. Should the routine use of atropine before succinylcholine in children be reconsidered? *Can J Anaesth.* 1995;42(8):724–9.

32. Kleinman ME, Chameides L, Schexnayder SM, et al. American Heart Association guidelines for cardiopulmonary resuscitation and emergency cardiovascular care science. *Circulation.* 2010;122:S876–S908.

## Chapter 40

# Neonatal Outcomes

Joseph P. Cravero

The study of healthcare *outcomes* is the study of the end result of care – and more specifically, the *most* important of these end results. When one considers neonatal surgical outcomes, the evaluation must look at both the important immediate outcomes as well as the longer-term outcomes that occur in this population. Since surgical intervention is occurring at the very beginning of a patient's life, a time in which there is rapid neurological development, we must evaluate later neuromotor and intellectual functioning as part of the outcomes evaluation for this patient population.

Given these considerations, the study of neonatal surgical outcomes is complex. Many surgical procedures occur in newborns that have a high risk for adverse short- and long-term outcomes because of coexisting morbidities unrelated to their surgery. Any study of outcomes must take into account the underlying comorbidities that are associated with a neonatal surgical patient. This chapter begins with a review of some concepts involved in evaluating outcome data (in general) and discusses some of the concepts that are involved in following neonatal outcomes specifically. Finally, we review some outcome data as they relate to specific neonatal surgical patients, with a focus on the types of outcomes that are chosen for evaluation.

## Outcome Research from Data Registries

Because of the nature of the patients involved and the acuity of their illnesses, prospective, randomized trials are particularly difficult to accomplish in a population of newborns. Instead, over the last ten years there has been an explosion in the use of observational registry research (databases) to evaluate outcomes in neonatal medicine, surgery, and anesthesiology. There are many reasons for this trend, most notably the complexity and prohibitive cost of conducting adequately powered randomized trials. In addition, many treatments

and exposures cannot be randomized based on ethical issues (such as exposure to a major surgery). In light of this, databases that are created from one or more institutions serve as the next best mechanism for evaluating different management strategies when it comes to neonates undergoing surgeries. Furthermore, collected outcomes from institutions that have different methodologies for accomplishing the same care can be compared in an effort to simulate a randomized trial. In fact, well-conducted observational research has been shown to result in similar findings when compared to randomized trials of the same clinical entities [1]. Finally, more than ever, anesthesiologists are working as perioperative physicians and need to evaluate patient-centered perioperative outcomes, quality improvement, resource utilization, risk-adjusted outcome reporting, and clinical prediction modeling – all of which are amenable to registry data outcome analysis.

Underpinning the adoption of outcome registry research is the switch from paper to electronic records (also known as the Electronic Medical Record [EMR]) – both for hospitalization and operating room data. The combination of data from many geographically distinct sources into common databases allows investigators the ability to produce an "n" that would otherwise be impossible to approach. There are innumerable examples of EMR collaboration to produce large data collaborations. The Anesthesia Quality Institute (AQI) and the National Anesthesia Clinical Outcomes Registry (NACOR), sponsored through the American Society of Anesthesiologists, is the largest and perhaps the most ambitious and notable to date (information available at http://aqihq.org). At this particular registry, data from hundreds of institutions are combined by sending specific data elements from EMRs directly to a central data repository that houses literally tens of millions of cases for review. In this way, no extra effort or time is required from the anesthesiologist providing care to the patient. The data collection goes on "in the background" – invisible to the care providers. The convenience of this type of data collection is undeniable and has garnered excitement from clinical researchers around the globe.

## Data Registry Concerns

Having noted some advantages of database-centered research, there are many issues that can lead to misinterpretation and undermine appropriate use and conclusions from data registry research [2].

(1) **Data mining:** In traditional clinical studies investigators begin with a hypothesis and test its validity. Data registries represent large cohorts of observational data that are collected – often from routine clinical care. In analyzing these data there is a temptation to search for interesting associations among them without strictly defining a hypothesis for data relationships. When embarking on such a study it is critical for investigators and clinicians to remember that the phrase "statistical significance" means a given result is unlikely to have occurred by chance. If one simply searches a large database for cause and effect between enough factors without a reasoned hypothesis, "significant" relationships will be found even in data that are unrelated. For instance, if we take $p < 0.05$ as the threshold for significant association, 1 out of 20 random data associations will appear to be related simply by chance.

Many methods attempt to account for this possible error. The simplest and most commonly employed is the Bonferroni correction [3]. With the Bonferroni methodology each additional test requires significance to be reached at $1/n$ times what it would be if one was testing only one hypothesis. For example, if one is trying to relate the rate of lung injury to major surgery in neonates and consider five possible factors in addition to a primary factor (such as postconceptual age), the threshold for significance should be held at $p < 0.05/5$ or $0.01$ rather than $0.05$ – as it would be for the original comparison.

Data mining is a major problem in database research. When considering outcomes derived from registry research, the analysis should be hypothesis-driven and planned before analyzing data.

(2) **Quality of data:** Data that are collected in the course of clinical care are not always consistent from one person (or institution) to another. Strict definitions for specific outcomes and metrics need to be explained and agreed upon by all participants. If this is not done, data collected can be inconsistent and conclusions inaccurate. Furthermore, data registries should establish a framework of procedures for data quality assurance [4]. The procedures in such a framework exist at the coordinating center level as well as at the centers where the data are collected. Procedures should be in place to prevent insufficient data quality, detect imperfect data, and define actions to be taken to correct insufficient data. Data systems that collect information for registries should be designed with automatic data "checks" that prevent the inclusion of spurious data.

In terms of anesthesia for newborns, consider the terms "respiratory distress," "bronchospasm," or "laryngospasm." The exact definition applied to each of these terms can vary greatly from one clinician to another. Do these terms imply change in physiological state or simply the appearance or sound of difficulty with air exchange? Unless registries have clearly defined outcome terminology, a great deal of uncertainty will be generated as the frequency and nature of these outcomes is encountered. Registries that restrict analysis to outcomes that are relatively unambiguous may largely avoid these issues.

(3) **Statistical methodology:** The use of multivariable regression with stepwise variable selection can lead to results that are difficult to replicate in other large data repositories. With these methodologies patient characteristics are considered as statistical variables unto themselves across a large population. Risk calculations are amended with respect to their cumulative known effect on a given outcome of interest. Newer and more sophisticated methods including propensity score techniques and mixed effects modeling are better suited for evaluating treatment effects in registries [5]. In the most general sense, these methodologies

require that the investigator identify populations of patients that share characteristics such as postconceptual age, presence or absence of neurological compromise etc., and then consider the effect of one variable that is not common to these cohorts – such as surgical exposure. When considering any of these sophisticated statistical methods, it is important to only consider confounders that are likely to affect final outcomes.

(4) **Missing confounders:** Outcome researchers can only compensate for those confounders that are known to exist or have been demonstrated in past studies. Unfortunately there may be a host of other influences that are not known or have not been identified. As an example, investigators may account for age of a neonate at the time of surgery or his/her diagnosis as a major influence on long-term outcome. On the other hand, it may be impossible to completely understand and codify the social context in which these neonates live after birth, or (perhaps) drug use by the patient's mother during gestation – even though these factors may heavily influence the long-term outcome for a given patient [6]. Since the patients in observational registries are not randomized, it is easy for these unknown issues to unevenly influence outcomes in groups that are being considered. Many authors will report the issues that were "controlled" for in their analysis of neonatal outcomes as if these represent a comprehensive list of all possible influences. Rarely is this the case, and caution is advised in considering the possible unknown influences on surgical results.

(5) **Confounders vs. mediators:** In any registry it is important to distinguish between variables that are potentially confounding but unrelated to the primary factor of interest (confounders) [7,8] and those that are actually related to the primary factor and work as mechanisms that change the outcome of interest (mediators) [9]. A mediator, therefore, plays a strong role in determining the relationship between a given attribute or variable and an outcome of interest. Statistically controlling for known confounders (as mentioned above) is necessary, but adjusting for mediators in the causal pathway can reduce or eliminate real associations. For example,

infants of diabetic mothers (IDMs) have multiple abnormalities in the newborn period, one of which is a propensity for hypoglycemia. If an investigator were to consider the outcomes from neonatal surgery in IDM newborns and control for hypoglycemia, this would underestimate the true impact that birth to a diabetic mother may have on overall risk in the newborn surgical patient. Registry researchers should clearly define confounders vs. mediators and only control for those factors that are not clearly linked to a fundamental aspect of a patient's state or diagnosis.

(6) **Selection and measurement bias:** Once again, registries are, by definition, not controlled comparison studies. Selection bias results when the study population is nonrandomly selected or distributed from the registry population [10]. For instance, neonatal patients who undergo surgical correction rather than conservative management for necrotizing enterocolitis (NEC) could be chosen for this therapy based on some assessment of their overall clinical appearance (i.e., more or less likely to be septic). If an investigator were to compare the outcomes from surgery for NEC vs. conservative treatment with medication or simple drainage and not appreciate that the two therapies were unevenly distributed, bias would be introduced and outcomes would not be comparable.

(7) **Interpretation issues:** Large observational trials with tens of thousands of patient records will often lead to findings of statistical significance when there is marginal clinical significance. For example, in a database evaluating 5000 postoperative neonatal patients, a difference at any one time point of 0.3 units on a neonatal pain scale (from 0 to 10) will have a $p$-value of 0.0001. The same difference would have a $p$-value of $>0.05$ in a cohort of 20 patients. Clinicians need to consider clinical vs. statistical significance in outcomes that are reported in such papers. The fact that a given data comparison results in statistical significance must be considered in the context of the clinical importance of the difference described.

Other statistical methods for looking at the issue of "significance" include the calculation of relative risk (RR), numbers needed to treat

(NNT), and absolute risk reduction (ARR) [11]. Relative risk is the ratio of the risks for a given outcome in a treated population vs. that in a control group. The RR is independent of the prevalence of an outcome and therefore (once again) can be confusing for clinicians. The RR may be significant, but if the prevalence of an outcome is very low, the clinical significance may be marginal. Measures such as the ARR and NNT vary with the rate of an outcome in a population. The ARR is calculated as the difference in the absolute risk rates between a treated cohort and the controls. The NNT is the number of patients that need to be treated in order to prevent one adverse outcome. This is numerically equivalent to 1/ARR. Both the NNT and ARR can be viewed as methods for avoiding the problem of overvaluing statistical vs. clinical significance in large registry studies.

Finally, when considering clinical significance of outcomes it is critical to consider the gravity of the outcome in question. In this way, neonatal surgical interventions that have a significantly higher survival rate are clearly of greater concern than those that may slightly decrease the length of hospitalization. When considering the literature resulting from data registry science, one cannot escape the conclusion that analysis of large sets of observational data yields associations, not "cause and effect" outcomes. These associations can be extremely helpful in the investigation of very rare conditions and may help in the design of controlled trials, but they do not prove "cause." Clinicians need to keep in mind the limitations (as well as the advantages) of this kind of study and base practice on a careful consideration of all aspects of this category of data.

## Immediate Outcomes and Risk Adjustment

While much of this chapter focuses on the issues of long-term outcomes related to neonatal surgery and anesthesia, there are significant issues to be addressed when considering shorter-term outcomes as well. Risk adjustment is the process of accounting for various cofactors in a patient population that could influence outcomes. Multiple investigators have stratified the risk associated with specific neonatal surgical interventions and looked for factors such as the underlying illness, surgical technique, and surgical setting that can

influence outcome in the short term as well as the long term [12–14]. This is critical in order to understand the variation in safety or efficacy results from various care settings. Several factors are known to affect the immediate outcomes involving neonatal surgery. When considering noncardiac surgery in neonates, in-hospital mortality for premature infants is five times higher than that of term neonates (10.5 percent vs. 2 percent). Associated clinical characteristics that predict increased mortality include serious respiratory conditions, NEC, neonatal sepsis, and congenital heart disease [15]. Any study that compares outcomes from neonatal surgery must consider these specific clinical cofactors that put newborns at risk.

Validated models aiding in risk adjustment for neonates are available and can be used to compare outcomes between institutions and care models. One such risk adjustment methodology was described by Lillehei et al. in 2012 [15]. In this study, International Classification of Disease (9th edn) codes were used to group surgeries into one of four risk categories based on previous data reported concerning these surgeries. Multiple covariates, including prematurity, were then considered in a logistical regression analysis. The resultant model was then validated in three distinct, large, national public health datasets. This type of validated risk adjustment tool is particularly important when considering the outcome of neonatal surgery since (in order to identify areas for perioperative improvement at any one institution) we must have the ability to understand the relative outcomes when compared to other organizations. When the Lillehei method was used to compare outcomes among 41 institutions, standardized mortality ratios ranged from 0.37 to 1.91 (Figure 40.1) [15]. The authors concluded that areas for improvement are most readily identified at institutions with high relative mortality rates that would not have been evident without risk adjustment.

## The Effect of Prematurity on Newborn Outcomes

As suggested in the risk adjustment analysis mentioned above, much of the medical and surgical care of newborns is caused by, and centers around, prematurity. In order to understand the surgical outcomes of patients in this age group, one must understand the impact of prematurity on outcomes – in general. There are many studies that evaluate the outcomes

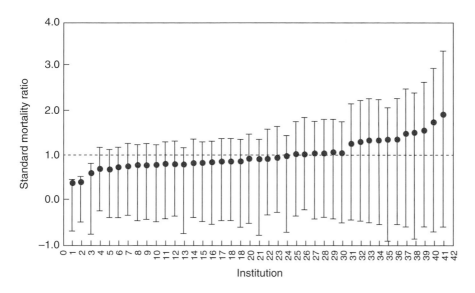

**Figure 40.1** Standardized mortality ratios from 41 free-standing children's hospitals participating in the PHIS 2006–2008. Bars represent 95 percent confidence intervals. Reproduced with permission.

of medical care in premature neonates. These studies are relatively consistent in their findings, with more extreme prematurity associated with more morbidity. Prematurity is divided into the very preterm newborn (born before 32 weeks' gestation) and the extremely preterm (born before 28 weeks' gestation). Survival is directly related to gestational age, ranging from 60 percent for those born at 24 weeks' gestation to over 90 percent for those born at 27 weeks or more [1]. These percentages showed considerable improvement from the mid-1990s to the late 2000s (increasing survival by 15 percent overall) due, in large part, to the adoption of evidence-based management strategies for these patients [16]. Unfortunately, significant morbidity continues to be evident – with 68 percent of survivors in the extremely premature group having bronchopulmonary dysplasia (BPD) and 13 percent displaying a significant intracerebral abnormality on head ultrasound at the time of discharge. Retinopathy of prematurity that was significant enough to require laser surgery was present in 16 percent of these babies.

Late neurocognitive development is a significant area of concern for former premature infants and children regardless of their surgical history. Results from the most recent national cohort study in England indicate that problems with neurological function are inversely related to gestational age at birth. Significant neurological impairment was discovered in 30 percent of infants born at 24 weeks compared with 20 percent for those born at 26 weeks (Figure 40.2) [11]. Cerebral palsy was present in 14 percent overall of extremely

premature neonatal survivors. Other investigators have documented a high rate of special educational needs in former premature infants at school age [17]. Behavior problems are also more common in this survivor group [18]. When one considers the outcomes from neonatal surgery, it is critical to control for factors that impact outcomes in this patient population (in general). Of these factors, none is more important than the presence and degree of prematurity of a given patient.

## Long-Term Neonatal Outcomes from Surgery and Anesthesia

In considering the long-term outcomes from neonatal surgery, neurological functioning is paramount. The effect of surgery on neonatal neurological outcomes has been the subject of debate and extensive investigation. In one of the most detailed evaluations of this relationship, Filan et al. reported the outcomes of 227 infants born at less than 30 weeks' gestation [19]. This convenience cohort was enrolled in a long-term follow-up study that included MRI imaging and serial developmental testing. Included in the cohort were 30 patients who underwent surgery and 178 who did not. Results of testing revealed that patients who had undergone surgery were found to have a greater degree of white matter injury and smaller total brain volumes. Mental development index scores were also found to be significantly lower in the surgical group, but this difference became non-significant when comparisons

**419**

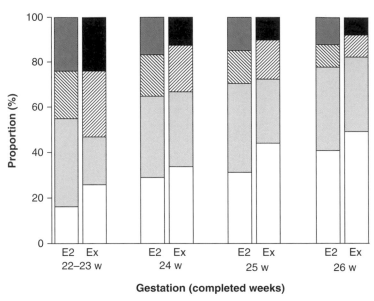

**Figure 40.2** Outcome of extremely low gestation newborns at age three years in two large national cohorts from England and Sweden. Reproduced with permission.

were done with correction for confounding variables. This study exemplifies the difficulty encountered in studying the effect of any one intervention in a population of premature infants. While issues that affect neonatal outcomes may be discovered, eliminating the effect of prematurity (itself) is often difficult to impossible. As mentioned above, when considering outcomes from neonatal anesthesia and surgery, prematurity remains a fundamental confounder.

Major surgery and anesthesia during the neonatal time period has also been associated with motor and intellectual development at 1–2 years of age [20]. Specific populations have been identified as particularly at risk. For instance, cardiac surgery and major abdominal procedures have been identified as significant areas of concern when it comes to cognitive outcomes in this age group [21]. Walker reported on the neurological outcome for cardiac and other major surgical patients who underwent procedures during the neonatal time period. Bayley scales of development were administered at one year of age to a registry group of 539 patients. Compared to nonsurgical patients, those who had cardiac surgery had lower mean scores in all five subscales of the evaluation

tool. Survivors of major noncardiac surgery had lower scores in four subscales of the same tool. Gross motor delay was found to be the area of greatest concern and consistent deficiency [21].

For noncardiac surgery, surgical patients with the highest risk for long-term cognitive delay include preterm neonates, newborns who have experienced intrauterine growth retardation, and patients with congenital anomalies (such as esophageal atresia, congenital diaphragmatic hernia, hypertrophic pyloric stenosis, and congenital heart disease). The exact reason for these associations is uncertain. Factors that have been implicated include the physiological stress of major surgery/exposure to multiple surgical interventions [22], anesthesia-induced neuroapoptosis [23], and the congenital anomaly itself [24].

## Data from Bowel Surgery

Neonatal bowel obstruction is the cause of a significant percentage of major surgeries in neonates. There are many causes of intestinal obstruction. Generally they are due to either a congenital abnormality such as intestinal atresia, or volvulus of the bowel or infection (NEC). Elsinga et al. evaluated school performance for children treated surgically for intestinal obstructions in the neonatal period [24]. In a cohort of 44 children (mean age nine years) they found that motor outcome was abnormal (less than the fifth percentile for age) in 22 percent of the children. Scores on selective attention were abnormal in 15 percent of the children. Both of these results are significantly different from the general population with $p < 0.01$. Lower birth weight and intestinal perforation were risk factors for worse motor outcomes, while intrauterine growth retardation and intestinal perforation were risk factors for deficiencies in selective attention. The authors also evaluated the educational setting that these infants were placed in. Of those studied, 85 percent were in a standard educational setting without receiving additional educational guidance, 4 percent attended a standard educational setting with additional guidance, and 7 percent were attending special education. The authors recommend that any patient with a history of bowel obstruction as a neonate deserves special attention when it comes to their education needs and should receive assessments on an ongoing basis as they mature from infants to toddlers and into school age.

Necrotizing enterocolitis is a serious and relatively frequent intestinal infection that affects premature infants. Over the last 20 years treatment of patients with NEC has shifted from early surgery to aggressively remove nonviable bowel to more conservative observation, decompression, and antibiotic therapy. The *immediate* outcomes of treatment for premature newborns with NEC or isolated intestinal perforation (IP) were described in a multicenter observation trial by Blakely et al. in 2005 [25]. This study included 156 infants with NEC. Of these patients, 80 underwent initial peritoneal drainage and conservative management, while 76 had laparotomy. The mortality rate in patients with NEC was 49 percent. The relative risk for death with a preoperative diagnosis of NEC was 1.4. The overall incidence of postoperative intestinal stricture was 10.3 percent, with wound dehiscence at 4.4 percent and intra-abdominal abscess at 5.8 percent. Immediate outcomes did not differ between those who underwent laparotomy vs. simple drainage as their initial procedure. These results largely support the profound shift to more conservative management of NEC that has occurred in the last 20 years. Specifically, immediate outcomes do not appear to be improved by extensive surgical intervention and resection when the diagnosis of NEC is made.

Few studies have followed the neurodevelopmental and growth outcomes of newborns with NEC. Some investigators have postulated that surgical intervention could be associated with poorer outcomes than patients treated medically because of the stress of surgery and exposure to general anesthesia. In 2005 Hintz et al. reported on the outcomes of extremely low birth weight premature newborns with NEC who had been managed surgically vs. those who had been managed medically [26]. These authors found that patients who had NEC and were treated surgically were more likely to have periventricular leukomalacia, BPD, and steroid therapy when compared to those patients who received medical therapy (only) for NEC and to those who did not have NEC. The fact that a patient was managed surgically was found to be an independent risk factor for Mental Developmental Index of <70 (OR 1.61), and neurodevelopmental impairment. This data is suggestive that surgical intervention is associated with adverse neurodevelopmental outcomes at 18 and 22 month's corrected age when compared to medically treated patients.

As outlined in the initial portion of this chapter, these data come from observational cohorts and the possibility that confounders that influence the late outcomes are not completely accounted for or understood must be considered. The conclusion that these patients have concerning long-term issues is, however, undeniable and early learning intervention for survivors is indicated.

## Data on Cardiac Surgery in Newborns

Cardiac surgery represents an area of extremely high risk for newborns. There is a rich literature following outcomes in this patient population. As with many other areas of outcome analysis in this age group, most of the papers produced in this area consist of observational reports of accumulated experience from one center or a limited number of centers. All such reports have to be considered in the context of the bias that is encountered when data are evaluated, reflecting the care from such a small group of providers and in one institution that will have its own bias for care factors and decision-making. In addition, studies of cardiac surgery in this age group are generally divided between those that look at immediate survival and major adverse events, and those that evaluate longer-term functioning and neurological outcomes. As with other areas of newborn surgery analysis, clinicians need to consider a combination of these types of outcomes to determine whether strategies or specific therapies are viable since neither (in isolation) yields a comprehensive answer to the outcome issues involved. The particularly high mortality of cardiac surgery requires a separate calculus since, in many cases, options are limited and surgery is urgently needed.

In considering the issue of outcomes after cardiac surgery we should evaluate some example reports that exist in the literature. Reports of overall mortality in neonatal cardiac surgery are often the primary outcome codified in these studies. Padley and colleagues reported the mortality associated with cardiac surgery over a five-year period spanning from 2005 to 2010 at their institution in Westmead, Australia [27]. These investigators determined that mortality was higher for neonates (6.8 percent) and low birth weight infants (12.1 percent) compared to that for the entire cohort (1.9 percent). Rates were reportedly no different between bypass and non-bypass cases. Not surprisingly, in multivariate analysis age, weight, and disease severity score were independent risk factors for mortality. The mortality rate did not change over the years studied, although the complexity of children who underwent surgery did increase with time. The authors suggest that their data highlight the risk factors involved in neonatal surgery.

Timing of neonatal cardiac surgery vs. outcome has long been debated. Should newborns undergo correction as soon as possible, or it is more prudent to wait a period of time prior to attempting correction? As an example of a study that focused on immediate outcomes to answer this question, in 2014 Kumar and colleagues reported outcomes from a retrospective series of 286 newborns undergoing a variety of major cardiac surgeries (arterial switch, stage 1 palliation, and systemic to pulmonary shunts) at the University of Michigan [28]. In this case, the primary outcome evaluated was that of mortality or 30-day out-of-hospital mortality and prolonged postoperative ICU stay. Secondary outcomes included ICU mortality, mechanical circulatory support, hospital-acquired infection, renal failure requiring dialysis, new neurologic injury, and NEC. The investigators found no relationship between the timing of surgery and composite outcomes. The only difference between the groups was that of stage 1 palliation patients in the oldest cohorts requiring a shorter duration of ventilation. From this relatively small sample the authors

concluded that early intervention was not associated with improved morbidity in neonatal cardiac surgery.

Efforts to follow the slightly longer-term outcomes from neonatal cardiac interventions have also been reported. These studies evaluate the durability of repair and the need to operate repeatedly on patients who have undergone a primary procedure. An example is a report from a single center evaluating the results of right ventricular outflow tract reconstruction in neonatal patients [29]. In this paper, Kaza et al. reported on 278 patients with various degrees of obstruction receiving a number of repair options. In this case, rather than mortality, the primary outcome evaluated was freedom from reoperation/reintervention. The results indicated that the durability of repair was diagnosis- and method-dependent. Anatomy that allowed right ventricular outflow tract patching provided an advantage compared to homograft repair.

In another effort to compare surgical outcomes in neonatal cardiac surgery, Ohye and colleagues evaluated the outcomes after two techniques for the Norwood Procedure [30]. In this study patients were randomized (unusual for neonatal studies) to receive either a modified Blalock-Taussig (MBT) shunt vs. a right ventricle-pulmonary artery (RVPA) shunt as part of their stage 1 repair. The authors considered the primary outcome to be that of death or cardiac transplantation within 12 months after randomization. Secondary outcomes of interest were unintended cardiovascular interventions as well as right ventricular size and function at 14 months of age. The results of the study are indicative of how difficult outcome analysis can be when considering this kind of intervention. As it turned out, the RVPA cohort had a better transplant-free survival rate at 12 months (74 percent vs. 64 percent, $p = 0.01$). On the other hand, the RVPA cohort had more unintended interventions ($p = 0.003$) and complications ($p = 0.002$) than the MBT group. Other outcomes were not different and analysis of the treatment effect after 12 months showed no difference in transplantation rate at that interval. This well-conducted study is an example of how the choice of outcome definitions affects the perception of treatment effect. If one focuses solely on the 12-month transplantation rate, the RVPA technique is superior. On the other hand, if any other metric is used, the MBT shunt is equal or superior. Clinicians need to appreciate that these choices can be arbitrary and must read the literature with regard to treatment of neonates with an eye toward the short-/intermediate-term outcomes they feel are most important for their patients.

Finally, there are a number of studies that have attempted to evaluate the long-term neurobehavioral outcomes in children who have undergone neonatal heart surgery [31–33]. By definition, these studies are longitudinal and look at cohorts of children who have had surgery for major congenital heart defects as neonates. Age of evaluation varies and ranges from 5 to 20 years. As such, the outcomes data are almost always out of date since they reflect practice that occurred in the remote past and likely do not reflect the outcomes that would be found from techniques/surgeries as they are practiced currently. Recognizing these limitations, the outcomes are very consistent. The frequency of neurological impairment in children who have had major cardiac surgery as neonates is higher than that in the general population, with 10–15 percent reporting significant developmental issues [31,32]. Deficits are centered on attention, behavior/adjustment problems, expressive language, and general academic performance. Investigators have also documented structural brain abnormalities on MRI scan in 32 percent of these patients [32]. Unfortunately, there is no generalized agreement on the outcome parameters that are of highest priority or greatest sensitivity/specificity. The preponderance of outcomes evidence in these cases, however, argues that neurodevelopmental delay is much more likely in survivors of neonatal cardiac surgery and early intervention is indicated.

## Pain Outcomes for Newborns

In 1987 Anand and colleagues published an intriguing study that compared the outcomes of patients who underwent ligation of patent ductus arteriosus utilizing anesthesia with and without fentanyl [34]. The investigators found that patients who received a dose of opiate in addition to nitrous oxide and relaxant had significantly less evidence of hormonal stress response. In terms of short-term outcomes, the non-opioid treated cohort had more circulatory and metabolic complications postoperatively. The impact of this study was immense as it alerted the anesthesia community to the need for appropriate analgesia for newborns during surgery. Many of these patients were previously thought to be too fragile for, or not requiring, such intervention. Subsequent practice around the world was altered to include appropriate doses of analgesia for newborns undergoing major surgery.

Data from animal studies have indicated that exposure to pain early in life can change behaviors to pain experienced later in life [35,36]. Human data on this issue has been developed by Grunau and colleagues as they evaluated the response of 32-week postconceptual age newborns to painful interventions [37]. These investigators found that higher cumulative (previous) exposure to pain was correlated with a blunted cortisol response to stress and less facial responsiveness to pain. Conversely, autonomic responses were not decreased. In another study, late outcomes for newborns who were exposed to painful stimuli were evaluated. Walker and colleagues demonstrated that there was altered sensory perception at 11 years of age in children who were born extremely premature. Notably, these alterations were most marked in babies exposed to surgical procedures during the newborn period [38].

Given the evidence for adverse long-term outcomes in patients exposed to pain as newborns, it would be logical to expect that the use of analgesics might improve these outcomes for newborns by blunting the painful stimulus. The use of preemptive opioids in newborns receiving intensive care (including mechanical ventilation and painful procedures) has been studied with exactly this strategy in mind. In the largest study of its kind, Anand and colleagues reported on 898 preterm newborn patients randomized to receive placebo vs. morphine infusion while ventilated [39]. Use of the opioid infusion decreased the clinical signs of pain in the treated group; however, it did not decrease the incidence of significant short-term adverse outcomes such as germinal matrix hemorrhages or death. Long-term follow-up on this cohort has not been provided to date. Clinicians need to balance the need to control pain for these patients in the immediate time frame while recognizing that this may not lead to short- or intermediate-term outcome improvement. The long-term impact of preventing pain with opioid medications in the acutely ill newborn is still a matter of investigation and debate.

## Summary

Neonatal outcome analysis is particularly important and challenging since surgery and anesthesia in this population occur in the context of a rapidly developing patient that often has coexisting pathology. Analysis of outcomes for neonatal patients is both straightforward and complex. While outcomes analysis can be defined simply as the analysis of the most important results of clinical work, the manner in which we obtain information on the results of work can be confusing and (at times) deceptive. With regard to data registries, consideration must be given to the possible pitfalls of large data analysis. Furthermore, studies can be divided into those that look at the short- and intermediate-term outcomes from specific interventions and those that look at the long-term effects on learning and behavior. Clinicians and investigators must keep in mind the special nature of this population and the wide-ranging impact of intervention as they consider the ways in which outcomes can be optimized around the perioperative time frame.

# References

1. Concato J, Shah N, Horwitz RI. Randomized, controlled trials, observational studies, and the hierarchy of research designs. *New Eng J Med.* 2000;342(25):1887–92.

2. Dalton J, Kurz A. Registry research: the new frenemy. *AUA Newsletter.* Winter 2011.

3. Shi Q, Pavey ES, Carter RE. Bonferroni-based correction factor for multiple, correlated endpoints. *Pharm Stat.*;11(4):300–9.

4. Arts DG, De Keizer NF, Scheffer GJ. Defining and improving data quality in medical registries: a literature review, case study, and generic framework. *J Am Med Inform Assoc.* 2002;9(6):600–11.

5. Senn S, Graf E, Caputo A. Stratification for the propensity score compared with linear regression techniques to assess the effect of treatment or exposure. *Stat Med.* 2007;26(30):5529–44.

6. Grzywacz JG, Daniel SS, Tucker J, Walls J, Leerkes E. Nonstandard work schedules and developmentally generative parenting practices: an application of propensity score techniques. *Fam Relat.* 2011;60(1):45–59.

7. Schneeweiss S. Sensitivity analysis and external adjustment for unmeasured confounders in epidemiologic database studies of therapeutics. *Pharmacoepidemiol Drug Saf.* 2006;15(5):291–303.

8. Sturmer T, Glynn RJ, Rothman KJ, Avorn J, Schneeweiss S. Adjustments for unmeasured confounders in pharmacoepidemiologic database studies using external information. *Med Care.* 2007;45(10 Supl 2):S158–165.

9. MacKinnon D. *Introduction to Statistical Mediation Analysis.* New York: Erlbaum; 2008.

10. Evans JM, MacDonald TM. Misclassification and selection bias in case-control studies using an automated database. *Pharmacoepidemiol Drug Saf.* 1997;6(5):313–18.

11. Leung WC. Balancing statistical and clinical significance in evaluating treatment effects. *Postgrad Med J.* 2001;77(905):201–4.

12. Bucher BT, Guth RM, Saito JM, Najaf T, Warner BW. Impact of hospital volume on in-hospital mortality of infants undergoing repair of congenital diaphragmatic hernia. *Ann Surg.* 2010;252(4):635–42.

13. Moss RL, Dimmitt RA, Barnhart DC, et al. Laparotomy versus peritoneal drainage for necrotizing enterocolitis and perforation. *New Eng J Med.* 2006;354(21):2225–34.

14. Abdullah F, Zhang Y, Camp M, et al. Necrotizing enterocolitis in 20,822 infants: analysis of medical and surgical treatments. *Clin Pediatr.* 2010;49(2):166–71.

15. Lillehei CW, Gauvreau K, Jenkins KJ. Risk adjustment for neonatal surgery: a method for comparison of in-hospital mortality. *Pediatrics.* 2012;130(3):e568–74.

16. Bhutta AT, Rovnaghi C, Simpson PM, et al. Interactions of inflammatory pain and morphine in infant rats: long-term behavioral effects. *Physiol Behav.* 2001;73(1–2):51–8.

17. Johnson S, Hennessy E, Smith R, et al. Academic attainment and special educational needs in extremely preterm children at 11 years of age: the EPICure study. *Arch Dis Child Fetal Neonatal Ed.* 2009;94(4):F283–9.

18. Johnson S, Marlow N. Preterm birth and childhood psychiatric disorders. *Pediatr Res.* 2011;69(5 Pt 2):11R–18R.

19. Filan PM, Hunt RW, Anderson PJ, Doyle LW, Inder TE. Neurologic outcomes in very preterm infants undergoing surgery. *J Pediatr.* 2012;160(3):409–14.

20. Walker K, Badawi N, Holland AJ, Halliday R. Developmental outcomes following major surgery: what does the literature say? *J Paediatr Child Health.* 2011;47(11):766–70.

21. Walker K, Badawi N, Halliday R, et al. Early developmental outcomes following major noncardiac and cardiac surgery in term infants: a population-based study. *J Pediatr.* 2012;161(4):748–52.

22. Anand KJ, Hansen DD, Hickey PR. Hormonal-metabolic stress responses in neonates undergoing cardiac surgery. *Anesthesiology.* 1990;73(4):661–70.

23. Bouwmeester NJ, Anand KJ, van Dijk M, et al. Hormonal and metabolic stress responses after major surgery in children aged 0–3 years: a double-blind, randomized trial comparing the effects of continuous versus intermittent morphine. *Br J Anaesth.* 2001;87(3):390–9.

24. Elsinga RM, Roze E, Van Braeckel KN, Hulscher JB, Bos AF. Motor and cognitive outcome at school

age of children with surgically treated intestinal obstructions in the neonatal period. *Early Hum Dev.* 2013;89(3):181–5.

25. Blakely ML, Lally KP, McDonald S, et al. Postoperative outcomes of extremely low birth-weight infants with necrotizing enterocolitis or isolated intestinal perforation: a prospective cohort study by the NICHD Neonatal Research Network. *Ann Surg.* 2005;241(6):984–9.

26. Hintz SR, Kendrick DE, Stoll BJ, et al. Neurodevelopmental and growth outcomes of extremely low birth weight infants after necrotizing enterocolitis. *Pediatrics.* 2005;115(3):696–703.

27. Padley JR, Cole AD, Pye VE, et al. Five-year analysis of operative mortality and neonatal outcomes in congenital heart disease. *Heart Lung Circ.* 2011;20(7):460–7.

28. Kumar TK, Charpie JR, Ohye RG, et al. Timing of neonatal cardiac surgery is not associated with perioperative outcomes. *J Thorac Cardiovasc Surg.* 2013;147(5):1573–9.

29. Kaza AK, Lim HG, Dibardino DJ, et al. Long-term results of right ventricular outflow tract reconstruction in neonatal cardiac surgery: options and outcomes. *J Thorac Cardiovasc Surg.* 2009;138(4):911–16.

30. Ohye RG, Sleeper LA, Mahony L, et al. Comparison of shunt types in the Norwood procedure for single-ventricle lesions. *New Eng J Med.* 2010;362(21):1980–92.

31. Hovels-Gurich HH, Konrad K, Wiesner M, et al. Long term behavioural outcome after neonatal arterial switch operation for transposition of the great arteries. *Arch Dis Child.* 2002;87(6):506–10.

32. Heinrichs AK, Holschen A, Krings T, et al. Neurologic and psycho-intellectual outcome related to structural brain imaging in adolescents and young adults after neonatal arterial switch operation for transposition of the great arteries. *J Thorac Cardiovasc Surg.* 2014;148(5):2190–9.

33. Hovels-Gurich HH, Seghaye MC, Ma Q, et al. Long-term results of cardiac and general health status in children after neonatal arterial switch operation. *Ann Thorac Surg.* 2003;75(3):935–43.

34. Anand KJ, Sippell WG, Aynsley-Green A. Randomised trial of fentanyl anaesthesia in preterm babies undergoing surgery: effects on the stress response. *Lancet.* 1987;1(8527):243–8.

35. Beggs S, Currie G, Salter MW, Fitzgerald M, Walker SM. Priming of adult pain responses by neonatal pain experience: maintenance by central neuroimmune activity. *Brain.* 2012;135(Pt 2):404–17.

36. Alvares D, Torsney C, Beland B, Reynolds M, Fitzgerald M. Modelling the prolonged effects of neonatal pain. *Prog Brain Res.* 2000;129:365–73.

37. Grunau RE, Holsti L, Haley DW, et al. Neonatal procedural pain exposure predicts lower cortisol and behavioral reactivity in preterm infants in the NICU. *Pain.* 2005;113(3):293–300.

38. Walker SM, Franck LS, Fitzgerald M, et al. Long-term impact of neonatal intensive care and surgery on somatosensory perception in children born extremely preterm. *Pain.* 2009;141(1–2):79–87.

39. Anand KJ, Hall RW, Desai N, et al. Effects of morphine analgesia in ventilated preterm neonates: primary outcomes from the NEOPAIN randomised trial. *Lancet.* 2004;363(9422):1673–82.

**Chapter**

# 41

# Research on Newborns and Infants

Patcharee Sriswasdi

## Ethics of Research on Infants and Newborns

Conducting neonatal and pediatric clinical research is often challenging. Obtaining Institutional Review Board (IRB) approval and informed consent can be particularly difficult in this age group. However, if approached correctly, neonatal research can provide evidence-based understanding and treatment of diseases unique to neonates. Parents of neonates and infants who have participated in clinical trials may view their research involvement as an exciting opportunity to improve the care of newborns [1,2].

Finding new effective treatments for newborns, infants, and children is dependent on the performance of clinical research in which newborns and infants participate. In the past, clinicians have often used knowledge gained from adult research and applied it to children. This can be problematic since pediatric physiology is different to that found in adults. This issue is more prominent in neonates. Newborns undergo profound physiological changes at birth. Most organ systems that are critical for growth and development undergo a maturation process during transition from the fetal to the extrauterine environment and continue to undergo further adaptive changes in the neonatal period. Additionally there are diseases and conditions that present most commonly during the neonatal period, such as gastroschisis or persistent pulmonary hypertension of the newborn. Information about the prognosis, progression, or new treatment options for diseases unique to neonates often depend on newborns recruited into research studies. Achieving a proper balance between the benefits of neonatal research and the obligation to protect newborns that participate in research can be a challenge.

When designing and implementing research protocols, it is important to consider legal and ethical requirements that govern research in humans. For research to satisfy ethical and legal requirements, it must be scientifically sound and significant, subject selection must be fair, and enrollment should be voluntary without any pressure on subjects or their families to enroll. The risks to participants must be minimized and cannot be excessive, and risks must be justified by the benefits of the research. Valid and voluntary informed consent must be obtained, enrolled subjects must be respected, and the protocol must have obtained approval of an independent ethical review board.

In practice, two sometimes challenging issues encountered in neonatal and infant studies include equipoise and informed consent.

Equipoise is a state of genuine uncertainty regarding the benefits or disadvantages of two therapeutic arms of a clinical trial. Clinical equipoise is also referred to as an honest null hypothesis and provides a basis for ethical enrollment of patients into clinical trials [3]. Equipoise is not simply a matter of whether or not a treatment works. Equipoise concerns a decision to act and to give a treatment without prejudice. Personal equipoise exists when the clinical investigator (or clinician) involved in the research study has no preference or is truly uncertain about the overall benefit or harm offered by the treatment to the patient. It is possible for a clinical investigator to develop a bias toward one therapy or arm of the study as it progresses. Once there is enough clinical evidence to prove or disprove the null hypothesis of the trial, then there is no genuine uncertainty about treatment arms and there is no longer clinical equipoise. There is then an ethical imperative for the clinical investigator to stop the study and offer the more beneficial treatments to all participants. Before this evidentiary threshold is reached, however, all investigators should continue to enroll patients blindly, despite their personal biases.

Investigators must also recognize the importance that parents may not be in equipoise because they may strongly desire that their baby receive an active treatment. Controversy is particularly likely when the trial investigates an intervention that is a potential treatment for a dangerous or debilitating condition for which current treatment is unsatisfactory.

This lack of equipoise leads to the creation of a "desperate volunteer" on the part of consenting parents. These are parents who agree to take part in the randomized trial only because it offers them a 50/50 chance of obtaining the treatment they desire for their baby. This situation must be recognized and the investigator should discourage participation in cases where parents are not able to make a decision with any level of equipoise.

Because newborns are not capable of assent, researchers need the consent of a person with parental responsibility in order to proceed with participation in the research protocol [4]. In order to obtain consent for medical treatment, the parent needs to understand the medical treatment being proposed. This same principle applies in the consenting process for clinical research. The research team must decide whether the parent thoroughly understands the nature of the study, the options, the risks involved, and the benefits.

Factors that cloud the informed consent process in this age group include time pressure, the moral obligation parents feel toward the clinicians who are caring for their child, and tendency of desperate parents to enroll in any trial that they believe has a chance to benefit their baby.

To further complicate this issue, parents are often emotionally overwhelmed, preoccupied with their baby, or unwell following labor, and thus their understanding of information given about a trial has been shown to be limited when approached for consent [5].

DeMauro et al. found that when done well, conversations about consent to research can empower and support families at a time of crisis and reassure them that healthcare professionals are committed to discovering the safest and most effective care for their baby [6]. For such consent discussions to occur, three conditions must be met. First, all clinical and study staff must thoroughly believe in the importance and safety of the research. Second, the research team must cultivate open, trusting relationships with the families of potential research participants. Finally, the goal must be not a signature on the consent form, but parents who are able to make a well-informed decision that is right for their baby and their family [6].

Children are widely recognized as a vulnerable population and deserve additional protections from research risk. Of particular concern is exposure of children to risk when there is no balancing prospect for benefit.

The Code of Federal Regulations (CFR) describes four categories of research involving children (Table 41.1). Federal regulations allow local IRBs to approve the research that poses the risk without the prospect for benefit only under those circumstances listed under 45 CFR, section 46.406, termed "category 406" (Table 41.1). There is a higher standard for the review and approval of this research category when it involves healthy children than when it involves sick children. To be locally approvable, the research protocol must also be found to pose only a "minor increase over minimal risk." Although the term "minor increase" is open to interpretation, it does preclude the conduct of significant risky research under category 406.

To improve neonatal care, it is sometimes necessary to perform research studies involving interventions in children that do not offer a compensating potential for clinical benefit.

For example, there are a number of recent studies in animal models and human observational trials studying the degenerative or toxic effects of commonly used general anesthetics on the developing human brain. The possibility of anesthesia-induced neurotoxicity during an uneventful anesthetic in neonates has led to questions and concerns about the safety of conducting a research in the field of neonatal anesthesia. However, there remains considerable uncertainty about the applicability of animal data to clinical anesthesia practice and the statistical significance of human observational and cohort studies. Leaders in this area of investigation agree there is no need to exclude neonatal studies that include anesthesia strictly because of this issue [7–9].

In recognition of the benefits of neonatal research, recommendation has evolved from a position of excluding newborns to one of cautious advocacy and acknowledging the critical role of neonatal research, accompanied by careful consideration of scientific context, evaluation of risks, benefits, and protection to participants. The regulatory agencies overseeing neonatal research are required to make careful ethical assessments that balance the newborn's safety and welfare with the need

**Table 41.1** Summary description of the types of research that can be funded by the Department of Health and Human Services under 45 CFR §46[a]

| Category | Description |
| --- | --- |
| 404 | Research not involving greater than minimal risk. |
| 405 | Research involving greater than minimal risk but leading to the prospect of direct benefit to the individual subjects, and the risk is justified by the anticipated benefit to the subjects. |
| 406 | DHHS will conduct or fund research in which the IRB finds that more than minimal risk to children is presented by an intervention or procedure that does not hold out the prospect of direct benefit for the individual subject, or by a monitoring procedure which is not likely to contribute to the well-being of the subject, only if the IRB finds that |
| | (a) the risk represents a minor increase over minimal risk; |
| | (b) the intervention or procedure presents experiences to the subjects that are reasonably commensurate with those inherent in their actual or expected medical, dental, psychological, social, or educational situations; |
| | (c) the intervention or procedure is likely to yield generalizable knowledge about the subjects' disorder or condition which is of vital importance for the understanding or amelioration of the subjects' disorder or condition; and |
| | (d) adequate provisions are made for soliciting assent of the children and permission of their parents or guardians, as set forth in 46.408. |
| 407 | Research not otherwise approvable that presents an opportunity to further the understanding, prevention, or alleviation of a serious problem affecting the health or welfare of children (requires specific DHHS approval). |

DHHS, Department of Health and Human Services
[a] US academic medical centers typically operate with a Federalwide Assurance, in which case these categories apply to all research within the institution.

to generate scientifically valid information concerning the health and welfare of newborns.

## Study Design [10–12]

### General Considerations in Clinical Research Design

The study population refers to the subjects who enter a study, regardless of whether they are treated, exposed, develop the disease, or drop-out after the study has begun. Usually a study population originates from some larger source population, which is then narrowed using both inclusion and exclusion criteria. The population is not fixed, but changes constantly. Researchers are usually interested not only in current patients with a specific condition, but also in future patients. Therefore, the population is sometimes considered infinite.

### Choice of Study Population and Generalizability of Study Findings

The choice of study population directly influences the generalizability of the study results. The population of interest is defined through inclusion and exclusion criteria.

- The *inclusion criteria* are the characteristics a subject/patient needs to have in order to belong to the population.
- The *exclusion criteria* are the characteristics a subject/patient is not allowed to have in order to belong to the population.

It would be ideal to be able to perform studies among the actual population, but that would be costly, time-consuming, and not necessarily feasible. Researchers usually select a sample from the population into each study. The strength of the evidence in the data and the validity of the conclusions based on the data depend entirely on both the definition of the population and the way the sample is drawn from the population. Ideally, the sample should be a perfect reflection of the total population of interest. In practice the only way to accomplish this is to test the entire population. However, it is possible to minimize sampling error by doing unbiased probability sampling (randomized) and by using a large sample size.

### Prospective Versus Retrospective Study

- *Prospective*: A group of people is followed for the occurrence or non-occurrence of specified endpoints, events, or measurements.

- *Retrospective*: Subjects having a particular outcome or endpoint are identified and studied. Often, measurements from the past are of interest.

**Incidence versus Prevalence.** Incidence and prevalence are both measures of the extent of disease in a population. Incidence tells us about a change in status from nondisease to disease, thus being limited to new cases. Prevalence includes both new cases and those who contracted the disease in the past and are still surviving. Incidence rates are favored if the rapidity with which new disease is occurring in the population is of interest. A measure of prevalence is preferred if the focus is on the overall number of cases surviving in the population.

**Incidence.** Incidence is a measure of change from nondisease to disease, which is the numerator in a "population-at-risk," which is the denominator over a specific time period. By "population-at-risk," we mean all persons in the population who have not been diagnosed with the disease of interest at the beginning of the observation period, but who are capable of developing the disease. Measures of incidence describe the occurrence of new disease in the population and have the units of either person-time-at-risk, i.e., total amount of time contributed by each individual while he/she remained at risk, or population-at-risk, i.e., the number of non-cases at baseline.

The *incidence rate* is a measure of the frequency with which a disease occurs in a population over a period of time. The formula for calculating an incidence rate is:

Incidence rate = new cases occurring during a given time period / population at risk during the same time period

*Cumulative incidence or incidence proportion* is a measure of disease frequency during a period of time. Where the period of time considered is an entire lifetime, the incidence proportion is called "lifetime risk." Cumulative incidence is defined as the probability that a particular event, such as occurrence of a particular disease, has occurred before a given time. It is equivalent to the incidence, calculated using a period of time during which all of the individuals in the population are considered to be at risk for the outcome. It is sometimes also referred to as the incidence proportion. Cumulative incidence is calculated by the number of new cases during a period divided by the number of subjects at risk in the population at the beginning of the study.

**Prevalence.** In contrast to incidence, prevalence is a static measure of the proportion of a population that is diseased, whether the disease cases occurred recently or at some time in the past. Prevalence measures reflect already-existing disease. The incidence and duration of the disease under study affect prevalence. The prevalence of a disease is a function of how often new cases develop and how long the disease state lasts.

## Exposure and Outcome

Clinical research often focuses on the relationship or association between an exposure and an outcome of interest.

*Exposure or predictor* is used to describe any factor or characteristic that may explain or predict the presence of an outcome. Predictor variables are sometimes referred to as independent variables.

*Outcome* refers to the factor that is being predicted. The outcome is often a disease or condition but can be any clinical characteristic. Outcome variables are sometimes referred to as dependent variables.

Effective clinical research requires well-defined definitions of exposure and outcome variables.

Once exposures and outcomes are specifically defined, they should be measured as carefully as possible. Error in measuring exposure and outcome data is common.

## Inferring Causation from Association Studies

Typically, clinical research involves analyzing the association between two or more variables. One or more variable is termed an outcome (dependent) variable, and the others are termed exposure/predictor (independent) variables. An association or correlation between the outcome and exposure/predictor variables is often interpreted as a cause-and-effect relationship.

### Importance of Distinguishing Causation from Association

Clinical research studies report associations between an exposure and outcome, because association and not causation is actually observed. Causes are termed *necessary* when they must always precede an effect, and *sufficient* when they initiate or produce an effect. Any of several factors may be associated with the potential disease causation or outcome, including predisposing factors, enabling factors, precipitating factors, reinforcing factors, and risk factors.

Assuming the causation between an exposure and outcome requires presuming a sequence of events was based on multiple lines of evidence, from clinical association studies to basic experimental work.

Many associations are not causal. Inferring causality from clinical research studies may not be easy. Causal inference is hampered in clinical research by the fact that multiple exposures often influence a single disease outcome and some exposures take a long time to influence the outcome.

## Factors Favoring an Inference of Causation

Even though researchers cannot be certain that a particular exposure causes a particular outcome, a number of factors can be used to help decide whether an exposure of interest is likely to be a cause of a disease, rather than just being associated with it.

- *Evidence arising from randomized studies*
  - Studies that randomly assign a subject to one treatment group versus another are generally the most powerful way to show that an exposure is a cause of an outcome. Large randomized trials are usually free from confounding factors since the characteristics of subjects assigned to one particular treatment are usually very similar to those of subjects assigned to another treatment. If the outcome differs between treatment groups, it is reasonable to conclude that the treatment is the cause of the difference.
- *Consistency*
  - The reproducibility of the association between the same outcome and exposure in multiple independent studies will increase the likelihood of its causal inference.
- *Strength of association*
  - For both interventional and observational studies, a strong association between exposure and outcome increases the likelihood that the exposure is a cause of that outcome. The strength of an association does not depend solely on the validity of observation, but is also based on the magnitude of the association estimate. The strength of association is not the same as statistical significance, such as

*p*-value, which evaluates chance as a possible explanation for the study findings. In general, a relative risk greater than 2.0 or less than 0.5 indicates a strong association.

- *Temporal relationship between exposure and outcome*
  - For an exposure to be considered as a cause of a disease, there should be evidence that the exposure was present before the disease developed.
- *Exposure-varying association*
  - If a primary association between exposure and outcome is observed, the case for causal inference may be strengthened by additional evidence that the association differs predictably across different levels of the exposure. This phenomenon is called "Biological Gradient."
- *Biological plausibility*
  - Causal inference relies on translational and basic science knowledge to make sense of observed epidemiologic associations. Associations that have proven biologic plausibility based on experimental data are more likely to be causal than those not supported by scientific evidence. The biological plausibility derives from scientific evidence obtained from other studies.

Specifically, establishing the causal link between a predictor and outcome variable involves evaluating the strength of the association and the validity of the observation, which means ensuring that the relationship is not attributable to bias, confounding, or chance.

*Chance* is the likelihood that the studied observation is the result of random variation. The role of chance in research is quantified through statistical tests (inferential statistics), and different study designs and data types require different statistical approaches.

*Bias* is a broad term for scenarios or processes in which systematic error in measurement of observations causes any deviation of results or inferences from the truth. Bias can result from several sources, including systematic variations in measurement from the true value (systematic error), flaws in study design, deviation of inferences, interpretations, and analyses based on flawed data or data collection. There is no sense of prejudice or subjectivity implied in the assessment of bias under these conditions.

Biases are generally categorized into one of two types: selection bias and information bias. Selection biases occur when subjects are selected for a study in a way that creates a false association. One common type of selection bias encountered in observational studies is "healthy user bias." This is based on the premise that subjects are not randomized to treatment groups and are self-selected; therefore, important differences in comorbidity and lifestyle may also be selected. This situation can create a nonrandom distortion of the true association between exposure/predictor variable and outcome variable.

Information bias occurs when the method of data collection is systematically different between study groups. In contrast to selection bias, information bias relates to systematic errors in how a variable is measured. One commonly cited type of information bias is recall bias, which arises when subjects have differential recollection of key variables that are related to their study group allocation. An example would be a case-control investigation of drug exposure in patients having a suspected adverse drug reaction. Those experiencing the adverse reaction may have a more heightened recall of everything they had ingested in the immediate past compared with those who did not have an adverse reaction. It is critical to note that, unlike chance and confounding, biases cannot be quantified easily and can only be eliminated or minimized in the design stage.

**Confounding.** Confounding occurs when the study association is partially or entirely mediated by a third factor. Confounding is typically depicted as the interplay among three variables – A, B, and C – where A is the exposure of interest, B is the outcome, and C is the potential confounder. For C to be a confounder, it must be associated with the exposure, be a true cause of B, and not be in the causal pathway (an intermediary) between A and B. Control of confounding is critically important in observational research, but it may also be problematic in nonrandomized, experimental research. Unlike biases, confounding is not necessarily introduced through a faulty study design, but rather is a result of complex relationships between observed and unobserved factors. Additionally, unlike bias, confounding can be analytically managed and adjusted for using different design or analytic strategies. The most powerful method for controlling confounding in experimental research is randomization. In theory, randomization equally distributes known,

unmeasured, and unknown subject characteristics that may confound associations of interest. While randomization greatly increases the likelihood of producing an equal distribution of potential confounders, it is not a guarantee and study group differences may persist. Because randomization is not always feasible, accounting and control of confounding in observational research are critical. There are four generally accepted methods to control for potential confounders in observational research: restriction, matching, stratification, and multivariate analysis. The first two methods must be implemented during the design stage, and the latter two can be handled during analysis.

Restriction, or exclusion, is a technique in which individuals with variables suspected to be confounders are excluded or restricted to a particular value from the study with the aim of producing a more homogeneous study sample. Matching is a procedure in which study patients are matched to controls on one or more potentially confounding variables. Confounding can also be minimized by stratifying by the confounding variable. This is similar to exclusion, except each level of the confounding variable is analyzed separately. Finally, multivariate analysis is one of the most commonly used techniques to control for confounders in observational research because it can statistically adjust for a multitude of variables simultaneously using regression techniques.

## Interventional Versus Observational Study Designs

Clinical research studies can be broadly categorized as interventional or observational. Interventional research entails any research in which the investigator intervenes in a population for the sole purpose of evaluation. Research that is observational makes no attempt to intervene in the study sample for exclusively investigational purposes. The difference is in the method by which study subjects are exposed. An interventional study assigns exposure to study subjects, usually at random, while an observational study observes the exposure, which occurred naturally.

Observational research can also be classified as retrospective or prospective with respect to the perspective of the investigator. For example, an observational cohort study is prospective if study subjects are followed in real time and data about exposures and outcomes are collected. In contrast, in a retrospective cohort study, all exposures and outcomes have occurred and the investigator recreates the time sequence using existing data, such as the medical record or administrative claims. All interventional research by nature is prospective.

## Type of Study Design (Table 41.2)

**Meta-Analysis.** A way of combining data from many different research studies. A meta-analysis is a statistical process using a quantitative method of combining the results of independent studies, usually drawn from the published literature, and synthesizing summaries and conclusions that may be used to evaluate therapeutic effectiveness and plan new studies. It is often an overview of clinical trials. It is usually called a meta-analysis by the author or sponsoring body and should be differentiated from reviews of literature.

**Systematic Review** . A systematic review is a critical assessment and evaluation of all research studies that address a particular clinical issue to provide a comprehensive review of all relevant studies on a particular clinical or health-related topic or question. The systematic review is created after reviewing and combining all the information from both published and unpublished studies using a set of specific criteria, focusing on clinical trials of similar treatments, and then summarizing the findings. The review typically includes a description of the findings of the collection of research studies. This may also include a quantitative pooling of data, called a meta-analysis.

**Randomized Controlled Trial.** A controlled clinical trial randomly assigns participants into an experimental group or a control group. There are various methods to randomize study participants to their groups. As the study is conducted, the only expected difference between the control and experimental groups in a randomized controlled trial is the outcome variable being studied.

**Cohort Study (Prospective Observational Study).** A cohort study refers to a clinical research study in which people who presently have a certain condition are followed over time and compared with another group of people who are not affected by the condition. Outcomes from participants are measured and relationships with specific characteristics are determined.

**Case-Control Study**. A case-control study compares patients who have a disease or outcome of interest (cases) with patients who do not have the disease or outcome (controls). Case-control studies begin with the outcomes and do not follow patients over time. Studies start with the identification of patients with a disease of interest and a control group without the disease. Researchers interview the groups or check their records retrospectively to compare how frequently the exposure to a risk factor is present in each group. They compare the odds of having an experience with the outcome to the odds of having an experience without the outcome. The relationship of an attribute to the disease is examined by comparing diseased and nondiseased persons with regard to the frequency or levels of the attribute in each group to determine the relationship between the risk factor and the disease.

Case-control studies are observational because no intervention is attempted and no attempt is made to alter the course of the disease. The goal is to retrospectively determine the exposure to the risk factor of interest from each of the two groups of individuals: cases and controls. These studies are designed to estimate odds.

**Case Reports and Series.** Case reports describe a series of patients with an outcome of interest. No control group is involved. Case reports often describe:

- unique cases that cannot be explained by known diseases or syndromes;
- cases that show an important variation of a disease or condition;
- cases that show unexpected events that may yield new or useful information; and
- cases in which one patient has two or more unexpected diseases or disorders.

Case reports are considered the lowest level of evidence, but they are also the first line of evidence, because they are where new issues and ideas emerge. If multiple case reports show similar findings, the next step might be a case-control study to determine if there is a relationship between the relevant variables.

## Levels of Evidence

The Evidence Pyramid (Figure 41.1) is often used to illustrate the development of evidence. The base of the pyramid is animal research and laboratory studies, where ideas are often first developed. As one progresses up the pyramid the amount of information available decreases in volume, but increases in relevance to the clinical setting.

**Table 41.2** Advantages and disadvantages of study types; see Table 41.3 for details of where to find each type of study

| Type of the study | Advantage | Disadvantage | Design pitfalls to look out for |
|---|---|---|---|
| (1) Meta-analysis | – Greater statistical power<br>– Confirmatory data analysis<br>– Greater ability for generalizability<br>– Evidence-based result | – Difficult and time-consuming<br>– Not all studies provide adequate data for analysis<br>– Requires advanced statistical techniques<br>– Heterogeneity of study populations | – The studies pooled for review should be similar in type<br>– The analysis should include published and unpublished results to avoid publication bias |
| (2) Systematic review | – Exhaustive review of the current literature and other sources<br>– Less costly to review prior studies than to create a new study<br>– Less time required than conducting a new study<br>– Results can be generalized and extrapolated into the general population more broadly than individual studies<br>– More reliable and accurate than individual studies<br>– Considered an evidence-based resource | – Very time-consuming<br>– May not be easy to combine studies | – Studies included in systematic reviews may be of varying study designs, but should collectively be studying the same outcome<br>– Some reviews may group and analyze studies by variables such as age and gender; factors that were not allocated to participants |
| (3) Randomized controlled trial | – Good randomization will "wash out" any population bias<br>– Easier to blind/mask than observational studies<br>– Results can be analyzed with well-known statistical tools<br>– Populations of participating individuals are clearly identified | – Expensive in terms of time and money<br>– Volunteer biases: the population that participates may not be representative of the whole<br>– Does not reveal causation<br>– Loss to follow-up attributed to treatment | – An RCT should be a study of one population only<br>– The variables being studied should be the only variables between the experimental group and the control group |
| (4) Cohort study | – Subjects in cohorts can be matched, which limits the influence of confounding variables<br>– Standardization of criteria/outcome is possible<br>– Easier and cheaper than an RCT | – Cohorts can be difficult to identify due to confounding variables<br>– No randomization, which means that imbalances in patient characteristics could exist<br>– Blinding/masking is difficult<br>– Outcome of interest could take time to occur | – The cohorts need to be chosen from separate, but similar, populations |
| (5) Case-control study | – Good for studying rare conditions or diseases<br>– Less time needed to conduct the study because the condition or disease has already occurred<br>– Allows for simultaneous examination of multiple risk factors<br>– Useful as initial studies to establish an association | – Retrospective studies have more problems with data quality because they rely on memory and people with a condition will be more motivated to recall risk factors (also called recall bias)<br>– Not good for evaluating diagnostic tests because it is already clear that the cases have the condition and the controls do not | – Care should be taken to avoid confounding, which arises when an exposure and an outcome are both strongly associated with a third variable<br>– Controls should be subjects who might have been cases in the study but are selected independent of the exposure |

(continued)

**Table 41.2** (continued)

| Type of the study | Advantage | Disadvantage | Design pitfalls to look out for |
|---|---|---|---|
| | – Can answer questions that could not be answered through other study designs | – Can be difficult to find a suitable control group | – Cases and controls should also not be "over-matched" |
| (6) Case report | – Can help in the identification of new trends or diseases<br>– Can help detect new drug side-effects and potential uses (adverse or beneficial)<br>– Educational – a way of sharing lessons learned<br>– Identifies rare manifestations of a disease | – Cases may not be generalizable<br>– Not based on systematic studies<br>– Causes or associations may have other explanations<br>– Can be seen as emphasizing the bizarre or focusing on misleading elements | – The patient should be described in detail, allowing others to identify patients with similar characteristics<br>– Case reports should include carefully recorded, unbiased observations.<br>– Case reports should explore and infer, not confirm or prove; they cannot demonstrate causality |

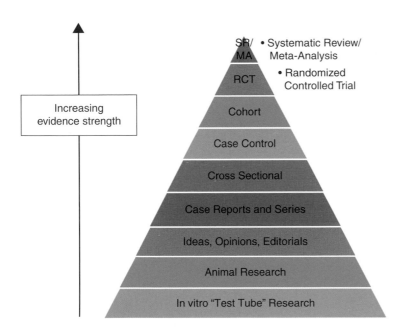

**Figure 41.1** Adaptation of the Evidence Pyramid diagram developed by the Medical Research Library of Brooklyn, SUNY Downstate Medical Center. http://libraryguides.unh.edu/health-literacy.

# Terminology of Clinical Research Design

**Control Groups.** Groups that serve as a standard for comparison in experimental studies. They are similar in relevant characteristics to the experimental group but do not receive the experimental intervention.

**Controlled Clinical Trials.** Clinical trials involving one or more test treatments, at least one control treatment, specified outcome measures for evaluating the studied intervention, and a bias-free method for assigning patients to the test treatment. The treatment may be drugs, devices, or procedures studied for diagnostic, therapeutic, or prophylactic effectiveness. Control measures include placebos, active medicines, no-treatment, dosage forms and regimens, historical comparisons, etc. When randomization using mathematical techniques, such as the use of a random numbers table, is employed to assign patients to test

**Table 41.3** Where to find each type of study

| Type of study | Where to find it |
| --- | --- |
| Systematic reviews or meta-analysis | Cochrane Library, MEDLINE, EMBASE |
| Critically appraised topics | DynaMed, UpToDate |
| Critically appraised articles | ACP Journal Club |
| Randomized controlled trials | Original articles (search MEDLINE, EMBASE) |
| Cohort studies | Original articles (search MEDLINE, EMBASE) |
| Case-controlled studies, etc. | Original articles (search MEDLINE, EMBASE) |
| Background info/expert opinion | Books, editorials |

or control treatments, the trials are characterized as *randomized controlled trials*.

**Cross-Over Studies.** Studies comparing two or more treatments or interventions in which the subjects or patients, upon completion of the course of one treatment, are switched to another. In the case of two treatments, A and B, half the subjects are randomly allocated to receive these in the order A, B and half to receive them in the order B, A. One criticism of this design is that effects of the first treatment may carry over into the period when the second is given.

**Single-Blind Method.** A method in which either the observer(s) or the subject(s) is kept ignorant of the group to which the subjects are assigned.

**Double-Blind Method.** A method of studying a drug or procedure in which both the subjects and investigators are kept unaware of who is actually receiving which specific treatment.

**Intention to Treat Analysis.** Strategy for the analysis of randomized controlled trials which are superiority trials and compares patients in the groups to which they were originally randomly assigned rather than the treatment they received.

**Lost to Follow-Up.** Study subjects in cohort studies whose outcomes are unknown – for example, because they could not or did not wish to attend follow-up visits.

**Matched-Pair Analysis.** A type of analysis in which subjects in a study group and a comparison group are made comparable with respect to extraneous factors by individually pairing study subjects with the comparison group subjects.

**Numbers Needed To Treat.** The number of patients who need to be treated in order to prevent one

additional bad outcome. It is the inverse of *absolute risk reduction.*

**Odds Ratio.** The exposure-odds ratio for case-control data is the ratio of the odds in favor of exposure among cases to the odds in favor of exposure among non-cases. The disease-odds ratio for a cohort or cross-section is the ratio of the odds in favor of disease among the exposed to the odds in favor of disease among the unexposed. The prevalence-odds ratio refers to an odds ratio derived cross-sectionally from studies of prevalent cases.

**Patient Selection**. Criteria and standards used for the determination of the appropriateness of the inclusion of patients with specific conditions in proposed treatment plans and the criteria used for the inclusion of subjects in various clinical trials and other research protocols.

**Random Allocation.** A process involving chance used in therapeutic trials or other research endeavors for allocating experimental subjects, human or animal, between treatment and control groups, or among treatment groups. It may also apply to experiments on inanimate objects.

**Retrospective Studies.** Studies used to test etiologic hypotheses in which inferences about an exposure to putative causal factors are derived from data relating to characteristics of persons under study or to events or experiences in their past. The essential feature is that some of the persons under study have the disease or outcome of interest and their characteristics are compared with those of unaffected persons.

**Cross-Sectional Study.** The observation of a defined population at a single point in time or time interval. Exposure and outcome are determined simultaneously.

**Sample Size.** The number of units (persons, animals, patients, specified circumstances, etc.) in a population to be studied. The sample size should be big enough to have a high likelihood of detecting a true difference between two groups.

# Principles of Biostatistics [13–15]

Biostatistics is the application of various methods of statistical analysis to biological data in the context of clinical trials and other forms of research. Biostatistics are useful for answering an array of questions about, for instance, the effectiveness of a particular drug or intervention, or the relative prevalence of adverse events associated with a drug or intervention. The correct application of sound biostatistical methods can help researchers avoid potential biases and inaccurate conclusions when answering the research questions.

## Data

Data are considered the result of an experiment. A rough classification is as follows:

- *Nominal data*: Numbers or text representing unordered categories (e.g., 0 = male, 1 = female).
- *Ordinal data*: Numbers or text representing categories where order counts (e.g., ASA classification).
- *Discrete data*: Numerical data where both ordering and magnitude are important but only whole-number values are possible (e.g., Apgar score).
- *Continuous data*: Numerical data where any conceivable value is, in theory, attainable (e.g., height, weight, drug dose, etc.).

## Type of Variable

Most variables used in clinical research studies can be classified into one of three categories:

(1) continuous variables which include discrete and continuous data;
(2) binary variables (e.g., smoking: 0 = yes, 1 = no);
(3) categorical variables which include binary and ordinal data.

There are four different types of measurement scales that can be used.

A *nominal scale* represents categories (e.g., males versus females). Each observation is required to fall into one of the mutually exclusive and exhaustive categories. Factors measured on nominal scales are sometimes referred to as discrete variables, and the outcomes are reported as frequency counts or percentages.

In contrast, *interval and ratio scales* represent quantitative data that can be measured, and there is relative positioning with no gaps or interruptions in the continuum (e.g., height, weight, percentages, cholesterol level, blood pressure). The difference between interval and ratio scales is that the former has no true zero value. Factors that are measured using interval and ratio scales are often referred to as continuous variables. For continuous variables, the most commonly used measures of central tendency would be the sample mean and standard deviation.

A fourth scale, *ordinal measures*, falls between discrete and continuous scales. This type of scale represents information that has ascending or descending order, but the difference between units is not necessarily the same. Examples of ordinal scales would include ASA classifications and 0–10 Apgar scores for assessing the health of newborns. When there is a large number of divisions on the ordinal scale or multiple subscales are combined, they may be treated as interval or ratio scales.

Continuous variables can be transformed into categorical or binary variables. For example, age, a continuous variable, can be transformed into an ordered categorical variable with response grouped by clinically accepted categories of "pediatric," "adult," and "geriatric."

For ordinal variables, the measures of central tendency would be the sample median (50th percentile) and dispersion as the 25th and 75th percentiles.

## Summary Measures in Statistics

Summary measure is a compact description of the data that conveys information about the distribution of a variable quickly. Summary measures that pertain to a single variable are called univariate statistics. One summary measure for a single variable is called a "histogram." A normal distribution means that the data appear to be shaped roughly like a typical bell-shaped curve. In addition to displaying the general shape of a distribution, the histogram also provides graphical information about "typical" values for a particular variable, and the range of possible values for that variable. The estimates of the "typical" value in a distribution are termed "measures of location," and estimates of how far apart the data are from this typical value are termed "measures of spread."

The most common measure of location is the arithmetic mean. The mean is calculated by summing all of the observed values of a variable and then dividing by the total number of observations.

$$\text{Mean} = x_i/N$$

The most common measure of spread is the standard deviation. High standard deviation represents the distribution of data that are very spread out, whereas low standard deviation represents the distribution of data that are tightly grouped.

Calculation of variance requires going through each data point in a distribution, calculating the squared distance between that data value and the mean, and then dividing this sum by the total number of data points.

The arithmetic mean is sensitive to extreme values of a distribution. For example, the mean age for children in a hospital may not reflect the "typical" age if the majority of the patients range between 0 and 21 years, but there are also some young adults.

The preferred options for describing typical values for highly skewed distributions are the median and the geometric mean. In terms of sensitivity to outlying values, the geometric mean is between the arithmetic mean, which is very sensitive to extreme values, and the median, which is completely unchanged by outlying values.

The geometric mean is calculated by taking the arithmetic mean of log-transformed data, and then converting back to the original scale by exponentiation. By taking the mean of the log-transformed data, the geometric mean is less sensitive to extreme values that are far away from most of the others. With categorical data, the mean is rarely scientifically meaningful, even if it is an ordered categorical variable. The primary interest is in the percentage of subjects in each classification.

Another common term used to describe the distribution of a variable is "quantiles," also called "percentiles." Quantiles describe specific values within a distribution that divide the data into groups. Continuous variables are commonly divided into categorical variables using quantiles.

Quantiles can be displayed graphically using "box plots." Box plot contain three main pieces of information:

(1) a shaded region representing the 25th and 75th percentiles, which is also called the interquartile range;
(2) a horizontal bar representing the median;
(3) "whiskers" that typically extend to 1.5 times the 25th and 75th quantiles or to the minimum and maximum observation, whichever is less extreme. Additional extreme observations are displayed as open circles beyond the whiskers.

## Summary

Conducting neonatal research presents unique ethical and study design challenges. However, research in this age group can offer the ability to provide improved understanding of diseases, as well as treatment for this fragile patient population.

## References

1. Sachdeva T, Morris MC. Higher-hazard, no benefit research involving children: parental perspectives. *Pediatrics*. 2013;132: e1302–9.

2. Wendler D, Jenkins T. Children's and their parents' views on facing research risks for the benefit of others. *Arch Pediatr Adolesc Med*. 2008;162:9–14.

3. Truog RD. Informed consent and research design in critical care medicine. *Crit Care*. 1999;3: R29–R33.

4. De Lourdes Levy M, Larcher V, Kurz R, Ethics Working Group of the Confederation of European Specialists in Paediatrics. Informed consent/assent in children: statement of the Ethics Working Group of the Confederation of European Specialists in Paediatrics (CESP). *Eur J Pediatr*. 2003;162:629–33.

5. Miller VA, Drotar D, Burant C, Kodish E. Clinician–parent communication during informed consent for pediatric leukemia trials. *J Pediatr Psychol*. 2005;30:219–29.

6. DeMauro SB, Foglia EE, Schmidt B. The ethics of neonatal research: a trialists' perspective. *Semin Fetal Neonatal Med*. 2015;20:431–5.

7. Psaty BM, Platt R, Altman RB. Neurotoxicity of generic anesthesia agents in infants and children: an orphan research question in search of a sponsor. *JAMA*. 2015;313:1515–16.

8. Olsen EA, Brambrink AM. Anesthetic neurotoxicity in the newborn and infant. *Curr Opin Anaesthesiol*. 2013;26:535–42.

9. McCann ME, Bellinger DC, Davidson AJ, Soriano SG. Clinical research approaches to studying pediatric anesthetic neurotoxicity. *Neurotoxicology*. 2009;30:766–71.

10. Long Q, Johnson BA. Variable selection in the presence of missing data: resampling and imputation. *Biostatistics*. 2015;16:596–610.

11. Nelson R, Staggers N. Privacy, confidentiality, security, and data integrity. In Nelson R, Staggers N, editors. *Health Informatics: An Interprofessional Approach*. St. Louis, MO: Mosby; 2013.

12. Hartung DM, Touchette D. Overview of clinical research design. *Am J Health Syst Pharm*. 2009;66:398–408.

13. Pagano M Gauvreau K, editors. *Principles of Biostatistics*. Pacific Grove, CA: Duxbury Press; 2000.

14. Glover T Mitchell K, editors. *An Introduction to Biostatistics*. Pacific Grove, CA: Duxbury Press; 2000.

15. Sharma AK, editor. *Textbook of Biostatistics: Volume 1*. New Delhi: Discovery Publishing; 2008.

# Index

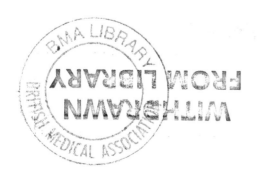